Diagnostic Medical Sonography

A Guide to Clinical Practice

SECOND EDITION

ECHOCARDIOGRAPHY

Diagnostic Medical Sonography

A Guide to Clinical Practice

SECOND EDITION

SERIES EDITORS

Mimi C. Berman, Ph.D., R.D.M.S.
Professor Emeritus
College of Health Related Professions
State University of New York
Health Science Center at Brooklyn
Brooklyn, New York

Diane M. Kawamura, Ph.D., R.T.(R), R.D.M.S.
Professor, Radiological Sciences
College of Health Professions
Weber State University
Ogden, Utah

Marveen Craig, R.D.M.S.
Author, Lecturer, Private Consultant
Dallas, Texas

Mark N. Allen, M.B.A., R.D.M.S., R.D.C.S., R.V.T.
Chief Cardiac Sonographer and Administrator
Echocardiography Laboratory and Mobile Cardiovascular
  Imaging Services
University of Rochester
Rochester, New York

ECHOCARDIOGRAPHY

SECOND EDITION

EDITED BY

Mark N. Allen, M.B.A., R.D.M.S., R.D.C.S., R.V.T.

Chief Cardiac Sonographer and Administrator
Echocardiography Laboratory and Mobile Cardiovascular Imaging Services
University of Rochester
Rochester, New York

With 25 additional contributors

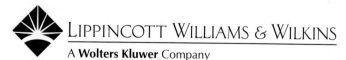

LIPPINCOTT WILLIAMS & WILKINS
A **Wolters Kluwer** Company

Philadelphia · Baltimore · New York · London
Buenos Aires · Hong Kong · Sydney · Tokyo

Acquisitions Editor: Lawrence McGrew
Editorial Assistant: Holly Chapman
Senior Production Editor: Virginia Barishek
Production Service: P.M. Gordon Associates, Inc.
Compositor: Maryland Composition Co., Inc.

Color Separator: Jay's Publishers Services
Insert Printer: The Sheridan Press
Printer/Binder: Quebecor/Kingsport
Cover Designer: William T. Donnelly
Cover Printer: Lehigh Press

Second Edition

Library of Congress Cataloging-in-Publication Data

Echocardiography.—2nd ed. / edited by Mark N. Allen, with
   additional contributors.
         p.   cm.—(Diagnostic medical sonography ; v. 2)
      Includes bibliographical references and index.
      ISBN 0-397-55262-9
      1. Echocardiography.   I. Allen, Mark N.   II. Series: Diagnostic
medical sonography (2nd ed.) ; v. 2.
      [DNLM: 1. Echocardiography—methods.   2. Heart Diseases—
ultrasonography. WN 208 D5355   1997 v.2]
      [RC78.7.U4D48   1997 vol. 2]
      [RC683.5.U5]
      616.07′543 s—dc21
      [616.1′207543]
      DNLM/DLC
      for Library of Congress   98–10883
                                                                          CIP

Care has been taken to confirm the accuracy of the information presented
and to describe generally accepted practices. However, the authors, editors,
and publisher are not responsible for errors or omissions or for any
consequences from application of the information in this book and make
no warranty, express or implied, with respect to the contents of the
publication.

   The authors, editors, and publisher have exerted every effort to ensure
that drug selection and dosage set forth in this text are in accordance with
current recommendations and practice at the time of publication.
However, in view of ongoing research, changes in government regulations,
and the constant flow of information relating to drug therapy and drug
reactions, the reader is urged to check the package insert for each drug for
any change in indications and dosage and for added warnings and
precautions. This is particularly important when the recommended agent is
a new or infrequently employed drug.

   Some drugs and medical devices presented in this publication have
Food and Drug Administration (FDA) clearance for limited use in
restricted research settings. It is the responsibility of the health care
provider to ascertain the FDA status of each drug or device planned for
use in their clinical practice.

9 8 7 6 5 4 3

For My Loving Wife,

Tamara

Contributors

Mark N. Allen, MBA, RDMS, RDCS, RVT
Chief Cardiac Sonographer and Administrator
Echocardiography Laboratory and Mobile
    Cardiovascular Imaging Services
University of Rochester
Rochester, New York

Benico Barzilai, MD
Associate Professor of Medicine
Department of Internal Medicine (Cardiology)
Washington University of Medicine
St. Louis, Missouri

Chris M. Baumann, RDCS
Sonographer
Cardiac Diagnostic Lab
Barnes-Jewish Hospital
St. Louis, Missouri

Raymond J. Carlson, MD, FACC
Director, Adult Echocardiography Laboratory
Department of Medicine
State University of New York
Health Science Center at Syracuse
Syracuse, New York

Judah A. Charnoff, MD, FACC
Assistant Attending Physician
Department of Cardiology
Maimomides Medical Center
Brooklyn, New York

Marveen Craig, RDMS
Author, Lecturer, Private Consultant
Dallas, Texas

Linda J. Crouse
Clinical Professor of Medicine
University of Missouri, Kansas City
Mid-America Heart Institute
Kansas City, Missouri

Cristy Davis, BS, RDCS, RCVT
President
Echo Training Corporation
Carmel, Indiana

Evalie DuMars, BS, RDCS
Adjunct Faculty
Long Beach State University
Orange Coast College
Costa Mesa, California
Senior Cardiac Sonographer
Hoag Memorial Hospital–Presbyterian
Newport Beach, California

Donna Ehler, BS, RDCS
Technical Director
Department of Cardiovascular Ultrasound
Mid-America Cardiology Associates, PC
Kansas City, Missouri

James P. Eichelberger, MD
Assistant Professor of Medicine
Cardiology Unit, Department of Medicine
University of Rochester School of Medicine &
    Dentistry/Strong Memorial Hospital
Rochester, New York

Alvin Greengart, MD
Director, Noninvasive Cardiology
Division of Cardiology
Maimonides Medical Center
Brooklyn, New York

Christopher L. Hare, BS, RDCS
Supervisor, Echocardiography Lab
Department of Medicine
State University of New York
Health Science Center at Syracuse
Syracuse, New York

Mark J. Harry, RDCS, RVT
Technical Director
Department of Ultrasound
The Iowa Heart Center
Des Moines, Iowa

Cynthia A. Hector, RDCS
Cardiac Sonographer
Department of Cardiology/Echocardiography
University of Rochester
Rochester, New York

Darrel Lewis, RDCS
Cardiac Sonographer
Department of Cardiology/Echocardiography
University of Rochester
Rochester, New York

Gerald Marx, MD
Associate Professor, Pediatrics
Department of Cardiology
Boston Children's Hospital
Harvard Medical School
Boston, Massachusetts

Natesa G. Pandian, MD
Director, Echocardiography Laboratory
Tufts New England Medical Center
Boston, Massachusetts

Priscilla J. Peters, BA, RDCS
Supervisor
Echocardiography Laboratory
The Methodist Hospital
Baylor College of Medicine
Houston, Texas

J. Charles Pope, III, BS, PAC, RDCS, RDMS, RVS
Director, Echocardiography Laboratory
Cardiovascular Associates of Augusta
Affiliate Clinical Instructor
Allied Health, Medical College of Georgia
Augusta, Georgia

Henny Rudansky, BS, RDMS
Supervisor of Echocardiography
Division of Cardiology
Maimonides Medical Center
Brooklyn, New York

Karl Q. Schwarz, MD
Director, Echocardiography Laboratory
Department of Cardiology
University of Rochester
Rochester, New York

Lissa Sugeng, MD
Research Fellow
Department of Cardiology
New England Medical Center
Instructor
Tufts New England Medical Center
Boston, Massachusetts

Susie C. Truesdell, PA
Division of Pediatric Cardiology
University of Rochester Medical Center
Rochester, New York

Alan D. Waggoner, MHS, RDMS
Chief Cardiac Sonographer
Barnes Jewish St. Peters Hospital
St. Peters, Missouri

Jiefen Yao, MD
Research Fellow
Department of Cardiology
New England Medical Center
Instructor
Tufts University School of Medicine
Boston, Massachusetts

Preface

Echocardiography has undergone revolutionary changes over the last dozen years. Technological advancements—from M-mode to two-dimensional echocardiography and then Doppler and color flow Doppler—have made echocardiography an essential tool in the diagnosis of cardiac disease. The advent of transesophageal echocardiography, three-dimensional echocardiography, and four-dimensional echocardiography demonstrate the incredible growth potential in the years ahead. Moreover, the use of contrast agents to aid in the visualization of Doppler signals, endocardial borders, and coronary perfusion represents a fascinating new era of research that will only result in an improvement of echocardiographic imaging results. With each new advance, additional information about cardiac structure and function is disclosed. As the new imaging equipment finds its way into large medical centers and small private practices, it is essential that those using this equipment are well grounded in proven echocardiographic techniques. The second edition of *Echocardiography* is intended as a usuable resource of echocardiographic techniques for the cardiac sonographer, echocardiographer, and student.

The format and content of this text vary considerably from the first edition. The book opens with two chapters devoted to basic concepts of cardiac (chest) anatomy and physiology, as a strong understanding of this material is essential before delving into the fundamentals of echocardiography. Novice echocardiographers should devote considererable time to the study of cardiac anatomy and physiology. Part II also focuses on basic concepts and provides an overview of the many modalities available in echocardiography today. Part III focuses on basic echocardiographic techniques and is intended to serve as a guide for those just beginning in the field. Because most techniques have variations, this section is meant to provide suggestions on how to begin scanning. Suggested procedures and protocols are provided as examples. Parts IV through IX are devoted to specific cardiac pathologies, with one whole section devoted to coronary artery disease. Part X examines the ever-puzzling realm of congenital disease and the associated echocardiographic findings. Part XI describes diseases of the aorta. The book concludes with a review of the ever-changing policies of training and quality assurance that are essential components of effective diagnostic testing. Besides the new chapters and new organization, the second edition is loaded with images (including an expanded color section) and summary tables that should enhance the reader's comprehension of the material.

The editors and the contributors of this book made every attempt to include the most up-to-date information. The main focus of this text, however, is on the fundamental principles and practices of echocardiography. I sincerely hope you find this text not only easy to read but also enjoyable, and I look forward to hearing your suggestions and comments.

Mark N. Allen, MBA, RDMS, RDCS, RVT
Mimi C. Berman, PhD, RDMS
Diane M. Kawamura, PhD, RT(R), RDMS
Marveen Craig, RDMS

Acknowledgments

When embarking on a project such as this, it becomes readily apparent that the support of family, friends, and coworkers is desparately needed in order to see the project through to completion. There are so many people I wish to thank for their encouragement and support.

First, the unconditional support and encouragement of my wife, Tamara, made it possible for me to complete the book. It is difficult to express my gratitude and appreciation for all that she has done—for her incredible patience and numerous sacrifices throughout this project and especially for her unwavering love. She is truly my best friend.

My children, Nicole, Joshua, and Christopher, kept me grounded throughout this process. They were a constant reminder of what is truly important in life. Their laughter and carefree way were a much-needed distraction. Even at their tender ages they gave support and encouragement and demonstrated a tremendous amount of understanding. Without a doubt they represent my most important achievement.

My parents, Bob and Leone, provided a loving environment in which to grow. The example they set and the values they bestowed provided the building blocks for taking on and completing projects like this. Their work ethic and determination have become great gifts to me. Words cannot express the admiration and gratitude that I have for these two very special people.

A speical thank you for my coworkers and colleagues Deborah Schwarz, Mike Michalko, Cindy Hector, Darrel Lewis, and Dale Martin, who not only supported me but also put up with me throughout the course of writing this book: For all the times they covered me in the lab so I could get away to the library or barricade myself in my office to write a few paragraphs, I thank them. To Peter Kapatos, thanks for helping with computer issues. To Mark Ott, Mark Sanchez, Susan Kirley, and Brenda Bott, thanks for providing secretarial support.

Thanks also to Dr. Karl Q. Schwarz, who continually sets challenges and provides inspiration to achieve goals, for the academic environment that he creates in our lab and his encouragement of projects like these. I could not have completed this book without his support, and I am very grateful to him.

To Gerson Lichtenberg, whose contagious enthusiasms for the field of echocardiography rubbed off on me. He is both a skilled cardiac sonographer and an excellent teacher, but above all he is a great friend.

Thanks go to Mimi Berman, Diane Kawamura, and Marveen Craig, who provided valuable guidance and insight to this project.

My thanks to the many contributors of this edition, whose valuable time and energy were devoted to complete their chapters. Their thoughts, ideas, and contributions were invaluable in putting this text together.

Special acknowledgment goes to those at Lippincott–Raven Publishers, especially Lawrence McGrew and Holly Chapman, for their incredible patience, expertise, encouragement, and friendship.

Even in the "darkest hours" of writing this book, they provided support and much-needed confidence.

And finally in memory of Edith Johnson, who had faith and confidence in that little third grader. She was a true educator who gave of herself willingly and unconditionally. She is sadly missed, and her many contributions as a teacher and friend will always be remembered.

MNA

Contents

List of Tables

PART I

Anatomy and Physiology of the Heart

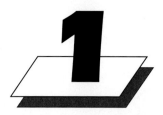

Anatomy of the Thoracic Cavity and Heart

MARK N. ALLEN

Introduction

Knowledge of the anatomy of the chest and heart is imperative in performing quality echocardiograms. It is important that the cardiac sonographer understand the physical relationships of the chest structures and the heart's orientation within the thoracic cavity. In order to better appreciate the echocardiographic views, one must be able to visualize the correct lie of the heart within the thoracic cavity. This chapter reviews the anatomy of the chest, as well as that of the heart.

ANATOMIC TERMS

In understanding the descriptive relationships of anatomy and even echocardiography planes, one must be familiar with some basic relational terms. Assuming that the body is in the anatomic position, that is to say, standing upright and facing forward, these terms are used to describe anatomical relationships and directions.[6] *Superior* (*cranial*) is used to describe those structures that are toward or near the head. It also describes a structure or part of a structure that is above another structure or part of a structure. For example, the left atrium is superior to the left ventricle or the left ventricular inflow tract is superior to the left ventricular apex. Those structures that are closer to the feet are *inferior or caudal*. For example, the inferior vena cava is closer to the feet or below the superior vena cava.

Medial refers to structures that are near the body's midline or the middle of a structure. For example, the heart is medial to the left lung. *Lateral* refers to structures that are farther from the body's midline or to the right or left of the center. An example of this would be the left ventricle, which is lateral to the right ventricle. *Anterior* refers to structures that are in front of or toward the ventral side of the body. The heart is anterior to the vertebrae. *Posterior* or *dorsal* refers to structures that are behind or in back of the body or organ. The esophagus is posterior to the heart.

Proximal is used to describe a structure that is close to its origin, such as blood vessels. *Distal* refers to an organ or structure that is far from its origin. The ascending aorta is proximal to the aortic arch; conversely, the aortic arch is distal to the ascending aorta (Fig. 1-1).

These terms are frequently used together in order to define anatomic relationships more clearly. For example, a structure that is superior and posterior to the heart would be a structure that is above but also behind the plane of the heart. These terms are used throughout the text in order to define anatomic relationships.

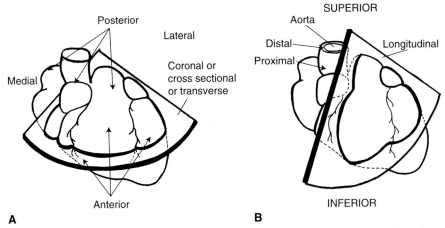

Figure 1-1. Anatomic planes of the heart demonstrating medial and lateral orientation, as well as posterior, anterior (**A**), superior, and inferior (**B**), orientation. The aorta is used to demonstrate proximal and distal descriptions.

Chest Anatomy

The chest or thorax constitutes the upper part of the body. The thoracic cavity proper occupies the upper portion of the thorax or thoracic cage. It is bound anteriorly by the sternum, laterally by the ribs, and posteriorly by the 12 thoracic vertebrae and the posterior portions of the ribs. Superiorly, the thoracic cavity is bordered by the clavicles, the first ribs, and the body of the first vertebrae. The superior border is not a true border, giving rise to the root of the neck. The inferior border of the thoracic cage is defined by the diaphragm. The diaphragm is a tough muscular organ which assists breathing and serves as the separation between the thoracic cavity and the abdominal or peritoneal cavity[1] (Fig. 1-2).

THE MEDIASTINUM

The mediastinum is an arbitrary subdivision of the thoracic cavity. Four sections are typically described, each containing specific organs or organ systems (Fig. 1-3). The superior mediastinum is formed by a plane drawn from the sternal angle to the level of the fourth thoracic vertebra. It contains the aortic arch, the brachiocephalic artery and veins, the proximal segments of the left common carotid and left subclavian arteries, the superior vena cava, the trachea, the esophagus, parts of the thymus gland, lymph nodes, and nerves.[2]

The inferior mediastinum is subdivided into three parts: anterior, middle, and posterior. The anterior mediastinum lies anterior to the heart. It contains some lymph nodes, muscles, and small blood

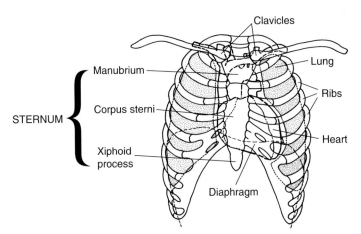

Figure 1-2. Thoracic cavity demonstrating the anatomic orientations relative to the heart.

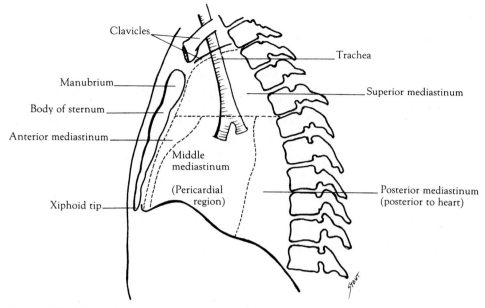

Figure 1-3. Lateral view demonstrating the four divisions of the mediastinum.

vessels. The middle mediastinum contains the heart, the pericardium, the ascending aorta, the terminal end of the superior vena cava, the pulmonary artery and its branches, the terminal parts of the right and left pulmonary veins, and the phrenic nerves. The posterior mediastinum contains the descending thoracic aorta, the bifurcation of the trachea, the right and left main bronchi, the esophagus, the azygous and hemiazygous veins, the splenic nerves, and the thoracic lymphatic duct[1,6] (Fig. 1-3).

Skeletal Structure

An understanding of the anatomic relationships of the heart, skeletal framework, lung, and musculature is important in cardiac sonography. The two main tissues within the body which interfere with the successful transmission and reflection of sound waves are bone and air-filled organs (i.e., lung). It is a wonder that the heart can be visualized at all, considering that it is surrounded by both of these obstacles. It is important, therefore, to understand the physical orientations of these systems relative to the heart and to understand how their presence can assist or interfere with visualization of the cardiac structures.

RIBS

The two main purposes of the bony structures of the thorax are (1) to protect the vital organs within the thoracic cage and (2) to prevent the collapse of the thorax during respiration. The rib cage is composed of several bony structures which articulate with one another. The sternum or breast bone is a flat, superficial structure that lies in the midline of the chest. It is composed of three distinct but adjacent parts: the manubrium, the corpus sterni, and the xiphoid process. The manubrium is the top portion of the sternum, the corpus sterni is the middle portion or body, and the xiphoid process is the bottom portion and smallest section (Fig. 1-2).

The clavicles connect or articulate with the upper border of the manubrium, forming a notch. This notch, called the *suprasternal notch*, serves as a landmark in one of the standard echocardiographic views. The thoracic cage is further made up of a pair of ribs, 12 on the right side and 12 on the left side of the body. The ribs articulate posteriorly with the thoracic vertebrae, and the first seven pairs articulate anteriorly with the sternum by costal cartilages which provide thoracic mobility and elasticity. The 8th, 9th, and 10th pairs join with one another but do not reach the sternum. The 11th and 12th pairs are rudimentary and small, ending in free cartilaginous tips.

The space between the ribs is called the *intercostal space*. This space is occupied by intercostal muscles, nerves, and blood vessels. The intercostal muscles arise from the lower border of the rib above and run obliquely downward and medially where they insert into the upper border of the rib below.[6] It is through these intercostal spaces that echocardiographic images are obtained.

Where the manubrium joins the body of the sternum, the sternal angle is formed. The sternal angle forms a small, palpable ridge on the anterior thorax. Laterally, the second ribs attach to the manubrium by cartilage. Clinically, this landmark is important because it serves as the starting point for counting the intercostal spaces. When discussing various echocardiographic views, it is important to know the starting point for counting these spaces (Fig. 1-4).

VERTEBRAL COLUMN

The vertebral column is composed of 33 vertebrae. There are six parts composing each vertebra, and each part serves a specific purpose. The *body* of the vertebra is the largest part. When piled on top of each other, the vertebral bodies provide strong support for the cranium and trunk. The *pedicles* are two short, rounded projections from the dorsal surface of the vertebrae, which form the body of the intervertebral foramen, which in turn functions as the articulating surface for ribs. The *laminae* are flattened areas of the vertebrae which are continuous with the pedicles, transverse process, and spinous process. This part of the bone helps form the vertebral foramen, which houses the spinal cord. The *spinous process* is a dorsal projection which functions as a lever for muscles which control body posture and movement. The *transverse processes* are lateral projections which provide attachments for muscles responsible for rotation and flexion. The *articulating surfaces* found superiorly and inferiorly on each vertebra are in contact with the vertebra above and below, allowing limited movement between vertebrae[2] (Fig. 1-5).

The vertebral column is formed by five regions: (1) the cervical, (2) the thoracic or dorsal, (3) the lumbar, (4) the sacral, and (5) the coccygeal. The cervical vertebrae make up the region of the neck. There are seven vertebrae in the cervical region. The major difference between the cervical vertebrae and the vertebrae in other regions is the size of the body, which in the cervical region is smaller. In addition, the cervical vertebrae possess a foramen in the transverse process. There are 12 thoracic or dorsal vertebrae. They are larger than the cervical vertebrae but smaller than the lumbar vertebrae and increase in size farther down the spine. They are distinguished

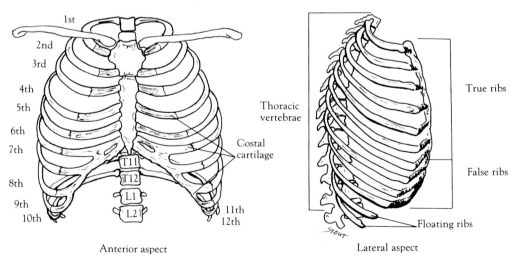

Figure 1-4. Anterior and lateral views of the bony thorax demonstrating the 1st through 10th ribs and the difference between true, false, and floating ribs.

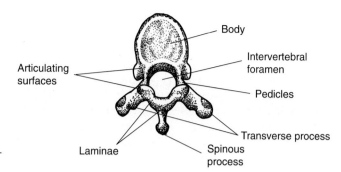

Figure 1-5. Thoracic vertebrae demonstrating various parts and articulating surfaces.

from other vertebrae by having facets on the side of the body that serve as attachment sites for the ribs. The spinal foramen housing the spinal cord is heart-shaped. There are five lumbar vertebrae. These vertebrae are the largest, and are further distinguished by the absence of a foramen in the transverse process (such as found in the cervical vertebrae) and by the absence of the lateral articulating facets (such as found in the thoracic vertebrae). There are five sacral vertebrae and four coccygeal vertebrae. In the adult, the sacrum is fused to form one large triangular bone. The coccygeal vertebrae are also fused in the adult and resemble the beak of a cuckoo, hence the name *coccyx*.

THORACIC MUSCULATURE

The major role of thoracic muscles is to assist respiration. Several groups of muscles are found in the thorax, but for the purpose of this text only the major ones will be discussed. The *diaphragm* is considered to be the primary breathing muscle. It accounts for the bulk of respiratory movement into and out of the thorax. In the normal adult, the vital capacity in the lungs is approximately 4.5 liters. The downward movement of the diaphragm during inspiration accounts for the intake of approximately 3 liters of air.[3] The diaphragm is attached to the surrounding thoracic structures on three sides. Anteriorly, the diaphragm is attached to the xiphoid process. Laterally, it is attached to the internal surface of the first six costal cartilages and their accompanying ribs. Posteriorly, it is attached to the first lumbar vertebra. The diaphragm possesses several apertures which allow the passage of various vessels and organs. The aortic aperture allows passage of the aorta, the esophageal aperture allows passage of

the esophagus, and the vena caval aperture allows passage of the inferior vena cava.

During inspiration the diaphragm contracts, moving downward and displacing abdominal organs. This downward displacement of abdominal organs is accomplished in part by the distensibility of the abdominal wall. The downward movement of the diaphragm also elevates the lower ribs and forces the sternum forward, which in turn forces the upper ribs outward. This increases the thoracic area, accommodating the intake of air by reducing intrathoracic pressure. During expiration when the diaphragm returns to its resting position, air is driven out by an increase in thoracic pressure.[1]

There are 11 pairs of internal and external intercostal muscles. The internal intercostal muscles are deep muscles which originate in the intercostal groove of the rib above and insert on the superior border of the rib below. They are continuous with the fibers of the internal oblique muscles of the abdominal wall. The internal intercostal muscles aid expiration by drawing the ribs together. The external intercostal muscles also attach between ribs, attaching to the lower border of the rib above and running to the upper border of the rib below. The fibers of these muscles run in an oblique direction and are mainly responsible for aiding inspiration. In addition to aiding inspiration and expiration, the internal and external intercostal muscles act together to stiffen the thoracic wall and provide uniform movement of the thoracic cage during descent of the diaphragm with inspiration.[5] The movement of these muscles can be exaggerated with deep respiration. An understanding of this mechanism is important to echocardiography because the physiologic changes as a result of muscular motion can hinder or enhance an echocardiogram. When imaging is difficult, having a patient take a deep breath and holding it may enhance the ability to image the heart by increasing the size of the intercostal space. Likewise, asking a patient to hold a breath out may enhance an image by preventing expansion of the lungs within the thoracic cavity. Taking advantage of the intercostal muscles' ability to affect the anatomic character of the thorax can be helpful (Fig. 1-6*A–C*).

ORGANS OF RESPIRATION

Trachea and Bronchi

The trachea is responsible for the exchange of gases into and out of the lungs. It is a long tube measuring 10–11 cm and is capable of changing in length with the effects of respiration. Its internal diameter varies from 1.0 to 2.5 cm.[6] Its internal lining is composed of various cell types, most of which vary in function.

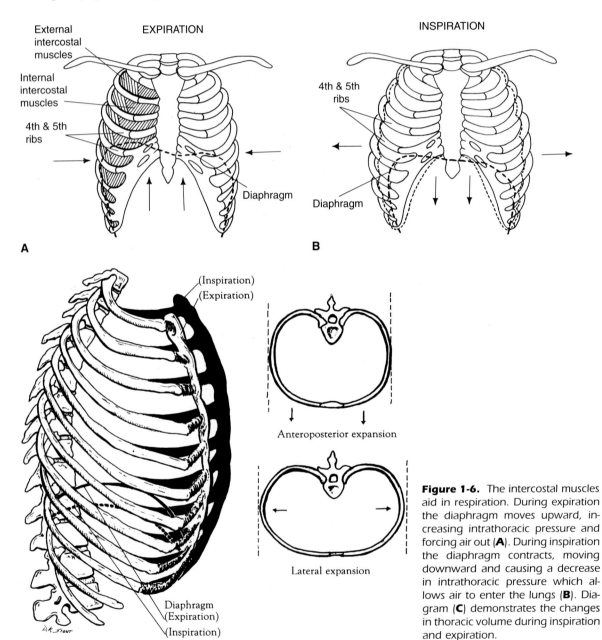

Figure 1-6. The intercostal muscles aid in respiration. During expiration the diaphragm moves upward, increasing intrathoracic pressure and forcing air out (**A**). During inspiration the diaphragm contracts, moving downward and causing a decrease in intrathoracic pressure which allows air to enter the lungs (**B**). Diagram (**C**) demonstrates the changes in thoracic volume during inspiration and expiration.

Besides moving gases into and out of the lungs, the trachea warms and moistens air. Some of the cells lining the trachea, called *pseudociliated columnar epithelium*, are responsible for moving trapped particles up toward the larynx, where they can be swallowed or expelled. The trachea contains incomplete rings of hyaline cartilage which lend support and flexibility to the trachea and are connected by smooth muscle and connective tissue. The trachea begins to branch at the level of the sixth cervical vertebra into left and right bronchi (Fig. 1-7).

The bronchi are a system of branches which decrease in diameter as they enter the lung tissue. Like the trachea, they are responsible for moving gases into and out of the lungs. They also warm and moisten air. There is a left and a right primary branch, each branching further to enter each lobe of each lung. The branches become increasingly small and eventually terminate in the alveolar ducts.

Lungs

The lungs are the vital organs of respiration. They are surrounded by a pleural sac consisting of a visceral and a parietal surface and containing pleural fluid in between. There are two lungs, located on opposite sides of the heart and termed the *right lung* and *left lung*. The right lung is composed of three lobes: superior, middle, and inferior. The left lung is composed of two lobes: superior and inferior. Each lobe is divided further into lobules. Each lobe is supplied by secondary bronchi. Tertiary bronchi supply the various segments within each lobe. The tertiary bronchi are supported by cartilaginous rings which disappear as the bronchi narrow further into smaller branches called *bronchioles*. The bronchioles are classified into three categories. The lobular bronchioles supply each lobule, where they divide into roughly six terminal bronchioles, which further divide into respiratory bronchioles. The respiratory bronchioles terminate in the alveolar ducts which lead to the alveolar sacs and alveoli[1,4] (Fig. 1-7).

The alveoli are exceedingly thin-walled pouches which allow gaseous exchange with capillaries. They are made up of several cell types, each serving a specific purpose. The main cell types are type I alveoli cells, which are simple squamous cells. These cells facilitate gaseous exchange from inside the alveoli to surrounding capillaries. Type II alveolar cells are responsible for producing surfactant, a chemical compound which helps to decrease cellular surface tension, thereby preventing the collapse of the alveolar sacs. Other cells are responsible for removing debris and other harmful particles within the alveolar sacs. Although the alveoli are microscopic, there are roughly 300 million in the average adult, for an

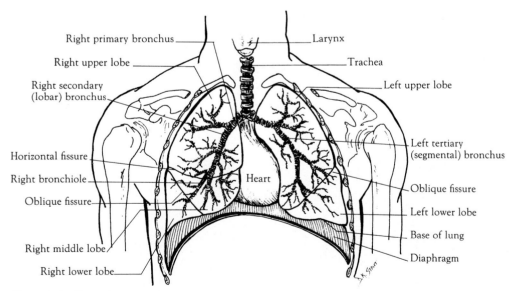

Figure 1-7. Frontal, exposed view demonstrating the bronchial tree, lobes of the lungs, and other thoracic structures.

estimated surface area of 143 m² (average body surface area ranges from 194 to 294 m² [1,2]) (Fig. 1-8).

CIRCULATION OF THE THORAX

Several major blood vessels supply the thorax. The thoracic aorta provides branches to the esophagus, bronchi, pericardium, lungs, and the thoracic walls. These blood vessels are named according to the organs they supply: bronchial artery, pericardial artery, and esophageal artery. The mediastinal arteries supply lymph nodes and other organs in the posterior mediastinum. The phrenic arteries supply the diaphragm. The intercostal arteries travel to the intercostal margins of the ribs, where they branch further to muscles and organs in the thorax and upper abdomen.

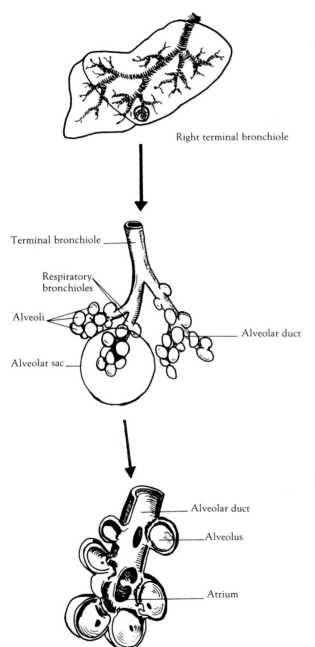

Right terminal bronchiole

Terminal bronchiole

Respiratory bronchioles

Alveoli

Alveolar duct

Alveolar sac

Alveolar duct

Alveolus

Atrium

Figure 1-8. Diagram of the alveoli, alveolar duct, and alveolar sac in relation to the terminal bronchiole.

The right and left brachiocephalic veins and the azygous vein are the principal veins returning blood from the thorax to the heart. The brachiocephalic veins drain the head, neck, upper extremities, mammary glands, and intercostal spaces. These vessels empty into the superior vena cava.

The thoracic cage is drained primarily from a network of veins called the *azygous network*. Blood drains from the thoracic wall into hemiazygous veins, which drain into the azygous vein, which drains into the superior vena cava (Fig. 1-9*A,B*).

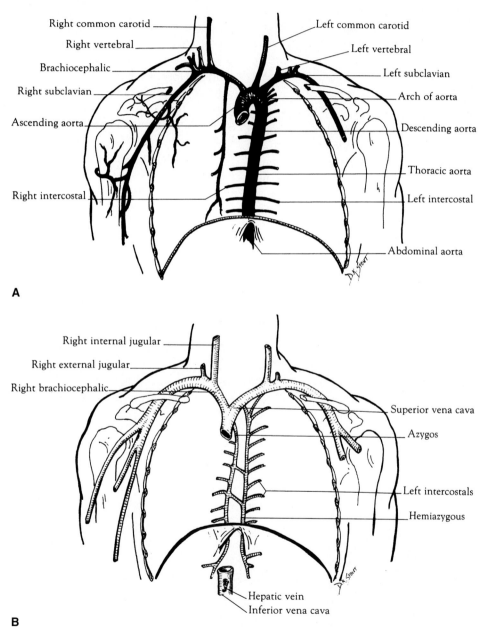

Figure 1-9. Exposed frontal view of the thoracic arterial system (**A**). Exposed frontal view of the thoracic venous system (**B**).

The Heart

CARDIAC BORDERS

The heart is a cone-shaped, hollow, muscular organ located in the middle mediastinum. It is surrounded laterally and posteriorly by the lungs, and anteriorly it is covered by the lower two-thirds of the sternum and the costal cartilage of the second through sixth ribs. The descending thoracic aorta and esophagus lie posterior to the heart. Inferiorly, the heart is bordered by the diaphragm. Within the chest, the heart extends roughly 3½ in to the left of midline (Fig. 1-10).

PERICARDIUM

The pericardium contains the heart and is made up of two components, fibrous and serosal. The fibrous pericardium is a tough outer sac made of connective tissue which completely surrounds the heart but does not adhere to or touch it. Superiorly, the fibrous pericardium is continuous with the adventitia of the great vessels. Anteriorly, it is attached to the posterior surface of the sternum. Laterally, the pericardium is bordered by the mediastinal surface of the lungs. The phrenic nerve descends between these two surfaces. Inferiorly lies the diaphragm, which separates the thoracic cavity from the abdominal cavity. Posterior to the pericardium lie the bronchi, esophagus, esophageal plexus, descending thoracic aorta, and part of the mediastinal surface of the lungs.[1]

The inner or serosal layer has two layers. The visceral or epicardial layer adheres to the surface of the heart and makes up the epicardium. At the base of the heart, at the origin of the great vessels, the serosal pericardium folds back on itself to form the outer or parietal layer. There are two major reflections of the serosal pericardium, one enclosing the aorta and pulmonary trunk and the other enclosing the superior and inferior vena cavae and the four pulmonary veins. Approximately two-thirds of the proximal ascending aorta and main pulmonary artery and half of the superior vena cava lie within the pericardium. Only 1 to 2 cm of the inferior vena cava lie within the sac. With two-thirds of the ascending aorta lying within the pericardium, type A aortic dissections or traumatic ruptures of the ascending aorta lead to rapid accumulation of fluid within the pericardial space, resulting in tamponade. Type B dissections, involving the arch and/or the descending thoracic aorta, can usually be contained by the tough parietal pleura which support the aortic adventitia and contain ruptures.[4] The parietal layer of the serosal pericardium lines the inside surface of the fibrous pericardium. Within the serosal layers is a thin film of pericardial fluid (Fig. 1-11).

The purpose of the pericardium is to (1) reduce friction with cardiac movement; (2) allow the heart to move freely with each beat, facilitating ejection and volume changes; (3) contain the heart within the mediastinum, especially during trauma; and (4) serve as a barrier to infection.[5]

CARDIAC SIZE AND EXTERNAL SURFACE

The heart has a base which is its most superior surface, from which the great vessels emerge, and an apex which extends toward the left of midline. From

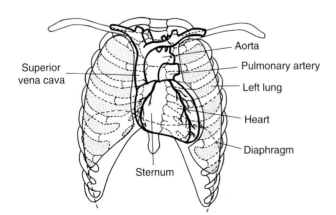

Figure 1-10. Frontal view of the heart in relationship to other thoracic structures.

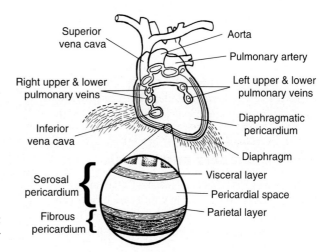

Figure 1-11. Frontal view of the pericardial sac with the heart removed. Enlarged view of the pericardium demonstrating the various layers.

base to apex, the average length of an adult heart measures 12 cm. Its width is 8–9 cm in its broadest diameter and 6 cm at its narrowest portion. Its weight is roughly 280–340 g in males and 230–280 g in females. Cardiac weight is approximately 0.45% of total body weight in men and 0.40% of total body weight in women.[4,6]

Due to the division of the heart into four chambers, the external surface of the heart has grooves or sulci. The *coronary* or *atrioventricular groove* separates the atria from the ventricles. Within this groove lie the main trunk of the coronary arteries

and the coronary sinus. The *interventricular groove* is formed from the separation of the right and left ventricles. There is an *anterior interventricular groove* which runs on the anterior surface of the heart. The anterior interventricular descending branch of the left coronary artery lies in this groove. The *posterior interventricular groove* runs on the diaphragmatic surface of the heart and contains the posterior interventricular descending coronary artery and the middle cardiac vein. The atria are separated externally by the *interatrial grooves*. The interatrial grooves are shallow and less pronounced

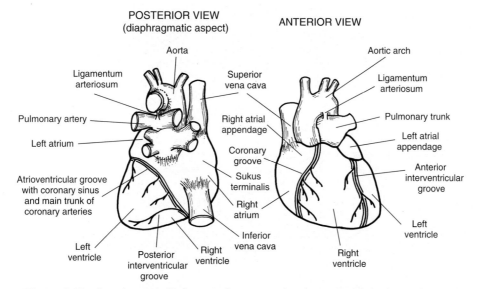

Figure 1-12. Anterior and diaphragmatic or posterior exposures of the heart demonstrating the external grooves or sulci demarcating the divisions of the cardiac chambers.

than the other grooves. The interatrial, atrioventricular, and posterior interventricular grooves meet to form the crux of the heart. The *terminal groove* or *sulcus terminalis* demarcates the true atrium and the venous component of the right atrium. These external grooves of the heart are filled with fatty tissue which varies with overall body fat and increases with age[4,6] (Fig. 1-12).

Cardiac Chambers and Vessels

The following discussion of cardiac anatomy will follow the course of an oxygenated red blood cell as it travels from the lung to the left side of the heart and returns to the right side of the heart from the body.

PULMONARY VEINS

The pulmonary veins carry oxygenated blood from the lungs to the left atrium. Four pulmonary veins enter the atrium on its upper posterolateral surface. Two vessels from each lung enter either side of the atrium. The orifices are smooth and oval, with the left pair frequently entering as a single channel. These veins are often referred to as the *right* and *left upper* and *lower pulmonary veins* (Fig. 1-11).

LEFT ATRIUM

The left atrium is located to the left of and posterior to the right atrium. It is smaller in volume than the right atrium but has thicker walls. It sits inferior to the right pulmonary artery and posterior to the aortic root and is therefore partially concealed by these structures. The endocardial surface of the left atrium is smooth except for the left atrial appendage, which contains numerous pectinate muscles. The left atrial appendage is a continuation of the upper anterior border of the left atrium. It is a long, narrow, and hooked appendage which lies anterior to and to the left of the pulmonary trunk. The posterior wall of the left atrium receives the pulmonary veins. Its anterior-inferior border adjoins the base of the left ventricle. The left side of the interatrial septum has a rough appearance, with the boundaries of the foramen ovale being defined as a crescent-shaped ridge[4,6] (Fig. 1-13).

Anatomically, the transverse or longitudinal axes are somewhat larger than the transverse or sagittal axes. This difference is noted on echocardiography and is most apparent from the parasternal long axis view compared to the apical four-chamber view.

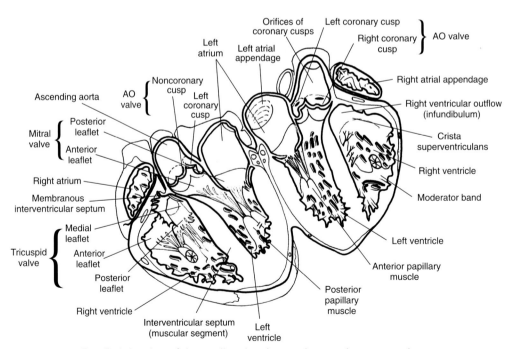

Figure 1-13. Detailed drawing of the cardiac chambers, valves, and great vessels.

MITRAL VALVE

The mitral valve is a very complex structure consisting of valve leaflets, chordae tendineae, mitral annuli, and papillary muscles. Each component contributes to the normal functioning of the mitral valve, and malformations or problems with any one component can lead to mitral valve dysfunction.

Mitral Annulus

The mitral valve orifice is a well-defined zone between the left atrium and ventricle. The annulus is composed of fibrocollagenous elements of varying consistency which make up the core of the valve leaflets.[4] To ensure proper functioning of the mitral valve, the annulus is capable of changing shape and dimension with cardiac function. The annulus is strongest at the left and right fibrous trigones, which also make up parts of the aortic and tricuspid annuli.

Mitral Valve Leaflets

The leaflets of the mitral valve are smooth, thin membranes which originate from the annulus fibrosus of the mitral annulus. The leaflets are roughly triangular in shape and resemble a bishop's miter, hence the name *mitral* valve.[3] Their edges are scalloped, with each leaflet possessing commissures or clefts which have fan-like projections of chordae tendineae. There are two major leaflets of the mitral valve, and since this is the only cardiac valve with this characteristic, the mitral valve is occasionally called the *bicuspid valve.*

The anterior leaflet guards one-third of the mitral orifice. This leaflet is sometimes called the *aortic, septal, greater,* or *anteromedial leaflet.* The main commissure of the anterior leaflet is the anterolateral commissure, and the majority of its chordae attach to the corresponding anterolateral papillary muscle. The posterior leaflet, (also called the *mural, ventricular, smaller,* or *posterolateral leaflet*), is longer and narrower than the anterior leaflet and guards two-thirds of the mitral annulus. It possesses three commissures: one large center one and two smaller ones, the anterolateral and the posteromedial commissural scallop.[4] This anatomic difference is important because in mitral valve prolapse any single commissural scallop can prolapse. Careful attention to valvular anatomy by echocardiography can also aid the surgical management of patients with valvular lesions. The chordae of each leaflet attach to the ventricular surface of the mitral valve. However, there are large areas of smooth surface which define the zones of apposition of the two leaflets when the valve is closed. There is also considerable overlap of the posterior leaflet to the anterior leaflet, forming a considerable barrier to the backflow of blood.

Chordae Tendineae

The valve closes as a result of increased pressure of the left ventricle, which exceeds left atrial pressure in systole. The valve is prevented from buckling into the left atrium by the chordae tendineae which arise from the anterolateral and posteromedial papillary muscles of the left ventricle and attach to the commissures of each leaflet. The chordae are formed from the embryonic ventricular trabeculae and are strong tendinous cords. They are subdivided into three groups, depending on their function and origin. The first-order chordae are thick and originate at the tips of the papillary muscles. As they approach the leaflets, they branch into several thinner strands and attach at the extreme edge of the leaflets. Their function is to prevent the leaflets from inverting during systole. The second-order chordae are stronger than the first-order chordae and also originate at or near the tips of the papillary muscle. They also branch as they approach the leaflets and attach on the ventricular surface of the leaflets. They function much the same way as the mainstays on an umbrella.[6,8] The second-order chordae are fewer in number than the first-order ones. The third-order chordae originate at the ventricular wall near the attachment of the leaflets. They attach primarily to the posterior leaflet of the mitral valve. These are usually single chordae that do not branch significantly.

Papillary Muscles

There are two primary papillary muscles in the left ventricle. The anterolateral papillary muscle is located on the sternocostal endocardial border, and the posteromedial papillary muscle arises from the diaphragmatic border. The papillary muscles may have a singular head or several. As these muscles contract, they exert tension on the chordae tendineae, preventing the mitral valve leaflets from prolapsing during systole. In the setting of myocardial infarction the papillary muscles can become damaged, creating valvular incompetence or rupture of the chordae (Fig. 1-14*A*).

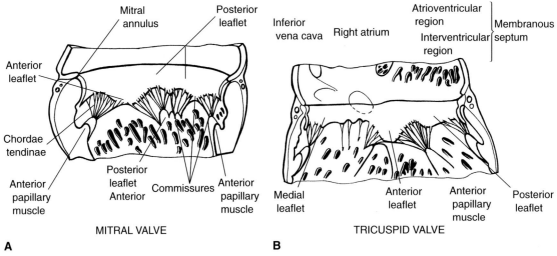

Figure 1-14. Detailed drawings of the mitral valve (**A**) and tricuspid valve (**B**) apparatus.

LEFT VENTRICLE

The left ventricle forms part of the sternocostal, left, and diaphragmatic or inferior surface of the heart. It is conical in shape and longer and narrower than the right ventricle. Its walls are approximately three times as thick as those of the right ventricle. Anatomically, the left ventricle is divided into several segments. There is an inlet region which is guarded by the mitral valve, an outlet region guarded by the aortic valve, and an apical region. The inlet and outlet portions of the left ventricle share a fibrous skeleton, causing the inflow and outflow sections of the ventricle to be separated only by the anterior leaflet of the mitral valve. The basal one-third of the ventricle tends to be smooth-walled, whereas the apical regions tend to have trabeculations.

The ventricular septum is composed of several anatomic regions. Simply, the septum is composed of a large inferior muscular portion and a small superior membranous portion which can be further subdivided. On the left, the membranous septum is located in the angle of the right and noncoronary cusps of the aortic valve. On the right, the anterior and septal leaflets of the tricuspid valve attach to the middle of the membranous septum. Therefore, part of the membranous septum lies above the tricuspid valve. This anatomic detail is important in ventricular septal defects of the membranous septum. The defect can be above the tricuspid valve, causing a left-to-right atrial tunnel. Alternatively, it can be below the tricuspid valve, causing an interventricular defect.

Anatomically, the left ventricle can be distinguished from the right ventricle by its (1) conical shape, (2) smooth basal and septal surface, (3) lack of a prominent apical trabeculation or moderator band, (4) bicuspid atrioventricular valve, (5) two prominent papillary muscles, (6) thicker walls, and (7) intimate association of the mitral and aortic valves.[1,2,8] Functionally, the left ventricle differs from the right ventricle in that it pumps oxygenated blood to the body or is responsible for systemic circulation.

AORTIC VALVE

The aortic valve is a semilunar valve and has three cusps, each named for the corresponding origins of the coronary arteries: right coronary cusp, left coronary cusp, and noncoronary cusp. The aortic valve cusps are folds of endocardium with a fibrous core attached to the aortic wall rather than the left ventricular wall. The base of the cusps is thicker, and the cusps themselves are thin and translucent. The cusps are crescent- and pocket-shaped and are equal in size. In diastole, the free margins of the cusps coapt tightly, preventing the backflow of blood into the ventricle. In systole, the cusps open in a triangular fashion, with flexion occurring at the base (Fig. 1-15).

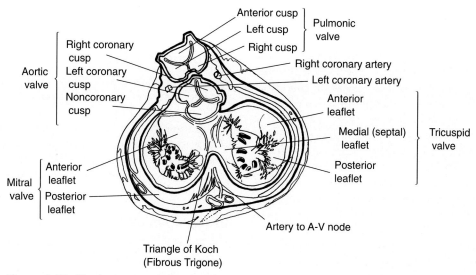

Figure 1-15. The heart viewed from the base with the atria removed. Note the open position of the AV valves and the closed position of the semilunar valves indicating diastole.

AORTA

The aorta begins below the origin of the aortic valve and dilates above the valve, forming the aortic sinuses or sinuses of Valsalva. The walls of the sinuses are made primarily of collagen, and the right and left sinuses contain the origin of the right and left coronary arteries, respectively. The aortic valve, when closed, supports the column of blood within the aorta. When open, the cusps remain open in a straight line and are not pressed against the walls of the sinuses. This arrangement is probably facilitated by blood filling the sinuses upon ejection, helping to maintain the cusp's straight-line orientation and allowing continued flow of blood into the coronary arteries. When the pressure within the aorta exceeds that of the left ventricle the valves close tightly, allowing for a rapid drop in left ventricular pressure in diastole. Above the sinuses the aorta becomes narrower.

INFERIOR AND SUPERIOR VENAE CAVAE

Once blood circulates through the body, it returns to the heart to be transported to the lungs for reoxygenation. The inferior vena cava (IVC) drains the trunk and lower extremities, while the superior vena cava (SVC) drains the head and parts of the upper extremities.

RIGHT ATRIUM

The right atrium is located to the right and anterior of the left atrium. It consists of three regions. Posteriorly, there is a smooth-walled venous component, which receives the inferior and superior venae cavae, as well as the coronary sinus. Anteriorly, there is a large oval vestibule which leads to the tricuspid valve. Within this region is a triangular zone lying between the attachment of the septal leaflet of the tricuspid valve, the anteromedial orifice of the coronary sinus, and the tendon of Todaro.[5] This region is of particular importance, as the atrioventricular (AV) node and its atrial branches are located here. This triangular region is referred to as the *triangle of Koch*. The final region consists of the atrium proper and the auricle. This region is separated from the posterior venous region by a ridge of muscle which runs from the anterior surface of the interatrial septum anteriorly to the opening of the SVC and to the right of the IVC opening. This ridge is the remnant of the embryonic venous valve, which directs oxygen-rich blood from the maternal circulation from the vena cava past the right ventricle and fetal lungs into the left atrium across the open foramen ovale. Within the superior region of this ridge lies the sinus or sinoatrial (SA) node. Externally, this ridge corresponds to the terminal groove.

Internally, the ridge is referred to as the *terminal crest.*[5,7]

Of particular importance for echocardiography are the structures noted in the venous region of the right atrium. The opening of the IVC enters the venous region in its lowest part, near the interatrial septum. The opening is guarded by a flap of endocardium called the *eustachian valve.* This valve is frequently noted on echocardiography and should not be confused with a thrombus or mass in the right atrium. In the fetus the eustachian valve, like the fetal venous valve, also serves to direct maternal blood from the placenta through the right atrium and patent foramen and into the left atrium, where oxygen-rich blood can be circulated to the fetus. In the adult, the eustachian valve serves no significant purpose. Also entering the venous region of the right atrium is the coronary sinus, which delivers venous blood from the heart itself. The opening of the coronary sinus is also guarded by a flap of tissue called *Thebesius' valve.* This valve is often continuous with the eustachian valve. Anterior and slightly inferior is the opening of the SVC, which has no flap at its opening.

The atrium proper and auricle are more anterior structures, with the auricle lying anterior and covering the right side of the ascending aorta. The auricle contains numerous strands of muscle called *pectinate muscles.* The septal wall consists of the fossa ovalis, septum primum, and septum secundum (Fig. 1-16).

TRICUSPID VALVE

The tricuspid valve is an atrioventricular valve which prevents the backflow of blood from the right ventricle into the right atrium. Like the mitral valve, the tricuspid valve is a complex structure composed of a tricuspid annulus, leaflet tissue, chordae tendineae, and papillary muscles. The integrity of any individual component has a direct effect on the function of the entire valve.

Tricuspid Annulus

The tricuspid annulus is the largest valvular orifice in the heart, measuring 11.4 cm in males and 10.8 cm in females.[4] The material found in the tricuspid annulus is similar to that of the mitral valve but is less strong. Its shape is roughly triangular.

Tricuspid Valve Leaflets

As the name implies, there are three leaflets to the tricuspid valve. They are named based upon their physical location in relation to the right ventricular walls. Like the mitral valve, the tricuspid leaflets are composed of collagenous material surrounded by endocardium. The basal zones are thicker than the tips, which possess indentations or commissures

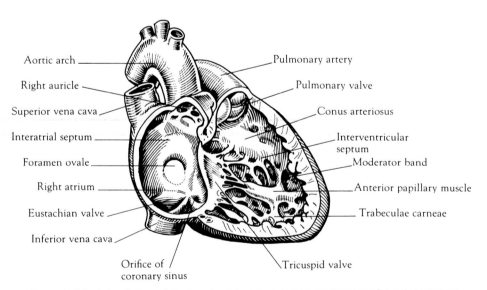

Figure 1-16. Lateral view of the heart removed, revealing the interior of the right atrium and ventricle, as well as the interatrial and interventricular septa.

which attach to chordae tendineae. There is an anterior, medial, or septal leaflet and an inferior (posterior) leaflet.

Chordae Tendineae

Chordae Tendineae support the leaflets and prevent them from prolapsing during systole. They are strong, fibrous, collagenous structures which arise from papillary muscles and insert on the ventricular side of the valve leaflets. They are also classified as primary, secondary, and tertiary, depending on their general relationship and their distance from the valve.

Papillary Muscles

The right ventricle possesses two major papillary muscles (which are less prominent than those of the left ventricle) named for their location within the ventricle. The anterior papillary muscle is the largest and is located on the anterolateral wall of the ventricle. The posterior (sometimes called *inferior*) papillary muscle is located on the inferoseptal wall. This muscle is smaller and frequently has two or three heads. The anterior papillary muscle supplies chordae to the anterior leaflet, and the posterior papillary muscle supplies the inferior leaflet. The medial or septal leaflet receives its chordae directly from the ventricular septum, a feature found only in the right ventricle.[5,7]

RIGHT VENTRICLE

The right ventricle makes up the bulk of the sternocostal surface of the heart and is the most anterior chamber of the heart, lying directly beneath the sternum. It is composed of three regions: an inlet region housing the tricuspid valve, a muscular outlet region supporting the pulmonic valve, and an apical region composed of heavy trabeculations. The right ventricle is below, slightly anterior to, and medial to the right atrium and is to the right of and anterior to the left ventricle. The right ventricle is crescent-shaped, with the anterior wall curving over the interventricular septum. There are several distinguishing features of the right ventricle that set it apart from the left ventricle: (1) The right ventricle is crescent shaped; (2) the walls are thinner than those of the left ventricle because the right ventricle ejects blood against relatively low resistance, its walls measuring 4–5 mm; and (3) the apical portion of the right ventricle possesses heavy trabeculations

called *trabeculae carneae*, the most prominent of which is the moderator band, which crosses from the septum to the anterior wall, where it joins the anterior papillary muscle. Knowledge of this band of muscle in the apex of the right heart is important since it should not be confused with thrombus (Figs. 1-13 and 1-16).

The inflow portion of the right ventricle supports the tricuspid valve and directs blood in a 60 degree angle to the outflow tract. The outflow tract is a smooth muscular region which forms the superior portion of the right ventricle. It is separated from the inflow tract by a thick muscular ridge called the *crista superventricularis*. The right ventricular outflow tract is also referred to as the *infundibulum* (Fig. 1-13).

PULMONIC VALVE

The pulmonic valve is a semilunar valve positioned in the right ventricular outflow tract. Its purpose is to prevent the backflow of blood into the right ventricle from the pulmonary circulation. The pulmonic valve is the most superior valve and is posterior to the other valves (Fig. 1-17). It is composed of three cusps named according to their relationship to other cardiac structures. There is an anterior cusp, a left cusp, and a right cusp (Fig. 1-15). No true annulus is found in the pulmonic valve; instead, there are fibrous semilunar attachments which support the cusps. The cusps themselves are made of endocardial tissue with a fibrous core.

MAIN PULMONARY ARTERY

The main pulmonary artery carries deoxygenated blood from the right heart to the lungs. The pulmonary artery begins just above the level of the pulmonic valve and courses superiorly and leftward. It lies posterior to and near the left medial aspect of the ascending aorta. The main pulmonary trunk is roughly 3 cm in diameter and 4–5 cm in length.[3,5] Above the level of the left atrium, the main pulmonary artery bifurcates into a left and a right branch. The left pulmonary artery continues in a superior and posterior course. It is attached to the descending thoracic aorta by the ligamentum arteriosus (Fig. 1-12), which in fetal life allows blood to flow from the right heart to the left. The left pulmonary artery eventually divides into four branches which continue to the left lung.

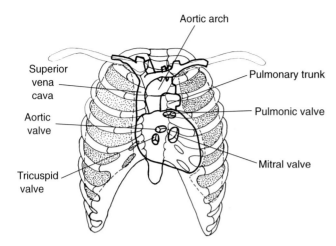

Figure 1-17. Frontal view of the heart demonstrating the anatomic relationships of the valves. Note the superior placement of the pulmonic valve.

The right pulmonary artery passes rightward, behind the ascending thoracic aorta and superior to the left atrium (Fig. 1-18). In a suprasternal view, the right pulmonary artery can be seen as a circular echolucent structure beneath the aortic arch. The right pulmonary artery also divides into four branches which travel to the right lung.

CORONARY ARTERIES

The coronary artery anatomy is covered in detail in Chapter 19. There are two major coronary arteries that arise from the sinus venosus region of the aorta. The left main coronary artery bifurcates into the left anterior descending and left circumflex arteries. The right coronary artery originates above the valve at the right sinus of Valsalva. There is considerable variation in the origins of the coronary arteries, but in this chapter the more usual anatomy will be covered. Although the coronary arteries originate at the sinus, their ostia are above the level of the aortic cusps when fully open; therefore, even in full systole, the aortic cusps do not flatten against the coronary ostia. Any particular coronary artery may be the dominant vessel, meaning that it supplies parts of the interventricular septum and posterolateral walls of the left ventricle. In 70% of cases, the dominant branch is the left coronary artery.[3,5]

The left coronary artery is usually the larger of the two main vessels. Its branches supply the majority of the left ventricle and atrium, including the interventricular septum. The right coronary artery

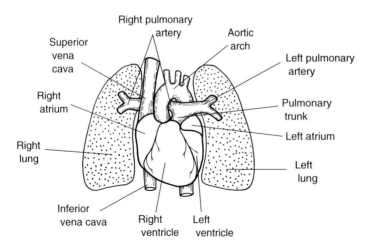

Figure 1-18. Anatomic relationship of the pulmonary artery and its branches.

supplies the right atrium, right ventricle, and segments of the interventricular septum.

CONDUCTION SYSTEM

The conduction system of the heart is made up of specialized myocardial cells called *myocytes*. These cells are capable of producing and transmitting to one another rhythmic waves of electrical excitation. The components of the conduction system are the sinus node, atrioventricular node, atrioventricular bundle or bundle of His, and subendocardial fibers or Purkinge fibers. The components of the conduction system are intimately related.

Sinus Node

The sinus node or SA node is located in the junction or terminal groove separating the venous region of the right atrium and the right atrium proper and just below the SVC. The node lies on the epicardial surface of the right atrial wall. It is the pacemaker of the heart because it initiates each cardiac cycle and sets the rate for the remainder of the conduction system. The electrical impulse spreads outward away from the SA node in all directions. The rate at which the pulses are sent ranges from 60 to 100 per minute. This event causes the atrium to contract and represents the P wave on an electrocardiogram (EKG).

Atrioventricular Node

The AV node lies in the junction of the atrioventricular cushion or septum on the floor of the right atrium. It is bordered by the septal leaflet of the tricuspid valve and the opening of the coronary sinus.[3,5,7] The top of the AV node is in continuity with the atrial myocardium, which transmits the impulses from the SA node.[3,5,7] The bottom part communicates with the ventricles by a common bundle of specialized tissue which are sometimes called the *bundle of His*. The bundle of His varies in length from 10 to 20 mm. The AV node is responsible for delaying the impulse from the SA node to the ventricles, thereby regulating the proper timing of atrial to ventricular contractions. This delay allows the ventricles to fill with blood.

Bundle Branches

From the bundle of His, two major branches run through the interventricular septum to the cardiac apex. These branches are referred to as the *left bundle branch* and *right bundle branch*. They are well-encapsulated fibers which eventually form Purkinje fibers.

Purkinje Fibers

The Purkinje fibers are the terminal branches of the bundle branches. They course through the endocardium of both ventricles, trabeculations, papillary

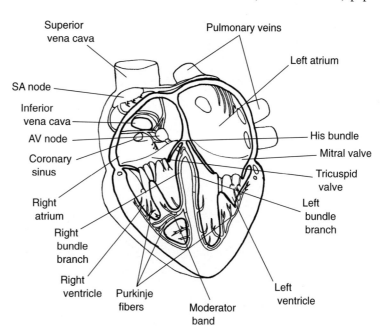

Figure 1-19. Intrinsic conduction system of the heart.

muscles, and moderator band. The fibers of the right bundle branch begin at the level of the anterior papillary muscle and invade the ventricular endocardium. The fibers of the left bundle branch begin as a wide sheet of fibers running down the interventricular septum, eventually reaching the apex and curving back up to reach all aspects of the ventricle. The impulses generated to the Purkinge fibers start in the cardiac apex and move upward toward the ventricular outflow tracts. This timing aids in the acceleration of blood toward the left and right outflow tracts. This excitation corresponds to the QRS complex on an EKG (Fig. 1-19).

REFERENCES

1. Cheitlin MD, Finkbeiner WE. Cardiology: An Illustrated text/Reference. Philadelphia and New York, JB Lippincott and Gower Medical Publishing; 1991.

2. Craig M, Kawamura D, Berman M. Diagnostic Medical Sonography: A Guide to Clinical Practice. Vol II: Echocardiography. Philadelphia, JB Lippincott; 1991.

3. Dubin D. Rapid Interpretation of EKG's. Tampa, FL, Cover Publishing Co; 1989;77.

4. Gabella G. Cardiovascular. *In* Williams P, Bannister I, Berry MM, et al: Gray's Anatomy. New York, Churchill Livingstone; 1995.

5. Hoerr NL, Osol A. Blakiston's New Gould Medical Dictionary, 2nd ed. New York, McGraw-Hill; 1956.

6. Netter FH. Anatomy. *In* The CIBA Collection of Medical Illustrations. Heart. New York, CIBA; 1981.

7. Silver MD, Lam JHC, Ranganathan N, et al. Morphology of the human tricuspid valve. Circulation. 1971;43:333–348.

8. Waller BF, Schlant RC. Anatomy of the heart. *In* Schlant RC, Alexander RW, O'Rouke RA, et al. (eds): Hurst's The Heart. New York, McGraw-Hill; 1994: 59–113.

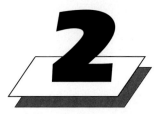

Normal Cardiac Physiology

EVALIE DuMARS

Knowledge of cardiac anatomy and the echocardiographic appearances of pathology are important to producing and recognizing diagnostic images, but the full value of such studies can be derived only by those with a sound understanding of cardiac function and hemodynamics. In this chapter, we explain the double circulation of the heart, the events of the cardiac cycle, and the normal hemodynamic pressures.

The heart is a muscular pump that is responsible for pumping blood to the body. In order for blood to be distributed adequately, blood pressure must be maintained. Both pressure and flow are governed by a complex control mechanism that responds to metabolic requirements of various parts of the body and their functional interrelationships.

The human heart consists of two fluid pumps that exist side by side anatomically but are connected in series functionally. The right side of the heart supplies the pulmonary (lung) circulation. The normal pressure in the right ventricle is about 22 mm Hg. From the lungs, the blood returns to the left side of the heart, which supplies blood to the body via the systemic circulation. The pressure in the left ventricle is about 120 mm Hg. The volume pumped by the two sides of the heart is the same to ensure the normal circuit of flow. This equality is balanced even when the volume pumped is increased as much as five times by exercise demand. The blood is pumped from the ventricles during systole, and the ventricles receive blood during the relaxation phase, diastole.

Right Heart Circulation

Venous blood returns from the body to the right atrium via the superior and inferior venae cavae. During atrial systole, blood travels through the tricuspid valve into the right ventricle, which is in diastole (Fig. 2-1). The blood returning from the body has a lower oxygen saturation (75%) than that pumped from the left side (95% to 100%).

The tricuspid valve is closed during right ventricular systole, and the blood contained in the right ventricle is propelled out of the right ventricular outflow tract (the conus arteriosus or infundibulum) through the open semilunar pulmonic valve to the pulmonic circulation.

Left Heart Circulation

The left atrium receives blood from the lungs through four pulmonary veins located in the back of the left atrial cavity. As left atrial systole occurs, the mitral valve (left atrioventricular {AV} valve) is in the open position, allowing the blood in the left atrium to be propelled down into the left ventricular cavity. The left atrium acts as a reservoir during ventricular systole and as a conduit during ventricular diastole. As ventricular systole occurs, the mitral valve is closed and the blood is propelled out of

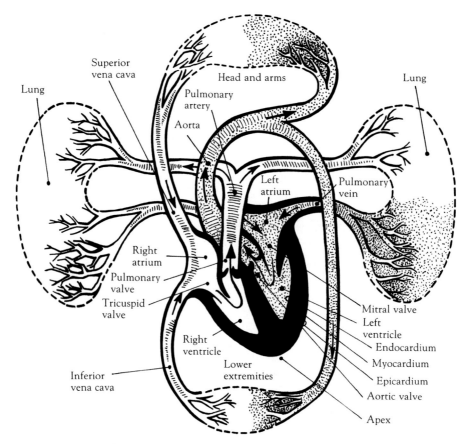

Figure 2-1. Plan of circulation.

the left ventricular outflow tract through the open semilunar aortic valve to the systemic circulation.

Blood Supply of the Heart

Two major arteries, the left and right coronary arteries, supply blood to the heart muscle and to the proximal portions of the great vessels. The coronary arteries arise from the base of the aorta, just above the valve leaflets at the sinus of Valsalva (see Chapter 1). The aortic valve cusps are named according to their specific location to the coronary arteries: right coronary cusp, left coronary cusp, and noncoronary cusp.

RIGHT CORONARY ARTERY

The right coronary artery courses in the coronary sulcus along the diaphragmatic surface of the heart before descending to the apex. Branches arise from this artery that supply the right atrium, the free wall

of the right ventricle, and, in approximately 70% of hearts, the posterior third of the ventricular septum and the posterior wall of the left ventricle.[4,17,24] An ascending coronary artery arises from the right coronary sinus approximately 50% of the time. This short vessel, the conus artery, supplies the outflow tract of the right ventricle at or near the level of the pulmonic valve.[24]

LEFT CORONARY ARTERY

The left coronary artery bifurcates into two major branches at or just beyond its origin. The left circumflex artery arises at right angles to the major vessel and courses through the AV sulcus before turning down to the apex. The left atrium and lateral wall of the left ventricle receive blood from this vessel. Both the right coronary artery and the circumflex artery supply blood to the posterior left ventricular wall (Fig. 2-2).[24]

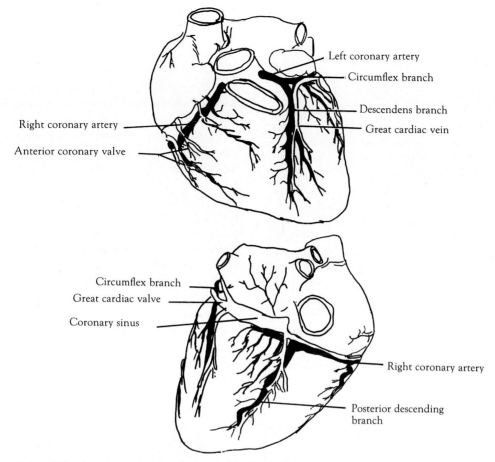

Figure 2-2. Coronary arterial and venous blood supply.

The left anterior descending artery continues as an extension of the main vessel before coursing downward in the interventricular groove toward the cardiac apex. The left ventricular free wall, ventricular septum, and, to a limited extent, the anterior wall of the right ventricle receive their blood supply from this artery.[24,26]

Approximately 50% to 60% of the time, a special branch of the right coronary artery supplies blood to the sinoatrial (SA) node. This artery is also the main source of blood for the atrial myocardium and the atrial septum. The AV node receives its blood supply from a branch of the right coronary artery in about 90% of persons and from the left circumflex artery in the remainder.[24,26] Some variations in vascular patterns exist and are not thought to be significant indicators of coronary insufficiency or predictors of the total amount of myocardium supplied by the right or left coronary artery system.[13,17,24,26]

VENOUS DRAINAGE

The coronary sinus, which lies in the posterior part of the AV groove, drains most of the blood from the heart walls into the right atrium to the left of the inferior vena cava. The coronary sinus is a continuation of the great cardiac vein, and the small and middle cardiac veins are tributaries of the coronary sinus. The anterior vein and some small cardiac veins return the remainder of the blood to the right atrium and cardiac chambers via direct openings.[17,26]

Intrinsic Innervation of the Heart

CONDUCTION SYSTEM OF THE HEART

To ensure that the chambers of the heart act in an orderly way, the heart possesses specialized conductive tissue responsible for the initiation, propagation, and coordination of the heartbeat. This conduction system consists of (1) the SA node, (2) the atrial internodal pathways, (3) the AV node, (4) the common AV bundle (bundle of His), (5) the right and left bundle branches, and (6) the Purkinje system (Fig. 2-3).

The SA node lies in the sulcus between the superior vena cava and the right atrium. It is referred to as the *pacemaker* of the heart because it is the source of bursts of electrical nerve impulses that spread through the walls of the heart. Because the SA node is located high in the right atrium, the first structures to contract in the normal activation sequence are the two atria. Once initiated, the impulse spreads throughout the atrial myocardium to the level of the AV node. The AV node is located in the lower part of the atrial septum just above the attachment of the septal cusp of the tricuspid valve. The electrical impulse coming from the atria slows somewhat at the AV node, and a delay occurs.[2,5,17,19]

From the AV node, the impulse is conducted to the ventricles by specialized conducting tissue, the AV bundle (or bundle of His) and its divisions, the right and left bundle branches. These structures ramify and become continuous with the fibers of the Purkinje network. At this time, the ventricles contract and the blood is ejected to the pulmonic and systemic circulations.

Extrinsic Innervation of the Heart

Although the heart possesses its own intrinsic rhythmicity (conduction system), its rate is modified by the autonomic nervous system. Fibers from both the sympathetic and parasympathetic nervous systems (which are divisions of the autonomic nervous system) are received by the heart (Fig. 2-4).

The *sympathetic nervous system* sends its fibers mainly to the atria via the right and left vagus nerves, thereby contributing to the control of the SA and AV nodes. These sympathetic fibers are derived from the upper thoracic sympathetic ganglia (and cord segments). They pass superiorly in the sympathetic trunk to the cervical region, where they are given off as the cervical sympathetic cardiac nerves, which then pass down through the neck to reach the cardiac plexus around the coils of the great vessels.[8,9,23,27,28,36] From here they are distributed to the atria and to the ventricular musculature. Stimulation of the sympathetic nervous system fibers to the heart causes four effects: it increases the heart rate, increases transmission between the atria and the ventricles, increases the force of contraction, and increases the conduction rate of nodes and atria.

The *parasympathetic* nerves are derived from the vagus and are given off in the neck as the vagal

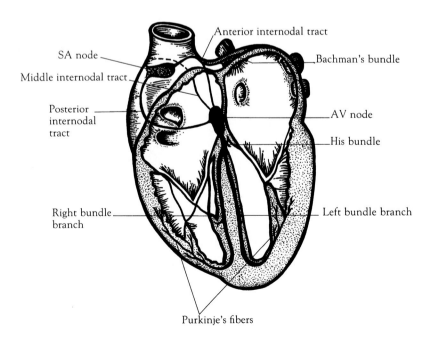

Anterior internodal tract

SA node

Bachman's bundle

Middle internodal tract

Posterior internodal tract

AV node

His bundle

Right bundle branch

Left bundle branch

Purkinje's fibers

Figure 2-3. Intrinsic conduction system of the heart.

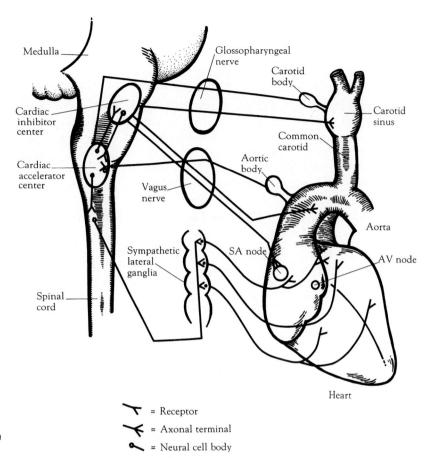

Medulla

Glossopharyngeal
nerve

Carotid
body

Cardiac
inhibitor
center

Carotid
sinus

Common
carotid

Cardiac
accelerator
center

Aortic
body

Vagus
nerve

Aorta

Sympathetic
lateral
ganglia

SA node

AV node

Spinal
cord

Heart

⊤ = Receptor

⫫ = Axonal terminal

⟍ = Neural cell body

Figure 2-4. Extrinsic innervation
of the heart.

cardiac nerves.[9,15,23] They enter the cardiac plexus and there connect to the SA node.

Stimulation of the parasympathetic nervous system fibers to the heart also causes four effects: it decreases the heart rate, retards transmission between the atria and ventricles, decreases the force of contraction, and decreases the conduction rate of nodes and atria.

It is now obvious that the sympathetic and parasympathetic nervous systems have basically opposite effects on the heart.[23,24] These two systems are reciprocally innervated, so increased activity in one is usually accompanied by decreased activity in the other. The reflex centers for both are in the medulla oblongata (Fig. 2-4).

Figure 2-4 shows the neural connections between the heart and various receptors via the central nervous system (CNS). Located in the medulla, the paired centers that influence the heart rate are the cardioaccelerator center (CAC) and the cardioinhibitor center (CIC). The CAC sends efferent (conducting away from the CNS) fibers to the heart by way of the sympathetic nervous system, and the CIC sends efferent fibers to the heart via the parasympathetic system. These two centers receive afferent (conducting toward the CNS) fibers from receptors located in one of four places: the carotid sinus, the aortic arch, the aortic bodies, and the carotid bodies. The CAC and CIC are also reciprocally innervated, so that when the activity in one increases, the activity in the other decreases.[8,9,15,16,23,27,31]

Events of the Cardiac Cycle

The cardiac cycle includes all of the electrical and mechanical events that occur during the cycle of one heartbeat. With each cardiac cycle or heartbeat there are two phases of passage of oxygenated and deoxygenated blood through the heart.

Cardiac contraction is preceded by electrical stimulation, which leads in turn to a series of events that are associated with the heart's function as a pump. These electrical and mechanical events are presented schematically in Figure 2-5. Representative pressure pulses from the left atrium (bottom hash line), left ventricle (solid line), and aorta (top hash line) are shown along with the scalar electrocardiogram (ECG). Heart sounds are presented below the ECG. Note also the timing of the echocardiographic representation of mitral valve (AV) and aortic valve (SL) patterns.

Our discussion of the cardiac cycle begins with

ventricular systole. Ventricular systole commences with the peak of the R wave of the ECG and the initial vibration of the first heart sound (lub; see Fig. 2-5).

The first phase of ventricular systole is *isovolumic contraction*, which begins with the start of ventricular contraction and ends with the opening of the semilunar valves (aortic and pulmonic). At the onset of ventricular contraction there is a rapid increase in ventricular pressure, which squeezes the blood inside the ventricle against the closed valves. During this time the circumference of the left ventricle increases, the apex-to-base length

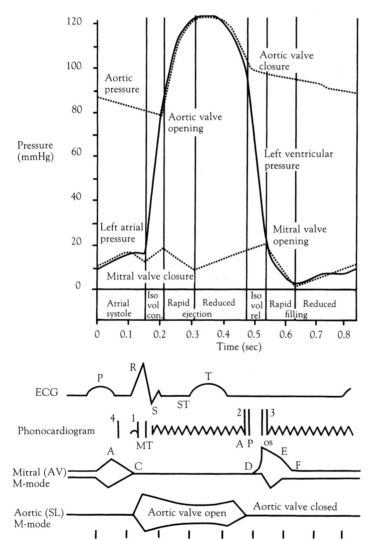

Figure 2-5. Events of the cardiac cycle. (Adapted from Netter FH. The CIBA Collection of Medical Illustrations, 1974; Little RC. Physiology of the Heart and Circulation, 1977; Rushmer RF. Cardiovascular Dynamics, 1961.)

decreases, and the left ventricle becomes more spherical.[7,20,26,29] These changes are well demonstrated in the normal left ventricular ECG comparing the apical and short axis views.[14,25]

The semilunar (aortic and pulmonic) valves open when the pressure within the respective ventricles exceeds the diastolic pressure of its great artery, i.e., the aortic valve opens when left ventricular pressure exceeds diastolic aortic pressure.[22] Under normal circumstances, this rise in ventricular pressure (to exceed the aortic diastolic pressure) occurs within approximately 0.06 to 0.08 sec after the onset of contraction.[13,17,19,20,24,32] Ventricular pressure continues to increase, and as it rises above aortic pressure, the aortic valve cusps are forced open and the period of *rapid ejection* begins, lasting until peak ventricular and aortic pressures are achieved. During this time (approximately 0.10 to 0.11 sec from the onset of ejection), 80% to 85% of stroke volume leaves the heart and the blood quickly reaches its maximal velocity (approximately 150 cm/sec or 1.5 m/sec).[14]

Near the end of the period of rapid cardiac ejection, ventricular pressure peaks and begins to fall, with *reduced ejection* occurring when aortic and left ventricular pressure closely approximate one another. The reduced ejection phase continues until the aortic valve closes (after approximately 0.17 sec). The reduced ejection phase represents the period during which runoff of blood from the aorta into the peripheral vessels exceeds ventricular output. Normally, about 50% of the blood contained in the ventricle before contraction is ejected.

Ventricular diastole commences with the closure of the aortic valve. This is indicated by the *incisura* (notch) on the aortic pressure tracing (see Fig. 2-5). This notch occurs as a result of the rapid deceleration of the fluid column and closure of the aortic valve, producing a sharp oscillation in the aortic pressure.

The second heart sound (dub) is now heard. It represents closure of the aortic and pulmonic valves. At this time, blood pours into the right atrium from the superior and inferior vena cavae and into the left atrium through the pulmonary veins.

The first phase of diastole, the *isovolumic relaxation* phase, commences with the closing of the semilunar valves (aortic and pulmonic) and continues until the opening of the AV valves (mitral and tricuspid). This period is characterized by a precipitous fall in ventricular pressure without a change in ventricular volume. As ventricular pressure drops below left atrial pressure, generating an AV pressure gradient, the AV valve cusps are forced open.[13,17,19,24]

The next phase in diastole is the *rapid filling phase,* which commences with the opening of the AV valves and the release of atrial blood into the ventricles, which are now in a relaxed state. The period of rapid filling lasts approximately 0.06 sec after the opening of the mitral valve, or until the left ventricular pressure reaches its lowest level and begins a rapid upward swing.

The rapid filling phase is followed by the *reduced filling* phase, during which blood returning from the periphery flows into the right ventricle and blood from the lungs flows into the left ventricle.

The final phase of ventricular diastole, *atrial systole,* occurs at the peak of the P wave on an ECG. This transfer of atrial blood to the ventricles by atrial contraction completes ventricular filling. The mitral and tricuspid valves close as a result of reduced blood flow against the atrial surface of these valves and increased eddy current forces on the ventricular surface of the valves. This marks the end of atrial systole and of ventricular diastole.[13,17,19,24]

The electrical events in the heart are visible on an ECG. The *P wave* represents atrial depolarization, or contraction. The *QRS complex* represents ventricular contraction. The time between the P wave and the QRS complex, the *PR interval,* represents slowing of the conduction through the AV node. The *T wave* represents repolarization of the ventricles. The isoelectric period between the S and T waves is the *ST segment,* during which the heart is refractory to electrical stimulation.[5,17,26]

REFERENCES

1. Arvidsson H. Angiocardiograph determination of left ventricular volume. Acta Radiol. 1961;56:321.
2. Badeer HS. "Contractility" of the non-failing hypertrophied heart. Am Heart J. 1967;73:693.
3. Berglund E. Ventricular function. VI. Balance of left and right ventricular output: Relation between left and right atrial pressure. Am J Physiol. 1954;178: 381.
4. Berglund E. The function of the ventricles of the heart. Acta Physiol Scand. 1955;33(suppl 119):1.
5. Bernreiter M. Electrocardiography, 2nd ed. Philadelphia, JB Lippincott; 1963:Chap. 1.
6. Blair HA, Wedd AM. The action of cardiac ejection on venous return. Am J Physiol. 1946;145:528.

7. Bowe AA. Radiographic evaluation of dynamic geometry of the left ventricle. J Appl Physiol. 1971;31: 227.

8. Bronk DW, Ferguson LK, Margaria R, et al. The activity of the cardiac sympathetic centers. Am J Physiol. 1936;111:237.

9. Bruce TA, Chapman CB, Baker O, et al. The role of autonomic and myocardial factors in cardiac control. J Clin Invest. 1963;42:721.

10. De Geest H, Levy MN, Zieske H, et al. Depression of ventricular contractility by stimulation of the vagus nerves. Circ Res. 1965;17:222.

11. Gebber G, Snyder DW. Hypothalamic control of the baroreceptor reflexes. Am J Physiol. 1969;218:124.

12. Guyton AC, Langston JB, Carrier O. Decrease in venous return caused by right atrial pulsation. Circ Res. 1962;10:188.

13. Guyton AG, Jones CE, Coleman TG. Circulatory Physiology: Cardiac Output and Its Regulation. Philadelphia, WB Saunders; 1973.

14. Hatle L, Angelsel B. Doppler Ultrasound in Cardiology: Physical Principles and Clinical Applications, 2nd ed. Philadelphia, Lea & Febiger; 1985.

15. Higgins CB, Vatner SF, Braunwald E. Parasympathetic control of the heart. Pharmacol Rev. 1973;25: 119.

16. Hockman CH, Taliesnic J, Livingston KE. Central nervous system modulation of baroreceptor reflexes. Am J Physiol. 1969;217:1681.

17. Hurst JW, Logue RB, Schlant RD, et al. The Heart. New York, McGraw-Hill; 1978.

18. James TN. The connecting pathways between the sinus node and the AV node and between the right and left atrium of the human heart. Am Heart J. 1963;66:498.

19. Katz AM. Physiology of the Heart. New York, Raven Press; 1977.

20. Katz LN. Relation of initial volume and initial pressure to dynamics of the ventricular contraction. Am J Physiol. 1928;87:348.

21. Kircheim HR. Systemic arterial baroreceptor reflexes. Physiol Rev. 1976;56:100.

22. Laniado S, Yellin E, Terdiman R, et al. Hemodynamic correlates of the normal aortic valve echogram: A study of sound, flow and motion. Circulation. 1976;54:729.

23. Levy MN, Ng M, Martin P, et al. Sympathetic and parasympathetic interactions upon the left ventricle of the dog. Circ Res. 1966;19:5.

24. Little RC. Physiology of the Heart and Circulation. Chicago, Year Book Medical; 1977:32–41.

25. Nanda NC, Gramiak R. Clinical Echocardiography. St Louis, CV Mosby; 1978.

26. Netter FH. The CIBA Collection of Medical Illustrations. Rochester, NY, Case-Hoyt Corporation; 1974:5.

27. Randall WC, McNally H. Augmentor action of the sympathetic cardiac nerves in man. J Appl Physiol. 1960;15:629.

28. Robinson BF, Epstein SE, Beiser GD, et al. Control of heart rate by the autonomic nervous system: Studies in man on the interrelationship between baroreceptor mechanisms and exercise. Circ Res. 1966;19: 400.

29. Rushmer RF. Length-circumference relations of the left ventricle. Circ Res. 1955;3:639.

30. Rushmer RF. Pressure-circumference relations of the left ventricle. Am J Physiol. 1956;186:115.

31. Rushmer RF. Autonomic balance in cardiac control. Am J Physiol. 1958;192:631.

32. Rushmer RF. Cardiovascular Dynamics. Philadelphia, WB Saunders; 1961:75–96.

33. Sonnenblick EH, Ross J Jr, Covell JW, et al. The ultrastructure of the heart in systole and diastole: Changes in sarcomere length. Circ Res. 1967;21: 423.

34. Spencer MP, Greiss FC. Dynamics of ventricular ejection. Circ Res. 1962;10:274.

35. Titus JL. Normal anatomy of the human cardiac conduction system. Mayo Clin Proc. 1973;48:24.

36. Zimmerman BG. Separation of responses of arteries and veins to sympathetic stimulation. Circ Res. 1966; 18:429.

PART II

Principles and Practical Applications of Echocardiography

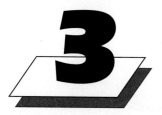

Physical Considerations in Ultrasound

MARK N. ALLEN

Waves

There are three basic classifications of sound: infrasound, audible sound, and ultrasound. *Infrasound* is defined as sound below the range of human hearing, *audible sound* is sound that falls within the range of human hearing, and *ultrasound* is sound above the range of human hearing. This classification is determined by the number of cycles per second that the sound waves travel through a medium, called its *frequency*. Frequency is measured in hertz (Hz).[24] Figure 3-1 demonstrates the various classifications and their frequencies.

Sound is a mechanical form of energy that travels through a medium by means of particle displacement or vibrations. The propagation of waves through a medium is accomplished by these vibrations. The more dense the particles in a medium, the higher the pressure within that area. This area of high pressure is also referred to as *compression*. Areas within the medium where the particles are less dense are referred to as *rarefaction*. The sound waves traveling parallel to the line of propagation are called *longitudinal waves* or *compressible waves*. Waves that travel perpendicular to the line of propagation are called *transverse waves*.[35] Ultrasound waves are longitudinal waves. Once waves hit particles within a medium, a vibration develops that, in turn, affects the surrounding particles within that medium. A simple analogy is that of a series of balls connected to one another by springs (Fig. 3-2). As mechanical pressure is applied to one ball, all the balls eventually begin to vibrate. This conduction of pressure is similar to what occurs as sound waves pass through tissue. In living tissue the propagation of sound occurs at the microscopic level and at a high rate, so no net particle displacement is observed[49] (Fig. 3-3).

A sound wave is characterized by a sine wave (Fig. 3-4). When viewed in this manner, the compressions are noted as peaks or antinodes and the rarefactions as nodes. Antinodes are the upward or downward peaks of the sine wave. The nodes depict no particle displacement. One complete node and one complete antinode represent one cycle or wavelength.[35] The wavelength is the distance between the onset of one compression to the onset of the next. The number of wavelengths per unit of time is equivalent to the wave's frequency. In diagnostic ultrasound, frequency is measured in megahertz (MHz). The typical range in cardiac work is 2.5 to 5 MHz. This notation indicates that the diagnostic wave produced has 2.5 million to 5 million cycles per second. The human ear is capable of hearing sound waves that have a frequency of 100,000 Hz.[35] Wavelength is a distance measurement that measures the distance covered by one complete cycle. This relationship between wavelength and

33

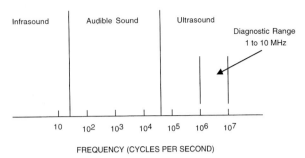

Figure 3-1. Classification of sound waves.

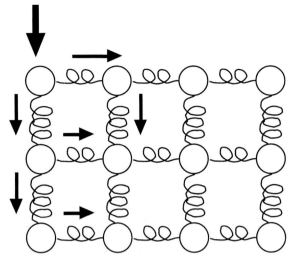

Figure 3-2. Propagation of sound waves through a medium. As pressure is applied to the first ball in the series, the pressure is exerted on all the balls as it is transferred via the springs. As in tissue, sound is propagated by transferring the pressure to surrounding tissue particles.

frequency can be expressed in the following formula:

$$c = F \times \int \qquad (3\text{-}1)$$

where c is the velocity of sound in a particular medium, F is the frequency, and $\int$ is the wavelength. Since velocity in any given medium is unchanging, c is constant; therefore, F and $\int$ have an inverse relationship. As the frequency increases the wavelength decreases, and vice versa. For soft tissue the velocity of sound propagation is 1540 m/sec. For the velocities of sound in other tissues[18,49] see Table 3-1. If the transducer or frequency is known, then the wavelength can be calculated using Eq. 3-1. Thus, at 2 MHz,

$$1540 = 2,000,000 \times \int$$
$$\int = 0.77 \text{ mm}$$

Similarly, at 2.5 MHz, $\int = 0.62$ mm; at 3.5 MHz, $\int = 0.44$ mm; at 5.0 MHz, $\int = 0.31$ mm; and at 10 MHz, $\int = 0.15$ mm. Note that as the frequency increases, the wavelength decreases. The distance between identical points on an ultrasound wave in soft tissue is on the order of 1 mm or less. Therefore, as frequency increases wavelength decreases, allowing more image detail at higher frequencies. This is

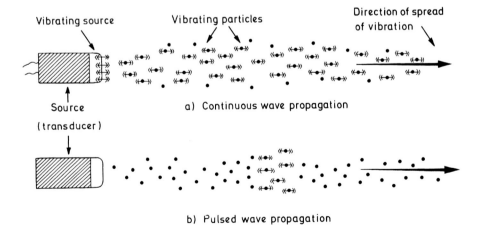

Figure 3-3. Propagation of sound waves through a medium, causing the particles to vibrate, which in turn affects all surrounding particles. (From McDicken WN [ed]. Diagnostic Ultrasonics: Principles and Use of Instruments, 2nd ed. New York, Wiley; 1981:Fig. 1-1. Reprinted with permission.)

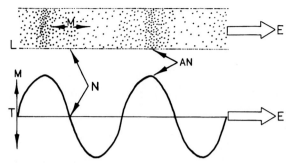

Figure 3-4. A sound wave can best be described as a sine wave with peaks and troughs. One complete cycle equals one wavelength. (From Ref. 35, Fig. 1-2. Reprinted with permission.)

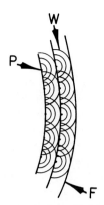

Figure 3-5. Huygen principle. Multiple waves (W) that are in phase will eventually merge to form a single wavefront (F). (From Ref. 35, Fig. 1-6. Reprinted with permission.)

a very important point, since the goal in echocardiography is to provide maximum detail.

To understand the physics behind sound propagation within a medium, a thorough understanding of the principles of wave properties is essential. The velocity of any sound wave is dependent on the wave's frequency and wavelength. Each material allows sound to travel through it at a particular velocity. The velocity of sound through a particular medium is determined by several factors, including the medium's density, elastic properties, and temperature.[35] The speed with which a sound beam travels is called its *propagation speed.*

The strength of a sound beam or ultrasound is defined by intensity and amplitude. Intensity is the power in a wave divided by the area over which the power is spread. It is measured in Watts per centimeter squared. It is represented by the following formula:

$$\text{Intensity} = \left(\frac{W}{\text{cm}^2}\right) = \frac{\text{Power (Watts)}}{\text{area (cm}^2)} \quad (3\text{-}2)$$

$$\text{or} \quad I = \frac{P}{A}$$

The wave's amplitude represents the maximum displacement of particles that occurs during the wave's cycle. Wave *amplitude* usually refers to the wave's peak amplitude. Amplitude is the value used to determine the amount of energy present in the wave and how disruptive that wave is to the material carrying it.[35]

So far, the discussion of waves has been limited to a simple wave. In diagnostic ultrasound, the waves are more complex and are usually multiple. As we will see, waves produced by cardiac transducers are multiple. There are several units, or transducer elements, all producing their own waves. Each wave produced travels at a constant velocity. If all the waves are in phase, then they begin to connect with one another. As the wave travels, its components begin to form a single wavefront. This principle is called *Huygen's principle*, named after its discoverer, Christian Huygen. This single product of multiple waves then propagates through a medium and is dictated by the physical properties of the material (Fig. 3-5).

Interaction of Sound in Soft Tissue

The manner in which sound waves interact with a particular material is highly dependent on many variables. The two most important factors are the

TABLE 3-1. The Velocity of Ultrasound in Selected Materials

Material	Velocity of Sound (m/sec)
Air	330
Bone	3500
Soft tissue	1540
Blood	1570
Muscle	1580
Fat	1450
Water (20°C)	1480

density and compressibility of a material. Temperature and frequency also influence sound waves, but to a lesser extent.

Several events can occur as sound energy passes through a material. In a homogeneous material, where all things are equal, sound waves propagate unobscured until they dissipate. However, in the body, all things are not equal, and so the propagation of sound through the material will change, depending on the properties of the material encountered. There are several physical phenomena that occur as the result of these encounters. The principal ones are refraction, diffraction, absorption, reflection, transmission, attenuation, and beam formation.

REFRACTION

Refraction occurs when sound crosses at an angle between two different materials where the velocity of sound within the materials differs. In this case, the sound waves deviate or bend. This occurs when a pencil is placed in a cup of water. When looked at above the water, the pencil appears to be straight. When looked at below the water line, it appears to bend. This demonstrates the refractive property of light. This phenomenon is explained by *Snell's law*, which states that the light rays, upon crossing between two different materials, refract, making the pencil appear to bend. This same principle holds when sound waves cross two media. Snell's Law is explained by the following formula:

$$\frac{\sin i}{\sin r} = \frac{c1}{c2} \qquad (3\text{-}3)$$

where sin *i* is the angle of incidence for the incident beam, sin *r* is the angle of the reflected beam, *c*1 is the velocity of sound in tissue 1, and *c*2 is the velocity of sound in tissue 2.

Large beam deviations are seen when the velocity differences are great or the angle is significant. In soft tissue the degree of refraction is relatively small, and because there are numerous angle differences, a certain amount of refraction is canceled out as the wave bends in different angles along its path. The amount of beam deviation between two typical human tissues will vary, depending on the tissues involved. Within a soft tissue to soft tissue interface the amount of deviation is 1 or 2 degrees, and since the area of interest is relatively small, the beam does not travel a great enough distance to make a signifi-

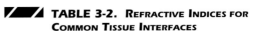

TABLE 3-2. REFRACTIVE INDICES FOR COMMON TISSUE INTERFACES

Tissue	Degree of Deviation
Fat/muscle	19.2
Muscle/blood	0.5
Muscle/fat	2.25
Muscle/fluid	1.05

Source: Ref. 24.

cant impact. Table 3-2 illustrates the degree of deviation between common tissue interfaces encountered in echocardiography.

In echocardiography, refraction is not a significant problem for the reasons stated above. However, when a soft tissue/bone interface is encountered, image degradation can occur. Refraction can produce artifacts, a topic discussed in more detail at the end of this chapter.

DIFFRACTION

Diffraction is the spreading of an ultrasound beam as it propagates through a medium. The mechanical vibrations generated by the mechanical wave diverge rapidly, causing degradation of the original wave.

ABSORPTION

Absorption accounts for most of the loss of sound waves as they pass through a medium. This fact raises the question of how any imaging can be accomplished at all. The mechanism of absorption is not completely understood; however, one explanation is that the cells absorb one form of energy and typically convert it into another form of energy. The mechanical sound waves are therefore converted into heat or internal molecular energy. The mechanism of absorption can be explained as a relaxation mechanism. An energy force applied to a molecule will set up stresses within that molecule. The molecule responds by converting that energy force into a form of energy that is more easily dissipated, such as heat. If we consider our ball and spring example, the force applied to the first ball creates stresses on that ball. The ball responds by transferring that energy to the next ball, thereby relaxing the initial stresses applied to it. A molecule acts much the same way when an external force is applied to it. The molecule relaxes from the stress applied to it by the sound wave by converting it to heat, which is more easily dissipated, thereby relaxing the stresses created.[24]

As an ultrasound wave passes through a medium, its intensity and amplitude are diminished, depending on the absorption characteristic of the material. The absorption characteristic of the material is defined by the material's absorption coefficient. The larger this coefficient, the greater the decrease in the wave's intensity. The amount of absorption that occurs in a given material is dependent on several factors, including the material's absorption coefficient, elasticity, viscosity, and temperature. The frequency of the transmitted wave also has an impact on the drop in intensity of the sound wave as it travels through a medium. The higher the frequency, the greater the degree of absorption. This physical finding can be demonstrated by the fact that a relatively narrow range of frequencies can be used for diagnostic testing purposes. The temperature of a material will also cause either a decrease or an increase in the amount of absorption, depending on the material.[16,17,48]

One must also keep in mind that in diagnostic ultrasound the effects of absorption are twofold. Absorption occurs not only as the beam enters the body, but also on the reflected waves going back toward the transducer.

REFLECTION

In a homogeneous medium, sound continues to propagate through until the mechanisms of absorption take their toll. In the human body this is not the case. In nonhomogeneous material, wave propagation is not equal in all directions. In the human body the mixture of material facilitates a process referred to as *reflection*. Reflection occurs as the result of the difference in wave-carrying capability between the two materials, such as density and propagation velocity. The product of a material's density and propagation velocity is called the *characteristic* or *acoustic impedance* of the material. Acoustic impedance can be expressed as

$$Z = pc \qquad (3-4)$$

where Z is acoustic impedance, p is density, and c is velocity of propagation.

The acoustic impedance mismatch between two neighboring materials will result in some of the

wave's energy being reflected. An interface exists between the two materials, resulting in reflection of the sound wave. As an incident wave encounters a change in acoustic impedance, a portion of that wave is reflected. The direction of the reflected wave will depend on the angle with which the incident wave encounters the surface. This angle is referred to as the *angle of incidence*. If the interface is laterally large relative to the wavelength, the reflection will be governed by the same rules that apply to light reflection at a mirrored surface. That is, the majority of the reflected wave will return to the source. This type of reflector is referred to as a *specular* reflector. Specular reflectors tend to be large, smooth surfaces whose angle of incidence is equal to and opposite the angle of reflection. Examples of specular reflectors in the body include the pericardium, diaphragm, and cardiac valves. These surfaces typically demonstrate bright reflections compared to other tissues. The amount of energy reflected will also depend on the magnitude of the acoustic impedance change between the two media. If the transition is from a lower to a higher impedance, the magnitude of the reflected wave will be high. Conversely, if the wave propagates from a higher to a lower impedance, the magnitude will be low.

In order to demonstrate some of these principles, refer to Table 3-3. In a bone/muscle interface the percentage of reflected energy is roughly 41%, compared to a muscle/blood interface, which reflects .07% of the energy. These differences account for the variations in appearance frequently observed when scanning the heart. If the wave encounters bone first, a high percentage of energy will be reflected, obscuring the structures beyond the bone. By contrast, a wave traveling through muscle that encounters blood will allow visualization of both tissues.

As stated earlier, the magnitude of the reflected energy is a function of the size and shape of the tissues encountered. Most biological materials have interfaces that are smaller than the ultrasound wavelength. Interfaces with dimensions less than one wavelength will reflect the wave differently than larger interfaces. As the incident wave strikes a small interface, a portion of the incoming wave will be redirected, depending on the angle of incidence. Some of the wave's energy will be reflected directly back toward the source, and some of it will be directed in numerous other directions[15] (Fig. 3-6).

TABLE 3-3. PERCENT OF ENERGY REFLECTED AT TYPICAL HUMAN TISSUE INTERFACES

Reflecting Interface	Percent of Energy Reflected
Fat/muscle	1.08
Muscle/blood	0.07
Bone/muscle	41.23
Soft tissue/air	99.9
Soft tissue/PZT*	80

* Material used to make transducer elements.
Source: Modified from Ref. 20.

These types of reflectors are called *scattering* reflectors and make up the bulk of what is seen in echocardiography.

TRANSMISSION

The mechanism whereby a wave continues to propagate through a material is referred to as *transmission*. A certain percentage of the wave will continue to be transmitted through the medium until forces cause the energy to dissipate. When the speed of sound through separate media is equal, the angle of incidence is the same as the angle of transmission when the sound is transmitted.

ATTENUATION

As ultrasound passes through a medium, its intensity is reduced due to the properties discussed above. This entire process is referred to as *attenua-* *tion*. The attenuation of sound waves from deep within the body is much stronger than the attenuation of sound waves received from more superficial structures. Another factor affecting attenuation is frequency. Attenuation significantly increases with an increase in frequency.[17] Mathematically, attenuation is the rate of intensity decrease in decibels (dB) per centimeter depth of tissue.[24] The attenuation of soft tissue can be expressed by the following formula:

$$\text{Attenuation} = 0.7 \times f \qquad (3\text{-}5)$$

where f is frequency, so at a transmit frequency of 3.5 MHz the attenuation of soft tissue would equal 0.7×3.5 MHz $= 2.45$ dB/cm.

The distance the ultrasound wave travels also affects the degree to which that wave is attenuated.[16] For each centimeter of tissue that the sound wave travels, its intensity is decreased by half for any given material. This value is known as the *half-value layer* or *half-power distance*. Generally, the attenuation of sound within soft tissue is roughly 0.7 dB/cm/MHz. Using the example above, if we wish to measure a structure that is 10 cm deep in the body at 3.5 MHz, the round trip attenuation would be

0.7 db/cm/MHz $\times$ 10 cm $\times$ 3.5 MHz
$$= 24.5 \text{ dB} \times 2 = 49 \text{ dB}$$

At 49 dB, the echo would be detectable at acceptable transmissions powers. At 10 MHz, however, the round-trip attenuation would be

0.7 dB/cm/MHz $\times$ 10 cm $\times$ 10 MHz
$$= 70 \text{ dB} \times 2 = 140 \text{ dB}$$

Current biomedical ultrasound equipment (transducers) have a dynamic range of 100 dB.[12] The amount of attenuation in this last example would be on the order of 140 dB, which would result in echoes that are too weak and therefore undetectable.

BEAM FORMATION

As the sound wave is propagated, it develops certain characteristics that are typical of all waves. The physical dimensions of the generated or incident wave are similar to those of the transducer that made it. For example, a simple disc transducer with a given diameter generates a wave; the wave's diameter is similar to that of the disc. As the beam moves away

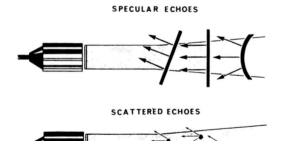

SPECULAR ECHOES

SCATTERED ECHOES

Figure 3-6. The two types of reflector found in the human body. Specular reflectors (top figure) are large, smooth surfaces; scattering reflectors (bottom figure) are small and irregularly shaped. (From Feigenbaum H [ed]. Echocardiography, 5th ed. Baltimore, Lea & Febiger; 1994:Fig. 1-3. Reprinted with permission.)

similar to that of the disc. As the beam moves away from its source, it begins to diverge. The area where the divergence begins is called the *transmit zone*. The area between the transducer and the transmit zone is called the *near field* or *Fresnal zone*. The area beyond the transmit zone where the beam begins to diverge is called the *far field* or *Fraunhofer zone* (Fig. 3-7).

The energy of the beam in the near field is more intense and decreases as the wave diverges. The length of the near field can be calculated from the formula

$$\ln = \frac{R^2}{\int} \qquad (3\text{-}6)$$

where *r* is the radius of the beam's source or the transducer radius and $\int$ is the wavelength of the transmitted wave. The length of the near field will then increase with an increase in the transducer radius or a decrease in the beam's wavelength. Since wavelength is inversely related to frequency, a higher-frequency transducer will also yield a longer near field. The significance of the near field is that the greatest signal amplitude occurs at this point, and the transducer can be focused only at or below this range.

At the far field the beam begins to diverge, which essentially weakens the beam's strength.

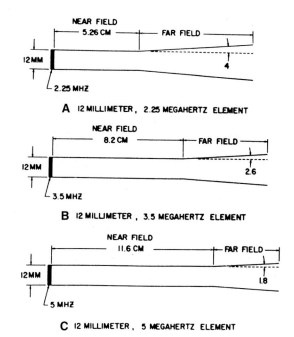

Figure 3-8. *The effects of transducer frequency. If transducer size is held constant but frequency is increased, the near field will be longer, resulting in a shorter far field with less divergence. (From Feigenbaum H [ed]. Echocardiography, 5th ed. Baltimore, Lea & Febiger; 1994:Fig. 1-7. Reprinted with permission.)*

Echoes returning from this region will be weaker due to the effects of attenuation. The far field can be calculated from the equation

$$\text{Sin } \theta = \frac{0.61}{r} \qquad (3\text{-}7)$$

where *r* is the radius of the beam at the transmit zone and θ is angle of incidence. Changes in transducer size will affect the far field. A smaller transducer will increase the far field, thereby increasing the amount of divergence. A larger, high-frequency transducer, on the other hand, will result in narrower, more intense beams. Higher frequencies create longer near fields, which in turn create less divergence in the far field. Conversely, lower-frequency transducers have shorter near fields, resulting in more beam divergence (Fig. 3-8).

Beam formation dictates to some degree the quality of the images, since the shape of the beam determines the area of the heart from which returning sound waves are received, the intensity of the beam within the beam path, and lateral resolution of

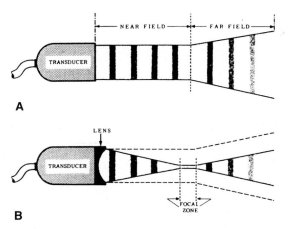

Figure 3-7. *The beam profile as it progresses from a transducer. The near field or Fresnel zone is the region closest to the transducer. The focal zone demarcates the change from the near field to the far field. In the far field or Fraunhofer zone the beam begins to diverge. (From Feigenbaum H [ed]. Echocardiography, 5th ed. Baltimore, Lea & Febiger; 1994:Fig. 1-9. Reprinted with permission.)*

the system. In cardiac applications, narrower beams have the advantage of providing less ambiguous echoes due to the smaller area imaged; the beam is more intense within that smaller area; and lateral resolution is improved, reducing artifactual information.

Resolution

Resolution of a system refers to its ability to discern two separate, distinct structures.[19,22] The greater the resolution, the higher the quality of the image. Sound beams are rather complex, especially when formed by phased array transducers. For multielement transducers, resolution can be categorized into axial, azimuthal, and lateral. *Axial resolution* defines the system's ability to differentiate two structures lying along the path of the beam.[22]

A systems' axial resolution depends on its frequency (wavelength) and the duration of the pulse. Remember that a higher-frequency transducer will have a shorter wavelength. An example will help illustrate this difference. The wavelength of a transducer can be calculated using the following equation:

$$c = F \times \int; \quad \text{solving for wavelength, } \int = \frac{c}{F}$$

If we consider a 2.5 MHz transducer and a 5.0 MHz transducer, $\int$ can be determined.

At 2.5 MHz

$$\int = \frac{1540 \text{ m/sec}}{2.5 \text{ MHz}} = 0.000616 \text{ m or } 0.616 \text{ mm}$$

At 5.0 MHz

$$\int = \frac{1540 \text{ m/sec}}{5.0 \text{ MHz}} = 0.000308 \text{ m or } 0.308 \text{ mm}$$

Therefore, the 2.5 MHz transducer will be able to discern two structures as separate if they are 0.616 mm or more apart. Structures that are less than 0.616 mm apart will appear as one structure. On the other hand, at 5.0 MHz, separate structures will be distinguishable at a distance of 0.308 mm or greater. Therefore, higher-frequency transducers will provide the greatest resolution.

Pulse length also plays a significant role in the system's ability to resolve separate structures. If we assume that a transmitted pulse is made up of five cycles, then the length of the pulse at 2.5 MHz will be 3.08 mm (0.616 mm × five cycles). At this pulse

length, the echo returning from the second structure will strike the transducer while the echo from the first structure is still hitting it. The system will therefore be unable to separate the two structures. On the other hand, at 5.0 MHz the pulse duration will be 1.54 mm, allowing the system to distinguish the first and second structures. Therefore, the structures will be seen as separate.

For multielement transducers the beam is more complex than for simple single-element transducers. The resultant beam has azimuthal as well as lateral dimensions. *Lateral* resolution enables the system to exclude structures that are outside the beam's path. Poor lateral resolution results in artificial echoes within the image. A system's lateral resolution is a function of the beam width. The wider the beam, the less the lateral resolution. In order for two structures lying side by side to be imaged separately, they must lie more than one beam width apart. If the two structures lie within one beam path, then the resultant image will appear as one (Fig. 3-9).

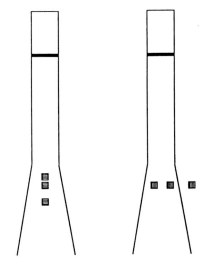

Figure 3-9. Axial and lateral resolution. *Left:* Reflectors that lie behind one another tend to blend into one signal if they are closer together than half the length of the ultrasound pulse. The shorter the pulse, the greater the ability of the system to sense the separation of two surfaces. This ability is called *axial resolution. Right:* Reflectors that lie next to each other will not appear as separate objects if they are both seen within the beam at the same time. The narrower the beam, therefore, the greater the chance that the system will be able to differentiate between the reflectors (i.e., the greater its lateral resolution capability). Since the length of an ultrasound pulse is much smaller than the width of the beam, axial resolution is usually better than lateral resolution.

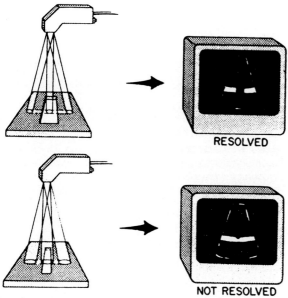

Figure 3-10. *Schematic illustration of the method for testing azimuthal resolution. The transducer is oriented with the scanning arc perpendicular to the axis of a defect in the tissue phantom. In the upper drawing, a relatively large defect appears as an echo-free space in the image of myocardium. In the lower drawing, the defect width is less than the effective beam width of the tranducer and is not resolved as a complete break in the image. (From Ref. 22, Fig. 1. Reprinted with permission.)*

Another factor affecting lateral resolution is the system's overall gain settings. High overall gain settings increase the beam width. In order to optimize the system's lateral resolution, the overall gain should be decreased.

Azimuthal resolution determines how well structures located at the same depth in the sound beam are separated.[22] The system's ability to discern structures that lie side by side and are perpendicular to the beam path describes azimuthal resolution. In Figure 3-10 a test phantom with a defect is imaged. If the system's azimuthal resolution is adequate, the defect will be identified. If it is inadequate, the defect will be missed. The axial and azimuthal resolutions of most systems are usually better than their lateral resolution.

Transducers

A *transducer* is anything that transforms one form of energy into another. This is accomplished in ultrasound with a piezoelectric crystal, which re-

sponds to any change in voltage by changing shape. The resulting change in pressure when applied to surrounding material causes a pressure wave or vibration. A piezoelectric transducer also functions as a receiver by responding to incoming sounds or pressure waves with a change in electrical potential across opposite crystal faces. The natural operating frequency of a transducer depends on its thickness. Thinner wafers vibrate at higher frequencies but are more difficult to produce because of the delicacy of thin crystals. Although a higher frequency offers better image quality, its ability to penetrate tissue is decreased. Frequencies above 3.0 MHz possess suboptimal characteristics for quantitative Doppler echocardiography. In most adults, good image quality is obtainable at 3.5 to 5.0 MHz, whereas pediatric studies require 5.0 MHz. Actual operating frequencies and usefulness vary greatly. Transducers are composed of several components, including the housing, damping material, matching layer, and piezoelectric element. The piezoelectric element is responsible for the production of the sound wave. Piezoelectric elements are made up of ferroelectric material, which consists of electric dipoles. Such elements have both a positive and a negative charge. In their natural state, dipoles are haphazardly arranged (Fig. 3-11). In order to make them functional, the dipoles must be organized. To do this, the material is heated to a temperature that allows the dipoles to move freely. This temperature is known as the material's *Curie temperature*. As this temperature is reached, an electrical field is applied to the material. The positive end of the ferroelectric material is attracted to the negative side of the field, and the positive side of the dipole is attracted to the negative

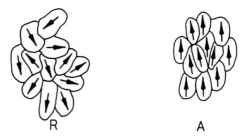

Figure 3-11. *Ferroelectric materials have dipoles that in their natural state are haphazardly arranged (left image). In order for the material to act as a transducer, the dipoles must be arranged in an orderly fashion (right image). (From Ref. 35, Fig. 3-1. Reprinted with permission.)*

side. The material is then cooled and fixed in this highly ordered fashion. The crystal is then capable of producing a mechanical sound wave when struck with an external force such as an electrical pulse (Fig. 3-12). This also explains why transducers cannot be heat sterilized, since heating the material will free the dipoles from their fixed position.

Quartz is a naturally occurring ferroelectric material. However, ceramics such as barium titanate and lead zirconate titanate are typical examples of manufactured ferroelectric materials and are the materials most commonly used in making the piezoelectric portion of the transducers. As an electrical pulse hits this material, the fixed dipoles expand and contract, establishing a mechanical field or sound wave. The piezoelectric materials used are cut exceedingly thin and must be handled with extreme care. Once the transducers are dropped, irreparable damage to the crystal usually results.

The frequency of the transducer is determined by its thickness. When the transducer is struck with a force such as an electrical pulse, it vibrates at a natural frequency that is determined by the physical dimensions of the crystal. This vibration occurs along the crystal's thickness and is called the *natural resonant frequency*. The time it takes for the sound wave to travel from one surface of the crystal to the other depends on the crystal's thickness and the speed of sound in that material. When the thickness of the material is exactly one-half of the wavelength, the transducer will resonant with a maximum dis-

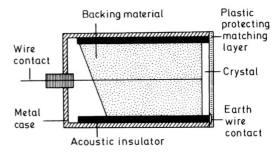

Figure 3-13. *An illustration of a simple transducer and its component parts. (From McDicken WN [ed]. Diagnostic Ultrasonics: Principles and Use of Instruments, 2nd ed. New York, Wiley; 1981:Fig. 1-2. Reprinted with permission.)*

placement amplitude. This is called the *fundamental resonant frequency*. Of course, there are numerous frequencies that are generated in between and that until now have been virtually ignored. But as we will see, these vibrations or intermediate harmonics have created quite a stir in the field of echocardiography.

TRANSDUCER DAMPING

Once the crystal begins to vibrate, sounds waves will be continuously generated until the vibrations cease. This continuous vibration is known as *ringing* and can produce an artifact known as *ring down*. Additionally, once a crystal is hit with an electrical pulse, a sound wave will be produced that travels forward into tissue, but will also be created at the back face and travel into the housing of the transducer. These sound waves then reflect off the internal housing, causing interference with returning echoes from tissue and generating an artifact. To prevent these two problems, a damping material with attenuating properties is placed within the housing of the transducer behind the crystals (Fig. 3-13).

The damping material in transducers also affects the pulse duration of the sound wave. A high damping material will shorten the pulse length, whereas a low or weaker damping material will allow a wave with an increased number of cycles. A wave with an increased number of cycles therefore provides greater resolution, but at the expense of range resolution. Figure 3-14 illustrates the various effects that damping material has on the pulse wave.

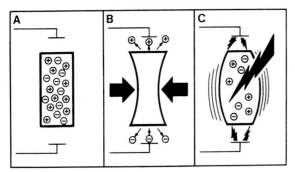

Figure 3-12. **(A)** The naturally occurring state of the piezoelectric element. **(B)** The element is heated and polarized by applying an electromagnetic field. **(C)** Once the crystal or element is organized it will vibrate, creating a mechanical sound wave when struck with an electrical current. (From Weyman AE [ed]. Principles and Practice of Echocardiography, 2nd ed. Baltimore, Lea & Febiger; 1994:Fig. 1-1. Reprinted with permission.)

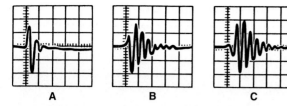

Figure 3-14. The effects of damping on the pulse configuration. (**A**) A highly damped transducer will result in a shorter "ring" or smaller number of cycles. (**B,C**) The damping is decreased, resulting in an increased number of cycles. The pulse duration is subsequently longer. (From Weyman AE [ed]. Principles and Practice of Echocardiography, 2nd ed. Baltimore, Lea & Febiger; 1994:Fig. 1-21. Reprinted with permission.)

MATCHING LAYER

The matching layer of the transducer serves two major purposes. First, it provides a protective layer for the delicate piezoelectric elements. Second, there is a large difference between the acoustic properties of the crystal material and those of human skin. In fact, when an echo hits a soft tissue/crystal boundary, as much 80% to 96% of the incident wave is reflected. By placing a matching layer between the skin and the crystal, it is possible to reduce the amount of mismatch at the skin level.[24] In order for a matching layer to allow transmission of sound waves at the skin level, it must be made of an appropriate acoustic impedance and must be equal to a quarter of the wavelength ($\int/4$) of the transmitted sound wave. If the matching layer meets these criteria, as much as 100% of the incident wave will be transmitted.

Matching layers that are a quarter of the incident wavelength will cause constructive interference, thereby increasing the amplitude of the wave. A portion of the initial wave will be transmitted through the matching layer. However, a portion of that wave will be reflected off the internal surface of the layer and reflect back off the piezoelectric surface. The resultant wave will then be transmitted, thereby adding itself to the initial waves generated. Multiple matching layers have the advantage of increasing amplitude even further.

TRANSDUCER TYPES

Two-dimensional echocardiography units automatically angle an ultrasound beam along one plane at a rate of 10 to 30 times per second. The information obtained in such a sweep can be compiled into a planar or cross-sectional image with up to an 80 or 90 degree arc, representing the relative positions of structures during that period. The two basic methods for steering the ultrasound beam in different directions are (1) automatically moving a single large (13 to 19 mm in diameter) crystal in different directions and (2) electronically sequencing voltage pulses to an array of 32 to 128 small crystals 13 to 19 mm in length (phased array). An illustration of each type of transducer is presented in Chapter 4.

MECHANICALLY STEERED TRANSDUCERS

Mechanical scanners consist of one to several crystals within a housing filled with sonolucent oil. The crystal or crystals are swept in a fixed plane by rapid oscillations that can be "wobbled" back and forth by either a motor or an electromagnetic system. As the axle spins, the machine activates the crystal that faces the patient. Mechanical transducers must be focused by applying a lens, a transducer curvature, or a mirror. For example, a lens forces light to converge toward a point. This point is the focal point where the light has its greatest intensity. Like light, ultrasound waves can be focused in this manner. As waves pass through a lens they are bent toward a common point, thereby focusing their energy.

Sound waves can also be focused by curving the transducer itself. As before, the waves converge on a common point where their energy is greatest. The use of a mirror can also generate a focused beam. These focusing techniques involve an external method in order to focus the beam. Transducers can also be focused internally, but they are entirely different. Earlier mechanical transducers tended to be large and bulky. Additionally, they tended to vibrate because of the motor and could be felt by both operator and patient. Some of these problems have been overcome with advanced technology. Some mechanical probes are as small as nonmechanical types of transducers, and through the use of magnetic drives rather than motors, the transducers function more smoothly.

ELECTRONIC TRANSDUCERS

The two major types of electronic transducers are linear and phased array. As their name implies, *linear transducers* arrange the piezoelectric elements in a linear fashion. The elements are activated sequentially, either individually or in small groups.

These transducers tend to be large and are best suited for large windows such as those used for abdominal or obstetrical ultrasound. The fields generated by these transducers are typically rectangular and do not provide a sector. Linear transducers do not have a role in cardiac work.

Phased array transducers are commonly employed in echocardiography. They are made up of a series of piezoelectric elements that are arranged in a square or rectangle so as to minimize the required space. The Huygen principle described earlier is well demonstrated here. Each element produces its own wave when struck with the electronic pulse. As the individual waves propagate forward, they eventually merge to form a single wavefront.

Like linear transducers, phased array transducers have the advantage of being both steered and focused electronically. As the excitation pulse arrives at the transducer, it passes through a delay system. Instead of firing all at once, certain crystals fire earlier than others. This delayed firing allows the beam to be steered and focused, depending on the delay sequence. On most phased array systems a transmit focus knob or button exists, allowing the operator to change the focus of the transducer. This delay also allows time for returning echoes. Should returning echoes or waves meet outgoing ones, they may cancel each other if they are in phase.

The shape of the beam generated by a phased array transducer will take on the physical characteristics of the transducer. Because the transducer has a square or rectangular shape, the resultant wave will have an elliptical shape. This shape provides another dimension to the wave, not seen with some other types of transducers. The characteristics of the resultant elliptical wave will be determined by the length and width of the array, the focus as well as the wavelength of the transmitted sound wave. Due to the elliptical shape of the beam, there will be not only lateral or axial resolution but also azimuthal resolution. The beam profile for a phased array transducer is more complicated than that for a simpler design. In the lateral beam dimension, the beam's near field is longer and diverges further from the transducer. In the thickness dimension, the near field is short and beam divergence begins closer to the transducer. This complex beam profile lends flexibility to the beam in terms of both angulation and depth of the field examined. Because of the large area of beam divergence Doppler and M-mode information can be obtained from a larger area.

ARRAY TRANSDUCERS

Annular array transducers are a combination of mechanical and electronic transducers. They consist of a round crystal cut into concentric rings. If the outer rings are fired first, a converging beam is created with the focal range electronically controlled. Because the crystals are round, focusing occurs in all directions perpendicular to the beam's axis. In this instance, the electronics control only the focus, not the steering. Steering is achieved mechanically using a motor or magnetic device. Dynamic (rapidly changing) focusing can be done to increase the effective length of the focal zone.

TRANSESOPHAGEAL TRANSDUCERS

Transesophageal transducers can be either mechanical (Fig. 3-15) or phased array. Commercially available transducers for examining the heart through the esophagus operate on the mechanical or phased array principle. The phased array is mounted on a flexible gastroscope long enough to be advanced down the esophagus. It travels behind the left atrium and is positioned behind the posterior wall of the left ventricle. The entire apparatus can be rotated or moved up or down to find an echocardiographic window. These probes are available with a single element, with two elements positioned in a lateral and transverse plane, or as a multiplane (Fig. 3-16) or omniplane design[3,29,32–34,38] (Fig. 3-17). The omniplane design allows the operator to rotate the transducer in an arc between 0 and 180 degrees.

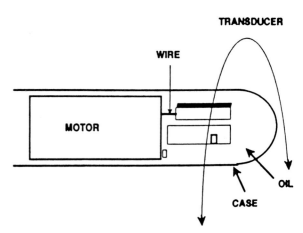

Figure 3-15. Mechanical TEE transducer with a motor to drive the transducer. (From Shu TL, et al. Panoramic transesophageal echocardiography. Echocardiography. 1991;8:677. Fig. 1-86. Reprinted with permission.)

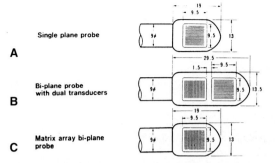

Figure 3-16. Phased array design TEE probes. (**A**) Mono-plane probe with a single element. (**B**) Multiplane probe with a longitudinal and a transverse element. (**C**) Matrix array biplane probe. (From Ref. 33, Fig. 1-82. Reprinted with permission.)

The optimal frequency of these transducers is usually 5.0 MHz, since greater resolution is more desirable and less penetration is needed. Such probes are capable not only of imaging but also conventional and color flow Doppler. The number of elements in current probes varies from 32 to 64. Transesophageal probes also vary in size and are available for adult as well as pediatric patients.[19,47]

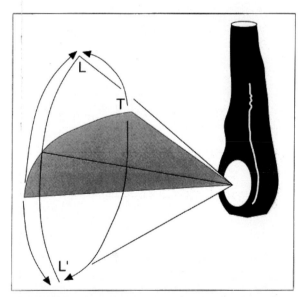

Figure 3-17. Diagram of an omniplane probe illustrating the rotational capabilities of the transducer. The elements rotate from 0 to 180 degrees. (From Roelandt J, et al. Multiplane transesophageal echocardiography with a vari-oplane transducer system. Thoraxcentre J. 1992;4:38. Fig. 1-84. Reprinted with permission.)

Signal Processing

So far, we have discussed the propagation of sound within the tissue. What happens to the sound waves when they return to the transducer is complex. Once the transducer receives the reflected sound, the ultrasound system must perform a series of manipulations in order to generate a diagnostic image. In recent years, new technologies have evolved that have helped to improve the images currently generated by systems. The first part of this section describes the path the raw signal takes from the transducer to the system monitor (Fig. 3-18).

AMPLIFICATION

In order for the system to create an image, the signal received must be converted from an analog to a digital format. The first step in the pathway from raw signal to image is for the signal to pass through the echo receiver. Because of attenuation, the signals received need to be amplified. Remember that the effects of attenuation will reduce the energy of the transmitted wave twice—once on the transmitted path and once again on the trip back to the transducer. Due to this dual effect of attenuation, the sound beam received by the transducer needs to be amplified. All signals received by the system will be amplified uniformly, regardless of the distance they traveled. Weak signals will be amplified, as will strong signals.

As previously discussed, the incoming or reflected sound wave returns to the transducer and strikes its piezoelectric elements. This generates the electrical signal, which is in the form of a radio frequency signal. This raw signal contains both amplitude and phase information. Until recently, only the amplitude component was processed by the system; the phase component was ignored. Recent technology is now taking advantage of both the amplitude and phase components, enabling image quality to be dramatically improved in some situations.

TIME GAIN COMPENSATION

Signals received from the near field or from structures closest to the transducer are expected to be stronger, since the effects of attenuation depend on distance. Therefore, signals received farthest from the transducer must be amplified in order to be properly manipulated for imaging. Time gain compensation enables the operator to increase the inten-

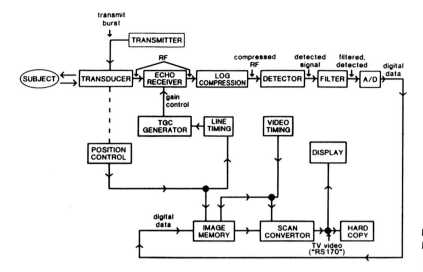

Figure 3-18. Block diagram of a basic echograph. (From Ref. 44, Fig. 1. Reprinted with permission.)

sity of the signals received from far distances or to decrease the intensity of the signals received from the near field. This process essentially reduces the dynamic range to levels better suited for digitization and storage.[37]

The time gain compensation provides increased amplification for echoes that originate from more distant structures. This is often displayed as a curve that represents the level at which the amplifier is operating at each distance from the transducer. It shows low power near the crystal (usually the top of the screen), gradually increasing gain as depth increases (moving down on the screen), and then peak amplification in the more distant field (Fig. 3-19).

The exact labeling and configuration of these controls vary from manufacturer to manufacturer, but they should be present in some form on all imaging instruments. It is important to understand how they operate in general and specifically on each machine. Proper application of this knowledge prevents incorrect display of the patient's anatomy, either by overlooking or by obscuring what is present. Some machines use knobs to control portions of the time gain compensation curve, some use slide potentiometers to control specific depths in the image, and still others use software controls.

COMPRESSION

Due to the wide range of echo intensities, the system or operator may have the ability to adjust the compression level of the system. Compression is

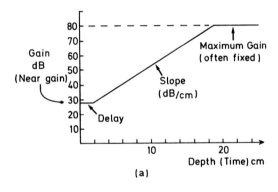

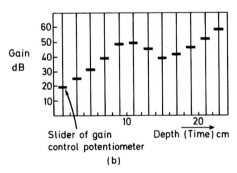

Figure 3-19. Time gain compensation slope (**A**) illustrating the gain settings for signals received from near field structures compared to signals received from far field structures. The variation of gain controls is accomplished by using gain control potentiometers (**B**). (From McDicken WN [ed]. Diagnostic Ultrasonics: Principles and Use of Instruments, 2nd ed. New York, Wiley; 1981:Fig. 6-2. Reprinted with permission.)

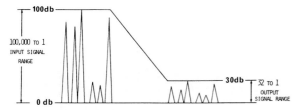

Figure 3-20. This diagram illustrates how 100 dB of ultrasound information can be compressed into 32 dB of ultrasound information. (From Feigenbaum H [ed]. Echocardiography, 5th ed. Baltimore, Lea & Febiger; 1994:Fig. 1-27. Reprinted with permission.)

useful in reducing the higher-intensity signals so that they are less likely to shadow those that are lower in intensity. The wide variety of analog signals returning to the system will eventually be converted into various shades of gray. Due to this wide variety, the resulting number of gray shades is too large for the human eye to appreciate, so the signal range is compressed. Once again, compression is carried out in a manner that allows the weaker signals to be preserved. In Figure 3-20, the raw signal coming from tissue may have a high signal to low signal ratio of 100,000:1. This range is too large, so it is compressed to a ratio of 32:1.[15]

DYNAMIC RANGE

The term *dynamic range* is frequently used to describe a variety of instrument functions and appears in seemingly unrelated topics. Dynamic range is simply a ratio of the highest signal amplitude, intensity, or voltage before the signal is saturated to the lowest perceived signal amplitude, intensity, or voltage just before it is eliminated by the system's reject control. It is used to evaluate the system's individual components. For example, the dynamic range of the system's gain control can be expressed by the following equation:

$$\text{Gain in dB} = 20 \log^{10} \left(\frac{V1}{V2} \right) \qquad (3\text{-}8)$$

where *V* represents voltage. Dynamic range is measured in decibels (dB). An amplifier that can process a maximum input signal of 100 to a minimum input signal of 1 has a dynamic range of 100:1 or 40 dB. Some systems allow the operator to adjust the dynamic range of the amplifier. In some current systems, the dynamic range of the amplifier can be adjusted to match that of the tissue, so that the tissue

signals are spread over the full maximum to minimum pulse voltage levels.[24]

PREPROCESSING

Preprocessing encompasses a variety of techniques designed to further optimize the image. These functions are called *preprocessing functions* because they affect the analog signal before they are digitized and stored in memory. Some examples of preprocessing include edge enhancement in which the signal is differentiated. Edge enhancement results in a new signal whose strength is proportional to the rate of change in the original signal.[44] This particular preprocessing function emphasizes endocardial borders.

Another form of preprocessing affects the manner in which the analog signal is mapped to a gray level value. The operator is able to modify the allocation of gray level values to the echo intensity, thereby changing the appearance of the final image. Because the number of gray levels is fixed, reallocating gray levels in one intensity range results in an increase of gray levels to the area of interest at the expense of gray levels from a different intensity range. The result will be an increase in detail with an increase in gray levels and a decrease in detail with the loss of gray levels. This is essentially a contrast-type function, which carries a variety of names depending on the manufacturer. This is useful in looking at the myocardium, for example, where an increase in gray levels will provide more detail.

FILTERS

Returning signals quickly become contaminated by electronic noise within the ultrasound unit itself. Therefore, both real and contaminating noise needs to be removed from the signal before it is presented in its final display. Signal features that are often filtered are amplitude (using a reject control), direction (by a manufacturer-programmed receive focus), and frequency (via an operator-controlled wall motion or high-pass filter).

Reject filtering is a way of removing the weak electronic noise from the display. When the reject level is set, all signals with powers below that level are removed from the image. Background "snow" that appears to be random can be eliminated this way, making real signals look sharper and easier to see (Fig. 3-21). It is important to note that increasing the amplifier gain tends to increase the strength of both real and noisy signals, negating the effect of the reject filter.

Direction filtering can be achieved with phased and annular array systems. Direction filtering is capable of removing signals that do not arrive from the desired angles. A flat wavefront approaching the crystals from other than a 90 degree angle reaches the nearer crystals slightly before it reaches the more distant crystals. The timing of the arrival is characteristic of the incident angle. The delay line of the processor can be programmed to accept only signals that come from the expected direction. With parallel processing technology applied to a phased array, multiple delay lines can be used to accept signals from more than one angle at a time, so more of the available information is used instead of being discarded.

Frequency filtering is used to help distinguish high-velocity signals from low-velocity signals. Red blood cells typically move at a higher velocity than the cardiac walls. In cardiac disease the high-velocity signals provide most of the clinically useful data, and this is much easier to display well if the lower-velocity but stronger signals are removed. This is done by filtering out the low velocities that give low Doppler frequency shifts by using a *high-pass* (often called *wall motion*) *filter*. There are usually at least three operator-selected settings for these filters. While the reject filter removes low-power signals, the wall motion filter removes low-frequency signals (Fig. 3-22). The display of any echocardiographic information concerning anatomic images or Doppler flow information is subject to a great deal of electronic manipulation.

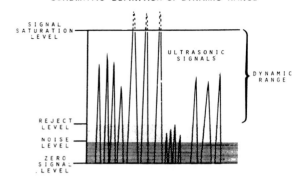

SCHEMATIC DEFINITION OF DYNAMIC RANGE

Figure 3-22. *Schematic of filtering. Signals below a particular reject setting will be eliminated, helping to display the desired signals clearly. Without such filtering, desired signals would be contaminated and would be displayed as fuzzy, ill-defined structures. (From Feigenbaum H [ed]. Echocardiography, 5th ed. Baltimore, Lea & Febiger; 1994:Fig. 1-26. Reprinted with permission.)*

SIGNAL STORAGE

The signals that return to the system are in an analog format. The signal must be converted to a digital format for proper processing and display. The returning signals are processed in an analog-to-digital scan converter allowing the analog signals to be stored for later processing. This step saves memory space. Analog signals occupy 8 to 10 times more memory space than digital signals. A number of steps are employed to convert the analog signal to a digital signal. The returning analog signal is a pressure wave with peaks and troughs. One of the initial steps in this sequence is to *demodulate* the signal, eliminating all negative components. The negative pressure waves are rectified and then smoothed. This process prepares the signal for digital signal storage.

Once the radio frequency arrives, it needs to be transformed into a video signal. A number of processes must occur in order to make the signal usable for imaging in a digital computer. The radio frequency signal will have positive as well as unrectified negative components. The negative signals are reversed and displayed above the baseline, a process referred to as *rectification* (Fig. 3-23). However, the rectified signal still demonstrates spikes of various frequencies. In order for the signal to be converted into a video signal, the spikes must be eliminated in a process called *smoothing*. This entire process of taking one form of signal, such as a radio frequency signal, and converting it into a more suit-

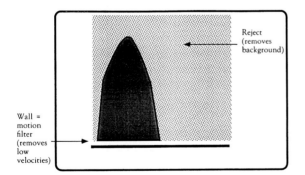

Reject (removes background)

Wall = motion filter (removes low velocities)

Figure 3-21. *Filters act to eliminate unwanted information, such as low-level signals from external sources. This process helps to clarify real images.*

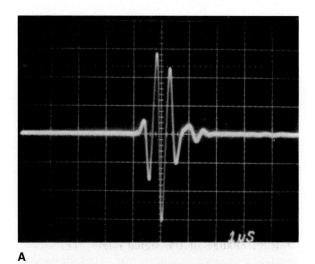

A

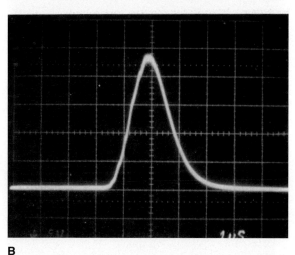

B

Figure 3-23. *Unrectified signals have positive as well as negative components (**A**). Rectified signals are all positive (**B**). (From McDicken WN [ed]. Diagnostic Ultrasonics: Principles and Use of Instruments, 2nd ed. New York, Wiley; 1981:Fig. 6-8. Reprinted with permission.)*

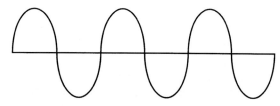

A. Raw RF signal

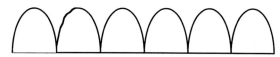

B. Rectified signal

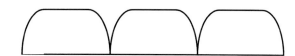

C. Smoothened

Figure 3-24. *The entire process of converting a raw radio frequency (RF) signal (**A**) into a video or digital signal is referred to as* demodulation = rectification *(**B**) and* smoothing *(**C**).*

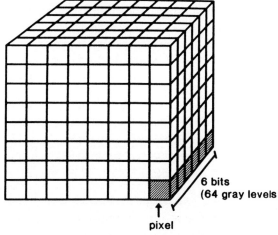

6 bits
(64 gray levels)

↑
pixel

Figure 3-25. *Once the analog signals are digitized, they are stored in a digital image matrix, with each signal being assigned to a pixel representing various shades of gray that correspond to the original echo intensity. (From Ref. 44, Fig. 3. Reprinted with permission.)*

able signal for display purposes is known as *demodulation* (Fig. 3-24).

Once the signal is changed from the analog to the digital format, it can be stored and retrieved for image processing. Within the digital scan converter are *random access memory (RAM)* devices. The resultant echo image is stored in a matrix of picture elements or *pixels*. Each of these pixels has a gray scale value (Fig. 3-25). A standard image matrix is 512 × 512 pixels, but this value may vary depending on the manufacturer. The image is stored as a word in RAM. Each word is stored as a sequence of these pixels or binary digits, also called *bits*. Each binary digit can have a value of 1 or 0, that is, on or off. A sequence of numerical information is stored in batches that can be displayed graphically. Shades of gray are used to represent the power of the signal returning from a location, white being a very strong signal and dark gray being a very weak one. Digital scanners offer a variety of ways of assigning these shades to the range of powers being shown, many of which are nonlinear. As discussed earlier, the precise selection of display parameters (often labeled *preprocessing*) is usually dictated by operator preference rather than by any scientific rule. Systems are capable of offering large numbers of gray shades in their displays; however, the eye is usually unable to detect and use more than eight shades in a real image.

DIGITAL SIGNAL PROCESSING

Imaging systems also batch distance information. Careful examination of a magnified image shows that it is made up of small rectangles or pixels, each of which is assigned a shade of gray. There may be multiple signals originating from within the tissue volume represented by that pixel, but all are assigned one shade. The size of the pixel represents the limit of the resolution (ability to display detail) of the display system. Other factors also limit resolution of the ultrasound system; the display components usually are not the limiting factor. Batching of directional information may occur in some systems.

Digital image storage can be broken down into three categories: (1) point, (2) spatial, and (3) temporal frequency domain processing.[44] Once the input signal is digitized, it is assigned an address within the complex digital matrix. As already discussed, this pixel will be of a particular gray level, which will in turn determine the gray level of the output signal. When the system is ready to display the signal at that particular address on the matrix, the resultant image will maintain the gray level characteristic of the original input signal. Once the signal is stored, the operator can manipulate the signals further using the postprocessing functions. These are considered postprocessing functions because they occur after the original signal has been converted to a digital format. Examples of such functions include inverse video display, postprocessing curve adjustments, and two-dimensional colorization.[44] The inverse video display allows the operator to display echo data as black on a white background.

This is seldom done in adult cardiac work because video display monitors have a tendency to "bloom" with high-intensity signals. Blooming results because the spot size actually increases due to overexcitation of phosphor, the material found on video display monitors.

Postprocessing curves allow the operator to adjust contrast by expanding a given range of echo intensities into a broader range of gray level values. The operator can also eliminate low-intensity gray levels caused predominantly by noise.

The two-dimensional image can also be viewed in color. In this situation, instead of mapping the input gray level to a particular output gray level, the input level is mapped to a particular color. The advantage of using a color format to display cardiac structures is that the human eye can more easily differentiate subtle variations in color compared to gray levels (Fig. 3-26).

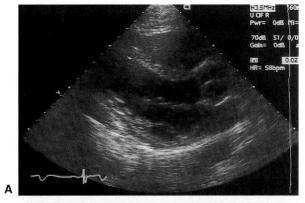

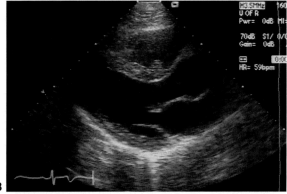

Figure 3-26. Two-dimensional colorized image of the left ventricle. Colorization can help to define endocardial borders and valvular detail (a) in technically difficult cases because the human eye is better able to detect shades of color (**A**) than shades of gray (**B**). (See also Color Plate 1.)

Another form of point processing is *histogram equalization.* A *histogram* represents the distribution of gray level values present in an image.[44] The histogram shows the number of pixels that possess a given gray level, but it does not give a location. The main purpose of the histogram is to show how well the available gray scale is being used. If a system is not using the gray scale appropriately, the contrast between various structures will not be appropriate. Ideally, the image should be spread over the entire range of the variable gray scale, but this seldom happens. The use of the histogram, sometimes called *edge enhancement,* better defines the endocardium by enhancing the contrast of the various structures (Fig. 3-27).

Spatial processing is an arithmetic process whereby a group of neighboring pixels are used to produce a single, modified pixel. The most common form of spatial processing is called *convolution* or *smoothing.* Smoothing involves replacing an original input pixel with the average of all its neighboring pixels. These new output signals are then stored on a different matrix and displayed as a smoothed image of the original signal.

Smoothing can also be used for edge enhancement. In this process, the original pixel is replaced by a linear or nonlinear combination of its original value with that of its neighbors. This allows a more dramatic differentiation between gray levels and helps to define tissue-blood interfaces.

Temporal processing operations include persistence and image subtraction. In *persistence* the input pixels are again averaged over several image frames. The net effect is an image that is softer in appearance and that theoretically reduces echo dropout and speckling. However, the image often appears too

| Mask Image | Contrast Image | Contrast Image Mask Image |

Figure 3-28. *Digital subtraction echocardiography. The original or mask image (left) and with contrast injection (middle). The mask image is removed, leaving only the contrast material (right). (From Ref. 44, Fig. 9. Reprinted with permission.)*

blurred to yield any diagnostic information. Image subtraction is used primarily in digital radiography, but its principles can be applied to echocardiography as well. In digital subtraction radiography an original image or *mask* image is obtained. A contrast agent is injected, and a series of images are acquired. Once these new images are obtained, the mask image is removed or subtracted, leaving the contrast images alone. Currently, work is being done in this field in the hope of better defining endocardial borders and calculating ejection fractions (Fig. 3-28).

DEPTH SETTINGS

With current systems, images can be magnified with little noticeable loss of information. The depth of the image field can also be manipulated so that specific regions of interest can be interrogated more closely. High depth settings allow the operator to visualize cardiac structures, aiding in image orientation, and also allow visualization of structures lying posterior to cardiac structures. Low depth settings allow the operator to "zero in" on specific structures, eliminating unwanted distractions (Fig. 3-29).

Harmonics

So far, we have discussed the frequency of a wave as a single entity, although in fact there are multiple integers of the incident or fundamental frequency.[7,9,13,14,41,42] *Harmonics* are components of the original frequency. Ultrasound waves act much the same way as musical notes. What gives a musical note its characteristic sound is the harmonics associated with it. Likewise, the same note played by two different instruments can be differentiated because of the harmonics characteristic of each instrument.

The term *harmonics* is used to describe two forms of image enhancement currently being used

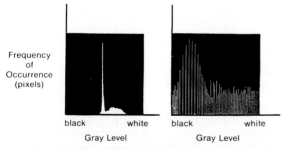

Frequency of Occurrence (pixels)

black   white   black   white
   Gray Level   Gray Level

Figure 3-27. *Histogram equalization. The left image shows the relative frequency of occurrence of all gray levels within the image. The right image has undergone histogram equalization and demonstrates greater relative uniformity among all gray levels, thus utilizing the entire range of possible gray levels. (From Ref. 44, Fig. 6. Reprinted with permission.)*

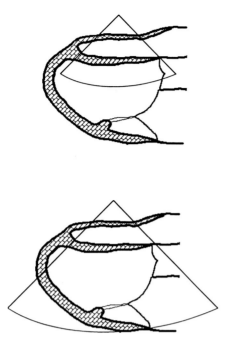

Figure 3-29. *Depth control illustrating the difference between a low depth setting (top image) and a high depth setting (bottom image). High depth settings allow a better overview of cardiac anatomy and structures beyond it, while low depth settings allow closer interrogation of structures.*

and further investigated in diagnostic ultrasound. The term describes a higher tone in a complex musical note[46] or, in the case of ultrasound, a complex frequency. Harmonics are generated from the fundamental or transmitted frequency or from another structure whose physical characteristics enable it to act as a sound source. In the first case the phenomenon is referred to as *native harmonics*, and in the second case it is referred to as *contrast harmonics*.

The two harmonics vary significantly in regard to the physical functioning of the sound waves and system processing. In our discussion of ultrasound so far, we have discussed linear propagation of waves. The harmonic component of a fundamental frequency wave represents nonlinear distortions[12] of that wave. The major advantages of the harmonic image are that (1) it provides better focus and (2) it has less clutter because there are fewer sidelobes, resulting in a clearer image. Image quality at fundamental frequencies suffers from losses associated with the divergence of the beam, as well as from attenuation such as scattering and resolution problems. The intensity of the fundamental, although greater than that of any of its harmonic compo-

nents, decreases rapidly and varies considerably with depth in an inhomogeneous medium (i.e., cardiac structures). Harmonic signals tend to be more steady and form a continuous and cumulative process, resulting in a more focused beam at a given point. For example, a boat traveling at a relatively low speed will create a wake. The wake will resemble a sine wave or slow, evenly spaced rolling waves that dissipate as they move away (K. Schwarz, personal communication, January 9, 1998). If the speed of the boat increases, the size of the waves will also increase but they will continue to resemble an even, rolling sine wave. Once the boat reaches a higher speed, the evenly spaced, slow, rolling sine waves begin to resemble turbulent waves that show signs of breaking as they move away due to their cumulative effect. Essentially, the power of these waves is greater than that of the slow, rolling sine waves created by lower speeds. In harmonic imaging, the amplitudes of the second and third harmonics exhibit relatively large gain in growth from near field to far field similar to the boat wave example. In essence, the amplitude increases as the beam travels away from the source toward the focal point. Once past the focal point, the decline in harmonic amplitude is similar to that of the fundamental wave[12] (Fig. 3-30).

The second advantage of second harmonics is the reduced effect of side lobes. Side lobes create low-level noise that degrades image quality. Sidelobes created by these nonlinear harmonics are much lower than their linear counterparts.[12] The effect is an image that has less clutter, resulting in clear endocardial borders (Fig. 3-31).

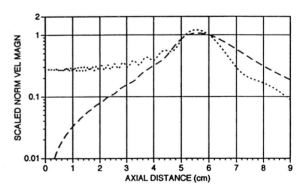

Figure 3-30. *Log-scaled axial amplitudes for a 4 MHz fundamental (dotted line) and 4 MHz second harmonic beam (long dashed lines). Note that the amplitude of the second harmonics continues to build, while the fundamental drops off. (From Ref. 12, Fig. 8. Reprinted with permission.)*

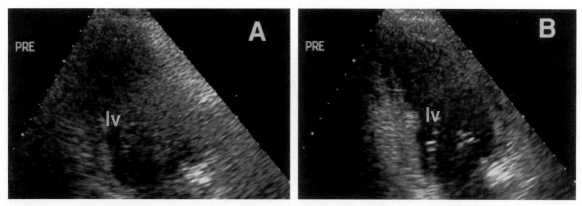

Figure 3-31. (**A**) An image of the heart with fundamental frequency at 3.5 MHz. (**B**) Represents the same image at a second harmonic frequency of 1.75 MHz. Note that the harmonic image has less clutter, allowing better definition of the endocardial borders.

Naturally, the fundamental signal would interfere with the harmonic signal from the tissue if both were to be received simultaneously. To overcome this obstacle, the fundamental signal must be separated from the harmonic signal and then filtered out so that only the harmonic image is accepted.[20] The result is an image with much higher resolution and less artifact or noise (Fig. 3-32).

Harmonic images are also created by small gas bodies or bubbles found within tissue. These bubbles act as a sound source. When a sound wave strikes them, they begin to oscillate or vibrate. These vibrations can result in resonation of the bubbles at a particular frequency. In addition to the fundamental resonating frequency, harmonic frequencies are also created. As long as the bubbles are oscillating, the fundamental and harmonic frequencies will be generated. In essence, the bubbles act as an amplifier, returning high-amplitude signals to the transducer and imager. When these signals are returned to the system, it filters the original signal,

which will possess only the fundamental frequency. The harmonic signals will remain.

This concept can be used by adding bubbles to the blood pool by injecting contrast agents rich in gaseous bodies. The higher signal-to-noise ratio of the contrast material can be enhanced by selecting and displaying only the harmonic signals[43] (Fig. 3-33).

Image Analysis

With advances in technology, it is now possible not only to improve image quality but also to provide some analytical information about the images displayed. Examples include complex calculation of chamber volumes, valvular areas, and regurgitant volumes, as well as simpler measurements such as diameter measurements. In addition, three-dimensional displays, tissue characterization, and measurements of myocardial perfusion are also possible using ultrasound systems. Obtaining accurate di-

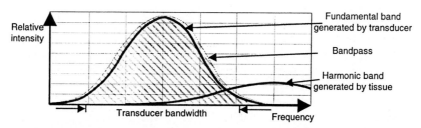

Figure 3-32. Harmonic and fundamental frequency bands are filtered and separated. Without filtering and separation, the fundamental image would overshadow the harmonic images. (From Thomas Jedrzejewicz, Acuson Corporation.)

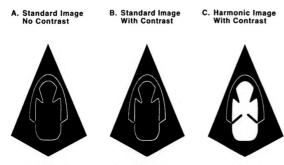

A. Standard Image No Contrast
B. Standard Image With Contrast
C. Harmonic Image With Contrast

Figure 3-33. *Example of contrast-enhanced images. (**A**) Cardiac image before contrast enhancement with fundamental frequency imaging. Endocardium and heart valves are modeled as the brightest echoes, followed by the myocardium and cardiac chamber as the lowest echoes but with overall gray tone simulating echo artifact. (**B**) Contrast-enhanced image with fundamental frequency imaging. The cardiac chamber is now equal to or exceeds the myocardium. Image brightness (or contrast) between the chamber and the myocardial/endocardial border has been lost. (**C**) Ideal second harmonic image before the contrast agent enters the myocardial circulation. Cardiac structures are not visible on the image, but contrast-filled cavities are seen clearly. (From Ref. 43, Fig. 1. Reprinted with permission.)*

mensions, volumes, valve areas, and other quantitative measures is of paramount importance, enhancing the advantage and utility to echocardiography. Various measurements can provide important information regarding cardiac structure and function. However, in today's health care environment, the need for accurate yet timely assessments is critical not only to patient management but to economical health care as well. Calculations that took countless off-line hours to make can now be done on-line during the course of an exam.

Calculations are often made using a bright spot called a *cursor*, which can be moved around an area of interest using either a marking or a tracing function. Some systems can automatically trace areas of interest. This process, referred to as *automatic edge detection*, traces the endocardial borders of a chamber in order to provide volume information on that chamber. Since the accuracy of many measurements is dependent on the operator, and since slight variations in measurements can occur between operator techniques, the use of standard procedures is invaluable to reduce variability and increase reproducibility. Still, the quality of the automated analysis is only as good as the images produced. As much detail as

possible is required in order for the analysis to be of good diagnostic quality.

Display Screens

Current echocardiography systems use either a black-and-white or a color television monitor for their display. These monitors are similar to a home television but do not have a channel selector. They cannot receive their own television signals and require an input from an external source. A monitor has the same basic structure as an oscilloscope. It has a screen that is clear but is coated on the inside with a phosphorescent material that glows in places where it is struck by a high-energy electron beam (Fig. 3-34). The beam is created by an electron gun at the rear of the television. The gun creates a cloud of electrons that are accelerated toward the screen

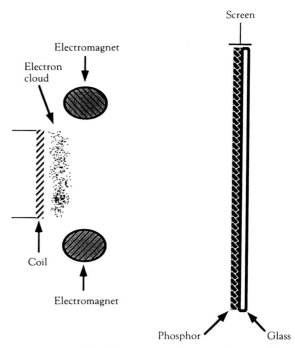

Screen
Electromagnet
Electron cloud
Coil
Electromagnet
Phosphor
Glass

Figure 3-34. *Television monitor. On the right side of the diagram is the screen: a sheet of glass coated with a phosphor, which glows when struck by high-energy electrons. On the left is a small coil that will produce a free cloud of electrons when heated by a small electrical current. These electrons gain a high level of energy because of acceleration toward an anode (not shown here) near the screen. The great voltage differential between the electron source and the anode (a positively charged plate) creates high acceleration. Electromagnets focus the electrons into a narrow beam as they travel toward the screen.*

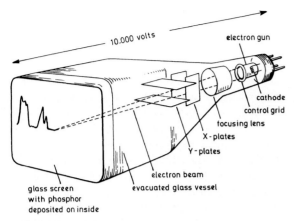

Figure 3-35. *Basic structure of a cathode ray tube. (From McDicken WN [ed]. Diagnostic Ultrasonics: Principles and Use of Instruments, 2nd ed. New York, Wiley; 1981: Fig. 1-10. Reprinted with permission.)*

by an anode (positive terminal) placed near it. The electron beam is steered through a raster pattern, consisting of horizontal lines, sweeping horizontally across the screen, moving down one line and sweeping again.

The pattern is created by a set of electromagnetic plates positioned in front of the tube near the electron gun. As the electrons are fired toward the phosphor screen, the plates are activated to attract or repel the electron beam, thereby "writing" a pattern on the phosphor coating. The plates are arranged in a vertical and horizontal pattern (Fig. 3-35). As the beam's position is steered, the incoming video signal modifies the force with which the electron beam strikes the screen, thereby creating dots of varying brightness. It does this by varying the voltage or potential difference between the electron gun and the plates near the screen, with greater voltage causing a brighter glow in that area of the phosphor. In order to create a coordinated raster pattern, a reference signal included in the video signal tells the television monitor when to begin a sweep. For color monitors, electron guns create combinations of red, green, and blue glowing phosphors on the screen. Combinations of color are created by subtracting and adding signals.[23]

Ultrasound Bioeffects

Diagnostic ultrasound has been used extensively in many medical disciplines without any significant ill effects. Organizations such as the American Insti-

tute of Ultrasound in Medicine (AIUM) have issued official statements on the clinical safety such as its March 1993 statement: "Although the possibility exists that such biological effects may be identified in the future, current data indicate that the benefits to the patient of the prudent use of diagnostic ultrasound outweigh the risks, if any, that may be present." A 1997 statement by the AIUM affirms that "There are no confirmed adverse biological effects on patients or instrument operators caused by exposures from diagnostic ultrasound instruments. Although the possibility exists that such biological effects may be identified in the future, current data indicate that the benefits to the patient of the prudent use of diagnostic ultrasound outweigh the risks, if any, that may be present."[4] Still, evidence of bioeffects of ultrasound on some types of tissue have been reported in both in vitro and in vivo experiments.[5,6,8,10,11,25–28,51]

The effects of diagnostic ultrasound on tissue depend on the total energy transmitted across a specific area, the frequencies used in the sound wave, the spatial distribution of the energy contained within the sound field, the amount of time that the tissue is exposed to the sound, and the sensitivity of the tissue to the sound wave. Before continuing, it is important to review a few terms commonly used to measure and describe the bioeffects of ultrasound on tissue.

Power is defined as the rate of work. In ultrasound it is defined as the rate at which energy is introduced into tissue. Power is measured in joules per second. Power creates an increase in temperature. If the amount of power introduced into tissue is doubled, the temperature of the exposed tissue will rise twice as rapidly.[45]

Energy is defined as the capacity to perform work and is measured in joules. In ultrasound, energy is found in the propagating pressure wave as the sum of the kinetic energy of the velocity of particles in tissue and the potential of the compressed or rarefied regions of the propagating wave.[45]

Pressure is defined as force per unit area and is measured in atmospheres or Pascals. Remember that as a wave propagates through tissue, it establishes areas of high and low pressure. The high-pressure areas cause compression within the tissue.[45]

Intensity is power per unit area and is measured in Watts per square centimeter. It is related to the square of the pressure amplitude. *Intensity* is the term used most frequently in discussing ultrasound transmission and is the topic of numerous measurements used to quantify diagnostic ultrasound equipment.[4]

The intensity of the sound wave is measured by its power divided by the area. Recall that the propagation of the sound in tissue is a function of acoustic pressure where the peak of the sound wave indicates the wave's highest amplitude and greatest pressure. Pressure is force and can be measured in Newtons (N) per square meter (m^2) or in Pascals (Pa) or atmosphere (atm). Where $1\ Pa = 1\ N/m^2$, or $1\ atm = 10^5\ Pa$. Since sound waves are emitted in pulses, there will be points along the sound beam that are at maximum pressure (p+) and minimum pressure (p−).

The amount of intensity in a given sound beam varies within that beam. The intensity of the sound beam within tissue varies depending on the particular location or point of measure, as well as the length of time the tissue is exposed. Numerous measurements are used to determine the effects of acoustic power on tissue, including spatial and temporal measurements.

Table 3-4 indicates some of the more common sound wave intensity measurements. The power output for any given system is a measure of when the system is on. Therefore, energy levels are described in terms of (1) when tissue is subjected to peak intensity at a given point or averaged over an area or (2) when tissue is subjected to peak intensity at a given point in time or over the time period that the system is on.

Temporal average intensity (I_{ta}) measures the intensity of the sound beam averaged over one pulse repetition. The intensity of the sound beam at any given point will vary with time. This measures the average time that the tissue is subjected to the sound beam when the system is on (45).

Spatial average temporal average intensity (I_{sata}) measures the temporal average intensity averaged over the cross-sectional area of the beam.[45] The significance of this measurement relates to the fact that the intensity of the beam will vary within the cross-sectional area of the beam. For example, tissue that lies directly in the path of the beam will be exposed to the highest intensity, while tissue that is not directly in the path of the beam (off axis) will not.

Pulse average intensity (I_{pa}) measures the intensity of the sound beam over the pulse duration.

Spatial average pulse average intensity (I_{sapa}) measures the pulse average over the cross-sectional area of the beam.[45]

Spatial peak pulse average intensity (I_{sppa}) measures the pulse average intensity at a particular location point where this measurement is at its highest.[50]

Spatial peak temporal average intensity (I_{spta}) measures the maximum spatial intensity when the system is on, averaged over the pulse repetition period. This is the most commonly reported measurement since it measures the peak energy level to which any of the tissue areas lying in the sound beam is exposed, averaged over the total time of the exposure.[50]

TABLE 3-4. COMMON MEASUREMENTS OF ULTRASOUND BEAM INTENSITY

Spatial peak, temporal peak intensity	The highest of all measured intensities, it is the point in space where the intensity is highest and occurs when the system is on.
Spatial average, temporal average intensity	Measures the peak intensity level to which any tissue is exposed in the sound beam, averaged over the total exposure time. This is the measurement most commonly used in discussing or measuring biologic effects on tissue.
Spatial average, temporal peak intensity	Measures the intensity over a particular area that occurs when the system is on.
Spatial peak, temporal average intensity	Measures the maximal spatial intensity occurring when the system is on, averaged over the pulse repetition period.

Spatial peak, temporal peak intensity (I_{sptp}) measures the peak intensity at a given point in space where the intensity of the sound beam is highest. This measurement yields the highest value of all intensity measurements.[50]

Spatial average, temporal peak intensity (I_{satp}) measures the peak intensity over a selected area that occurs when the system is on.[50]

The importance of these various measurements comes from the fact that the intensity of a sound wave has the potential to cause biological effects on tissue. In order to provide a safe yet diagnostic test, it is important to establish guidelines and regulations regarding these systems.

BIOEFFECTS

Bioeffects is a general term used to describe the potential for tissue damage as a result of using ultrasound on humans. There are three mechanisms that can result in tissue damage.[30,31,36] These mechanisms may create various biological effects on tissue, including (1) local heating, which causes an increase in the temperature of the tissue being exposed; (2) cavitation, a process in which the sound wave causes bubbles to develop or causes existing bubbles to react in a violent manner, causing damage to surrounding cells; and (3) mechanical stresses, which include all other potentially damaging forces or events, such as radiation forces or microstreaming.[45]

THERMAL CHANGES

As discussed earlier, when a sound wave passes through tissue, much of it is absorbed by that tissue. This absorbed energy must be converted into another form of energy, such as heat. The amount of heat generated or the temperature increase is directly related to the intensity of the sound beam and the absorption of the material. The higher the intensity of the sound beam, the higher the temperature in the exposed tissue region. If the exposure of the tissue is fixed but its absorption is high, then the temperature will increase in proportion to the absorption rate for that material or tissue. Temperature changes are inversely related to tissue density. In dense materials, temperature changes are not as rapid. Bone and muscle are more dense than fat, so temperature rises will be slower in these tissues when exposed to sound waves.

The process of scattering can redirect the sound energy to other areas not intended to be observed with the sound waves. This can result in the intensity of the sound wave being directed to a more confined region, ultimately increasing the temperature in that region. Scattering of sound occurs most noticeably in inhomogeneous tissues such as lung. However, scattering plays a relatively minor role in the overall attenuation of sound waves.

In diagnostic use, heat does not cause noticeable discomfort to the patient. Within the human body, an increase in heat in a particular location can be diffused by the perfusion of blood to that area. This process is referred to as *convection*. Heat is actually carried away by the flow of blood, which helps to maintain a steady internal temperature.[36] Should heat be allowed to increase, surrounding cells would be destroyed by the increase in temperature.

Another mechanism that serves to maintain a constant temperature is *conduction*—the transfer of heat, which helps to regulate temperature.[36] Many materials, including tissue cells, have this property.

CAVITATION

Cavitation is a term used to describe a number of events that result from sound waves encountering compressible bodies within the exposed tissue, such as gas, bubbles, or cavities.[1] Within body tissues, dissolved gases can produce small bubbles that exist throughout interstitial spaces. When these bubbles are struck by sound waves they may begin to vibrate, sometimes violently, or they may function as a secondary sound source.[36]

These interactions between sound and bubbles can create several potentially adverse effects on surrounding tissue. First, gas bodies may begin to oscillate around a resonant frequency. These oscillations are caused when the pressure inside the gas bubble differs from the pressure of the sound wave. As a result, these oscillations can become severe and violent, causing damage to surrounding cells from shearing and streaming forces. Second, bubbles may grow in a sound field.[36] This growth is a result of the diffusion of gases into and out of the bubbles. If the exchange of gases into and out of the bubbles is equal, the net change is the same. If the change is asymmetric, then the bubbles continue to grow if the energy within them is not dissipated. Cavitation occurs when the pressure within gas bubbles changes dramatically. If the change is too great the bubbles may collapse, creating an enormous amount of pressure within a very localized spot, causing shear stresses sufficient to disrupt surrounding cell membranes. Third, bubbles may also absorb a tremendous amount of the sound energy. Similarly, if tissue absorbs a lot of the energy, this energy is converted into heat. In tissue areas consisting of a high density of bubbles or other gas bodies, the temperature in those areas can increase exponentially relative to surroundings areas. This heat increase will result in damage to surrounding tissue. Fourth, these drastic changes in bubbles can create high-velocity gradients around their surfaces. These high-velocity gradients, referred to as *microstreaming*, can ultimately cause damage to surrounding cells by fragmenting them.[45]

MECHANICAL EFFECTS

Mechanical effects include all other potentially damaging events that can create shear stresses sufficient to damage cell membranes. These include acoustic microscopic streaming, effects of microscopic streaming, viscous stresses, radiation forces, and radiation torque. Many of these mechanisms are not clearly understood, and further investigation is needed to clarify their effects on biologic tissue.

Artifacts

Artifacts are caused most commonly by operator errors but may also be the result of foreign material and the physical nature of the sound wave. Operator errors result in improper scanning techniques and positions, improper instrument setup, and improper transducer selection. Artifacts are signals that are displayed in such a way that they do not accurately represent the anatomic or flow characteristics of the subject. Many types of artifacts are possible, and when viewing sonographic information, it may be difficult to be sure which type of artifact is present. In echocardiography, as in other diagnostic modalities, accurate diagnoses depend on knowledge of normal patterns and the changes that are likely to occur in disease states. The operator must also be aware of the physical interaction of sound waves with tissue and how this interaction affects the image.

Artifacts can be classified into three main categories: (1) artifacts that distort the size, shape, position, or brightness of a structure; (2) artifacts that remove or mask real structures from the display; and (3) artifacts that suggest the presence of structures that are not really there.[2] Many of these artifacts can be identified by the sonographer since most of them do not move with surrounding cardiac structures or can be seen to be continuous throughout the heart, as well as outside the heart. There are many other signs that one needs to look for in determining true form false structures.

ARTIFACTS THAT DISTORT SIZE, SHAPE, POSITION, OR BRIGHTNESS

Propagation Speed Errors

The most common of these in echocardiography is *speed of sound artifacts or propagation speed errors.* These artifacts are caused when the sound wave strikes tissue or structures where the velocity of sound differs from the value assumed by the system.[2] This results in a longer transmit time for the ultrasound signal. Consequently, this longer transmit time is interpreted by the system as a more distant target and therefore is misplaced.

The machine determines the axial location of a reflector according to the time of echo return and the assumed speed of ultrasound travel in soft tissue or 1540 m/sec. Not all materials found in the body are soft tissue; hence, the speed of sound will vary, depending on the material. This phenomenon is commonly seen in patients with ball-and-cage prosthetic valves. The speed of sound within the ball is often much slower than in the average soft tissue, causing the echo from the far surface of the ball to appear farther away than it really is.

Multipath Artifacts

The system assigns spatial location on the basis of round-trip time. Some echoes may bounce off multiple surfaces or back and forth between two highly reflective surfaces before returning to the transducer. They appear on the display at a depth where no real interface exists. Many mechanisms can produce incorrect displays in the axial dimension, but these are usually recognizable because they do not make anatomic and physiologic sense.

An excellent common example of multipath artifacts can be seen in TEE imaging of the thoracic aorta in cross section (Fig. 3-36). In this case, a linear artifact mimicking an intimal flap is seen in

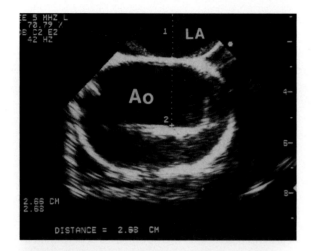

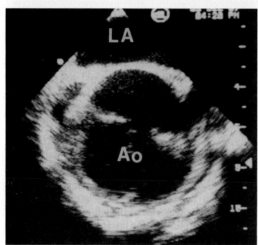

Figure 3-36. A transesophageal image of the ascending aorta at the level of the left atrium obtained in the transverse imaging plane. An ascending artifact in the middle of the aorta mimics an intimal flap. (From Ref. 2, Fig. 3. Reprinted with permission.)

linear echo is seen beyond the farther structure (Fig. 3-37). This is a common occurrence in TEE imaging of the aorta.[2] Knowledge of the diameter and distance relationship of these artifacts is important in distinguishing real from false structures.

Linear artifacts can be distinguished from intimal flaps by several key characteristics: (1) linear artifacts typically have fuzzy borders; (2) the artifact can usually be seen extending beyond the aortic wall; (3) artifacts lack the rapidly oscillating mobility of intimal flaps; and (4) the distance of the artifact is equal to the diameter of the anterior structure.[2]

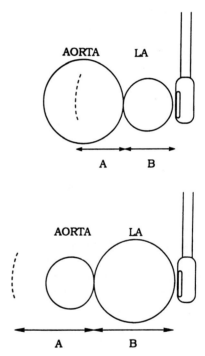

Figure 3-37. Diagram of the in vitro model of the ascending aorta linear artifact. Two latex balloons, one representing the aorta and one the left atrium (LA), were placed side by side in a water bath. An artifact was consistently present within the aortic balloon when the diameter of the aortic balloon exceeded the diameter of the left atrial balloon (top). The artifact was projected outside the aorta when the left atrial balloon was larger than the aortic balloon (bottom). By altering the diameter of the balloons, it was shown that the distance from the aorta-left atrium interface to the artifact (arrow A) equaled the diameter of the left atrial balloon (arrow B). This finding demonstrates that the linear artifact is due to reflection of ultrasound with the atrium. (From Ref. 2, Fig. 1. Reprinted with permission.)

the center of the aorta. The sound waves bounce off two highly reflective surfaces, such as the left atrial and aortic walls. If two fluid-filled objects are adjacent to one another, as is the case in this particular TEE view, with the left atrium seen anterior to the aorta, the stage is set for this type of artifact. If the structure closest to the transducer is smaller in diameter than the structure behind it, a linear artifact is seen within the larger-diameter structure at a distance roughly equal to the diameter of the anterior structure. If the structure closest to the transducer is larger than the structure farther away, a

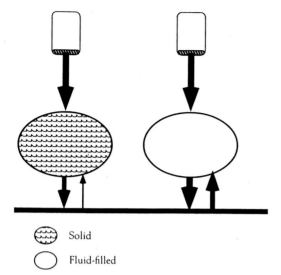

Figure 3-38. Power or enhancement artifacts. The strength of a reflection from an interface is partially determined by the amount of energy that reaches the interface. In the diagram, the echo from the part of the interface that is behind a fluid-filled structure (right) is much stronger than the signal that had to pass through a solid structure with internal reflectors (left). While time gain compensation gives greater amplification to more distant structures, it does not account for differences along different image lines. Identical interfaces may have different appearances, depending on the structures that lie in front of them.

Enhancement Artifacts

These artifacts result in areas distant to low-attenuation structures or regions such as fluid-filled chambers. Due to the low attenuation properties of fluid, the signals from a solid structure distal to fluid regions will be enhanced, causing the structure to appear larger or thicker than it actually is[2] (Fig. 3-38). An example of enhancement artifact can be seen in patients with circumferential pericardial effusions. In this case, the walls of the left ventricle appear thicker than they actually are. Proper gain settings are critical in measuring left ventricular walls in this setting.

ARTIFACTS THAT DISTORT OR OBSCURE REAL ECHOES

Shadowing Artifacts

Shadowing artifacts result when sound waves strike a highly reflective surface such that structures distal to that surface are not seen. Such is the case with prosthetic valves or calcified valves, where structures distal to these highly reflective surfaces are obscured.[2] In Figure 3-39, the left ventricular cavity and walls are not clearly seen because of masking or shadowing from the prosthetic valve. Another common example of this artifact can be seen in transthoracic imaging where a mitral valve prosthesis shadows the left atrium, making the diagnosis of mitral regurgitation difficult.

Shadowing artifacts are also observed at the edges of curved surfaces.[40] Shadowing created in this situation may be due to refraction and reflection properties of the boundaries encountered by the sound wave.[21,52] This is particularly true when the angle of incidence to the boundaries is perpendicular. The speed of sound at these curved interfaces will vary, allowing some portions of the sound waves to travel at faster or slower speeds, depending on the material encountered. Since the system is assuming a speed of sound of 1540 m/sec, signals being received at speeds different from this speed may in fact cancel one another when they meet. This will result in the loss of a signal and consequently will produce a shadow.[40]

ARTIFACTS THAT CREATE FALSE STRUCTURES

Reverberation Artifact

Reverberation artifact results when an echo reflects off of two highly reflective surfaces that are parallel to one another. Multiple sound waves will be reflected back to the transducer at different times.

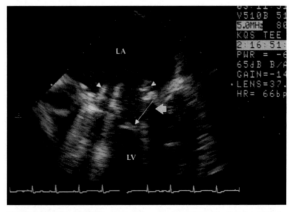

Figure 3-39. TEE image of a prosthetic mitral valve. Note the shadowing distal to the mitral prosthesis (large arrow). The left ventricle is obscured.

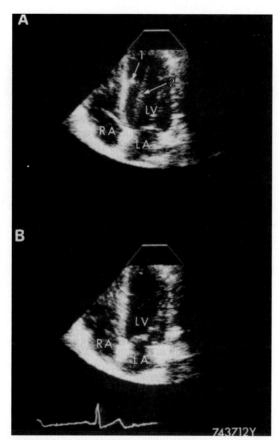

Figure 3-40. Reverberation artifact seen in an apical four-chamber view. The false echoes are reflection from the left ventricular (LV) wall and transducer housing. RA, right ventricle; LA, left ventricle. (From Feigenbaum H [ed]. Echocardiography, 5th ed. Baltimore, Lea & Febiger; 1994:Fig. 1-46. Reprinted with permission.)

Since some of the signals will be received later in time, the resulting image will be displayed at a different location, creating a false image. This type of artifact can also be seen in the apical four-chamber view (Fig. 3-40).

Reverberation artifacts usually appear as separate parallel lines occurring at regular intervals. Since the system automatically compensates for echoes returning from a farther distance by increasing their intensity, this artifact is further enhanced. *Mirror image* artifact is an example of reverberation artifact. Mirror image artifact usually results when the sound beam strikes a highly reflective surface. The sound beam returning from the far wall of the surface will be reflected by the near surface, essentially doubling the return time to the transducer.

The resultant image appears to be on the other side of the surface. Reverberation artifact can be reduced or eliminated by repositioning the transducer or changing the scan angle.

Side Lobe Artifact

In addition to the central ultrasound beam, most transducers, especially phased array transducers, also produce peripheral ultrasound beams that are usually lower in intensity. These extra skirts of ultrasound energy around the central beam create side lobe artifacts. When echoes from interfaces within these lobes are very strong, they are also displayed and greatly degrade the lateral resolution of the system. When discussing cross-sectional image lateral resolution, one must realize that it is difficult to separate reflectors next to each other both within the plane of the section and perpendicular to that plane (Fig. 3-41). In other words, the "slice" of the heart that is looked at also has thickness.

Refraction Artifact

As stated earlier in this chapter, refraction of sound waves is a phenomenon whereby the sound beam

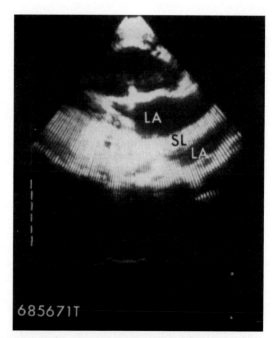

Figure 3-41. Two-dimensional echocardiogram demonstrating a side lobe (SL) within a dilated left atrium (LA). (From Feigenbaum H [ed]: Echocardiography, 5th ed. Baltimore, Lea & Febiger; 1994:Fig. 1-42. Reprinted with permission.)

is bent so that targets outside the main axis of the beam are displayed in the image.[2] Again, these artifacts can be eliminated by changing the transducer's angle and position.

Near Field Clutter or Speckle Artifact

These artifacts are seen near the top of the image closest to the transducer surface. They are created by high-amplitude oscillations of the transducer elements, also called *ring down*.[15] As a result, bright echoes are noted in the near field, obscuring or creating echoes in superficial structures. This is particularly troublesome for the apical views when attempting to interrogate the left ventricular apex for clot. These extra echoes can resemble clot or obscure a real clot. Careful gain and focus adjustments can reduce or eliminate these artifacts. In addition, the use of a higher-frequency transducer can better illuminate this area.

Like most artifacts, speckle artifacts are not observed from all views, but usually from only one, whereas actual structures are seen from a variety of acoustic windows. If an artifact is suspected, the operator should attempt to eliminate it by adjusting gains, transducer angle, and transducer position. Real structures are reproducible or can be seen from multiple windows, while artifacts usually are not.

REFERENCES

1. Apfel RE. Acoustic cavitation. *In* Edmonds PD (ed): Method of Experimental Physics: Ultrasonics. San Diego, Academic Press, 1981;355–411.
2. Appelbe AF, Walker PG, Yeoh JK, et al. Clinical significance and origin of artifacts in transesophageal echocardiography of the thoracic aorta. J Am Coll Cardiol. 1993;21:754–760.
3. Bansal RC, Shakudo M, Shah PM, et al. Biplane transesophageal echocardiography: Technique, image orientation and preliminary experience in 131 patients. J Am Soc Echocardiogr. 1990;3:348.
4. Bioeffects Committee of the American Institute of Ultrasound in Medicine. Safety Considerations for Diagnostic Ultrasound in Medicine. AIUM Publication 316. Bethesda, MD: American Institute of Ultrasound in Medicine; 1984.
5. Brayman AA, Azadniv M, Makin IRS, et al. Effects of a stabilized microbubble echo contrast agent on hemolysis of human erythrocytes exposed to high intensity pulsed ultrasound. Echocardiography. 1995;12:13–21.
6. Brayman AA, Church CC, Miller MW. Re-evaluation of the concept that high cell concentrations "protect" cells *in vitro* from ultrasonically induced lysis. Ultrasound Med Biol. 1996 (in press).
7. Burns PN, Powers JE, Simpson DH, et al. Harmonic imaging and Doppler using microbubble contrast agents: A new method for contrast imaging. Ultrasound Med Biol. 1994;20:S72.
8. Carstensen EL, Kelly P, Church CC, et al. Lysis of erythrocytes by exposure to CW ultrasound. Ultrasound Med Biol. 1993;147–165.
9. Chang P, Shung KK, Wu S-J, et al. Second harmonic imaging and harmonic Doppler measurements with Albunex. IEEE Trans UFFC 1995;42:1020–1027.
10. Child SZ, Carstensen EL. Effects of ultrasound on *Drosophila*. IV. Pulsed exposure of eggs. Ultrasound Med Biol. 1982;8:311–312.
11. Child Z, Hartman C, Shery LA, et al. Lung damage from exposure to pulsed ultrasound. Ultrasound Med Biol. 1990;16:817–825.
12. Christopher T. Finite amplitude distortion-based inhomogeneous pulse echo ultrasonic imaging. IEEE Trans Ultrason Ferroelectrics Frequency Control. 1997;44:125–139.
13. de Jong N, Cornet R, Lancee CT. Higher harmonics of vibrating gas-filled microspheres, part one: Simulations. Ultrasonics. 1994;32:447–453.
14. de Jong N, Cornet R, Lancee CT. Higher harmonics of vibrating gas-filled microspheres, part two: Measurements. Ultrasonics. 1994;32:455–459.
15. Feigenbaum H. Instrumentation. *In* Feigenbaum H (ed): Echocardiography, 5th ed. Philadelphia, Lea & Febiger, 1994:2, 26.
16. Goldman DE, Hueter TF. Tabular data of the velocity and absorption of high-frequency sound in mammalian tissues. J Acoust Soc Am. 1956;28:35–37.
17. Goss SA, Frizzell LA, Dunn F. Ultrasonic absorption and attenuation in mammalian tissues. Ultrasound Med Biol. 1979;5:181–186.
18. Goss SA, Johnston RL, Dunn F. Comprehensive compilation of empirical ultrasonic properties of mammalian tissues. L Acoust Soc Am. 1978;64:423–457.
19. Helmcke F, Mahan EF III, Nanda NC, et al. Use of smaller pediatric transesophageal echocardiographic probe in adults. Echocardiography. 1990;7:727.
20. Jedrzejewicz T. Lecture Mountain View California, September 1997 (unpublished article).
21. LaFollette PS, Ziskin MC. Geometric and intensity distortion in echocardiography. Ultrasound Med Biol. 1986;12:953–963.
22. Latson LA, Cheatham JP, Gutgesell HP. Resolution and accuracy in two dimensional echocardiography. Am J Cardiol. 1981;48:106–110.

23. Lichtenberg GS. Echocardiography instruments and principles. *In* Craig M, Kawamura D, Berman M (eds): Echocardiography, Diagnostic Medical Sonography: A Guide to Clinical Practice, vol. II. Philadelphia, JB Lippincott; 1991:58–59.

24. McDicken WN. Introduction to diagnostic ultrasound. *In* McDicken WN (ed): Diagnostic Ultrasonics: Principles and Use of Instrumentation, 2nd ed. New York, Wiley; 1981:3, 60, 64–67, 98, 311.

25. Miller DL. Cell death thresholds in Elodea for 0.4–1.0 MHz ultrasound compared to gas body resonance theory. Ultrasound Med. Biol. 1979;5: 351–357.

26. Miller DL, Reeses JA, Frazier ME. Single strand DNA breaks in human leucocytes induced by ultrasound *in vitro*. Ultrasound Med Biol. 1989;15: 765–771.

27. Miller DL, Thomas RM, Frazier ME. Single strand breaks in CHO cell DNA induced by ultrasound cavitation in vitro. Ultrasound Med Biol. 1991;17: 401–406.

28. Miller DL, Thomas RM. Ultrasound gas body activation in Elodea leaves and the mechanical index. Ultrasound Med Biol. 1993;19:343–351.

29. Nanda JC, Pinheiro L, Sanyal RS, et al. Transesophageal biplane echocardiographic imaging: Technique, planes and clinical usefulness. Echocardiography. 1990;7:771.

30. National Institutes of Health Consensus Development Conference. Diagnostic ultrasound imaging in pregnancy. NIH Publication No. 84-667. Bethesda, MD: U.S. Department of Health and Human Services; 1984.

31. Nyborg WL. Physical mechanisms for biological effects of ultrasound. HEW Publication (FDA) 78-8062. Rockville, MD: U.S. Department of Health, Education and Welfare; 1977.

32. Omoto R, Kyo S, Matsumura M, et al. Future technical prospects in biplane transesophageal echocardiography: Use of adult and pediatric biplane matrix probes. Echocardiography. 1991;8:713.

33. Omoto R, Kyo S, Matsumura M, et al. New direction of biplane transesophageal echocardiography with special emphasis on real-time biplane imaging and matrix phased array biplane transducer. Echocardiography. 1990;7:691.

34. Pandian NG, Hsu T-L, Schwartz SL, et al. Multiplane transesophageal echocardiography. Echocardiography. 1992;9:649.

35. Powis RL, Powis WJ. A Thinker's Guide to Ultrasonic Imaging. Baltimore, Urban & Schwarzenberg; 1984:3, 8.

36. Proceedings of the Workshop on Interaction of Ultrasound with Biological Tissues, November 8–11, 1971. DHEW Publication (FDA) 73-8008. Seattle, Battelle Seattle Research Center, 1972.

37. Pye SD, Wild SR, McDicken WN. Adaptive time gain compensation for ultrasonic imaging. Ultrasound Med Biol. 1992;18:205–212.

38. Roelandt J, Brommersma P, Bom N, et al. Multiplane transesophageal echocardiography with a varioplane transducer system. Thoraxcenter J. 1992;4: 38.

39. Roelandt J, van Dorp WG, Bom N, et al. Resolution problems in echocardiography: A source of interpretation errors. Am J Cardiol. 1976;37:256–262.

40. Rubin JM, Adler RS, Fowlkes JB, et al. Phase cancellation: A cause of acoustical shadowing at the edges of curved surfaces in B-mode ultrasound images. Ultrasound Med Biol. 1991;17:85–95.

41. Schrope BA, Newhouse VL, Dubin SE, et al. Second harmonic ultrasonic blood perfusion measurement. Ultrasound Med Biol. 1993;19:567–579.

42. Schrope BA, Newhouse VL, Uhlendorf V. Simulated capillary blood flow measurements using a nonlinear ultrasonic contrast agent. Ultrason Imaging. 1992; 14:134–158.

43. Schwarz KQ, Chen X, Steinmetz S, et al. Harmonic imaging with Levovist. J Am Soc Echocardiogr. 1997;10:1–10.

44. Skorton DJ, Collins SM, Garcia E, et al. Digital signal and image processing in echocardiography. Am Heart J. 1985;110:1266–1283.

45. Skorton DJ, Collins SM, Greenleaf JF, et al. Ultrasound bioeffects and regulatory issues: An introduction for the echocardiographer. J Am Soc Echocardiogr. 1988;1:240–251.

46. Webster's II New Riverside Dictionary. New York, Berkley Books; 1984:319.

47. Weintraub R, Shiota T, Elkadi T, et al. Transesophageal echocardiography in infants and children with congenital heart disease. Circulation. 1992;86: 711.

48. Wells PNT. Absorption and dispersion of ultrasound in biological tissue. Ultrasound Med Biol. 1975;1: 369–376.

49. Wells PNT. Biomedical Ultrasound. New York, Academic Press; 1977.

50. Weyman AE. Physical principles of ultrasound. *In* Weyman AE (ed): Principles and Practice of Echocardiography, 2nd ed. Philadelphia, Lea & Febiger; 1994;24.

51. Wood RW, Loomis AL. The physical and biological effects of high-frequency sound waves of great intensity. Phil Mag. 1927:4:417–436.

52. Ziskin MC, LaFollette PS, Blathras K, et al. Effect of scan format on reflective artifacts. Ultrasound Med Biol. 1990;16:183–191.

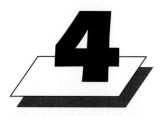

M-Mode and Two-Dimensional Echocardiography

CHRISTOPHER L. HARE

Introduction

Ultrasound has become a useful clinical tool since it was first described.[5] Its ability to show the structures and function of the heart has made it invaluable in cardiac diagnosis. M-mode and two-dimensional echocardiography were early formats for displaying this information, and remain current and helpful today. M-mode was the first modality to become commercially available for routine use in the heart. Imaging cardiac structures with this format created the opportunity to diagnose noninvasively diseases that earlier could only be viewed with invasive procedures or directly with surgery. The capabilities of M-mode were quickly realized, however, and its shortcomings in demonstrating the three-dimensional structures of the heart in a one-dimensional format were apparent. Two-dimensional imaging eliminated many of the shortcomings of M-mode. The medical community has shown great enthusiasm for this technique. With each year that has passed since its introduction, the technique has been improved and refined. In its present format, two-dimensional imaging has become a basic tool in the cardiologist's ability to diagnose and monitor diseases of the heart quickly and accurately.

Both modalities have strengths and weaknesses in resolving normal anatomy and pathologies. It is through a careful examination of cardiac structures with all modalities that a comprehensive echocardiographic exam is accomplished.

M-Mode: An Image from Ultrasound

To understand M-mode imaging, one must start with the physics of sound propagation. Sound travels through a homogeneous medium at a constant velocity. The velocity of sound will vary with the density and elasticity of the medium through which it travels. For example, sound travels faster through water than it does through air due to the higher density of water. In the human body, sound travels through the soft tissues at a fairly constant velocity of 1540 m/sec.[16] If the velocity of the sound wave in a medium is known, it becomes possible to determine how far an object, or interface, is from the transducer. To determine this distance, the time needed for the sound wave to leave the transducer, strike the interface, and return is multiplied by 1540 m/sec and then divided by 2. It is divided by 2 since it must travel to the interface and back again.

If two objects are along the sound beam's path, the location of both may be determined if they are far enough apart. The wavelength, or distance between sound packets, will determine this.[16] The sound beam must be able to strike each object individually if both are to be seen. If the wavelength is long enough to strike both objects at the same time, then they will appear as one object. If the wavelength is short enough to strike each object separately, each will reflect some of the sound energy back and allow its location to be documented separately (Fig. 4-1).

Because sound travels so fast in soft tissue, and the distances that are of interest in imaging the body are relatively limited, a transducer with a very high frequency can be used. Thus, ultrasound transducers in the 1,000,000-Hz or 1 MHz range are used for diagnostic purposes. A transducer with a frequency of 1 MHz can resolve structures that are

1.5 mm apart.[17] With the ability to resolve such small structures, an image can be formed demonstrating the distances from the transducer of the interfaces that the beam crosses. The interfaces can be represented as a series of points or dots that are perpendicular to the transducer. The simplest way to display this information is known as *amplitude mode* (*A-mode*)[16] (Fig. 4-2). In A-mode, the signal from each interface is represented as an amplitude at a distance from the transducer. If the strength of the signal at each interface is represented as varying in brightness instead of amplitude, different structures can be more usefully displayed. This format is known as *brightness mode* or *B-mode*. These formats display an image with a single dimension of information. In *motion mode* or *M-mode*, this single perpendicular axis of information is repeatedly displayed. The resulting image can demonstrate the motion of cardiac structures.

M-mode echocardiography was quickly adapted for early ultrasound units. It is still standard equipment on most echocardiography units today. M-mode is a display of depth (its only dimension), which is updated continuously over time. The resulting images are diagnostically useful in observing the function of cardiac structures. While M-mode can display only a single line or dimension of information, it can update this information rapidly. It is not uncommon for frame rates to be as high as 1000 to 2000/sec.[6] Fast-moving structures like the mitral or aortic valves can be accurately displayed over time. When recorded simultaneously with an electrocardiographic (EKG) signal, the precise timing of events can be documented. This ability remains M-mode's greatest strength. The opening and closing of cardiac valves can be accurately timed. Contraction and expansion of the chambers can easily be seen and measured.

Historically, M-mode images have been recorded on various paper strip chart systems. These systems have done well in displaying the resolution available from M-mode. High-quality strip chart recorders are capable of displaying the high frame rates of M-mode.[2] Control of paper speed allows the sonographer to demonstrate the timing of events by enlarging the time aspect through increasing the paper speed. Typically, a paper speed of 25–100 m/sec is used for common measurements of chamber size, wall thickness, or valve opening. When the timing of events such as differences in

Transducer 1   Transducer 2

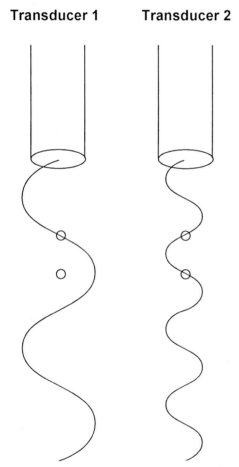

Figure 4-1. The first transducer demonstrates how the sound wave with a low frequency may be unable to strike two objects that are close together. The second transducer demonstrates how a higher frequency will intersect each object in the sound beam's path.

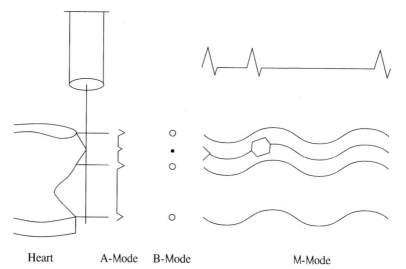

Figure 4-2. Ultrasound information can be displayed in different formats. The earliest format was A-mode. The amplitude of each interface varies with the strength of the returning signal and is demonstrated as a single dimension of depth. B-mode uses shades of gray to depict the strength of the returning signal. M-mode takes the B-mode points and demonstrates the changes in location of these points by graphing them horizontally to represent time.

mitral and tricuspid valve openings or isovolemic periods is measured, increasing the paper speed to 100–200 mm/sec allows for clear visualization of these events.

Storage and maintenance of these paper tracings have become issues in many labs. Paper tracings tend to fade over time, and the volume of paper can be large and requires extensive storage space in crowded labs. Videotaped images display the M-mode format reasonably well but lack the high resolution of paper systems. Video monitors are limited in the number of frames or lines of M-mode information that can be displayed since there is a finite number of pixels on the monitor screen to display them. Even so, many labs record M-mode images on video.

Two-Dimensional Echocardiography

Two-dimensional imaging started as a variation of B-mode technology. It has been accepted as a major advance in echocardiography and has seen constant improvements over the years. Although B-mode scanning allowed two-dimensional imaging of other human structures, it was not useful in the heart. Different transducer designs were developed that have allowed imaging of the heart. There are three types of two-dimensional scanners today: mechanical, phased array, and annular array. Each has taken a different approach to imaging, and each has strengths and weaknesses.

MECHANICAL SCANNERS

Mechanical scanners were among the first instruments to attempt real-time two-dimensional imaging of the heart. The basic principle in two-dimensional imaging using a mechanical scanner is to display a series of B-mode images on the same screen. Early two-dimensional transducers attempted to move the single B-mode image from side to side across a plane or sector to give the image both depth and width. This could be done by physically moving the transducer over the skin or angling it back and forth from a single location. For the heart, this format was not useful due to the small intercostal spaces and relatively long time required to obtain a single image. A transducer design was developed to allow it to be held in place and be moved mechanically over an arc or sector to create the image (Fig. 4-3). These scanners are driven by an electric motor that is used to oscillate or rotate the transducer head through the image plane.[6] To ensure that the B-mode images were correctly spaced in the sector image, a potentiometer was fixed to the transducer. As the transducer head moved, its location was noted and the corresponding B-mode image was placed on the appropriate spot on the composite image being displayed on the screen. Axial resolution and signal-to-noise ratios

Heart   A-Mode   B-Mode   M-Mode

Transducer 1   **Transducer 2**

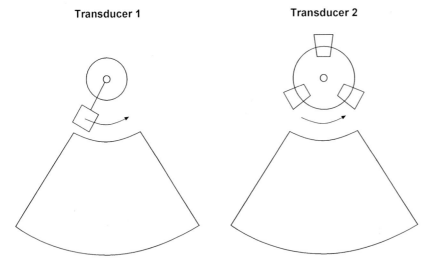

Figure 4-3. The first transducer demonstrates a single element that is angled from one side of the image sector to the other. Once the arc is completed, this element will reverse its direction and travel back to its starting point. The second transducer has three elements that spin like a wheel. As the first element completes its sweep across the image sector, it stops sending and receiving sound waves and the next element begins to cross the arc.

for this type of system are high. Lateral resolution was dependent on how accurately the potentiometer could track the current location of the transducer, as well as how many lines of information made up the image.

Two types of mechanical scanners have been employed. The first type rotates a single transducer head over a sector in one direction. As it moves to each angle in the sector, an ultrasound pulse is sent out and received, creating the composite image. Once the transducer has completed its arc, it is reversed and sent back in the other direction to repeat the process and update the image. The wider the sector, the longer it takes to complete the arc and the slower the rate at which the images can be updated. To compensate for this slow rate, a narrower sector can be selected. In some cases, a sector as narrow as 30 degrees is chosen to allow for a reasonable frame rate. There is clearly a trade-off between the narrowness of the image sector and the speed with which the image can be updated.

To avoid the problems of a narrow image sector and to increase the frame rate, a second type of mechanical scanner was employed. This has multiple elements mounted at intervals in a wheel-type format and rotated. As the first transducer completes its sector, the next one comes into the starting position and is ready to travel on the same path. Three or four separate elements were commonly used. On these early mechanical scanners, one could distinctly see the individual scan lines, or B-mode lines, on

the image. Subsequent improvements in mechanical scanners have allowed for much better control over the number of scan lines and have improved image quality.

PHASE ARRAY SCANNERS

Phased array scanners are the most commonly used transducer type today. They are sophisticated, electronically steered systems which can create a beam that is shaped or tailored by the operator for each task. Instead of using a single element, like the mechanical scanners, these systems use multiple elements lined up side by side to create an ultrasound wavefront that can be steered electronically across the sector to create the image. The typical system has between 64 and 128 elements that make up the transducer scan head. When the individual elements are fired at slightly different times, a series of small wavefronts are created[10,11] (Fig. 4-4). As these wavefronts move away from the transducer, they begin to combine to form one large wavefront. If the timing of these small wavefronts is changed, the direction of the large wavefront that they ultimately combine to form can be steered at any number of angles away from the transducer (Fig. 4-5). This process is known as *beam steering*.[11] The beam can be oscillated over an arc which is determined by the operator. With such precise control over the direction of the sound beam, the quality of the image can be improved.

Figure 4-4. This illustration depicts a phased array transducer. Note the multiple elements lined up next to each other at the face of the transducer.

The sound beam can also be focused by manipulating the firing sequence of the elements.[17] For example, if a structure lies 10 cm away, the beam can be focused to obtain its best lateral resolution at that depth (Fig. 4-6). This is accomplished by altering the sequential firing of the elements so that when they combine to form a single wavefront, it is concave as it moves away. If the concave shape is dramatic, the beam will continue to narrow as it moves away. Eventually, there comes a point at which the beam no longer narrows but starts to diverge. This point is known as the *focal point*. If a shallower concave wavefront is created, the narrowest point of the beam will be elongated; this is known as the *focal zone*.

Thus, with a phased array system, the operator can select several characteristics of the beam and image. Each of these variables will allow the operator to maximize the sound beam characteristics to best image a specific structure. Mastery of each variable will allow the operator to select the correct beam shape for each structure or function. These variables are commonly changed throughout the ultrasound exam.

ANNULAR ARRAY SCANNERS

Annular array technology is a variation in the element design of the phased array system. In this type, the elements are circular rather than rectangular. Instead of several dozen elements, only a few elements are used (Fig. 4-7). Each circular element or ring is placed inside the other, giving the transducer itself a circular shape.[17] This unique design allows

Figure 4-5. If the timing of the sound waves coming from each element is changed, some waves begin to travel away from the transducer earlier than others. The waves start as a series of individuals but end by combining to form a larger single wavefront. This single wavefront can travel at an angle to the transducer. If the timing of each series of wavefronts is changed, an image sector can be created.

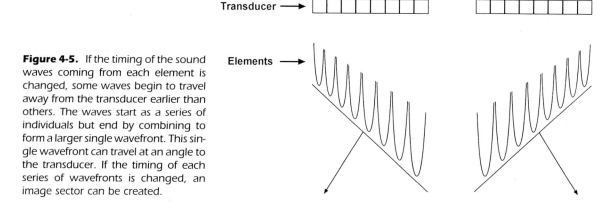

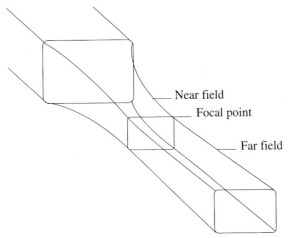

Figure 4-6. This illustration shows the elements of the sound beam along the axial plane. The first part is the near field. In this field, the beam becomes increasingly narrow as it moves farther from the transducer. The focal point represents the area where the beam has reached its narrowest point and will no longer converge. The far field is the last part of the sound beam as it travels along the axial plane. In the far field the sound beam diverges.

focusing of the ultrasound wavefront as it is sent as well as received. This gives much greater flexibility of the focal zone in terms of its location along the beam and the length of the zone itself. The circular nature of the transducer does not allow electronic beam steering. Therefore, the transducer must be mechanically moved over an arc to create the sector image. These elements are typically housed in a plastic sphere or cover and filled with an oil solution. The mechanical rotation is easily viewed on most commercial systems. The frame rate and sector image can be altered merely by limiting the arc over which the elements are allowed to move.

Principles of Imaging

With any transducer type, there are general limitations to ultrasound. Because sound travels at a known speed in soft tissue and because the depth of interest is limited, these basic parameters represent physical limits within which images can be created over time. Consider that a sound wave must be sent out and received back at each scan line in which the image is constructed. Then each image must be updated rapidly enough to demonstrate the motion of the heart. Clearly, a tremendous amount of information is being processed in each second of image acquisition. A discussion of how these parameters are defined follows.

PULSED REPETITION FREQUENCY

The number of ultrasound pulses that can be sent out each second is limited by the speed of sound in soft tissue and by the location of the farthest point of interest. Each pulse must be sent out and the reflected information received before the next pulse is sent. Therefore, only a limited number of pulses can be sent in each second.[10,11,17] This number of pulses is known as the *pulsed repetition frequency*. As the depth of the image is increased, the length of time allowed for each pulse of reflected information to return from the farthest depth is also increased. The increase in depth limits the pulse repetition information available to form each image. Fortunately, several thousand pulses can generally be made available for images.

FRAME RATE

With pulse repetition frequency limited to a specific number at any given depth, the next issue is how many pulses are committed to each image that is

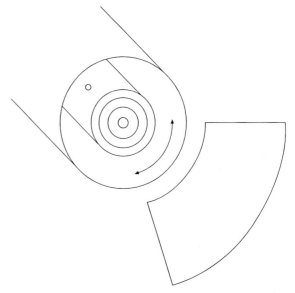

Figure 4-7. An annular array transducer combines features of the mechanical and phased array technologies. Note the concentric rings within the transducer. These rings allow the sound beam to be shaped and focused similar to a phased array transducer. The rings are mechanically moved across the arc of the sector image in the same fashion as a mechanical transducer.

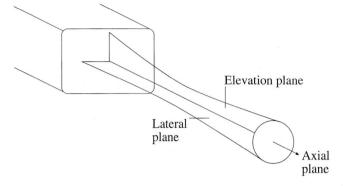

Figure 4-8. There are three planes that can be used to describe a sound beam, as demonstrated in this illustration. The lateral plane is defined along the width of the transducer. The elevation plane is defined along the height of the transducer. The axial plane is defined along the direction of the sound beam's path and is away from the transducer.

produced. Since the heart is a constantly moving structure, the ability to resolve that motion over time is important. (For example, if there are 4000 pulses available for demonstrating ventricular contractility, a frame rate of 20 frames per second would give each image 200 lines of information [4000/20 = 200].) For a faster-moving structure such as a valve, a frame rate of 40 or 60/sec may be required. At these frame rates, the number of pulses of information would be limited to 100 and 66, respectively (4000/40 = 100; 4000/60 = 66). When the frame rate is increased, there is a loss of information dedicated to each image.

IMAGE SECTOR ANGLE

The width of the sector image will determine how close together the lines of sound information, or scan lines, will be. If the depth of the image field is significant, the number of lines is limited. When the sector angle is wide, individual lines may be seen. In an effort to produce a clinically acceptable image, the scan angle can be reduced to bring these scan lines closer together and reduce the apparent space between them. In a typical acceptable clinical image, there would be two or more scan lines per degree.

In a sector image of 90 degrees, at least 180 scan lines will be required to obtain two lines per degree. In situations with high frame rates and large depths of field, the line density may fall below this level. Many scan systems are set up to produce high-quality images by maximizing the pulse repetition frequency at any given depth and sacrificing the frame rate. The operator can then reduce the scan angle to bring the frame rate back to an acceptable range.

RESOLUTION

The ability to resolve finite structures in the heart is defined at two primary levels: at the transducer and at the sector image being displayed. Axial resolution at the transducer is determined by the frequency and therefore the wavelength. The higher the frequency, the shorter the wavelength and the smaller the structure that can be demonstrated. The length and width of the elements determine the size of the ultrasound beam and therefore the initial lateral and elevation resolution (Fig. 4-8). Focusing the sound beam can further improve the lateral resolution.

At the scan system level, the apparent resolution of the entire system can be seen. Time resolution can be changed by increasing or decreasing the frame rate. Increasing the depth will reduce the pulse repetition frequency and the amount of sound information available to form the image. Changing the sector image angle will change the line density (Table 4-1).

TABLE 4-1. Principles of Imaging

Width of the image sector	Inc. sector size	Dec. frame rate
Depth of image sector	Inc. depth	Dec. frame rate
Location of the focal point	Short focus	Dec. far-field res.
	Deep focus	Dec. near-field res.
Frequency of the transducer	Inc. freq.	Inc. res.
		Dec. penetration
Line density	Inc. res.	Dec. frame rate

Advantages and Limitations of the Ultrasound Techniques

The value of ultrasound to the clinician is in its ability to differentiate normal from abnormal anatomy and function. Both M-mode and two-dimensional modalities can resolve cardiac anatomy and function under ideal circumstances. Both, however, have limitations.

M-MODE

The sonographer must take great care to orient the probe perpendicular to the minor axis of the heart when collecting parasternal images. Placing the probe one or two interspaces too low will create an M-mode image that distorts the cardiac anatomy and provides false information. An improper transducer position can falsely enlarge cardiac chambers and cause exaggerated motion of the walls.[15] Furthermore, the mitral valve can be made to appear prolapsed by erroneous placement of the probe. The orientation of the heart to the chest wall can vary due to several factors, including body habitus, age, and the presence of regurgitant valvular lesions or congenital abnormalities such as atrial or ventricular defects, making the use of a standard transducer position all the more important.

To perform an M-mode exam properly, the sonographer must evaluate multiple sites to determine the proper location of the minor axis of the heart. Most current ultrasound systems will provide an updated two-dimensional image with a cursor line demonstrating the location of the M-mode information. If the M-mode cursor line is not perpendicular to the minor axis, then the information is suspect and a new interspace or location needs to be attempted.

Once the proper axis is found, the M-mode image demonstrates precise information on a very small area of the total cardiac anatomy. For example, an M-mode scan from the minor axis will cross through the interventricular septum and the left ventricular posterior wall. This may demonstrate normal contraction of these areas but give no information on the apical or lateral regions. Consequently, M-mode has no real application in the evaluation of left ventricular wall motion abnormalities. Similarly, M-mode can provide useful information in the evaluation of mitral stenosis by demonstrating

restricted leaflet motion. Its ability to provide information on mitral regurgitation on the same patient is limited.

The most useful function of M-mode today is in imaging valvular motion when timing is important and in measuring chamber diameter and wall thickness. For most measurements like cardiac output, left ventricular mass, ejection fraction, and valve area, the two-dimensional and Doppler techniques have proven to be superior.[1,3,9,12,14]

TWO-DIMENSIONAL IMAGING

Two-dimensional imaging overcomes the limitations of M-mode by assessing cardiac anatomy and function in a global or regional fashion. Because its image presentation has both depth and width, parameters such as ventricular wall motion and chamber size become much more apparent. Imaging planes from the apical and subcostal approaches become useful adjuncts to the parasternal orientation. Combined, these areas give the sonographer the ability to demonstrate the anatomy throughout all three dimensions.

This advantage of two-dimensional imaging creates some limitations when specific parameters are evaluated. Two-dimensional imaging becomes problematic when the object being imaged is parallel to the transducer. In the short axis view, the left ventricle has a circular shape. The lateral wall and the corresponding portion of the septum tend to "drop out" or fail to reflect the ultrasound because they are parallel to the sound beam. Complete visualization of the entire circumference of the left ventricle can be obtained in most but not all patients. Similarly, the lateral wall will again become parallel to the sound beam in the apical window. In both cases, this is a limitation of the lateral resolution of the system. To properly image as much of the left ventricle as possible, multiple windows are required. On occasion, off-axis images will be collected by the sonographer to specifically document a wall that may have not been imaged from the traditional planes.

A second limitation of two-dimensional imaging is that its frame rate can be relatively slow in certain circumstances. For example, calculating left ventricular volume from the apical window becomes difficult when a large depth setting is required. Obtaining an image at exactly the right time during both diastole and systole may be impossible if too few frames are acquired. Similarly, small, fast-moving structures such as torn chordae, valvular vegetations, or small, pedunculated tumors may be difficult to diagnose if the frame rate is low. Improved technology in some systems allows for increased frame rates, which have overcome some of these limitations.

A related limitation of two-dimensional imaging is its recording modality. Video recording has a set frame rate of 30/sec. Small, fast-moving structures may be seen well at a rate of 40–60 frames per second and are discernible by the sonographer. When recorded on videotape at nearly half the initial rate, much of the diagnostic image information may be lost. A second limitation of the video format is that the images are displayed as two interlaced fields. Each field is made up of every other line of horizontal information. The video monitor interlaces two fields of information in each frame that is displayed in the play mode. Only a single field or every other line of information is displayed in a pause or freeze frame mode. Pausing an image on video in order to study detail creates a significant loss of information. Sonographers can avoid this pitfall by pausing an image on the ultrasound unit and recording the paused image on the videotape for detailed viewing.

Many ultrasound systems have some type of limited digital memory that allows the user to record a short digital movie of several cardiac cycles, enabling the viewer to replay specific cycles.[7] Again, pathology that is fast-moving or images that are of great interest can be captured in digital memory and replayed at slower rates or paused at intervals to make the pathology more apparent when recorded on videotape.

Computer technology offers the promise of digital storage of all the information created during the ultrasound exam. Many exercise stress echocardiograms are recorded and stored this way today. With expanded digital memory and larger memory storage capacities on computers, more types of ultrasound exams will be stored this way.

Measurements

As ultrasound has improved, various methods of measuring and quantifying cardiac structures have evolved. Several different methods or criteria for making these measurements are currently used (Fig. 4-9). The major methods differ from each other in whether they include or exclude the image border or "echo" in the measurement. The leading edge of a structure is defined as that portion that is closest to the transducer. As a sound wave travels toward a structure, its "leading edge" will contact first. Some borders appear as a thin, distinct line, while others may be several millimeters thick. When one considers that some of these measurements involve area

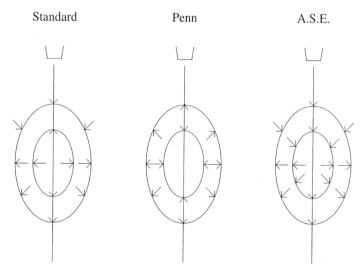

Figure 4-9. The three methods depicted here vary from one another by which side of the interface is included in or excluded from the measurement. The standard method switches from including to excluding the interface, depending on which structure is being measured. The Penn method measures from an anatomic point of view. The entire endocardial and epicardial interface is excluded from the measurement. The American Society of Echocardiography (ASE) method references all interfaces the same way. The leading edge of any interface, as referenced from the transducer, is the point where the measurement is taken.

and volume, this small difference can be raised to the second or third power, depending on the calculation, and the results can be significantly different.

The major methods for making measurements are the standard convention, the Penn convention, and the American Society of Echocardiography convention. The standard convention was developed for M-mode and allowed measurement of the left ventricle, septum, and posterior wall.[8] This method demonstrated good correlation with autopsy and angiography findings. It defines the septum as including the area from the leading edge to the trailing edge. The posterior wall is defined as running from the leading edge of the endocardium to the leading edge of the pericardium. This method, however, is difficult to translate into two-dimensional images.

The Penn convention was first developed to provide a correlation with the left ventricular mass.[4] This method excludes the thickness of the endocardial echo from the septum, as well as the posterior wall. It includes the thickness of the endocardial echo on the septum and posterior wall when measuring the left ventricular mass.

The American Society of Echocardiography recommended that a single convention be used so that results reported from different labs can be standardized.[13] The society recommended that the leading edge, as referenced from the transducer location, to the next leading edge of the next structure be used as the convention. This standard can be used by both M-mode and two-dimensional techniques. This method does tend to be difficult when measuring structures that are parallel to the sound beam. For example, in the short axis view when measuring the left ventricle's area, one must cross over the thickness of the endocardial border when tracing the endocardium from the top of the image to the bottom.

The heart is a dynamic structure, and one must be concerned with the timing of the measurements during the cardiac cycle. The high sampling rate of M-mode can demonstrate the difference in electrical signals of diastole or systole on the EKG, as well as delay in the mechanical contraction or relaxation of the heart. This high degree of precision has led to the proposal of numerous methods. There have been many reported methodologies of standardization, either on the mechanical movement of the heart or precise time marks based on EKG events. Each lab must adapt a measurement criterion for M-mode from the many reported in the literature. Once a criterion is accepted, it is important for everyone in the lab to follow the same protocol.

Timing of two-dimensional images for measurements is less crucial since there are fewer points in time (video frames) in which to make measurements. With the relative number of frames to measure being limited to 30 on video, one must make measurements from the image as close to the end of diastole and systole as possible. Computer image capture allows the sonographer to acquire images based on precise EKG timing. Since the computer can be set to wait for an EKG event to occur, the image can be stored in computer memory at exactly that point in the cardiac cycle.

REFERENCES

1. Albin G, Rahkop S. Comparison of echocardiographic quantitation of left ventricular ejection fraction to radionuclide angiography in patients with regional wall motion abnormalities. Am J Cardiol. 1990;65:1031–1032.
2. Chang S. M-Mode Echocardiographic Techniques and Pattern Recognition, 2nd ed. Philadelphia, Lea and Febiger; 1981.
3. Collins HW, et al. Reproducibility of left ventricular mass measurement by two dimensional and M-mode echocardiography. J Am Coll Cardiol. 1989;14:672–676.
4. Devereux RB, Reichek N. Echocardiographic determination of left ventricular mass in man: Anatomic validation of the method. Circulation. 1977;55:613–618.
5. Edler I: Diagnostic Use of Ultrasound in Heart Disease. Acta Med Scand. 1955;32:308–311.
6. Eggleton RC, et al. Visualization of cardiac dynamics with real-time B-mode ultrasonic scanner. *In* White D (ed): Ultrasound in Medicine. New York, Plenum Press; 1975.
7. Feigenbaum H. Echocardiography, 5th ed. Philadelphia, Lea and Febiger; 1994.
8. Feigenbaum H, et al. Left ventricular wall thickness measured by ultrasound. Arch Intern Med. 1968;121:391–395.
9. Force J, Parisi AF. Quantitative methods for analyzing regional systolic function with two dimensional echocardiography. Echocardiography. 1986;3:319–331.
10. Hedrick WR, Hykes DL, Starchman DE. Ultrasound Physics and Instrumentation, 3rd ed. St Louis, Mosby Year Book; 1995.
11. McDicken WN. Diagnostic Ultrasonics: Principles

and Use of Instruments, 3rd ed. Edinburgh, Churchill Livingstone; 1991.

12. Recheck N, et al. Anatomic validation of left ventricular mass estimated from clinical two dimensional echocardiography: Initial results. Circulation. 1983; 67:348–352.

13. Sahn DL, et al. Recommendations regarding quantitation in M-mode echocardiography: Results of a survey of echocardiographic measurements. Circulation. 1978;58:1072–1083.

14. Schiller NB, et al. Recommendations for quantitation of the left ventricle by two dimensional echocardiography. J Am Soc Echocardiol. 1989;2:358–367.

15. Waggoner AD, et al. Quantitative echocardiography: Part III. J Diagn Med Sonographers. 1995;11: 285–299.

16. Wells PNT. Biomedical Ultrasonics. New York, Academic Press; 1977.

17. Weyman A. Principles and Practice of Echocardiography. Philadelphia, Lea and Febiger; 1994.

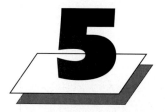

Spectral and Color Flow Doppler

MARK N. ALLEN

Doppler ultrasound varies significantly from two-dimensional ultrasound both in the information produced and in the manner in which it is obtained. Doppler ultrasound allows the evaluation of moving targets; in the case of echocardiography, this target is blood. Bats and dolphins use this principle in finding food. These animals emit a sound that travels through air or water until it encounters a reflector such as an insect or a fish. The reflected sound waves are received by the bat or dolphin. Several very important pieces of information are provided, including the distance of the potential meal, as well as the direction and speed in which the meal is traveling. With this information, the bat or dolphin can adapt its own behavior to overcome its prey (Fig. 5-1).

A sound source that is fixed will generate a sound wave with a constant frequency and wavelength. Once the sound source begins to move, its wavelength and frequency will be affected. To illustrate this point, consider the siren of a fire truck. Even though we may not be able to see the truck, we can hear it. Additionally, we can tell when the truck is getting closer or farther away from us and therefore can tell the general direction in which it is heading, even though we cannot see it. What allows us to know all this about the truck is that as the siren moves closer to us, its wavelength decreases and its frequency increases, causing a higher pitch or a louder sound. As the siren moves away from us, the wavelength increases and the frequency decreases, causing a lower pitch or a softer sound. This

phenomenon, first observed by Christian Johann Doppler in 1842, is referred to as the *Doppler effect*.

In diagnostic ultrasound this same information can be obtained, interpreted, and displayed by ultrasound systems. The sound wave generated by the system is emitted at a particular frequency and wavelength. If the target is stationary relative to the transducer, the reflected sound wave will return with the same characteristics as the transmitted one—in other words, the same frequency and wavelength. If the structure begins to move, the returning sound wave will have a different frequency and wavelength. The system will detect that the sound wave is being returned faster if the target is moving toward the transducer or sound source or the system will detect an increase in the amount of time it takes for the signal to return, indicating that the reflecting surface is moving away from the transducer.

This Doppler effect can be demonstrated using the following equations:

$$f_d = f_r - f_t = 2f_t \frac{v \cdot \cos \theta}{c} \tag{5-1}$$

$$v = \frac{f_d \cdot c}{2 f_t (\cos \theta)}$$

where f_d = Doppler frequency
f_r = reflected frequency
f_t = transmitted frequency
c = velocity of sound in soft tissue (constant)

v = velocity of the moving target

θ = angle between the direction of the moving target and the path of the sound wave

In this equation, c is constant and the transmitted frequency is known; therefore, the velocity of the target is a function of the cosine of the angle between the target and the sound wave. If we plug a few numbers into the equation, it becomes obvious how important the angle becomes in performing a Doppler exam. For example, suppose that the transmitted frequency is 3.5 MHz, f_d = 3.0 MHz, c = 1540 m/sec, and θ = 90 degrees.

$$v = \frac{3.0 \times 1540 \text{ m/sec}}{2\,(3.5 \text{ MHz} \times \cos 90)};$$

$$\cos 90 = 0$$

Therefore

$$v = \frac{4620}{\theta} = 0$$

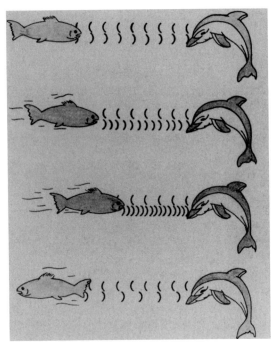

Figure 5-1. Dolphins use Doppler to detect the presence, direction, and speed at which their prey moves. This same technique is used in Doppler ultrasound to evaluate the direction and speed of blood as it moves through the heart. (From Hagan AD, DeMaria AN (eds). Clinical Applications of Two-Dimensional Echocardiography and Cardiac Doppler, 2nd ed. Boston, Little Brown and Company; 1989:11, Fig. 1-8.)

Angle	0	10	20	30	45	60
Cos	1	.98	.93	.86	.70	.50
Error	0%	2%	7%	14%	30%	50%

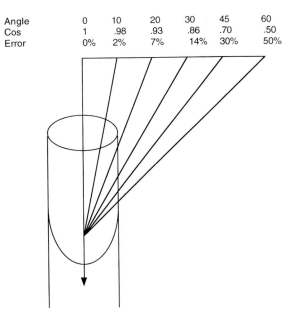

Figure 5-2. The effects of angle on the Doppler shift. At an angle of 0 degrees, the error is 0%. As the angle increases, so does the percent error. Doppler signals are best detected at less than 20 degrees. (Modified from Harry M: Cardiac Doppler Hemodynamic Workbook: An Illustrated Guide for Doppler Echocardiography. Iowa Heart Institute; 1995, Chap. 1. Reprinted with permission.)

or no effect; in other words, no signal will be detected.

The cos θ of 0 degrees is equal to 1, demonstrating that the ideal signal will be detected if the angle between the target and the sound wave is parallel rather than not perpendicular (90 degrees). For Doppler exams of the heart, the ideal angle is anything less than 20 degrees (Fig. 5-2).

A great advantage of Doppler is that, due to the frequencies used (i.e., 1–10 MHz), the Doppler shifts generated from human blood fall within the audible range of human hearing, which ranges from 250 to 25,000 cycles/sec.[14]

Doppler Modes

There are two basic modes of Doppler: pulsed wave (which includes color flow Doppler) and continuous wave Doppler. Each mode has particular advantages and limitations. The two modes are typically used together in order to obtain the most information regarding hemodynamics. Pulsed wave Doppler uses one transducer requiring the transmitted signals to be timed so that it does not interfere with the received signals. Continuous wave Doppler requires two transducers, one to send or transmit the signal and one to receive them.

PULSED WAVE DOPPLER

Pulsed wave Doppler has the advantage of range resolution. It uses range gates or a sample volume that allows signals to be received from one particular location. This provides very specific information regarding blood flow from a particular area of interest. For example, if one wishes to know what the velocity of blood is from the left ventricular outflow tract, the range gate from the pulsed wave Doppler would be placed within the left ventricular outflow tract and only signals from that location would be obtained. Velocity samples would then be received and displayed from that point. The operator controls the distance at which the sample volume is placed, as well as the width of the sample. The system calculates the distance and therefore allows signals returning from that location to be processed. Signals returning from other locations are not processed, nor are they displayed. This allows a precise assessment of velocities in a particular area.

The disadvantage is that pulsed wave Doppler is limited in the velocities that can be measured. The system is limited by its pulsed repetition frequency (PRF). The PRF determines how high a Doppler shift can be detected. For regions with high velocities such as stenotic valves, regurgitation, or shunts, the Doppler shifts typically exceed the PRF, resulting in a phenomenon called *aliasing* or *range ambiguity*. Aliasing is the major disadvantage of pulsed wave Doppler.[1,2] Aliasing occurs when the Doppler shift exceeds the system's Nyquist limit. The Nyquist limit is equal to one-half of the PRF.

To illustrate this point, consider a car commercial. As you watch the car of your dreams cruising down an open road, you will note, if you watch carefully, that the tires of the car appear to be going backward. This is due to the fact that the camera filming the moving car can take only a limited number of frames or cycles per second. Thus the tire rotations will exceed the camera's frame rate, resulting in artifact. Figure 5-3 also helps to illustrate aliasing. In pulsed Doppler the same phenomenon occurs and results in a wraparound effect, as illustrated in Figure 5-3. Blood flow velocity that exceeds this Nyquist limit will therefore not be properly displayed.

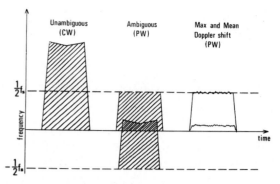

Figure 5-3. *Aliasing caused by flow velocities above the Nyquist limit. Flow appears both above and below the baseline. To correct this, the baseline may be shifted or continuous wave Doppler may be needed in order to display the signal properly. (From McDicken WN (ed): Diagnostic Ultrasonics: Principles and Use of Instrumentation, 2nd ed. New York, Wiley; 1981.)*

Clinical Applications

Despite this apparently staggering limitation of pulsed wave Doppler, there are many clinical settings for which it is ideal. In normal hearts, the velocity or frequency shift generated by blood traveling across all four of the valves or vessels will normally be well within the system's Nyquist limit. Therefore, not only velocity information but also direction of flow is displayed. It is important to align the pulsed system gate properly in order to obtain the relevant information. The size of the gate is important and will affect the spectral display. Larger gates are used when searching for flow or a vessel, whereas smaller gates are more desirable when displaying and measuring the spectral display. Smaller gates improve the signal-to-noise ratio and the quality of the spectrum.[9]

Pulsed wave Doppler has many clinical applications, including the assessment of aortic stenosis, diastolic measurements, pulmonary vein flow, Qp/Qs calculations, and regurgitant orifice areas. The specific calculations are discussed in subsequent chapters. For example, the area of a stenotic aortic valve can be calculated using a formula called the *continuity equation*. Part of the equation requires the determination of flow in the left ventricular outflow tract. This information is very specific and must be obtained only from this region. Only pulsed wave Doppler will provide velocity information in a small area, allowing the valve area to be calculated using the equation. Pulsed wave Doppler can also be used to help map the severity of regurgitation, although this is seldom done since the advent of color Doppler. Any situation in which the velocity or flow from a specific location is to be measured or evaluated requires the use of pulsed wave Doppler.

CONTINUOUS WAVE DOPPLER

Continuous wave Doppler requires the use of two transducers, one to transmit the sound waves and one to receive them. The sound waves are sent out in a continuous stream of pulses that do not allow enough time between the transmitted signals for the received signals. The Doppler sample volume of the continuous system is quite large, and the system receives signals anywhere along the intersection of the transmitted and received signals. Therefore, the exact location of the signals is never known. In addition, the signals can be confusing if the reflectors within the sound beam are moving at varying velocities and in different directions.[8]

The advantage of continuous wave Doppler is that there are no limitations due to pulse repetition frequency. This allows high-frequency shifts or velocities to be detected and displayed. Its advantage is also its disadvantage in that although reflectors traveling at high velocities can be detected and the velocities evaluated, their exact location is not known. It is assumed and explained by fluid dynamics that the highest velocities are typically seen in smaller orifices, while lower velocities are typically from larger orifices.

In our aortic stenosis example, a high-velocity

signal is assumed to come from the narrow opening of the stenotic valve. However, a supravalvular obstruction could also generate a high-velocity signal. In this scenario it is difficult to determine where the highest velocity originates.

Figure 5-4 demonstrates the difference between continuous and pulsed wave Doppler.

Clinical Applications

As with all Doppler techniques, it is important to align the Doppler sample volume parallel to blood flow. Angles greater than 20 degrees usually result in a poor or no spectral display. The clinical applications of continuous wave Doppler include any situation in which the peak velocity is required. In diseased states such as valvular stenosis or regurgitation, coarctation of the aorta, ventricular septal defects, or other shunts, continuous wave Doppler is usually required in order to measure peak velocities. In situations where there is aortic stenosis, continuous wave Doppler is used to determine the peak velocity across the stenotic aortic valve. In the presence of tricuspid regurgitation, the pulmonary artery pressures can be calculated if the peak trans tricuspid gradient is obtained. Velocities obtained from regurgitant lesions such as those causing tricuspid and mitral regurgitation are typically high and are beyond the Nyquist limit, causing range ambiguity for pulsed wave systems.

Signal Analysis and Display

Doppler instruments today use spectrum analyzers to detect the various frequencies within a wave. There are various types of spectral analyzers, but the most commonly used types today are the Fourier analyzers.[16] These analyzers resolve waveforms into their component frequencies. The use of fast Fourier analyzers permits a very rapid computation of the various frequencies within the wave. The resultant display is an array of the components of a sound wave separated and arranged in order of increasing frequency.[12] The *fast Fourier transform (FFT)* is a mathematical process that analyzes the Doppler signals at a rate of 25,600 times per second.[15] Each spectrum can include the amplitudes of 128 frequencies, which can then be displayed in a two-dimensional format.[16] At this rate, the spectral display generated is clear enough to provide the necessary information.

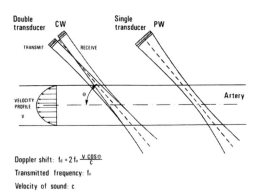

Doppler shift: $f_d = 2 f_0 \frac{v \cos\Theta}{c}$

Transmitted frequency: f_0

Velocity of sound: c

Figure 5-4. Illustration of pulsed and continuous wave Doppler echocardiography. Pulsed wave (PW) Doppler requires only one transducer, while continuous wave (CW) Doppler requires two. (From McDicken WN (ed): Diagnostic Ultrasonics: Principles and Use of Instrumentation, 2nd ed. New York, Wiley; 1981.)

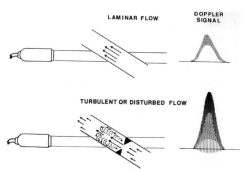

Figure 5-5. *(Top)* Spectral display of a Doppler signal from laminar flow. Note the thin border and large, anechoic region under the curve. *(Bottom)* Spectral display of a Doppler signal from an area of turbulent flow. Note the large border or spectral broadening *(arrow)* and relatively small, anechoic region under the border. This pattern is typical of disturbed flow such as aortic stenosis or ventricular septal defects. (From McDicken WN (ed): Diagnostic Ultrasonics: Principles and Use of Instrumentation, 2nd ed. New York, Wiley; 1981.)

Signals generated from regions of normal flow will not have a wide range of frequencies, so the resultant spectrum will be narrow. This results in a display that is well defined (Fig. 5-5, *top*). In turbulent flow, where there is a wider range of frequencies, the spectral display will demonstrate *spectral broadening* (Fig. 5-5, *bottom*). The borders of the display are wide and, depending on the background used, will be white or black. The area under the border will be anechoic. In turbulent flows this area is small. Thus spectral broadening indicates disturbed or turbulent flow. Proper gain settings are important in evaluating spectral displays. Gain settings that are too high may result in the appearance of spectral broadening.

In addition to identifying the presence of turbulent versus laminar flow, the spectrum can be traced using the system's on-line calipers to determine peak and mean velocities by measuring the peak spectrum or tracing the spectrum, respectively. From this information, peak and mean gradients, and ultimately the degree of severity of the lesion, can be ascertained.

The peak information is represented by the highest point on the spectrum where the mean information is derived by averaging all the frequency shifts in the display. This information is obtained by tracing either along the outside border of the spectral display or within the spectral border. The latter technique is referred to as *modal velocity*. This area represents the velocity with which the greatest number of reflectors

are traveling. The modal velocity on the spectral display is typically the brightest region on the display because it reflects the greatest number of reflectors. The trace is typically done within the brightest region. Whether tracing the outside border or the modal region, one should be consistent, since each technique yields different values.

Types of Flow

Within the human heart there are essentially two basic types of flow: laminar and turbulent. Laminar flow is uniform, with all blood cells moving at a relatively uniform speed and in the same direction. Flow within a tube demonstrates laminar flow; blood flow is fastest toward the center and slowest toward the tube walls. This difference is due to the frictional forces from the walls acting on the blood. The effects of friction on the blood are overcome by the pressure differences within the tube. Similarly, in the heart, the blood is driven by the pressure differences between the chambers. Figure 5-6 demonstrates laminar flow. Such flow is encountered in the normal heart and across normally functioning valves. The spectral display is usually uniform, without spectral broadening.

Turbulent flow is characterized by random, chaotic swirling, in which the particles or reflectors within the vessel are moving in all directions but typically have a net forward flow. Such flow is typically seen in stenotic valves, regurgitation lesions, or shunts. In order to understand this concept, it is important to understand the conservation of mass. In a closed system such as the circulatory system, the volume flow rate of blood must be constant

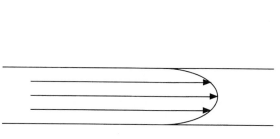

Figure 5-6. Profile of laminar flow. All reflectors are moving in a forward direction and at a relatively uniform speed. The reflectors closest to the vessel walls move more slowly due to frictional forces.

proximal to, at, and distal to a narrowing. Since fluid within a closed system is neither destroyed nor changed, the same volume that goes into the system must also go out of it. For every heartbeat, the volume of blood going into the left ventricle must also go out. When there is aortic stenosis, for example, the volume of blood crossing the mitral valve equals that going across the aortic valve. Therefore, in order for the same volume of blood to move across a narrowed opening, the blood must move faster. Turbulent flow is usually generated distal to the stenosis because of the pressure drop due to the loss of energy. Figure 5-7 demonstrates turbulent flow. Turbulent flow is characterized by reflectors (blood cells and other particles) traveling in various directions and at various velocities. The resultant chaotic flow generates eddy currents[7] (Fig. 5-8).

Flow Dynamics

There are two very important concepts to consider in discussing flow dynamics. First, as was mentioned above, at a stenosis the blood must accelerate in order to follow the law of continuity, which states that, for fluids, the volume that goes in must equal the volume that comes out. If the area of stenosis is half that of the vessel proximal and distal to it, then the average speed of the blood must be double that of blood in the proximal and distal vessels. If the diameter of the stenosis is half that of the diameter of the proximal and distal vessels, then the average speed of blood traveling through the stenosis must quadruple.

The second point to consider is the effect on flow speed as an entire vessel decreases in diameter and therefore in area. In situations where there is vasoconstriction, the average flow speed decreases.

Turbulent flow

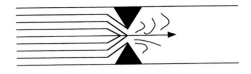

Figure 5-7. Profile of turbulent flow. Reflectors are moving in a wide variety of directions and speeds.

Eddy currents - flow is in various directions and speeds

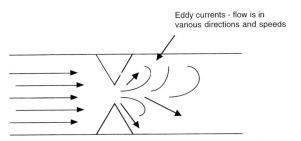

Figure 5-8. In turbulent flow eddies are generated, particularly distal to a stenosis.

This may seem contrary to the previous discussion. In this scenario, resistance increases along the entire length of the vessel, causing a decrease in flow speed. This is referred to as *Poiseuille's law*. A stenosis in a small region of a vessel does not have the same resistance effect that a decrease in an entire vessel has on flow speed.

Another important concept is the relationship between speed or velocity and pressure. The driving forces of blood within the heart are pressure differences between chambers and between the proximal and distal ends of vessels. What moves the blood from the left atrium into the left ventricle is the pressure difference generated between the two chambers. In order for the blood to move from the left atrium to the left ventricle, the pressure within the left ventricle must at some point in the cardiac cycle become less than the pressure in the left atrium. Velocity and pressure are related and can be described by the *Bernoulli effect*. In aortic stenosis the pressure in or at the stenosis decreases. If the pressure was high, then the speed of the blood would have to decrease due to the loss of energy as a result of the increased pressure. The pressure in a stenosis will be greatest proximal to the stenosis and less distal to the stenosis. To illustrate this, let's consider an example. Anyone waiting to see a popular sports competition has experienced the Bernoulli effect. Before the gates to the sports complex open, the lobby is crowded with enthusiastic fans. Everyone is standing shoulder to shoulder, waiting to get in. At this point, the pressure is the greatest. When it is your turn to enter the turnstyle, you and only you enter at that particular point, so the pressure is relieved. After you enter the complex, the pressure is reduced further because there is more room to move around. If everyone tried to enter the turnstyle at the same time, your speed would be reduced because the pressure would impede your progress. The Bernoulli effect is illustrated by the following equation:

$$P_1 - P_2 = 4v^2 \qquad (5\text{-}2)$$

where v is the velocity of blood in meters per second and $P_1 - P_2$ is the pressure drop across the stenotic valve.

Color Flow Doppler

Color flow Doppler or color flow mapping displays both anatomic and flow in a spatially correct two-dimensional image.[4,13,15] Color flow systems analyze the Doppler shifts of the sound waves reflecting and returning from moving targets such as blood cells. The typical colors used are red and blue. Red typically identifies blood flow moving toward the transducer, and blue represents blood flow moving away from the transducer. However, other colors are also seen, especially in turbulent flow. In situations such as stenosis, shunts, and regurgitant lesions, a mosaic of colors can be seen if the flow is turbulent and blood cells travel in a variety of directions at varying speeds. The process by which ultrasound systems generate color images is complex. The system must be able to process a tremendous amount of information in order to display color images. Color flow Doppler information must be combined with the two-dimensional, M-mode, and conventional Doppler in order to be displayed with these other modalities.

Color flow Doppler is a form of pulsed wave Doppler and is therefore subject to the same limitation as the pulsed wave mode. As with pulsed wave Doppler, the pulse repetition of the system will affect the display of the color signals. At blood flow velocities above the Nyquist limit, aliasing occurs. Flow that would normally be displayed as red may be displayed as blue. This is best seen across the aortic valve (normal or diseased). The velocity across even a normal aortic valve may exceed the Nyquist limit, resulting in a color flow pattern that may be confusing. In Figure 5-9, systolic flow across the aortic valve would appear blue since flow is away from the transducer in this apical "five-chamber" view; however, a red jet can be noted. This red jet may cause some confusion and should not be interpreted as aortic insufficiency (AI). The fact that AI

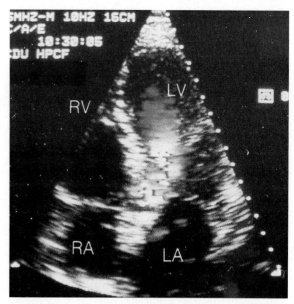

Figure 5-9. *Effects of aliasing in color flow Doppler. Because color flow Doppler is a pulsed wave technique, velocities above the Nyquist limit will result in aliasing of the color display. In this example of normal flow across the aortic valve (blue is away from the transducer), a red jet is also noted. This jet denotes aliasing and should not be confused with aortic insufficiency. (From Ref. 4, Fig. 6-9b. Reprinted with permission. See also Color Plate 2.)*

is seen only in diastole will also help identify this signal as an alias. The color jets, when aliased, will wrap around the baseline and be displayed according to their relative direction to the transducer.

The Doppler-shifted signals received by the ultrasound system are detected using mathematical autocorrelation technique that rapidly detects the mean and the variance of the received signals along each scan line.[3,10] The autocorrelation detects the mean magnitude of the Doppler shift, the sign (above or below the baseline), and the variance for each location. This information is stored in memory and displayed later at the appropriate location on the display.

COLOR MODES/MAPS

There are a number of color modes that can be used in most systems. These modes provide more than directional information. Three of them are variance, velocity, and power. Velocity maps display the mean velocity of the sampled blood flow area at a particular point in time.[5] For normal flow, the mean and peak velocity are nearly the same. Since the primary colors used in color Doppler are red or blue, the displayed patterns in a velocity mode will be red or blue, depending on the direction of blood flow relative to the transducer. In abnormal flow such as turbulent flow, the peak and mean are very different because the blood cells are moving at very different velocities. If you recall, blood cells in turbulent flow move at a wide range of velocities and in differing directions. The display will therefore demonstrate a mosaic of colors.

Variance is used to help express the degree to which the velocities in a turbulent flow region differ from the mean velocity within that region.[6] The more turbulent the flow region, the more variance will be displayed. The color green is added to this mode to help identify areas of turbulence. When green is added, yellow and blue-green colors are also produced. The result is a turbulent jet that is more vivid and therefore more easily recognized. The color green can be displayed alone in this mode, but for practical purposes this is seldom done.

Power mode displays the amplitude of the Doppler shift signal.[16] The colors used are typically red toward and blue away from the transducer, and only these colors are displayed. The shades of these colors will vary, depending on the amplitude of the Doppler shift.

The color maps can be changed with most systems, and the maps used are largely a matter of personal preference. Maps are normally defined by a number or letter and are controlled by the operator.

Color Flow Doppler Controls

There are several controls on the ultrasound systems that allow the operator to optimize the color image. These controls include the color gain, color sector length and width, depth gain compensation, color inversion, wall filter, baseline shift, velocity range, color map, variance, smoothing, and ensemble length.[11] The color gain increases the strength of the signals displayed. The gray scale gains should be decreased when displaying color since most systems give priority to the gray scales. High gray scale gain and depth gain compensation can mask the color display (Fig. 5-10). In order to optimize the color gain, the gray scale gain is reduced and the color gain is increased to the point when color specs or flashes are observed. The gain is then reduced until

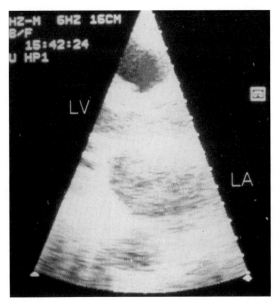

Figure 5-10. *Overall gain set too high, masking the color jets. (From Ref. 4, Fig. 5-6b. Reprinted with permission.) (See also Color Plate 3.)*

these artifactual signals disappear (Fig. 5-11). The color sector can and should be adjusted in order to increase frame rate and "zero in" on the area of interest. A system's zoom or res function can also be used to help define the color display. Normally, for cardiac work, red denotes flow toward the transducer, while blue denotes flow away from the transducer. Usually this format is not changed in echocardiography. Wall filters eliminate noise in the image due to wall motion. Too high a wall filter setting, however, can eliminate low-flow color information (Fig. 5-12). Baseline shifts allow adjustment of the zero line either up or down. This may be done in order to eliminate aliasing and to better define color flow areas such as flow within the left ventricular outflow tract or for certain regurgitant lesion measurements. Color velocity range sets the Nyquist limit on the color bar. A lower velocity range facilitates the observation of slower flows.

The color maps can be altered from a number of choices and vary from system to system. Smoothing is analogous to persistence on the gray scale. This is an averaging of frames in order to fill in mixing pixels of information, providing a "smoother" image. Similar to the persistence control of two-dimensional imaging, this setting is normally set on a minimal level. Ensemble length is the number of pulses required for each color scan line. Large ensemble lengths provide better detection of low flow rates but at the expense of frame rate (lower frame rate). Smaller ensemble lengths provide faster frame rates but at the expense of lower flow rates.

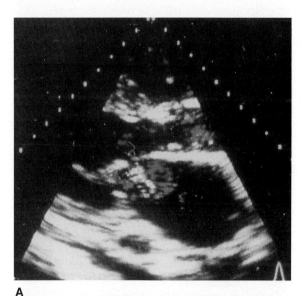

A

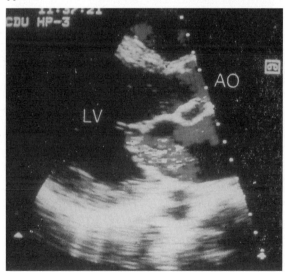

B

Figure 5-12. Reject or wall filters help eliminate background noise but can also eliminate "real" low flow states. A proper wall filter setting is needed to establish a balance between the two. (**A**) Demonstrates a higher color reject, in turn eliminating some of the real signal. (**B**) Demonstrates proper reject controls and best defines the mitral regurgitation. (**A** from Ref. 4, Fig. 5-13a; **B** from Ref. 4, Fig. 5-13b. Reprinted with permission.) (See also Color Plates 6 and 7.)

A

B

Figure 5-11. Parasternal long-axis view illustrating mitral regurgitation. (**A**) The effects of color gain setting on the color display. A setting that is too low will not reveal the severity of the mitral regurgitation. In (**A**) the severity of the mitral regurgitation would be underestimated. (**B**) Demonstrates the proper gain settings and better defines the severity of the regurgitation. (**A** from Ref. 4, Fig. 5-5a; **B** from Ref. 4, Fig. 5-5b. Reprinted with permission.) (See also Color Plates 4 and 5.)

CLINICAL APPLICATIONS

As you will notice in this text, color flow Doppler has many applications in the clinical setting. It has added a spatial dimension to blood flow imaging not previously available. This, in turn, more readily identifies blood flow patterns within the heart. One can easily see valvular regurgitation and identify the direction and pattern of flow of the lesion. Stenotic valves typically produce a turbulent color pattern. An important advantage of color Doppler is the identification of shunts that would typically take much longer to identify using pulsed or continuous wave Doppler. Defects across the ventricular and atrial septa can be more readily identified. In addition, color Doppler can be used to identify the direction of flow across a valve in order to help guide a continuous or pulsed wave Doppler cursor (Fig. 5-13).

Color is also applied to other aspects of cardiac imaging in addition to blood flow. Colorization of the two-dimensional image (Fig. 5-14) can be helpful in identifying endocardial borders. A more recent technique using color focuses on the amplitude of wall motion. This technique helps to identify hypokinetic walls. Various hues of red or blue are assigned to the moving walls. Red denotes wall excursion toward the transducer and blue denotes wall excursion away from the transducer. In a normally functioning left ventricle the colors are well demonstrated. With wall motion abnormalities the colors are not as bright (Fig. 5-15).

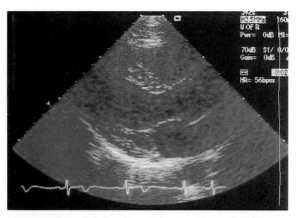

Figure 5-14. Colorization of the two-dimensional image can be helpful in identifying endocardial borders. This parasternal long-axis view demonstrates one of the many colors used to colorize the two-dimensional image. (See also Color Plate 9.)

Color Doppler can also be used to help enhance contrast agents, which in turn help identify endocardial borders (Fig. 5-16).

As with conventional Doppler techniques, the advantage of color Doppler can also be its disadvantage: the spatial information is provided at the ex-

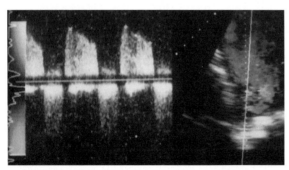

Figure 5-13. The use of color Doppler to guide the placement of a continuous wave Doppler cursor. By observing the direction of flow by color, the continuous wave cursor can be placed nearly parallel to the direction of flow. This helps eliminate the need to optimize cursor placement. (See also Color Plate 8.)

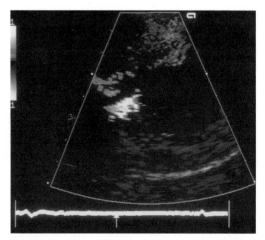

Figure 5-15. Tissue Doppler demonstrating the effects of color in identifying the amplitude or excursion of the endocardium. This technique may help to quantitate the severity of left ventricular dysfunction and to identify regional wall motion abnormalities. (From McDicken WN, Color Doppler velocity imaging of the myocardium. Ultrasound Med Biol. 1992;18(6,7):653. Reprinted with permission.) (See also Color Plate 10.)

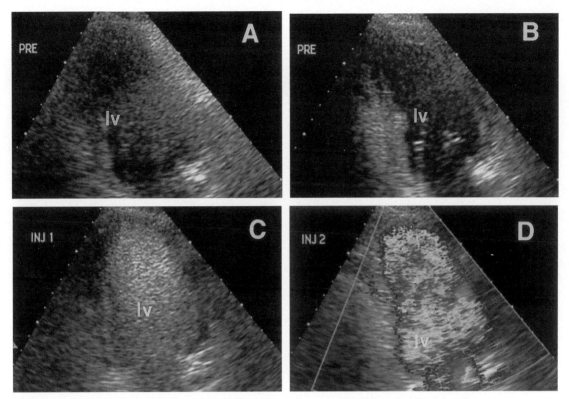

Figure 5-16. Color flow Doppler enhancement of contrast agents. This apical four-chamber view demonstrates fundamental imaging (**A**). The endocardial borders are not well delineated. With harmonic imaging (**B**), the endocardial borders are better defined but still lack some detail. Intravenous contrast is given which further defines endocardial borders (**C**). With the addition of color flow (**D**) the endocardial borders are even better defined. (See also Color Plate 11.)

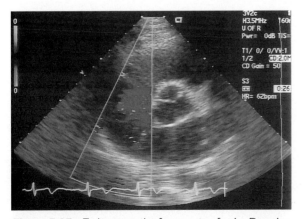

Figure 5-17. To improve the frame rate of color Doppler, a narrow sector is used to sample the area of interest. This parasternal short-axis view demonstrates normal flow across the tricuspid valve. (See also Color Plate 12.)

pense of the frame rate. This problem can be overcome by narrowing the color sector or using the magnification or zoom function, which limits the area of view to a small region of interest (Fig. 5-17).

Summary

Since the heart is a dynamic organ, the use of two-dimensional and Doppler echocardiography has made echocardiography a very useful diagnostic technique since it provides not only structural but also hemodynamic and functional information. The two techniques should be used together in order to provide an integrated look at the heart. As you will see throughout this text, the combination of imaging and Doppler is necessary in order to provide a thorough exam of the heart.

REFERENCES

1. Bom K, deBoo J, Rijsterborgh H. On the aliasing problem in pulsed Doppler cardiac studies. J Clin Ultrasound. 1984;12:559.
2. Hatle L, Angelsen B. Doppler Ultrasound in Cardiology: Physical Principles and Clinical Applications, 2nd ed. Philadelphia, Lea & Febiger; 1984.
3. Kasai C, Namekawa K, Koyano A, et al. Real-time two-dimensional blood flow imaging using an auto-correlation technique. IEEE Trans Son Ultrasound SU. 1985;32:458–464.
4. Kisslo J, Adams DB, Belkin RN. Doppler Color Flow Imaging. New York, Churchill Livingstone; 1988.
5. Kisslo J, Adams DB, Belkin RN. Doppler Color Flow Imaging. New York, Churchill Livingstone; 1988:29.
6. Kisslo J, Adams DB, Belkin RN. Doppler Color Flow Imaging. New York, Churchill Livingstone; 1988:39.
7. Kremkau FW. Doppler Ultrasound: Principles and Instruments. Philadelphia, WB Saunders; 1990:71.
8. Kremkau FW. Doppler Ultrasound: Principles and Instruments. Philadelphia, WB Saunders; 1990:105.
9. Kremkau FW. Doppler Ultrasound: Principles and Instruments. Philadelphia, WB Saunders; 1990:109.
10. Kremkau FW. Doppler Ultrasound: Principles and Instruments. Philadelphia, WB Saunders; 1990:182.
11. Kremkau FW. Doppler Ultrasound: Principles and Instruments. Philadelphia, WB Saunders; 1990:186.
12. Kremkau FW. Doppler Ultrasound: Principles and Instruments. Philadelphia, WB Saunders; 1995:141–142.
13. Meritt CRB (ed). Doppler Color Imaging. New York, Churchill Livingstone; 1992.
14. Weyman AE. Doppler signal processing. *In* Weyman AE (ed): Principles and Practice of Echocardiography, 2nd ed. Philadelphia, Lea & Febiger; 1994:202.
15. Weyman AE. Doppler signal processing. *In* Weyman AE (ed): Principles and Practice of Echocardiography, 2nd ed. Philadelphia, Lea & Febiger; 1994:218.
16. Weyman AE. Principles of color flow mapping. *In* Weyman AE (ed): Principles and Practice of Echocardiography, 2nd ed. Philadelphia, Lea & Febiger; 1994:229–230.

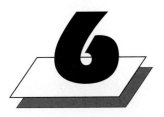

Transesophageal Echocardiography

MARK N. ALLEN

Introduction

Over the last two decades, echocardiography has benefited from technological advances which has allowed it to become one of the most widely used diagnostic tools in cardiac disease. Transesophageal echocardiography (TEE) is the latest technological advance to gain widespread clinical use. Frazin and associates described their initial experience in esophageal ultrasound as early as 1976 with a single-element transducer attached to a coaxial cable.[125] These early devices were problematic; they did not allow adequate contact, they tended to be large and difficult to pass, and they provided views in only a single plane. Over the years, TEE has gone through a series of advances including the attachment of multiple elements to more flexible gastroscopes; the use of phased array technology; more flexible, smaller, and more versatile scanning devices which allow for multiple-plane imaging through 180 degrees; and the addition of Doppler and color flow Doppler.

Unlike transthoracic echocardiography, TEE is considered an invasive procedure and should not be used for routine screening. Only physicians with special training in TEE performance and interpretation should perform these exams.[87] The American Society of Echocardiography has established guidelines for training in TEE (see Chapter 11).[234] TEE can be used in a variety of settings including inpatient, outpatient, emergency room, operating room, and mobile service, as long as necessary equipment and appropriately trained staff are available.

A TEE study should, with few exceptions, include a complete evaluation of all regions of the heart and great vessels, regardless of the indication. Many laboratories will evaluate the area of interest first in the event that the exam needs to be interrupted.[87]

Contraindications to and Complications of TEE

Contraindications to TEE can be divided into two general categories, absolute and relative (Display 6-1). Absolute contraindications preclude the use of TEE and include known esophageal conditions such as tumors, stenosis or strictures, diverticulum, advanced varices, perforated viscus, gastric volvus or perforation, and active gastrointestinal bleeding. Patient refusal or unwillingness to cooperate is also an absolute contraindication. Relative contraindications often can pose a dilemma for the physician, and the benefits of TEE must be weighed against the potential for complications. Relative contraindications include prior esophageal surgery, radiation therapy, oropharyngeal distortion and cervical

---

Display 6-1.   Contraindications to TEE

ABSOLUTE

Esophageal tumors
Esophageal stenosis
Esophageal strictures
Esophageal diverticulum
Advanced esophageal varices
Perforated viscus
Gastric volvus or perforation
Gastrointestinal bleeding
Unwilling patient

RELATIVE

Prior esophageal surgery
Radiation therapy
Oropharyngeal distortion
Cervical spondylosis
Severe cervical arthritis
Severe cardiopulmonary distress
Suspected esophageal varices

The complications of TEE are summarized in Display 6-2. Serious complications are extremely rare.[59,85,125,168,237,276] Complications are minimized by taking a careful history, using sedation and local anesthesia, and careful monitoring of the patient during and following the procedure. Complications of TEE range from mild sore throat to death.[328] The incidence of serious complications is less than 1% percent in major studies.[87,276,328] These complications include laryngospasm, sustained ventricular tachycardia, congestive heart failure, and death. A drop in oxygen saturation among patients undergoing endoscopy with intravenous midazolam sedation has also been noted.[33] The incidence of hypotension and arrhythmias is low with TEE exams, even in the setting of cardiac disease.[134]

Bacteremia is rarely associated with TEE.[207,208,221,299] Still, TEE has the potential to induce gingival, pharyngeal, and esophageal mucosal trauma and subsequently to induce bacteremia, which could lead to endocarditis in susceptible patients.[208] Generally, prophylaxis of endocarditis is not recom-

spondylosis or severe cervical arthritis, which can make passing the probe difficult, severe cardiopulmonary distress, and suspected esophageal varices.[87,242,328]

The risks of TEE are very low when the exam is performed by a trained physician.[87] In the European Multicenter Study, which analyzed 10,419 TEE examinations, probe insertion was unsuccessful in 201 cases, or 1.9%. These failures were due primarily to one of two reasons. First, 98.5% of the failures were due to lack of patient cooperation or to lack of experience on the part of the operator. The remaining 1.5% of the failures were the result of anatomic conditions such as tracheotoma or esophageal diverticulum.[85] Most conscious patients in this series did not receive general sedation. Of the 10,218 cases in which the probe was successfully passed, 90 studies could not be completed due to the patient's inability to tolerate the probe (65 cases); because of pulmonary, cardiac, or bleeding-related complications (18 cases); or because of other reasons. In this series, one patient with a malignant lung tumor with esophageal infiltration died of a bleeding-related complication (mortality rate, 0.01%).[85,87] Similar results have been reported by others.[59,167]

Display 6-2.   Complications of TEE[87,276,328]

MECHANICAL COMPLICATIONS

Probe buckling
Probe compression of surrounding structures
Probe interference with other esophageal or nasogastric devices

PROCEDURE-RELATED COMPLICATIONS

Patient intolerance
Sore throat
Transient hypoxia
Supraventricular tachycardia
Transient hypertension
Transient hypotension
Blood-tinged sputum
Normal sinus (NS) supraventricular tachycardia
Laryngospasm
Parotid swelling
Bradycardia
Congestive heart failure
Sustained ventricular tachycardia
Death (0.02%)

mended in procedures with a low risk of induced bacteremia.[17,83] Patients in intensive care units may be at higher risk of developing bacteremia than those in an outpatient setting. Regardless of the setting, TEE is considered to pose a very low risk of induced bacteremia; therefore, routine antimicrobal prophylaxis is, in general, not recommended.[208]

Buckling of the tip of the TEE probe has been reported and may result in resistance to withdrawal, poor imaging, and fixation of the probe in the extreme anteflexion position. This situation is corrected by advancing the probe into the stomach and straightening it before withdrawal.[324] In addition to esophageal perforations, a case of gastric laceration has been reported.[183] This may be due to the extreme anteflexion of the probe necessary to obtain apical four-chamber views. To obtain this view, the probe comes into direct contact with the gastric mucosa. The use of a TEE probe in conjunction with other devices may also theoretically cause some complications. Frequently when the probe is removed, nasogastric tubes are displaced. Esophageal stethoscopes can also be displaced with simultaneous use of a TEE probe, presenting a potential for esophageal damage.[342]

There is also an increased risk of radionuclide contamination of the TEE probe in patients who have recently undergone nuclear imaging studies.[101] In these patients it is advisable to use a protective sleeve, which significantly reduces contamination.

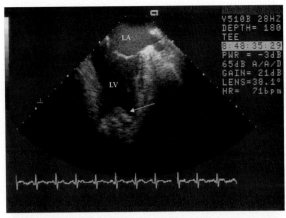

Figure 6-1. Two-chamber view of the left ventricle demonstrating a thrombus (arrow) in the left ventricular apex. LA, left atrium; LV, left ventricle.

Transthoracic imaging can be problematic in patients who are obese, have chest deformities, or suffer from chronic obstructive lung disease.[129] In these cases, because the esophagus lies in close proximity to the cardiac structures, TEE has proven very useful. The role of TEE in the operating room to monitor left ventricular and right ventricular function during and after open heart surgery is also well documented.[89,313]

All left ventricular segments can be imaged using a combination of horizontal and longitudinal views.[223] Using the American Society of Echocardiography recommendations for wall segments,[265] all segments can be seen by either biplane or mul-

Evaluation of Left Ventricular Function and Ischemia

One of the primary indications for adult echocardiography is the assessment of global and regional left ventricular function. The extent and location of regional wall motion abnormalities can be well documented using echocardiography.[206,283,323,325] High-risk patients can be identified using semiquantitative wall motion scoring to express the extent of myocardial function.[222,283] Additionally, complications associated with myocardial infarction, such as ventricular septal defect, free wall or papillary muscle rupture, true and false aneurysms, left ventricular thrombus, and pericardial effusions can be identified by echocardiography[223,290] (Figs. 6-1 and 6-2).

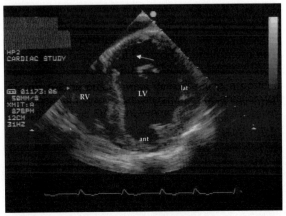

Figure 6-2. Short-axis view demonstrating a posterior wall aneurysm (arrow). lat, lateral wall; ant, anterior wall; LV, left ventricle; RV, right ventricle.

tiplane imaging. Longitudinal long-axis views allow visualization in a two-chamber orientation of the inferior and anterior walls, while transgastric long-axis views allow visualization of the anteroseptum and inferior or inferolateral segments. The transgastric transverse plane displays excellent short-axis views of the basal and middle segments of the left ventricle, as well as the right ventricle. With lateral probe advancement and angulation, the left and right ventricular apices can be seen in 70–80% of patients. From a transverse four-chamber view, the inferoseptal and anterolateral walls are imaged. From these views, the probe can be angled anteriorly toward the left ventricular outflow tract to display the anteroseptal and inferolateral segments.[223] The transgastric view at the level of the papillary muscles allows visualization of segments supplied by all three major coronary arteries and is therefore the view of choice in intraoperative monitoring of the left ventricle[2] (Fig. 6-3).

Stress echocardiography is highly accurate in the diagnosis and assessment of coronary artery disease. However, transthoracic imaging is difficult in some patients. In these situations,[18,19,129,263] TEE allows better delineation of endocardial borders. Development of regional wall motion with exercise, an increase in left ventricular volume, or a decrease in overall ejection fraction is an indicator of coronary artery disease. Several stress echocardiography and TEE combinations have been used.[205] Since upright or supine exercise with TEE monitoring is impractical, atrial-paced TEE[181,344] or pharmacologic stress TEE[129] echocardiography are the methods of choice.

With atrial-paced TEE, a flexible, silicone-coated pacing catheter is attached to the TEE probe for transesophageal pacing of the left atrium.[223] Pacing is increased incrementally to 85% of the patient's age-predicted maximal heart rate. Left ventricular function is monitored by TEE at baseline, as well as during and immediately after maximal pacing. This technique has shown high sensitivity and specificity for the detection of coronary artery disease and has been successful in 90–100% of patients.[181,344]

The use of pharmacologic agents with TEE to assess for coronary artery disease has proven to be both feasible and accurate.[7,129] In one study, overall sensitivity for single-vessel stenosis was 76%, with a specificity of 91%. In patients with double-vessel disease, sensitivity was 90% and specificity was 91%.[129] Studies using other pharmacologic agents have demonstrated similar results.[7] At each stage of dobutamine infusion, it is important to use both longitudinal and transverse planes in order to optimize visualization of all wall segments.[129] Still, some potential limitations do exist with this technique.

With the improved resolution of TEE, visualization of the proximal coronary arteries is now possible (Fig. 6-4). Coronary arteries can be observed in both horizontal and longitudinal planes.[233,274,277]

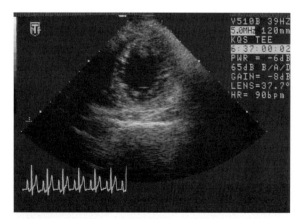

Figure 6-3. *Short-axis view of the left ventricle. This view is ideal in continuous monitoring of left ventricular function intraoperatively because it allows visualization of segments supplied by all three coronary arteries.*

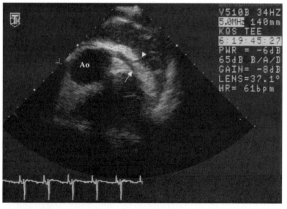

Figure 6-4. *Short-axis view at the level of the aortic sinus of Valsalva. Note the left main coronary artery and its bifurcation of the left circumflex (arrowhead) and left anterior descending branches (arrow). Ao, aorta.*

In the horizontal position, the arteries can be seen in the basal short-axis plane.[223] From a short-axis view of the aortic cusps, mild anteflexion of the transducer tip will reveal the left main coronary artery. The length of the left main coronary artery and its bifurcation can be seen. Starting with a view of the left atrial appendage the probe is slightly flexed inferiorly, allowing delineation of the course of the left main coronary artery. Visualization of the right coronary artery is more difficult since it lies in a different topographic plane. From a longitudinal plane, the proximal portions of the coronary arteries are imaged from a short-axis view of the aortic root with superior and inferior angulation. The left circumflex coronary artery is best visualized by lateral rotation of the transducer in the two-chamber view.[223]

Some studies have attempted to quantitate the severity of coronary artery stenosis by TEE.[10,233,343] Severity is quantitated as a percentage of the largest diameter of the normal-appearing segment of the

artery just distal or proximal to the lesion. The location and severity of the stenosis are then correlated with coronary angiographic findings.[10] Some studies have reported 100% positive predictive accuracy and 98% negative predictive accuracy of TEE in patients with left main coronary artery disease.[343] Still, there are practical considerations that may limit the visualization of the coronary arteries. Characteristic cardiac motion can make it difficult to locate and follow a vessel. Improper gain settings can underestimate lumen diameter. Calcium in the wall of the vessel can interfere with visualization of the vessel. In addition, visualization of the coronary artery is generally limited to the proximal or ostial region and provides information on the vessel in more distal regions.

TEE may provide information about coronary artery disease by measuring coronary flow reserve.[251,306,311,340,348] Coronary flow reserve can be measured from either the coronary sinus or directly from the coronary arteries using Doppler scanning

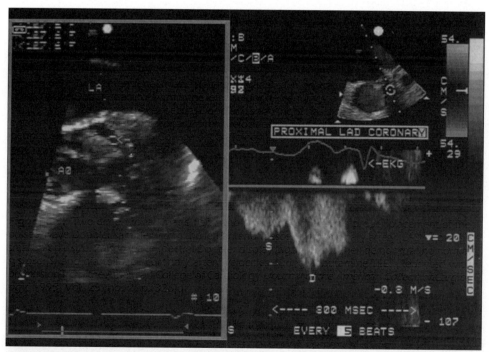

Figure 6-5. Two-dimensional image (left-hand panel) demonstrating proper placement of the pulsed wave Doppler sample within the left anterior descending coronary artery (LAD); note the small sample size. Pulsed wave spectral Doppler display (right-hand panel) demonstrating normal systolic (S) and diastolic (D) coronary artery velocities during dobutamine TEE. (Reprinted with permission from the American College of Cardiology [*Journal of the American College of Cardiology*, 1995, Vol. 25, no. 2, p. 326].)

to measure the difference between maximal and baseline flow.[251,348] To obtain coronary flow reserve from the coronary sinus, a modified four-chamber view with dorsal angulation is used. From this approach, the coronary sinus is visualized entering the right atrium. In this view the diameter of the coronary sinus can be measured. The Doppler sample volume is positioned within 10 mm of the coronary opening, and the velocity time integral (VTI) is measured during prolonged expiration.

Measurements from the coronary arteries are obtained using a basal short-axis view of the aorta. The probe is slowly withdrawn to the level of the left atrial appendage, revealing the opening of the left main coronary artery. The course of this artery can be followed to the bifurcation of the left circumflex and, with slight rotation, to the left anterior descending coronary artery.[251] From this view, di-

ameter as well as Doppler measurements using a small sample size (6 mm) can be made (Fig. 6-5).

Doppler measurements of the coronary arteries include peak and mean diastolic velocities and velocity time integrals, as well as peak systolic velocities.[251] Doppler measurements of the coronary sinus include peak systolic and diastolic velocities and VTI.[348] This technique is used in conjunction with pharmacologic agents such as dipyridamole[348] or adenosine.[251] Baseline measurements of coronary artery flow reserves are made and compared to measurements made following pharmacologic infusions. In the absence of significant left anterior descending coronary artery disease, the velocities obtained by Doppler will increase with maximal infusion of the pharmacologic agents. In the presence of significant disease, the velocity increases will not be significant with maximal infusion (Fig. 6-6).

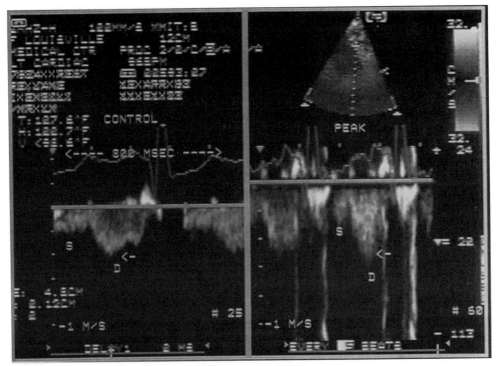

Figure 6-6. Pulsed wave spectral Doppler display of the left anterior descending coronary artery with ≥70% stenosis. The left panel is taken at base infusion and the right panel is taken at peak infusion. In the presence of significant disease, velocities at peak will not significantly increase. (Reprinted with permission from the American College of Cardiology [*Journal of the American College of Cardiology*, 1995, Vol. 25, no. 2, p. 329].)

This technique provides a seminoninvasive method to evaluate patients with coronary artery disease. However, there are some limitations to this technique. Measurements of coronary sinus flow do not assess regional stenoses since flow in the coronary sinus comes from the left coronary artery (left anterior descending and left circumflex); therefore, the precise location of the stenoses cannot be assessed. The diameter of the coronary sinus may vary throughout the cardiac cycle, making precise flow calculations difficult.[348] At this time the effects of collateral circulation on these measurements are not known. Additionally, technical problems with sample volume placement and angle of flow relative to the Doppler beam have adverse effects on these measurements.[251,348]

Despite these limitations, some studies have shown that this technique offers a safe, reliable, and reproducible means of evaluating flow in the coronary circulation. Studies have shown that it is feasible in identifying patients with significant coronary artery disease.[251,348]

Evaluation of the Aorta

TEE has become an important diagnostic tool in the evaluation of the aorta and in some clinical situations is the diagnostic test of choice.[180,331] Pathologic processes of the aorta are frequently very serious, sometimes life-threatening. A number of diagnostic tests allow visualization of the aorta, including aortography, chest radiography, computed tomography, echocardiography, and magnetic resonance imaging. Naturally, each of these has advantages and disadvantages, and not all of them are well suited to all clinical situations. An echocardiogram can be done quickly, relatively inexpensively, and portably, making it one of the ideal diagnostic tools. However, transthoracic imaging is limited by attenuation of the chest wall, as well as by limitations due to body habitus, chest deformities, bandages, and interference due to the lungs.

With the advent of TEE, especially multiplane TEE, all segments of the aorta can be interrogated. Difficulties in imaging the aorta from a transthoracic approach are overcome using TEE because the aorta lies close to the esophagus and attenuation by the esophagus is minimal. Multiplane TEE allows close, unobscured views of the entire thoracic aorta. There is only one small section at the junction of the ascending and transverse aortas which may be obscured by the trachea.[100] TEE can be used to evaluate the aorta for a number of pathologic conditions, including abnormalities of the left ventricular outflow tract, aortic valve disease, atherosclerotic disease, aortic aneurysms and dissections, pseudoaneurysms, congenital aortic disease, and traumatic rupture of the aorta.

ATHEROSCLEROTIC DISEASE

Atheromatous disease of the aorta has been shown to be a risk factor in systemic embolization.[4,161,174,310] Embolization from the heart can occur in 15–20% of patients with ischemic stroke.[312] The physical characteristics of the plaque have been shown to contribute to the risk of embolization.[4,15,310] Ulcerated plaques have been found in 39–61% of patients with cryptogenic stroke.[13,312] Furthermore, atheromas protruding 5 mm or more into the lumen and mobile lesions are more strongly correlated with embolic symptoms and events.[323]

These findings support the importance of detecting and accurately diagnosing aortic plaques as a source of thromboembolism leading to neurologic deficits. TEE allows detailed visualization of the ascending arch and descending thoracic aortas. Consequently the extent and morphologic characteristics of the atheromatous plaque can be clearly seen. Atherosclerotic disease of the aorta can be classified as either (1) simple, in which the plaque extends from the aortic wall into the lumen less than 5 mm, with a smooth intimal surface (Fig. 6-7), or (2) complex, which is identified by extension of more

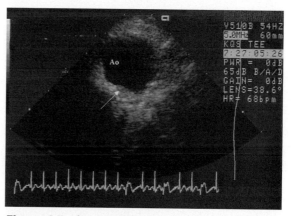

Figure 6-7. An example of a simple atherosclerotic plaque in the aorta. Ao, aorta.

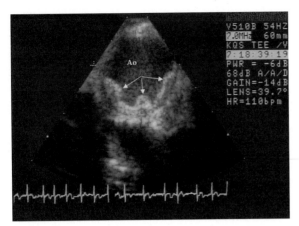

Figure 6-8. Complex atherosclerotic plaque in the aorta. Note the irregular borders. Ao, aorta.

than 5 mm into the lumen, with disruptions and irregularities of the intimal surface[161] (Fig. 6-8).

Multiplane TEE in particular allows visualization of the ascending and descending aortas as well as the aortic arch. Identifying the location of the atheromas is critical. The presence of atheroma in the ascending aorta and aortic arch has been associated with 50% of patients over 60 years of age presenting with cerebral infarcts without an obvious cardiac or arterial source of embolus.[14] Furthermore, autopsy studies have revealed that atheroembolus from the ascending aorta is a major etiologic factor in stroke in patients who have cardiac surgery.[41] Detection by TEE and avoidance of these diseased areas may reduce the risk of perioperative stroke.[335]

TRAUMATIC AORTIC RUPTURE

Only 15% of patients with traumatic rupture of the aorta survive to reach the hospital.[116,232] These injuries are frequently the result of abrupt deceleration injuries such as those occurring in motor vehicle accidents. Shearing forces act principally in the area of the aortic isthmus where the mobile aortic arch attaches to and becomes fixed to the thoracic cage by the ligamentum arteriosum, the intercostal arteries, and the left subclavian artery.[105] Over 90% of traumatic rupture cases involve this region.[173]

In a large number of these cases, immediate death results due to massive hemorrhage.[331] Early diagnosis and immediate surgical repair of traumatic

rupture are imperative to improve survival rates in these patients.[173] A number of diagnostic exams can be used to evaluate for traumatic rupture. Display 6-3 summarizes these exams and lists their disadvantages and advantages.

Although aortography is currently considered the gold standard in this clinical setting,[176,331] TEE is fast becoming the preferred diagnostic tool for several reasons and in some cases may be the primary diagnostic test.[23,70,293] Aortography needs to be performed in a cardiac or radiologic suite; however, some patients are too unstable to be transported. Furthermore, aortography is difficult to perform in patients with multiple traumatic injuries or in hemodynamically unstable patients[331] and may delay surgical repair for an average of 50 to 75 min.[163,293] Some patients are too unstable for surgical repair of their rupture and may be medically managed[8,21,334]. TEE is well suited to follow these patients.

TEE is portable, allowing the exam to take place at the patient's bedside. The personnel can be assembled and perform the exam relatively rapidly, and the exam is cost effective and safe. TEE findings of traumatic aortic rupture may include asymmetric isthmus diameter, the presence of a mediastinal hematoma, a mobile linear or circular medial flap

Display 6-3. Indications for Aortography/TEE[70]

MECHANISM OF INJURY

Ejection
Same-car occupant death
Fall from height (>20 ft)
Associated pelvic fracture

CHEST ROENTGENOGRAM WITH EVIDENCE OF AORTIC INJURY

Widened mediastinum
Blurred aortic knob
Left pleural effusion
Depression of the left mainstem bronchus

SIGNIFICANT KINETIC ENERGY TRANSMISSION

Multiple rib fractures
First and second rib fractures
Scapular fractures
Thoracic spine fractures

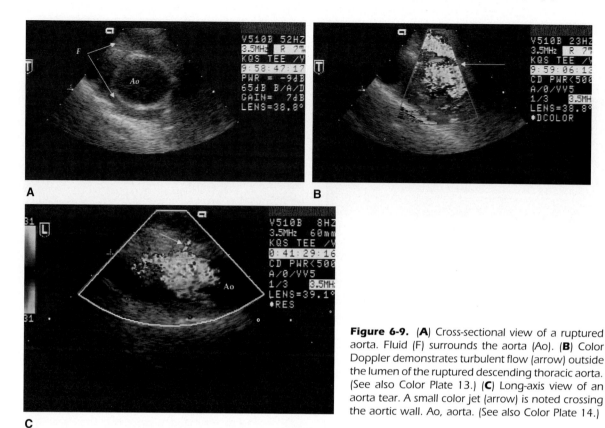

Figure 6-9. (**A**) Cross-sectional view of a ruptured aorta. Fluid (F) surrounds the aorta (Ao). (**B**) Color Doppler demonstrates turbulent flow (arrow) outside the lumen of the ruptured descending thoracic aorta. (See also Color Plate 13.) (**C**) Long-axis view of an aorta tear. A small color jet (arrow) is noted crossing the aortic wall. Ao, aorta. (See also Color Plate 14.)

within the lumen, evidence of color flow on both sides of the medial flap, and turbulent blood flow[70,293,331] (Fig. 6-9A–C). The presence of a crescent-shaped atherosclerotic plaque may lead to a false-positive diagnosis of traumatic aortic disruption, so caution is warranted and each institution using TEE should validate its studies internally using the gold standard.[229,293,333]

AORTIC DISSECTIONS

Dissection of the thoracic aorta is a potentially life-threatening condition requiring immediate diagnosis and treatment.[26,180,332] Dissection occurs when the intima of the aorta is disrupted and the blood leaks into the medial layer of the vessel.[100] The manifestation of dissection is degeneration of the media,[77] which is most commonly caused by hypertension.[26] Other factors that can lead to dissection include connective tissue diseases such as Marfan's syndrome, congenital bicuspid aortic valve, coarctation of the aorta, and pregnancy.[77,96,105]

Aortic dissections can be classified based on their location. There are two common classification systems. One is the Stanford Classification, which designates all dissections of the proximal aorta, regardless of the site of the intimal tear, as type A (Fig. 6-10). All dissections that do not involve the ascending aorta are classified as type B[82] (Fig. 6-11). The second classification system is the DeBakey system, including types I, II, and III. DeBakey type I dissections begin in the aortic root and involve the entire length of the transthoracic aorta. DeBakey type II dissections involve only the ascending aorta. DeBakey type III dissections begin beyond the arch of the aorta, usually at the origin of the left subclavian artery.[90,118]

Stanford type A (DeBakey types I and II) dissections require surgical repair, while Stanford type B (DeBakey type III) dissections may be treated medically.[77,90,96,104,339] A major concern in type A dissections is the level of involvement of the coronary arteries. From a management point of view, it

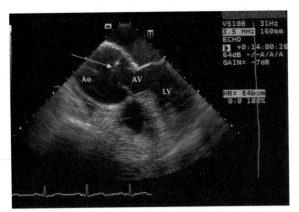

Figure 6-10. Type A dissection of the aorta. The tear begins in the proximal aorta. An intimal flap (arrow) can be seen in the sinus venosus region of the aorta. Identification and interrogation of the coronary arteries are critical in these patients. AV, aortic valve; LV, left ventricle; Ao, aorta.

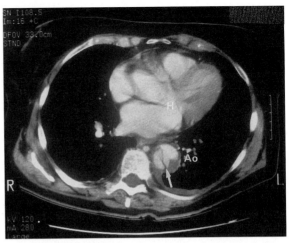

Figure 6-12. CT scan demonstrating an aortic dissection. Ao, aorta.

is important to know if the coronary arteries come off the true or false lumen.[118]

The diagnosis of aortic dissection is currently made using contrast-enhanced computed tomography (CT) (Fig. 6-12), magnetic resonance imaging (MRI) (Fig. 6-13), and/or TEE (Table 6-1). These techniques have been shown to be comparable to one another and equal to or better than the previous gold standards of contrast-enhanced cineangiography and conventional or digital subtraction aortography[108,180,220] (Table 6-2). However, there are pitfalls with CT[136] and MRI,[297] primarily the time required for image acquisition, which makes them unsuitable for these typically unstable patients. Ad-

ditionally, these technologies are relatively expensive and, like TEE, may not always be readily available at all facilities.

The classic TEE finding of aortic dissection is the presence of an intraluminal intimal flap.[26,113,180,288,332] The intimal flap resembles the aortic wall in appearance but is clearly independent, is hyperreflectile, and oscillates throughout the cardiac cycle. Artifacts, on the other hand, do not demonstrate the rapid oscillating motion of a true flap and have poorly defined walls which typically extend through the aortic wall[113] (Fig. 6-14). Further, the true lumen will expand with systole, while the false lumen will demonstrate variable compression[127]

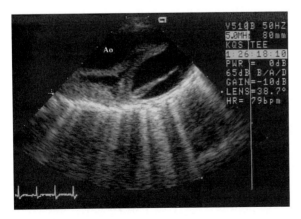

Figure 6-11. Long-axis view of the descending aorta demonstrating numerous flaps in this type B dissection. Ao, aorta.

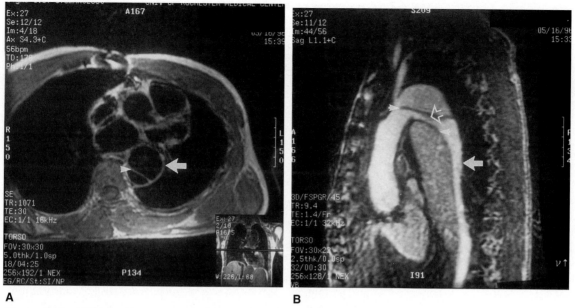

A   **B**

Figure 6-13. MRI scan of an aortic dissection. Cross-sectional view (**A**) at the level of the base of the heart. The descending thoracic aorta is noted (arrow) with an intimal flap (arrowhead). A sagittal view (**B**) demonstrating the aorta. Two intimal flaps (arrowheads) and the true lumen (open arrow) are noted.

(Fig. 6-15). Doppler, particularly color Doppler echocardiography, further delineates dissections and aids in identifying entry and exit sites of the dissection. In the normal aorta blood flow is laminar, while in dissections it is typically turbulent. In addition, there may be several turbulent, high-velocity jets communicating between the true and false lumens.[26,180,127] In systole a high-velocity jet can be seen moving from the true lumen to the false lumen, while in diastole a low-velocity jet is seen moving back to the true lumen.

Type A dissections are best seen in a longitudinal plane and can be traced from their origin near the aortic root to the aortic arch. This view also allows visualization of the aortic root, which may demonstrate varying degrees of dilatation, depending on the acuity of the disease.[127] TEE can identify secondary findings associated with aortic dissections such as thrombus formation within the false lumen, the degree of aortoannular involvement, and the presence of aortic regurgitation and aortic valvular involvement. All of these factors are important in determining surgical management since associated aortic regurgitation may require valve replacement.[127] TEE can also detect the presence of coronary artery dissection associated with aortic dissection. Right and left coronary dissections occur with almost equal frequency.[25]

The classic pattern of dissection is not always detected on TEE, particularly when there is an intraluminal hematoma displacing the intimal flap.[108,127,212] Intraluminal hematomas may increase the wall thickness from 5 to 40 mm, with longitudinal extension averaging 7–11 cm.[127,212]

TABLE 6-1. Current Diagnostic Tools in the Evaluation of Aortic Dissection[220]

	TEE (%)	CT (%)	MRI (%)
Sensitivity	98	94	98
Specificity	77	87	98
Accuracy	90	91	98
Pos. pred. value	88	92	98
Neg. pred. value	95	90	98

TABLE 6-2. COMPARISON OF TECHNIQUES USED TO DIAGNOSE AORTIC DISSECTIONS[108]

	TEE (%)	Cineangiography (%)	Aortic Angiography (%)
Sensitivity	99	83	88
Specificity	98	100	94
Pos. pred. value	98	100	96
Neg. pred. value	99	86	84

Localized intraluminal hematomas are an early sign of dissection and can be a prognostic indicator of the progression of aortic dissection[211] (Fig. 6-16).

Other complications of aortic dissection can also be identified by TEE. Roughly 20–25% of patients studied by TEE for aortic dissection have associated pericardial effusions.[25,108] Cardiac tamponade can also be assessed by TEE. The free wall of the right atrium and ventricle can be visualized with a modified four-chamber or transgastric view to evaluate for diastolic collapse, a frequent finding in cardiac tamponade. In addition, pulsed Doppler scanning of the pulmonic and mitral valve can be used to look for respiratory variation.[47,127] Pleural effusion is also detected by rotating the transducer adjacent to the descending thoracic aorta.[127] TEE detection of false aneurysms with thrombus has also been reported in the literature.[25]

Several investigators advocate using TEE as the diagnostic method of choice in patients with suspected aortic dissections.[108–110] Further, many of these investigators advise that in cases where the diagnosis of dissection is clear by TEE, the patient should go directly to surgery, when indicated, and that no other noninvasive imaging be done.[5] TEE is also useful in diagnosing conditions that mimic aortic dissections such as ischemic syndromes, extrinsic masses adjacent to the aorta, and acute pulmonary embolus.[58] With its portability, availability, and further improvements in technology, TEE is fast becoming the gold standard in the diagnosis of aortic dissection.

NONDISSECTING AORTIC ANEURYSMS

TEE is also very useful in identifying nondissecting aortic aneurysms. Dilatation of the aorta can be seen at any level from the sinus to the descending aorta. As the diameter increases, flow within the lumen decreases and spontaneous contrast is frequently

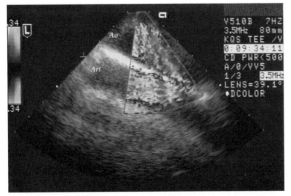

Figure 6-14. Artifact (Art) mimicking an aortic dissection. Note the poorly defined walls. In addition, artifacts such as these do not demonstrate the independent motion typical of a dissection. Ao, aorta. (See also Color Plate 15.)

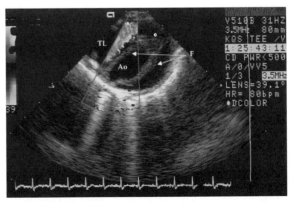

Figure 6-15. Cross-sectional view of the aorta (Ao) demonstrating two false lumens (F). Note the compression of the false lumens during systole. TL, true lumen. (See also Color Plate 16.)

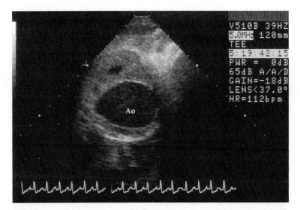

Figure 6-16. Cross-sectional view of the aorta with thrombus. Thrombus can mask intimal tears. Ao, aorta.

noted. Mural thrombus is not uncommon in these conditions. Using a variety of longitudinal and transverse planes, localized dilatation of the aorta can be identified.

Evaluation of the Source of Embolus

A major indication for TEE is in evaluating the source of embolism. At the University of Rochester in New York, 48% of the TEE studies ordered in 1996 were performed for this purpose (Display 6-4). The percentage of embolism from the heart ranges from 6% to 23% of all ischemic strokes.[55,56,281] Approximately 75% of cardiac emboli lodge in the brain[6]; the remainder embolize peripherally, and many are silent. The most common cause of a cardiac source of emboli is left atrial thrombus resulting from atrial fibrillation, followed

Display 6-4. Transesophageal Indications

Lv function	5%
Endocarditis	25%
Valvular disorders	7%
Pericardial abnormalities	2%
Aortic abnormalities	7%
Shunts	4%
Source of embolism	48%
Right heart function	2%

less frequently and with nearly equal prevalence by acute myocardial infarction, ventricular aneurysm, rheumatic heart disease, and prosthetic valves.[55]

There are two major classifications of embolus: direct source and indirect source. Direct sources of emboli include those lesions which have a high probability of causing stroke. These lesions include thrombus, tumor, vegetations, and aortic atheroma. Lesions which can cause stroke, but with a lower probability, are indirect sources. These include valvular disease, dilated cardiomyopathy, atrial septal defect, patent foramen ovale, and spontaneous echocardiographic contrast.[68] Transthoracic echocardiography is insensitive in detecting intracardiac sources of embolism.[189,262] However, it may still have a role in identifying patients at risk for potential embolic events and can be used as a screening tool for TEE in patients following stroke or systemic embolic events.[189]

TEE is useful in detecting potential sources of embolism.[27,30,38,57,95,106,121,126,140,147,148,179,189,214,239,246,308,309,319] It is still undecided whether all patients suffering from stroke or other systemic embolic events should undergo TEE. The American Society of Echocardiography has established guidelines on the appropriate use of TEE. Further, many insurance companies have established reimbursement protocols for TEE in this clinical setting. Still, embolic sources continue to be a major indication for TEE. Many of the limitations of transthoracic echocardiography are overcome with TEE. TEE provides a better look at the left atrium, left atrial appendage, atrial septum, and thoracic aorta. Specifically, TEE can identify lesions that pose a risk of thromboemboli such as left atrial spontaneous contrast, patent foramen ovale, thrombus within the left atrium or left atrial appendage, native valvular and prosthetic valve vegetations, atrial septal aneurysms, and atherosclerotic plaque within the thoracic aorta.[68,79,84,189,308]

LEFT ATRIUM AND LEFT ATRIAL APPENDAGE

One of the major benefits of TEE is its ability to interrogate the left atrium, particularly the left atrial appendage. Predisposing factors for thrombus in the left atrium or its appendage include rheumatic valve disease[22,246,267,285] and atrial fibrillation.[3] TEE has the ability to evaluate the entire atrium and the appendage, which is seldom seen by trans-

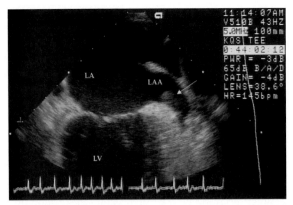

Figure 6-17. Two-chamber view demonstrating a small thrombus (arrow) in the left atrial appendage (LAA). LA, left atrium; LV, left ventricle.

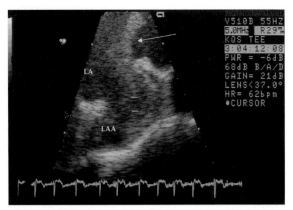

Figure 6-19. Enlarged view of the left atrial appendage (LAA) with spontaneous contrast or "smoke" (arrow). LA, left atrium.

thoracic echocardiography. Thrombus within the atrium or the appendage can range in appearance from large lobular masses (Fig. 6-17) to string-like projections or "sludge."[68]

Thrombus in the atrial appendage can be defined if there are clear borders, independent mobility, and a difference in echogenicity from surrounding structures[106,270] (Fig. 6-18). Associated findings in patients with atrial fibrillation and a history of an embolic event include left atrial/appendage thrombi, spontaneous contrast, and an enlarged left atrial appendage.[37,86,91,321,330]

Other masses in the atrium which may cause embolus are myxomas. TEE is helpful in differentiating these from thrombus by demonstrating the location and site of attachment.

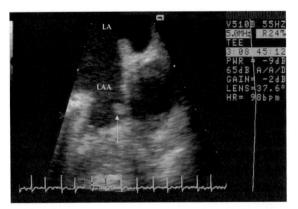

Figure 6-18. Enlarged view of the left atrial appendage (LAA) demonstrating a small clot (arrow). Note the well-defined borders. LA, left atrium.

SPONTANEOUS ECHO CONTRAST

Spontaneous echo contrast is diagnosed by the presence of dynamic echoes within the left atrium and appendage which resemble swirling smoke[34,106] (Fig. 6-19). Spontaneous echo contrast is best seen at higher frequencies. When it is suspected, the gain settings should be decreased so as to better distinguish echo contrast from low-level noise artifact.

Spontaneous echo contrast is manifested by erythrocyte and platelet aggregates in regions of low blood flow.[209] It has a significant correlation with previous embolic events.[115,179] In addition, it may serve as a marker for increased risk of embolism.[40,52,88,179,209] TEE is ideal for identifying spontaneous echo contrast because of the higher frequencies used for imaging and the proximity of the left atrium and appendage to the transducer.

ATRIAL SEPTUM

Embolic events caused by abnormalities of the atrial septum can result from two different mechanisms: atrial septal aneurysms and patent foramen ovale. Atrial septal aneurysms are rare and are defined by a protrusion of the interatrial septum into the left or right atrium by more than 10 mm beyond the plane of the interatrial septum[214,237,287] or by phasic excursions of the atrial septum during the cardiorespiratory cycle of more than 15 mm at its base[146] (Fig. 6-20). Aneurysms of the interatrial septum result from interatrial pressure differences or congenital malformation of the fossa ovalis section of the interatrial septum.[144,287] Atrial septal aneurysms can

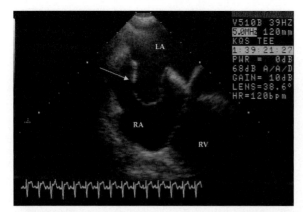

Figure 6-20. Four-chamber view demonstrating an interatrial septal aneurysm (arrow). Note the jumprope appearance. RA, right atrium; LA, left atrium; RV, right ventricle.

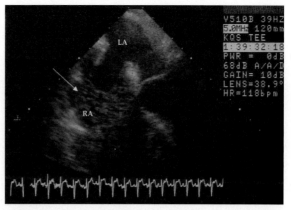

Figure 6-21. Four-chamber view of an interatrial septal aneurysm with contrast (arrow). Agitated saline is frequently used to identify interatrial shunting. LA, left atrium; RA, right atrium.

be isolated abnormalities or can occur in association with mitral valve prolapse[156,254] or atrial septal defects.[32]

Several studies have suggested the potential association between isolated atrial septal aneurysms and cardiogenic embolism in patients with no other obvious risk factors.[31,98,132,146,214,240,268,346] The incidence of cardiogenic embolism in patients with atrial septal aneurysm ranges from 20% to 52%.[31,98,132,146,214,268,346] Whether an atrial septal aneurysm is a direct source of thrombus formation or if the morphologic characteristics of the aneurysm may serve as a predictor of embolic events is unclear.[214]

TEE is much more sensitive in identifying atrial septal aneurysm than transthoracic echocardiography because the former allows an unobstructed view of the atrial septum. In the past, there was no reliable method to identify atrial septal aneurysms. Now TEE is the method of choice in demonstrating these lesions. Contrast echocardiography used in conjunction with TEE can identify the presence of a shunt (Fig. 6-21).

Patent foramen ovale (PFO) is another atrial septal lesion which can be seen well using TEE. The foramen ovale is a remnant flap between the septum primum and septum secundum which in fetal life allows blood to flow from the right atrium into the left atrium.[121] Shortly after birth this communication closes, but in roughly 25–34% of patients the foraman ovale remains patent[145] (Fig. 6-22). The communication between the right and left atria can potentially serve as a pathway for thrombotic

emboli from a venous site to the cerebral circulation.[121,147,309] However, the definitive diagnosis can be made only in cases where the thrombus is seen crossing the atrial septum.[147,218,256] The relationship between a PFO and embolic events is unclear[121] and may depend on the size of the shunt.[147,309]

Color flow Doppler and peripheral venous contrast injection are typically used in conjunction with transthoracic echocardiography as well as TEE to confirm the presence of a PFO. When a PFO is present, microbubbles from the contrast can be seen traversing the atrial septum (Fig. 6-23A,B). Since

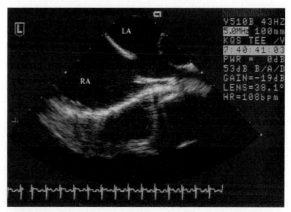

Figure 6-22. Enlarged four-chamber view illustrating a PFO. The break in the interatrial septum occurs at the level of the foramen. This region typically closes shortly after birth but may remain open, allowing paradoxical embolism. RA, right atrium; LA, left atrium.

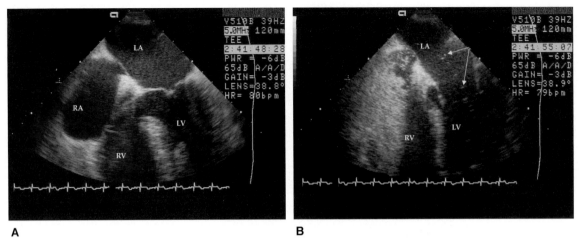

A   **B**

Figure 6-23. Four-chamber view (**A**) Four-chamber view with contrast (**B**) The right atrium and right ventricle are obliterated with contrast. A few bubbles are noted in the left side of the heart (arrow) immediately after injection, indicating a biatrial shunt at the atrial level. LA, left atrium; LV, left ventricle; RA, right atrium; RV, right ventricle.

left atrial pressure is slightly higher than right atrial pressure, microbubbles can cross the PFO only when pressure in the right atrium exceeds that in the left atrium. In the absence of pulmonary hypertension or right ventricular failure, transient elevation in right-sided pressure can be achieved by having the patient cough or perform the Valsalva maneuver.[121] A PFO is confirmed when three or more bubbles are seen traversing the atrial septum into the left atrium immediately after contrast reaches the right atrium.[121,140,309]

The presumptive mechanism for paradoxical emboli in patients with PFO is thrombus from a venous source that enters the right atrium, crosses the PFO, and travels to the cerebral circulation.[309] There is an association between PFO and venous thrombosis in patients with cerebrovascular accident (CVA).[99,159,186,335] TEE is helpful in assessing for PFO.[121,147,309] Using a biplane device, the best planes for visualizing the atrial septum are the longitudinal or transverse four-chamber planes.[68,121] These views allow the thinnest portion of the interatrial septum to be visualized.[121] Although contrast and color Doppler aid in the detection of PFO, it can also be imaged as an interruption in the superior portion of the fossa ovalis membrane.[68] PFOs can be large or barely detectable.[182]

In patients with a PFO and a history of CVA but no other potential cause for neurologic events, TEE can provide important information on the morphologic and functional features of the PFO.[336] Significant right-to-left shunting or a large opening are associated with embolism. Smaller PFOs have a lower association with embolism.

VALVULAR ABNORMALITIES

Vegetations of the heart valves, mitral valve prolapse, and aortic sclerosis may be precursors to embolic events. A more detailed description of valvular disease is presented later in this chapter. TEE is helpful in identifying valvular abnormalities that may lead to embolic events.

Valve strands seen on native as well as prosthetic valves pose a potential risk of embolic events.[126,187] Valve strands are defined as highly mobile, fine, thread-like structures typically less than 1 mm in width and 0.5 to 3.0 cm in length[126] (Fig. 6-24). In a large retrospective study,[126] strands were observed to be more prevalent on the mitral valve than on the aortic valve. Strands have been associated with embolization in patients with both native and prosthetic valves in the absence of other sources of embolism.[126,157,227,187,302] In several studies[157,227] there was a higher prevalence of strands on mechanical prostheses compared to tissue prostheses, and in one study[302] there was a 75% prevalence of strands on St. Jude prostheses in the mitral prostheses.

The cause of valvular strands is unclear. In some cases these strands are filamentous processes first

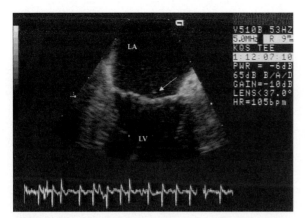

Figure 6-24. Two-chamber view demonstrating mitral valve strands (arrow). LA, left atrium; LV, left ventricle.

described as Lambl's excrescences.[126] These filamentous processes may represent fibrin deposits over damaged endocardial valvular tissue that eventually become detached and fibrosed.[196] Whatever their cause, they represent a potential source of emboli, either in themselves or as fragments, platelet aggregation, or clot formation.[126] TEE affords a detailed look at the valves, particularly prosthetic valves, where shadowing poses a major obstacle to transthoracic imaging.

PULMONARY EMBOLI

Pulmonary embolism results in roughly 50,000 deaths each year in the United States.[247] Rapid diagnosis is important to plan therapy or intervention. Echocardiographic signs of pulmonary emboli include dilatation of right heart chambers, dilated pulmonary artery, small left ventricular cavity, paradoxical septal motion, and visualization of thrombi in the pulmonary arteries.[68] Ventilation-perfusion scans and pulmonary angiography are the two diagnostic tests used to diagnose pulmonary emboli. However, these scans are helpful when they are entirely negative.[68] Pulmonary angiography, although, the gold standard, is costly, not always available, and cannot be performed on all patients.[155] TEE is a good adjunctive test because it can be done at the bedside, is noninvasive, provides detailed images, and generates important information immediately.

The presence of thromboembolism within the right heart strongly supports the diagnosis of pulmonary embolism (Fig. 6-25). In addition, TEE can sort out the possible causes and can define the problem as cardiac or noncardiac.[68] The use of TEE with other tests can also aid in diagnosis and therapy.[27,148,319] Treatment of patients with pulmonary emboli includes thrombolytic therapy, surgical embolectomy, or a combination of diagnostic catheterization and therapeutic embolectomy/fragmentation.[43,137,148] This last technique is best suited for patients with large proximal clots.[71] TEE is used to demonstrate the pulmonary emboli and guide the catheter.

Catheter fragmentation as therapy for pulmonary emboli is relatively new. A large-diameter ensnaring catheter is used to withdraw the thrombus from the proximal pulmonary vessel. Smaller catheters can be used to break apart the proximal clot,

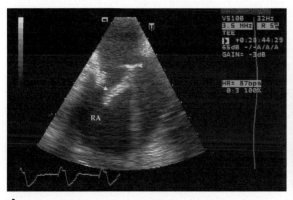
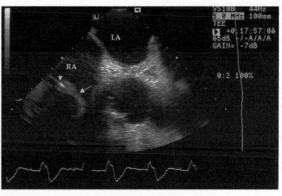

A   B

Figure 6-25. (**A, B**) Images of the right atrium with a thrombus (arrow) attached to a pacemaker wire (arrowhead). RA, right atrium; LA, left atrium.

causing it to disperse to more distal vessels. This improves pulmonary flow because of the increased vascular area of the distal vessels relative to the proximal vessels.[43] TEE is used to locate these proximal clots and view the advancing catheter. Patients with large proximal emboli are ideally suited for catheter fragmentation. In addition to confirming the presence of clot, confirmation of its absence or persistence by TEE following the procedure will help the clinician decide on further management.[135]

Heart operations such as coronary artery bypass and valvular surgery can be complicated by cerebral emboli, resulting in stroke.[27,319] Because of the highly reflective properties of emboli, TEE can be used to identify them during cardiac operations. The size of detectable emboli by ultrasound varies between 2 and 125 μm.[319] The ability to detect these emboli depends on several factors, including the ultrasound frequency, the composition of the emboli (air versus particles), and varying acoustic properties. Transcranial Doppler (TCD) is the standard technique used in monitoring emboli during coronary bypass surgery.[27,67,230,250] TEE has been shown to be as reliable as TCD in detecting emboli during surgical procedures.[27,319] Unlike TCD, TEE can provide information on the size and composition of emboli.[27] However, compared to TCD, TEE is more expensive, labor intensive, and more invasive.[27]

Atrial Fibrillation

Thromboembolism as a consequence of atrial fibrillation is a major cause of morbidity and mortality.[201] It is the most common cardiac rhythm disturbance, with a prevalence of about 2% in the general population.[102] Atrial fibrillation occurs in 5% of patients over 60 years of age.[160,171] In untreated patients with chronic atrial fibrillation, the risk of stroke is 5%.[269] The risk of stroke is also higher in patients with atrial fibrillation and valvular heart disease.[102] In patients with atrial fibrillation and other nonvalvular heart diseases such as coexisting hypertension, recent congestive heart failure, or a prior history of arterial thromboembolism, the annual risk of stroke is greater than 7%.[315] In patients less than 60 years of age with isolated atrial fibrillation, the annual risk is 0.5%.[175]

Treatment of atrial fibrillation includes conversion to sinus rhythm by DC cardioversion, treatment with antiarrhythmic drugs, and anticoagulation therapy.[269] Cardioversion is performed on patients with atrial fibrillation to prevent thromboembolism and to improve left ventricular function.[141,169,198,243,279] The success rate of conversion to a normal rhythm depends significantly on the duration of the atrial fibrillation. In patients with atrial fibrillation of less than 2–3 day's duration the conversion rate is high, but in patients with prolonged atrial fibrillation the success rate drops.[120] The initial success rate of conversion from atrial fibrillation to a sinus rhythm by DC cardioversion is 90%.[13] The number of patients remaining in sinus rhythm after 6–12 months following cardioversion depends largely on the duration of the atrial fibrillation and may be less than 50%.[75] Successful cardioversion carries a 5–7% chance of embolization in patients without anticoagulation therapy.[193,252] The incidence of stroke is reduced to 1.6% in patients treated with anticoagulation.[20,33,337] The American College of Chest Physicians recommends that patients undergoing cardioversion for atrial fibrillation lasting for more than 2 days should be given anticoagulation for 3 weeks before the procedure.[185] In patients with atrial fibrillation for less than 48–72 hrs, anticoagulation may not be necessary.[33] Following successful cardioversion, the normal function of the left atrial appendage may not be restored for weeks or months.[200,206] Therefore, the American College of Chest Physicians recommends anticoagulation for 4 weeks following cardioversion.[185]

TEE has an important role in patients who are candidates for DC cardioversion.[236] It offers an excellent view of posterior cardiac structures and is particularly well suited for the evaluation of left atrial pathology including left atrial tumors, atrial septal defects, PFO, and left atrial thrombus.[22,60,213,216] TEE has been proven to be safe and well tolerated.[85,345] Its use in conjunction with cardioversion has gained widespread attention, and its feasibility has been well documented.[39,199,201,228,304] TEE is highly sensitive in detecting clots in the left atrium and left atrial appendage[22] and in evaluating left atrial function following the procedure.[198] However, to date the minimal size of clots detectable by TEE has not been systematically determined.[269]

The standard practice of care for patients with atrial fibrillation lasting for more than 2 days is prophylactic anticoagulation prior to cardioversion.[36,102,248] However, anticoagulation is associated with an increased risk of hemorrhage.[74,337] In addition, this practice delays cardioversion for up to 1 month.[201] If the left atrium and left atrial appendage are clearly seen by TEE and no thrombus are visualized, precardioversion anticoagulation therapy may not be necessary and may even be contraindicated in some patients.[201] In these cases cardioversion could be done sooner, allowing earlier return of sinus rhythm and atrial mechanical function.[46] For inpatients this would eliminate the need for a second hospital admission for cardioversion.[201]

Evaluation of Native Heart Valves

FLAIL MITRAL VALVE LEAFLETS

The use of TEE in the evaluation of heart valves is widespread. Some of its many uses include quantification of mitral and aortic valve diseases including mitral and aortic stenosis, mitral and aortic regurgitation, flail mitral valve leaflets, and aortic valve abscesses. TEE is more specific and sensitive than transthoracic echocardiography in the setting of flail mitral valve leaflets.[12,151,286] TEE provides higher resolution of posterior cardiac structures of the mitral valve and left atrium. Flail mitral valve leaflets are characterized on TEE by a fluctuating chord in the left atrial cavity during systole (Fig. 6-26). The flail leaflets appear as a linear echo with high-frequency fluttering.[286] In addition, the presence of eccentric regurgitant jets may be a marker of flail

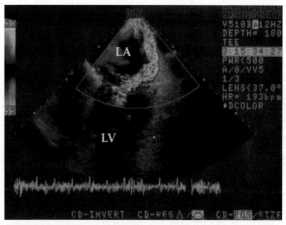

Figure 6-27. Color Doppler demonstration of an eccentric mitral regurgitant jet. TEE is helpful in identifying the pathology associated with eccentric jets. LA, left atrium; LV, left ventricle. (See also Color Plate 17.)

mitral valve.[151] However, an eccentric mitral regurgitant jet can be caused by other valvular lesions such as marked mitral valve prolapse.

The mechanism for eccentric jet formation may be caused by abnormal mitral leaflets coaptation, which does not allow the leaflet to coapt properly during systole. The unsupported leaflet moves into the left atrium, creating a channel that directs the flow of blood toward the opposite leaflet.[151] Therefore, a flail or ruptured chordae of the posterior leaflet will result in a regurgitant jet directed toward the interatrial septum. A ruptured chorda of the anterior leaflet will result in a regurgitant jet directed toward the posterolateral atrial wall[286] (Fig. 6-27). The combination of high-frequency linear echoes and an eccentric color jet of mitral regurgitation is a good indicator of ruptured chordae tendineae.

Using a variety of standard and nonstandard TEE views in the long axis, four chamber, and short axis of the left ventricle, the mitral valve can be well appreciated. Images can be optimized by gently advancing and withdrawing the probe. The anteroposterior and lateral flexion controls are also used to optimize the mitral valve. Color frame rate and image resolution are optimized to best delineate the mitral valve structures.[151] The use of multiplane TEE further enhances imaging of the mitral apparatus because of the various intermediate imaging planes available.

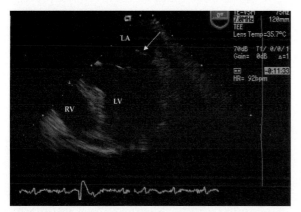

Figure 6-26. Four-chamber view illustrating a flail mitral valve leaflet (arrow). During systole the posterior leaflet is seen prolapsing into the left atrium. LA, left atrium; LV, left ventricle; RV, right ventricle.

MITRAL STENOSIS

Although transthoracic echocardiography is currently the technique of choice for the evaluation and quantification of mitral stenosis, in some cases TEE may be more appropriate. In cases where transthoracic imaging is difficult or suboptimal, TEE can better define the extent and distribution of fibrosis and calcification at the free margins and commissures of the leaflets.[72,184,265,341,347] In addition, the ability to assess the subvalvular apparatus can lead to more reliable judgment of the suitability of valvuloplasty or commissurotomy.[1,73,76,93,204,285,317] Myxomatous versus rheumatic thickening can also be better diagnosed using TEE.[93]

The restriction of mitral valve leaflets in patients with mitral stenosis is demonstrated in various planes and is similar in appearance to that seen from a transthoracic approach (Fig. 6–28). The leaflets demonstrate the typical diastolic doming pattern caused by fusion of the commissures. With the probe advanced to the gastric level, cross-sectional views of the mitral valve can be obtained. With small angulations of the scanning plane the valve orifice can be positioned to achieve a true cross-sectional view, allowing the operator to trace along the free margins of the valve in order to estimate the valve area by planimetry.[93,305] As with transthoracic echocardiography, improper gain settings, heavy valvular calcification, and irregular orifice shape due to mitral commissurotomy pose limitations for this method.[92,203,294,316]

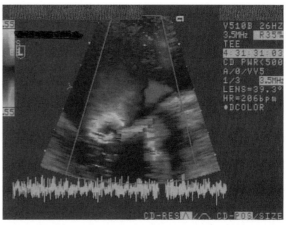

Figure 6-29. In moderate to severe cases of mitral stenosis an area of flow convergence can be seen on the atrial side of the valve. Flow convergence or PISA can be used to calculate mitral valve areas. Under the principles of flow, blood passing through any given hemisphere must also pass through the stenotic region. Using this principle, the instantaneous flow rate through the stenotic orifice can be calculated. The flow radius (r) is measured from the narrowest point of the convergence to the first aliased hemisphere. Since the mitral valve is domed, the angle of the convergence must be determined and corrected by dividing by 180 degrees. The velocity at which the first aliased hemisphere occurs (V1) is used in the calculation and can be obtained from the ultrasound system. The flow rate in cubic centimeters per second is calculated by multiplying $2\pi r^2 \times V1 \times$ the corrected angle. The flow rate is then divided by the peak mitral inflow velocity obtained by continuous Doppler to yield the mitral valve area. This calculation is covered in more detail in Chapter 13. (See also Color Plate 18.)

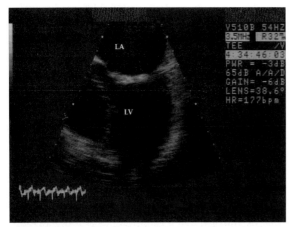

Figure 6-28. Four-chamber view of mitral stenosis. The leaflets are thickened and dome in diastole. Using TEE, the level of subvalvular involvement can be better defined. LA, left atrium; LV, left ventricle.

Estimation of mitral valve area by the pressure half-time or a continuity equation can also be performed using TEE.[294,307] These methods are outlined in detail in Chapter 13. The same potential errors that can occur from the transthoracic approach can also result from TEE.[122,139,162,194] Velocities obtained by either method depend on the alignment of the cursor with the stenotic jet. The angle between the jet and the cursor should be as close to zero as possible. Multiplane TEE is particularly well suited to these measurements since it provides a wide range of positional changes, facilitating proper alignment.[93]

Another method of mitral area calculation employed by TEE uses flow convergence of the field proximal to the obstruction (Fig. 6-29). As flow from the atrium converges on the obstructed mitral valve, a proximal isovelocity surface area or hemisphere develops. The radius of this hemisphere is measured in early diastole from the tips of the mitral valve to the first aliasing boundary. This technique assumes a flat surface, and since the stenotic mitral valve domes, the surface is angle corrected by dividing the funnel angle by 180 degrees. The angle created by the funnel is obtained using an offline analysis package. The peak forward flow rate across the mitral valve is calculated as a product of $2\pi r^2$ and the corrected angle multiplied by the aliasing velocity, which is obtained from the color scale bar on the system. The mitral valve area is then obtained by dividing this product by the peak mitral inflow obtained from continuous Doppler scanning. The angle, radius, and peak mitral inflow are measured and averaged 5 beats for patients with normal sinus rhythm; an average of 10 beats is used for patients with atrial fibrillation.[257]

MITRAL REGURGITATION

Color flow Doppler by transthoracic echocardiography has proven to be a useful and accurate means of assessing and semiquantifying mitral regurgitation. The correlation of the severity of mitral regurgitation by TTE color Doppler scanning and angiographic severity has been well documented.[51,150,298] Assessment by color flow Doppler scanning of mitral regurgitation is highly operator and instrument dependent. Several factors affect the clear delineation of the mitral regurgitant jets. Instrument gain settings, available windows,[128] frame rate, and scan depths[292] all affect the duration of color flow jets that are visualized. Regurgitant volumes, orifice areas, left ventricular pressures and compliance, and mitral leaflet malcoaptation also affect the configuration and trajectory of the mitral regurgitant jet.[128] Eccentric jets which may adhere to atrial walls as a result of the Coanda effect may diminish the apparent size of the regurgitant jet.[50,61]

With TEE the left atrium and mitral valve are placed closer to the probe, reducing the scan depth and allowing an increase in frame rate. The number of color flow frames produced is increased within a given sector size.[292] The increased number of planes available by TEE also allows better, unimpaired visualization and more thorough interrogation of the left atrium as well as the mitral valve anatomy. As a

result of these factors, color jets appear larger by TEE than by transthoracic echocardiography.[219,295]

TEE has another advantage: its success rate in establishing the cause of mitral regurgitation and in discovering other unsuspected lesions is high.[128,280,292] In patients with acute, severe mitral regurgitation, the pressure gradient between the left ventricle and atrium is dissipated early in systole as a result of a high volume and high pressure within the noncompliant left atrium.[142,292] This results in a relatively brief time in which the mitral regurgitant flow occurs. By transthoracic echocardiography this may appear as a brief flash of mitral regurgitation, and therefore the severity of the regurgitation may be underestimated. By TEE the regurgitant flow can be seen originating from the mitral valve orifice throughout most of systole.[292] The advantage of multiplane imaging with color flow Doppler is that it greatly enhances the assessment of patients with mitral regurgitation, determining the cause and predicting the severity of the regurgitation.[24,292]

The most widely accepted grading criteria by TEE are the extension of the regurgitant jet, viewed from multiple views, and the amount of filling within the left atrium. More recently, investigators have suggested that the width of the regurgitant jet measured at the orifice or vena contracta width is a more precise measure of the severity of regurgitation, because, unlike the jet extension or volume, the width at the orifice is not dependent on loading conditions.[117,138,320] Vena contracta width is best suited to distinguish patients with and without severe mitral regurgitation.[138]

Other techniques, such as flow convergence and detection of systolic pulmonary venous flow, can also be used to grade the severity of mitral regurgitation using TEE. TEE is particularly well suited for evaluation of flow within the pulmonary veins because it allows better visualization of the pulmonary veins (Fig. 6-30) with improved positioning of the sample volume within the lumen of the vessel.[93] The normal flow pattern within the pulmonary veins demonstrates a biphasic pattern of forward flow toward the atrium in systole and a smaller diastolic forward component as well as a retrograde flow away from the atrium during atrial contraction.[28,94] In mitral regurgitation the systolic component is reversed and occurs away from the transducer (Fig.

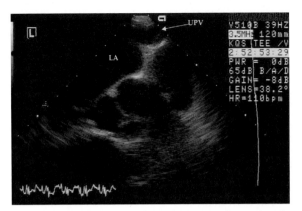

Figure 6-30. TEE view of the left upper pulmonary vein (UPV). TEE greatly increases the visibility of the pulmonary veins. LA, left atrium.

6–31*A–C*). However, these findings are not always conclusive evidence of severe mitral regurgitation. While some investigators have noted a pronounced backward systolic component in severe mitral regurgitation,[53,177,238] others have noted this pattern in mild degrees of mitral regurgitation or not at all, regardless of the severity of mitral regurgitation.[53,158,172] In addition, this backward systolic pattern may be seen in patients with other disease processes, in which elevated left atrial pressure and reduced left atrial compliance exist, such as in patients with prosthetic mitral valves, aortic valve disease, congestive heart failure, and hypertrophic cardiomyopathy.[318]

The quantification of mitral regurgitation by proximal flow convergence using TEE has proven to be highly accurate.[249] The required measurements and formula are discussed in detail in Chapter 13. This technique requires careful measurements, but when done correctly it is highly accurate.

The mechanism of mitral regurgitation frequently determines the feasibility of mitral valve repair.[103,300] TEE accurately assesses the mitral valve apparatus for anatomic, annular, and papillary muscle abnormalities, as well as differentiation of ischemic mitral regurgitation.[244] With this information, surgical procedures for mitral valve repair or replacement can be predicted and planned.[49,244]

AORTIC STENOSIS/REGURGITATION

Calculation of the aortic valve area by echocardiography has proved to be reliable and invaluable in assessing the clinical and surgical implications for patients with aortic stenosis. Doppler measurements across the stenotic aortic valve can be obtained by transthoracic echocardiography in most patients. The role of TEE in assessing aortic stenosis is primarily limited to patients who have poor transthoracic windows, in cases where the outflow obstruction is unclear, or in cases where there are other associated abnormalities ill defined by transthoracic echocardiography. Due to the variety of high-quality acoustic windows by TEE, the aortic valve can be seen well from longitudinal and short-axis views. Planimetry of the aortic valve from two-dimensional TEE has proved to correlate well with both cardiac catheterization and continuity equation methods.[152,153,301,314]

To obtain the optimal position of the aortic valve, a longitudinal view is first obtained. Using a multiplane device, the longitudinal view of the aortic valve can be obtained with the transducer rotated to 110 to 160 degrees. The probe is then steered to between 30 and 60 degrees.[314] Minimal manipulation of the probe is then performed to obtain the smallest orifice area. With all three cusps visualized, the aortic valve is then traced along the borders during its maximal excursion in systole (Fig. 6-32). With biplane devices, imaging also begins from a longitudinal view. The probe is advanced to the upper to middle esophagus in the neutral position. With rightward rotation and left lateral flexion of the transducer tip, the left ventricular outflow tract and aortic valve cusps can be visualized. The short-axis view is then obtained by further flexion of the probe toward the right[225] (Fig. 6-33*A,B*).

A significant advantage of anatomic planimeterization of the aortic valve over other methods is that the valve area does not seem to change with a change in cardiac output or stroke volume.[314] A decrease or increase in flow does not significantly change the valve area. Another advantage of TEE in the assessment of the aortic valve is that it allows a more detailed assessment of the valve cusps. The identification of discrete membranes is also more likely with TEE than with transthoracic echocardiography. Doppler measurements can also be made across the valve using TEE, but currently they have no significant advantage over a transthoracic Doppler exam.

Aortic regurgitation is also best assessed using the views just described for aortic stenosis. Quantification of aortic insufficiency is described in subse-

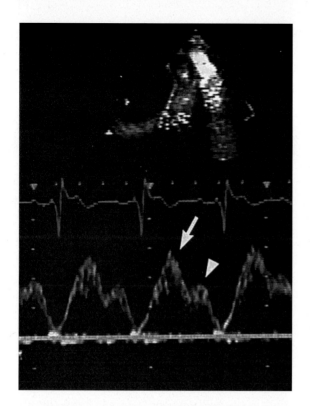
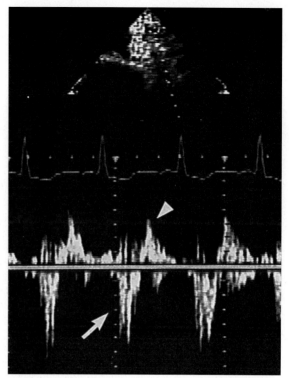
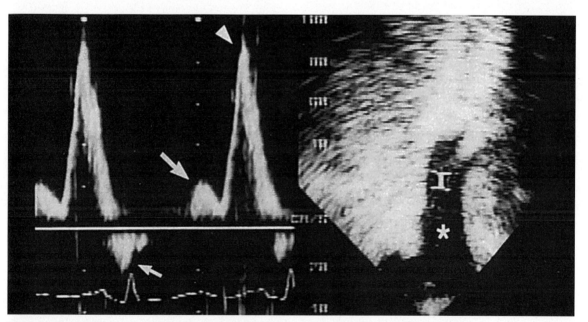

Figure 6-31. Pulsed wave spectral Doppler display of pulmonary venous flow in various degrees of mitral regurgitation. In mild mitral regurgitation (**A**), normal systolic (arrow) and lower-velocity diastolic (arrowhead) antegrade pulmonary venous inflow are noted. In moderate to severe mitral regurgitation (**B**), the systolic component is significantly reduced and the diastolic component is increased due to an increase in left atrial pressure. The low-velocity end-diastolic signal noted (small arrow) below the baseline is caused by atrial contraction. (See also Color Plates 19 and 20.) In severe mitral regurgitation (**C**), the systolic component is reversed (arrow) due to direct reflux of the mitral regurgitation into the pulmonary vein and an increase in atrial pressure. The increased diastolic component is due to the systolic regurgitation.

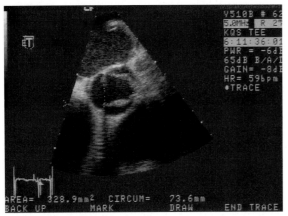

Figure 6-32. Cross-sectional view of the aortic valve. Due to increased visualization of the valve by TEE, the area can be calculated by tracing the borders of the cusps at their maximal opening in systole.

quent chapters and may be achieved using the transesophageal approach. Aortic regurgitation appears as a mosaic signal extending into the left ventricle during diastole. Currently the most widely accepted method used to quantitate the severity of aortic insufficiency is the ratio of the immediate subvalvular width of the regurgitant jet to the width of the left ventricular outflow tract. Eccentric jets can also be well documented using the transesophageal approach.

TRICUSPID AND PULMONIC VALVES

Disease of the right-sided valves is much less frequent than that of the left-sided valves. TEE allows excellent visualization of both the tricuspid and pulmonic valves. The most common pathologic condition of the right-sided valves is tricuspid regurgita-

tion. Using a number of tomographic planes, thorough assessment of the regurgitant lesions can be made.

Rheumatic tricuspid stenosis can occur and is usually accompanied by mitral stenosis. Tricuspid stenosis caused by carcinoid heart disease usually occurs by itself or with pulmonic valve disease. TEE can help make these distinctions in patients with technically difficult transthoracic echocardiograms. Pulmonic valve disease, although rare, can be assessed by TEE.

Evaluation of Prosthetic Valves

The evaluation of prosthetic heart valves is performed largely by transthoracic echocardiography. Using a combination of two-dimensional imaging and pulsed, continuous, and color Doppler interrogation, assessment of valve structure and function can be done. The major pitfall with transthoracic echocardiography in evaluating prosthetic heart valves is the acoustic shadowing and artifactual imaging created by some of the prosthetic material. In conjunction with the transthoracic exam, TEE is useful in eliminating some of the problems associated with transthoracic imaging.

Perhaps the most important questions to be answered by TEE concern valve structure and the presence or absence of regurgitation. Close attention should be paid to the sewing ring and then to the mobile components of the prosthetic valve. Given the close proximity of the TEE probe to most cardiac valves, assessment of the tissue or mechanical components of the valve can be made. In assessing tissue-type valves, the echocardiographer should evaluate for thickening, calcification, coaptation,

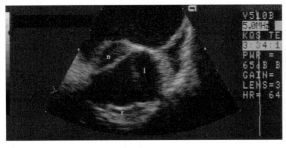

A

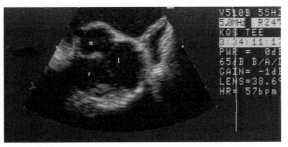

B

Figure 6-33. Cross-sectional views of the aortic valve in systole (**A**) and diastole (**B**). n, noncoronary cusp; 1, left coronary cusp; r, right coronary cusp.

and restriction of motion of the valve leaflets or cusps.[210] In evaluating mechanical valves, the timing and motion of the mobile components are crucial factors. M-mode can be used to help time occulder motion.[80]

Transthoracic echocardiography and TEE complement one another since shadowing and artifacts are viewed on opposite sides (Fig. 6-34*A,B*). Aortic regurgitation can be identified by transthoracic echocardiography because clear views of the left ventricular outflow tract are usually obtained from conventional apical views. Since vegetations tend to form on the ventricular side of the aortic valve, TTE can usually detect them.[329] However, with the higher resolution provided by TEE, the presence of thrombus or vegetations can be identified more easily, particularly where the mass is small. In assessing the mitral valve TEE has the advantage, since the left atrium is usually obscured by shadowing from the mitral prostheses.[144] Due to the image orientation of TEE, the left atrium can be more thoroughly viewed, allowing for assessment of regurgitation and vegetations.

In patients with prosthetic valves and embolic events, TEE can help alter clinical management by identifying the presence of vegetations, strands, or thrombus[107,144,227] (Fig. 6-35). Associated findings, such as abscess formation, fistulas, and pseudoaneurysms, are also seen by TEE. Additionally, TEE provides ancillary information regarding ven-

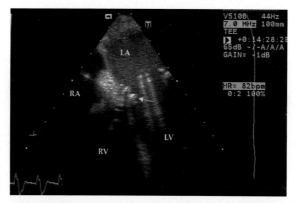

Figure 6-35. TEE four-chamber view of a disk valve in the mitral position. Vegetations (arrow) on prosthetic valves are frequently missed by TTE because of masking by the prosthetic material. TEE enables these small, mobile masses to be identified. LA, left atrium; LV, left ventricle; RA, right atrium; RV, right ventricle.

tricular size and function, atrial size, native valve function, and the presence of pericardial effusions.

Evaluation of Thrombus and Masses

Transthoracic two-dimensional echocardiography has been the technique of choice to evaluate the heart for masses. TEE, with its close proximity to cardiac structures and its increased resolution, has

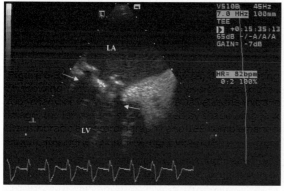

A

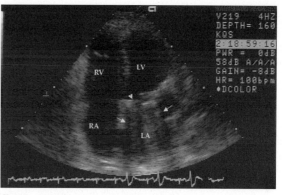

B

Figure 6-34. TEE two-chamber view (**A**) demonstrating a St. Jude valve in the mitral position. Shadowing (arrows) from the prosthesis can mask the left ventricle (LV). Transthoracic apical four-chamber view (**B**) of a St. Jude valve in the mitral position. Due to the orientation of the image, the left atrium is now masked by shadowing (arrows) from the prosthesis (arrowhead). Transthoracic echocardiography and TEE complement one another in these situations. LA, left atrium; RA, right atrium; RV, right ventricle.

enhanced the ability to assess the heart for masses.[11,45,78,97,114,143,188,195,303] TEE is more sensitive in diagnosing cardiac masses than transthoracic echocardiography.[11] TEE can provide information about the location of the mass, its size and appearance, the presence of attachment and the site, as well as the extent of involvement of other cardiac structures and the amount of compromise present. With its increased resolution, abnormal masses can be differentiated from normal variants.[11]

The most common intracardiac mass is thrombus, which may occur in any of the cardiac chambers, but is more frequently found in the left ventricle.[271] Transthoracic echocardiography often detects thrombus in the left ventricle, but imaging may be difficult in patients with poor acoustic windows; in these patients, TEE is a better choice. It is particularly suitable for evaluating the left atrium for thrombus. The left atrial appendage is the most common site of thrombus formation within the left atrium, particularly in patients with atrial fibrillation, mitral stenosis, or prosthetic mitral valves. TEE is able to interrogate the left atrial appendage and is therefore extremely useful. Thrombus can also occur in the right-sided chambers but is more likely to be found on the left side of the heart. Still, thrombi on the right side of the heart may occur as the result of thromboemboli from systemic veins, or they may form in the right atrium or ventricle. Other intracardiac masses can be primary benign or malignant tumors or metastases.[271]

Evaluation of Endocarditis and Its Complications

Embolic events are a common complication of bacterial endocarditis. The mortality rate from infective endocarditis ranges from 19% to 46%.[29] Vegetation size, extent, and mobility are predictors of these complications.[261] Clinically, infective endocarditis is suspected when the following features are present: (1) predisposing valvular disease, (2) embolic phenomena, (3) bacteremia, and (4) evidence of an endocardial process.[83,112] TEE is superior to transthoracic echocardiography because vegetations as small as 1 to 2 mm can be detected using TEE; transthoracic echocardiography is less sensitive in detecting smaller vegetations.[111,165] TEE is a recommended diagnostic test in patients suspected of having endocarditis.

The echocardiographic appearance of vegetations varies widely, from globular or polypoid to frond-like, shaggy, or linear [35,221,261] (Fig. 6-36A–D). Whatever their appearance, they can all be described as discrete, variably mobile echogenic foci with mobility distinct from that of the rest of the cardiac surface. Vegetations can be sessile and adherent to endocardial surfaces or they can be highly mobile masses which can prolapse into and out of chambers with the cardiac cycle.[166] Vegetations typically occur wherever there has been damage to the endocardium. The typical sites of vegetation formation are the cardiac valves, particularly the left-sided valves. Diseases that compromise the valves range from congenital defects to rheumatic disease and trauma. Vegetations usually form on the atrial side of the atrioventricular valves and on the ventricular side of the semilunar valves.

Right-sided endocarditis is less common than left-sided endocarditis and is usually associated with intravenous drug use, mechanical devices in the right side of the heart such as pacemaker leads,[69] and immunocompromise.[255] TEE is particularly useful in visualizing the pulmonic valve (Fig. 6-37), which can be difficult to see with transthoracic echocardiography. From a longitudinal short-axis plane the pulmonic valve can be well visualized.[166] Problems in identifying vegetations on prosthetic valves are largely overcome with TEE since acoustic shadows and other artifactual images are lessened with biplane and multiplane devices. With TEE, vegetation location and attachment site are better delineated.

Another complication of bacterial endocarditis is abscess.[42,258] Abscess formation can be expected in 5–30% of patients with vegetations confirmed by echocardiography.[258] Identifying the site and extension of the abscess is important for surgical management of patients with this complication. Because TEE allows better visualization of cardiac structures and is more reliable than transthoracic echocardiography, it is invaluable in detecting these lesions (Fig. 6-38).

Caution must be exercised when diagnosing vegetations or any other mass echocardiographically since many of these lesions have a similar appearance. There are several potential pitfalls in diagnosing vegetations using TEE. In the presence of prosthetic valves, an echogenic mass could represent a thrombus, suture material, part of the native valve, or sewing ring cloth.[166] Another potential problem

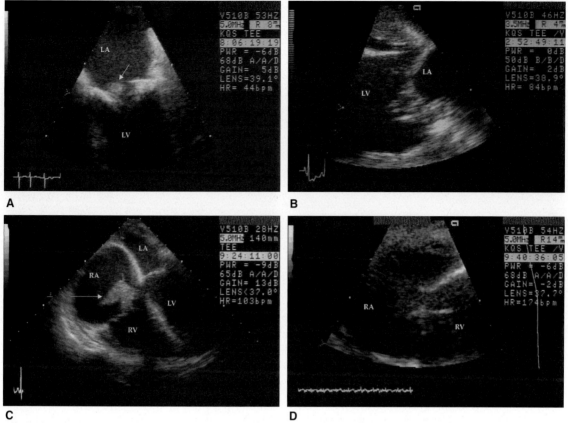

Figure 6-36. Vegetations can have a variety of appearances and are seen on all valves, although left-sided involvement is more prevalent than right-sided involvement. **A** demonstrates a polypoid vegetation on the mitral valve (arrow). **B** demonstrates another mitral valve vegetation which is more complex and globular in appearance. **C** demonstrates a tricuspid valve vegetation. Note the shaggy appearance. **D** demonstrates another tricuspid valve vegetation which appears linear in shape. LA, left atrium; LV, left ventricle; RA, right atrium; RV, right ventricle.

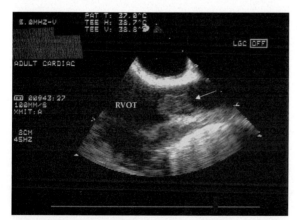

Figure 6-37. The pulmonic valve is not always visualized easily by transthoracic echocardiography. TEE allows better interrogation of the pulmonic valve and is ideal for identifying vegetations on the pulmonic valve (arrow). RVOT, right ventricular outflow tract.

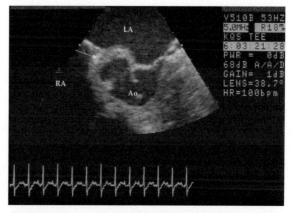

Figure 6-38. Aortic root abscess (arrow) is a serious complication of endocarditis. Involvement of the valve and surrounding tissue is important information in determining surgical management in these cases. RA, right atrium; LV, left ventricle; Ao, aorta.

is that old vegetations cannot always be distinguished from new vegetations. Additionally, myxomatous degeneration of valvular tissue, particularly in the mitral valve, can lead to false-positive and false-negative study results, especially if there are torn leaflets or chordae tendineae.[215,284] It is therefore important to consider the patient's clinical setting with any echocardiographic findings.

Congenital Heart Disease

The use of TEE to assess congenital defects has become critical in a variety of clinical settings.[16,44,130,192,217,224,226,253,309,326] To be successful, the operator needs a sound understanding of normal anatomy and pathophysiology. In examining adults with congenital abnormalities, it is important to understand the changes that can occur over time, the operative procedures, and the sequelae, complications, and residua that can occur. When performing echocardiography in patients with congenital heart disease, a segmental approach is used. This approach involves identification of atrial and ventricular situs, as well as the connections and relationships of the atria to the ventricles and of the ventricles to the great arteries.[63]

A detailed description of congenital abnormalities is presented in Chapter 29. The purpose of this chapter is to highlight some of the uses of TEE in congenital heart disease. In addition, TEE has been useful in identifying unsuspected or incidental conditions as well as residual defects during or following surgical repair,[224] in addition to providing guidance for surgical procedures[326] and postoperative follow-up.[63] The TEE exam in patients with congenital conditions should start by identifying the crux of the heart.[272] The right-sided atrioventricular valve or morphologic tricuspid valve inserts lower on the crux than does the left-sided atrioventricular valve or morphologic mitral valve. Once this relationship is identified, the orientation of the ventricles and valves can be established.[272,278] Another landmark that helps establish the cardiac situs is the characteristic thin, triangular pouch of the left atrial appendage.[63]

ATRIAL SEPTAL DEFECTS

Atrial septal defects (ASDs) are common congenital anomalies that can present as PFO or as primum, secundum, or sinus venosus defects. The

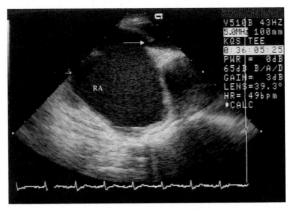

Figure 6-39. *Primum atrial septal defect (arrow) in a modified four-chamber view. RA, right atrium.*

interatrial septum is well visualized with TEE, using a longitudinal plane[133] (Fig. 6-39). The use of color Doppler or contrast echocardiography enhances TEE in this clinical setting (Fig. 6-40). Identification of sinus venosus type ASDs has been greatly increased by TEE because these defects are located high in the atrial septum, an area not well seen by transthoracic imaging. Roughly 30% of sinus venosus ASDs are missed by transthoracic echocardiography.[272] Sinus venosus ASDs may be associated with partial pulmonary venous connections. Primum and secundum ASDs are usually visualized easily using transthoracic echocardiography. TEE is helpful in cases where confidence of the diagnosis is low.

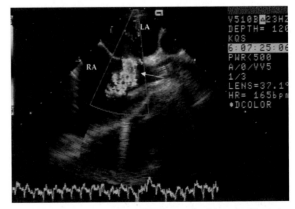

Figure 6-40. *Secundum ASD (arrow) with color Doppler demonstration of a left-to-right shunt. Four-chamber view. LA, left atrium; RA, right atrium. (See also Color Plate 21.)*

VALVULAR AND OUTFLOW TRACT ANOMALIES

Assessment of the cardiac valves by TEE allows detailed evaluation of the severity of regurgitation, chordal attachments, and leaflets or cusp anatomy. This information is particularly useful in making surgical decisions.[63,272] By using a variety of imaging planes all the cardiac valves may be visualized, allowing a thorough investigation of valve anatomy. Congenital bicuspid aortic valves are a common congenital defect. TEE allows visualization of the aortic valve and the left ventricular outflow tract. Longitudinal views using a biplane probe or a 120- to 130-degree long-axis view using a multiplane probe allow visualization of the left ventricular outflow tract. The 45- to 60-degree multiplane short-axis view provides a detailed picture of the aortic valve cusps[63] (Fig. 6-41). These views aid in the evaluation of aortic or subaortic stenosis (Fig. 6-42). In cases of aortic valve abnormalities, the valve area can be determined using the same formula used from a transthoracic approach. Associated findings in bicuspid aortic valves include perimembranous ventricular septal defects, coarctation of the aorta, and possibly ascending aortic dissection.[63,241]

Other congenital valve abnormalities identified using TEE include Ebstein's anomaly[282] and pulmonic stenosis (Fig. 6-43A,B). In the latter case the stenosis may be subvalvular, valvular, or supravalvular and may have other associated findings such as ASD or ventricular septal defect (VSD). TEE is invaluable in identifying the location of the stenosis,

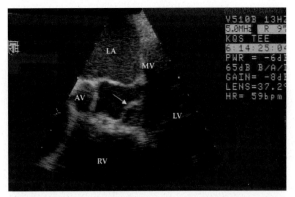

Figure 6-42. Longitudinal view of the left ventricular outflow tract demonstrating a subaortic membrane (arrow). LA, left atrium; LV, left ventricle; AV, aortic valve; MV, mitral valve; RV, right ventricle.

its degree, and any associated findings which aid surgical decision making. Using a multiplane device, the obstruction can be seen in the midesophageal region at angles between 60 and 80 degrees.[63]

Ebstein's anomaly is characterized by apical displacement of the septal tricuspid valve leaflet with atrialization of the right ventricle. With multiplane TEE the tricuspid valve can be seen best in the midesophageal region at an angle of 0 degrees, revealing a four-chamber view.[65,66,202,273]

VENTRICULAR SEPTAL DEFECTS

VSDs are another common congenital abnormality which can be diagnosed by TEE. The most common site of VSD is the membranous septum, followed by the muscular, inlet, and outlet septa. Membranous VSDs tend to be easier to detect because of their location (Fig. 6-44). Muscular VSDs can be more difficult to image. TEE is particularly useful in identifying residual defects and is helpful in defining the surgical management of these cases.[224] Interrogation of VSD patches immediately following surgery while the patient is in the operating room is important since residual defects can be re-repaired at that time.

VSDs are classified based on their location, but are also described as being aligned or malaligned and restrictive or nonrestrictive. Due to the curvature of the septum, no one plane allows complete visualization of the entire septum. The perimembranous region is best seen using a multiplane device

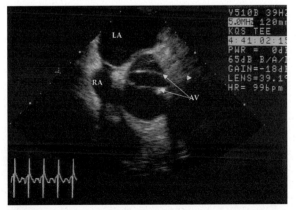

Figure 6-41. Cross-sectional view of a bicuspid aortic valve (arrows). LA, left atrium; RA, right atrium; AV, aortic valve.

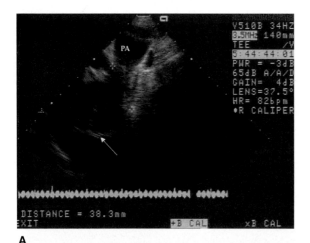

A

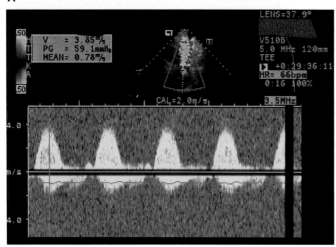

B

Figure 6-43. Longitudinal view of the right ventricular outflow tract (**A**) demonstrating the pulmonic valve (arrow) and narrowed main pulmonary artery (PA). Color Doppler (**B**) demonstrates turbulent flow, and conventional Doppler shows increased velocity across a stenotic pulmonic valve. (See also Color Plate 22.)

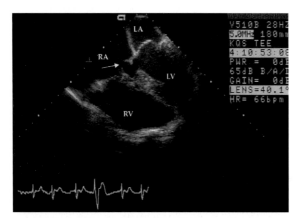

Figure 6-44. Four-chamber view of a membranous VSD (arrow). The muscular portion of the interventricular septum is hypertrophied. LA, left atrium; LV, left ventricle; RA, right atrium; RV, right ventricle.

in a 90- to 100-degree angle from the middle to low esophageal position.[63] Imaging VSDs using biplane devices can be more difficult. Shadowing or echo dropout can mimic VSDs, so multiple views should be used to fully interrogate the septum. Using continuous Doppler scanning, pressure gradients across the defect can be determined. The gradients obtained will help determine if the defect is restrictive or nonrestrictive. In tetralogy of Fallot and other great artery overriding conditions, the VSD can be visualized in a vertical plane in biplane TEE or in a 0-degree position using multiplane devices.[63]

The use of TEE in evaluating VSD aids in identifying other associated abnormalities and the effects of the VSD on other surrounding structures. In some cases, an aortic valve cusp may prolapse into the defect, causing aortic insufficiency.

PATENT DUCTUS ARTERIOSUS AND COARCTATION OF THE AORTA

Patent ductus arteriosus and coarctation of the aorta can also be diagnosed with TEE. Although patent ductus arteriosus is usually detected in childhood, it is occasionally found in the adult. Color Doppler scanning helps identify these lesions. With multiplane devices, interrogation of the main pulmonary artery is possible. Once the color lesion is identified, the orifice of the duct can usually be seen.[63] Visualization of aortic coarctation by transthoracic imaging is difficult. The diagnosis is usually made using Doppler scanning where the location and peak gradients can be determined. Color Doppler can also help assess the severity of the lesion.[81,289] TEE allows more detailed imaging of the stenotic region. Coarctations are best seen in a longitudinal position using a biplane device or at 150 degrees using a multiplane system[63] (Fig. 6-45).

CORONARY ARTERY ANOMALIES

Anomalies of the coronary arteries include abnormal origins and abnormal connections or fistulas.[131] Most of these abnormalities are benign, but some can cause myocardial ischemia, ventricular dysfunction, arrhythmias, and sudden death.[241] Anomalies of the coronary arteries are frequently associated with other congenital conditions, such as transposition of the great arteries, and can occasionally be seen in tetralogy of Fallot. It is important to identify these abnormalities in order to plan appropriate surgical treatment. TEE helps identify the coronary

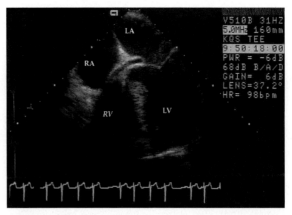

Figure 6-46. Four-chamber view demonstrating an anomalous coronary artery. LA, left atrium; LV, left ventricle; RA, right atrium; RV, right ventricle.

ostia, the initial course of the artery, and the presence of fistulas.[63]

Coronary fistulas occur rarely.[190,191] Clinically, patients with fistulas usually have no symptoms but, on auscultation, present with a continuous murmur at an atypical precordial site. The right coronary artery is involved in approximately 50% of the cases, the left in approximately 42%, and both in roughly 5%. The most common drainage sites, in order of frequency, are the right ventricle, the right atrium, the pulmonary artery, the coronary sinus, the left atrium, the left ventricle, and the superior vena cava.[192] The diagnosis of coronary artery fistula is made on coronary angiography; however, transthoracic echocardiography, with or without color Doppler, has been useful in identifying these lesions.[178,291,327] Single and biplane TEE has allowed improved imaging of the coronary arteries with regard to vessel origin and drainage site (Fig. 6-46).[48,192,233,260,264,268,322] With multiplane TEE the delineation of these abnormalities is further improved since multiplane TEE allows 180 degree rotation around the region of interest.[231,266,275]

TETRALOGY OF FALLOT AND TRANSPOSITION OF THE GREAT ARTERIES

Although tetralogy of Fallot and transposition of the great arteries can be identified by transthoracic echocardiography, TEE can provide more detail and is helpful in identifying residual defects following sur-

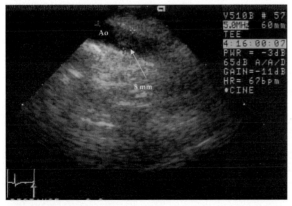

Figure 6-45. Longitudinal view of the descending thoracic aorta (Ao). The descending aorta in this patient measured 8 mm. In the adult the aorta normally measures 2.5 to 4.0 cm.

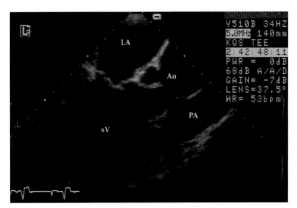

Figure 6-47. Four-chamber view of a single ventricle (sV). The aorta (Ao) and pulmonary artery (PA) are seen running parallel to one another. LA, left atrium.

gery. Tetralogy of Fallot is characterized by VSD with an overriding aorta, and infundibular narrowing with associated right ventricular hypertrophy. Multiplane TEE can be used to locate and determine the degree of right ventricular obstruction, as well as demonstrating the VSD and aortic override. Perhaps the most important role of TEE is in evaluation of the surgical repair. Tetralogy of Fallot repairs include VSD patch closure and relief of right ventricular outflow tract obstruction by resection or conduit (valve) placement.[64,241] TEE helps identify any residual leaks across the VSD patch. A deep transgastric approach of 0 to 90 degrees allows visualization of the ventricular side of the patch.[63] Because TEE can be performed in the operating room, identification of these leaks can be followed by immediate repair.

Transposition of the great arteries occurs when each of the great arteries comes off the "wrong" ventricle. The aorta comes off the right ventricle, while the pulmonary artery comes off the left ventricle (Fig. 6-47). TEE is helpful in identifying and following the course of the great vessels. In addition, TEE helps identify associated lesions such as VSD, valvular regurgitation, right ventricular outflow tract obstruction, and any other conditions that may be present.[63]

TEE in Critically Ill and Trauma Patients

TEE is useful in assessing critically ill patients[9,119,123,149,235,245,296] and trauma patients.[54,62,154,164,259,338] The availability, portability, and ease of per-

forming the exam in a timely manner are very important in assessing these patients. Transthoracic imaging is frequently difficult due to mechanical ventilation, patient position, and chest injuries.

Indications for TEE in the critically ill patient include native and prosthetic valve dysfunction, aortic dissection, endocarditis, cardiac embolism, pulmonary embolism, intracardiac shunt, complications of myocardial infarction,[9,235,245,296] and hypotension.[149] In one study, TEE correctly identified a prominent cardiovascular abnormality responsible for hemodynamic compromise in 52% of the patients studied.[296]

The most significant impact of TEE in the critically ill patient is in confirming the cause of the hemodynamic compromise, allowing immediate medical or surgical treatment. Prompt bedside TEE exams facilitate diagnosis and hence management decisions. Negative studies are also helpful in excluding cardiac sources of compromise.

In trauma patients injury to the thorax or to pulmonary, cardiac, and aortic structures by blunt forces requires immediate diagnosis and treatment. Because TEE can be performed at the bedside and is a relatively quick exam, it has become the technique of choice in many trauma situations. TEE is invaluable in assessing the heart for transplant since many of the donors are victims of motor vehicle accidents and transthoracic imaging can be difficult. As many as 15% of patients with blunt chest trauma suffer from myocardial contusion.[170] Since only a normally functioning heart can be considered for transplant, it is important to determine cardiac function. Evaluation of the right ventricle is also important. One study revealed that right ventricular contusion occurs twice as often as left ventricular contusion.[338]

Tears to the great vessels can also occur and are a life-threatening situation. As discussed previously, TEE is the technique of choice in diagnosing aortic tears. TEE can also diagnose vena caval and pericardial tears.[164] The presence of pericardial effusion has been documented in 20%[54] to 44%[124] of patients with blunt chest trauma. The rapid identification of pericardial fluid by TEE can facilitate treatment and avoid potential cardiac tamponade. Coronary artery dissection, although rare, can also occur as a result of chest trauma. TEE's improved resolution and close proximity to cardiac structures can identify coronary artery abnormalities such as dissection.[62]

Other cardiac problems and conditions associated with chest injuries can also be diagnosed with TEE, including valvular lesions and hemodynamic compromise.[54]

Summary

TEE is well suited to a number of clinical situations and provides a unique look at cardiac structures not always available on transthoracic imaging. Although still considered a semi-invasive technique, its portability, ease of performance, and low cost have made it the technique of choice in diagnosing many conditions.

REFERENCES

1. Abascal VM, Wilkins GT, O'Shea JP, et al. Prediction of successful outcomes in 130 patients undergoing percutaneous balloon mitral valvotomy. Circulation. 1990;82:448–456.
2. Abel MD, Nishimura RA, Callahan MJ, et al. Evaluation of intraoperative transesophageal two-dimensional echocardiography. Anesthesiology. 1987;66:64–68.
3. Aberg H. Atrial fibrillation. Acta Med Scand. 1969;185:373–379.
4. Acarturk E, Ozeren A, Sarica Y. Detection of aortic plaques by transesophageal echocardiography in patients with ischemic stroke. Acta Neurol Scand. 1995;92:170–172.
5. Adachi H, Omoto R, Kyo S, et al. Emergency surgical intervention of acute aortic dissection with rapid diagnosis by transesophageal echocardiography. Circulation. 1991;84(Suppl):3:14–19.
6. Adams RD, Victor M. Principles of Neurology, 4th ed. New York, McGraw-Hill; 1989:617–692.
7. Agati L, Renzi M, Sciomer S, et al. Transesophageal dipyridamole echocardiography for diagnosis of coronary artery disease. J Am Coll Cardiol. 1992;19:765–770.
8. Akins CW, Buckley MJ, Daggett W, et al. Acute traumatic disruption of the thoracic aorta: A ten year experience. Ann Thorac Surg. 1981;31:305–309.
9. Alam M. Transesophageal echocardiography in critical care units: Henry Ford Hospital experience and review of the literature. Progr Cardiovasc Dis. 1996;38(4):315–328.
10. Alam M, Gabriel F, Khaja F, et al. Transesophageal echocardiographic evaluation of left main coronary artery. Angiology. 1995;46(12):1103–1106.
11. Alam M, Rosman H, Grullon C. Transesophageal echocardiography in evaluation of atrial masses. Angiology. 1995;46(2):123–128.
12. Alam M, Sun I. Superiority of transesophageal echocardiography in detecting ruptured mitral chordae tendineae. Am Heart J. 1991;121:1819–1821.
13. Albers GW (moderator). Stroke prevention in nonvalvular atrial fibrillation. Ann Intern Med. 1991;115:727–736.
14. Amarenco P, Cohen A, Baudrimont M, et al. Transesophageal echocardiographic detection of aortic arch disease in patients with cerebral infarction. Stroke. 1992;23:1005–1009.
15. Amarenco P, Duyckaerts C, Tzourio C, et al. The prevalence of ulcerated plaques in the aortic arch in patients with stroke. N Engl J Med. 1992;326:221–225.
16. Andrade A, Vargas-Barron J, Rijlaarsdam M, et al. Utility of transesophageal echocardiography in the examination of adult patients with patent ductus arteriosus. Am Heart J. 1995;130(3):543–546.
17. Simmons HA, Cawson RA, Eykyn SJ, et al. Antibiotic prophylaxis of infective endocarditis. Lancet. 1990;335:88–89.
18. Armstrong WF. Stress echocardiography for detection of coronary artery disease. Circulation. 1991;84(Suppl)I:43–49.
19. Armstrong WF, O'Donnell J, Dillon JC, et al. Complementary value of two-dimensional exercise echocardiography to routine treadmill exercise testing. Ann Intern Med. 1986;105:829–835.
20. Arnold AZ, Mich MJ, Mazurek RP, et al. Role of prophylactic anticoagulation for direct current cardioversion in patients with atrial fibrillation or flutter. J Am Coll Cardiol. 1992;19:851–855.
21. Aronstam EM, Gomez AC, O'Connell TJ, et al. Recent surgical and pharmacological experience with acute dissecting and traumatic aneurysms. J Thorac Cardiovasc Surg. 1970;59:231–238.
22. Aschenberg W, Schlüter M, Kremer P, et al. Transesophageal two-dimensional echocardiography for the detection of left atrial appendage thrombus. J Am Coll Cardiol. 1986;7:163–166.
23. Azevedo J. Results of transesophageal echocardiography used to detect aortic rupture. N Engl J Med. 1995;333(7):458.
24. Bach D, Deeb M, Bolling S. Accuracy of intraoperative transesophageal echocardiography for estimating the severity of functional mitral regurgitation. Am J Cardiol. 1995;76:508–512.
25. Ballal RS, Nanda NV, Gatewood R, et al. Usefulness of transesophageal echocardiography in assessment of aortic dissection. Circulation. 1991;84:1903–1914.

26. Bansal R, Chandrasekaran K, Ayala K, et al. Frequency and explanation of false negative diagnosis of aortic dissection by aortography and transesophageal echocardiography. J Am Coll Cardiol. 1995; 25(6):1393–1401.

27. Barbut D, Yao-FS, Hager DN, et al. Comparison of transcranial Doppler ultrasonography and transesophageal echocardiography to monitor emboli during coronary artery bypass surgery. Stroke. 1996;27(1):87–90.

28. Bartzokis T, Lee R, Yeoh TK, et al. Transesophageal echo-Doppler echocardiographic assessment of pulmonary venous flow patterns. J Am Soc Echo Cardiogr. 1991;4:457–464.

29. Bayliss R, Clarke C, Oakley CM, et al. Incidence, mortality and prevention of infective endocarditis. J R Coll Physicians Lond. 1986;20:15–20.

30. Belkin R, Chaudhry S, Chung J, et al. Detection of ascending aorta thrombi with transesophageal echocardiography in patients with systemic embolization. Am Heart J. 1995;130(6):1294–1295.

31. Belkin RN, Hurwitz BJ, Kisslo J. Atrial septal aneurysm: Association with cerebrovascular and peripheral embolic events. Stroke. 1987;18:856–862.

32. Belkin RN, Waugh RA, Kisslo J. Interatrial shunting in atrial septal aneurysm. Am J Cardiol. 1986;57:292–297.

33. Bell GD, Reeve PA, Moshiri M, et al. Intravenous midazolam: A study of the degree of oxygen desaturation occurring during upper gastrointestinal endoscopy. Br J Clin Pharmacol. 1987;23:703–708.

34. Beppu S, Nimura Y, Sakakibara H, et al. Smoke-like echo in the left atrial cavity in mitral valve disease: Its features and significance. J Am Coll Cardiol. 1985;6:744–749.

35. Berger M, Gallerstein PE, Benhuri P, et al. Evaluation of aortic valve endocarditis by two-dimensional echocardiography. Chest. 1981;80:61–67.

36. Bjerkelund CJ, Orning OM. The efficacy of anticoagulant therapy in preventing embolism related to DC electric cardioversion of atrial fibrillation. Am J Cardiol. 1969;23:208–216.

37. Black IW, Chesterman CN, Hopkins AP, et al. Hematologic correlates of left atrial spontaneous echo contrast and thromboembolism in nonvalvular atrial fibrillation. J Am Coll Cardiol. 1993;21: 451–457.

38. Black IW, Hopkins AP, Lee LC, et al. Role of transesophageal echocardiography in evaluation of cardiogenic embolism. Br Heart J 1991;66:302–307.

39. Black IW, Hopkins AP, Lee LCL, et al. Evaluation of transesophageal echocardiography before cardioversion of atrial fibrillation and flutter in nonanticoagulated patients. Am Heart J. 1993;126:375–381.

40. Black IW, Hopkins AP, Lee LCL, et al. Left atrial spontaneous contrast: A clinical and echocardiographic analysis. J Am Coll Cardiol. 1991;18: 398–404.

41. Blauth CI, Cosgrove C, Webb BW, et al. Atheroembolism from the ascending aorta. J Thorac Cardiovasc Surg. 1992;103:1104–1112.

42. Blumberg E, Karalis D, Chandrasekaran K, et al. Endocarditis-associated paravalvular abscesses: Do clinical parameters predict the presence of abscess? Chest. 1995;107(4):898–903.

43. Brady AJ, Crake T, Oakley CM. Percutaneous catheter fragmentation and distal dispersion of proximal pulmonary embolus. Lancet. 1991;338: 1186–1189.

44. Brili S, Mcclements B, Castellanos S, et al. Significance of an atrial septal aneurysm in the presence of an ostium secundum atrial septal defect. Cardiology. 1995;86:421–425.

45. Brown R, Khandheria B, Edwards W. Cardiac papillary fibroelastoma: A treatable cause of transient ischemic attack and ischemic stroke detected by transesophageal echocardiography. Mayo Clin Proc. 1995;70:863–868.

46. Bryan A, Barzilai B, Kouchoukos T. Transesophageal echocardiography and adult cardiac operations. Ann Thorac Surg. 1995;59:773–779.

47. Burstow DJ, Oh JK, Bailey KR, et al. Cardiac tamponade: Characteristic Doppler observations. Mayo Clin Proc. 1989;64:312–324.

48. Calafiore PA, Raymond R, Schiavone WA, et al. Precise evaluation of a complex coronary arteriovenous fistula: The utility of transesophageal color Doppler. J Am Soc Echocardiogr. 1989;2: 237–241.

49. Caldarera L, Van Herweden LA, Taams MA, et al. Multiplane transesophageal echocardiography and morphology of regurgitant mitral valves in surgical repair. Eur Heart J. 1995;16:999–1006.

50. Cape EG, Yoganathan AP, Weyman AE, et al. Adjacent solid boundaries alter the size of regurgitant jets on Doppler color flow maps. J Am Coll Cardiol. 1991;17:1094–1102.

51. Castello R, Lenzen P, Aguirre F, et al. Variability in the quantitation of mitral regurgitation by Doppler color flow mapping: Comparison of transthoracic and transesophageal studies. J Am Coll Cardiol. 1992;20:433–438.

52. Castello R, Pearson AC, Labovitz AJ. Prevalence and clinical implications of atrial spontaneous contrast in patients undergoing transesophageal echocardiography. Am J Cardiol. 1990;65:1149–1153.

53. Castello R, Pearson AC, Lenzen P, et al. Effect of mitral regurgitation on pulmonary venous velocities

derived from transesophageal echocardiography color-guided pulsed Doppler imaging. J Am Coll Cardiol. 1991;17:1499–1506.

54. Catoire P, Orliaguet G, Liu N, et al. Systematic transesophageal echocardiography for detection of mediastinal lesions in patients with multiple injuries. J Trauma. 1995;38(1):96–102.

55. Cerebral Embolism Task Force. Cardiogenic brain embolism. Arch Neurol. 1986;43:71–84.

56. Cerebral Embolism Task Force. Cardiogenic brain embolism. The second report of the Cerebral Embolism Task Force. Arch Neurol. 1989;46: 727–743.

57. Chammas E, Trinca M, Goullard L, et al. Multiple cerebral infarcts associated with an atrial septal aneurysm: Superimposed thrombus detected by transesophageal echocardiography. Angiology. 1995; 46(4):327–331.

58. Chan KL. Usefulness of transesophageal echocardiography in the diagnosis of conditions mimicking aortic dissection. Am Heart J. 1991;122:495–504.

59. Chan KL, Cohen GI, Sochowski RA, et al. Complications of transesophageal echocardiography in ambulatory adult patients: Analysis of 1500 consecutive examinations. J Am Soc Echocardiogr. 1991; 4:577–582.

60. Chan S, Kannam J, Douglas P, et al. Multiplane transesophageal echocardiographic assessment of left atrial appendage anatomy and function. Am J Cardiol. 1995;76:528–530.

61. Chao K, Moises V, Shandas R, et al. Surface adherence (the Coanda effect) reduces regurgitant jet size: Studies by color Doppler in an in-vitro model (abstract). J Am Coll Cardiol. 1990;15:121A.

62. Cherng W, Bullard M, Chang H, et al. Diagnosis of coronary artery dissection following blunt chest trauma by transesophageal echocardiography. J Trauma. 1995;39(4):772–774.

63. Child JS. Congenital heart disease. *In* Roelandt JRTC, Pandoan NG (eds): Multiplane Transesophageal Echocardiography. New York, Churchill Livingstone; 1996:173–198.

64. Child JS. Echocardiographic assessment of adults with tetralogy of Fallot. Echocardiography. 1993; 10:1–12.

65. Child JS. Echo-Doppler and color flow imaging in congenital heart disease. Cardiol Clin. 1990;8: 289–313.

66. Child JS, Marelli AJ. The application of transesophageal echocardiography in the adult with congenital heart disease. *In* Maurer G (ed): Transesophageal Echocardiography. New York, McGraw-Hill, 1994:159–170.

67. Clark RE, Brillman J, Davis DA, et al. Microemboli during cardiopulmonary bypass grafting: Genesis and effect on outcome. J Thorac Cardiovasc Surg. 1995;109:249–258.

68. Click RL, Espinosa RE, Khandheria BK. Source of embolism: Utility of transesophageal echocardiography. *In* Freeman WK, Seward JB, Khandheria BK, et al (eds): Transesophageal Echocardiography. Boston, Little, Brown; 1994:469–499.

69. Cohen GI, Klein AL, Chan KL, et al. Transesophageal echocardiographic diagnosis of right-sided cardiac masses in patients with central lines. Am J Cardiol. 1992;70:925–929.

70. Cohn S, Burns G, Jaffe C, et al. Exclusion of aortic tear in the unstable trauma patient: The utility of transesophageal echocardiography. J Trauma. 1995;39(6):1087–1090.

71. Come PC. Echocardiographic evaluation of pulmonary embolism and its response to therapeutic interventions. Chest. 1992;151–62S.

72. Come PC, Riley MF. M-mode and cross-sectional echocardiographic recognition of fibrosis and calcification of the mitral valve chordae and left ventricular papillary muscles. Am J Cardiol. 1982;49: 461–466.

73. Condit JR, Benoit SB, Gottdiener JS. Transesophageal echocardiography is of no additional diagnostic value to transthoracic echocardiography in the evaluation of mitral stenosis for balloon mitral valvuloplasty. Circulation. 1993;88:I–351.

74. Coon WW, Willis PW. Hemorrhagic complications of anticoagulant therapy. Arch Intern Med. 1974; 133:386–392.

75. Coplen SE, Antman EM, Berlin JA, et al. Efficacy and safety of quinidine therapy for maintenance of sinus rhythm after cardioversion. A meta-analysis of randomized controlled trials. Circulation. 1990;82: 1106–1116.

76. Cormier B, Vahanian A, Michel PL, et al. Transesophageal echocardiography in the assessment of percutaneous mitral commissurotomy. Eur Heart J. 1991;12:61–65.

77. Crawford ES. The diagnosis and management of aortic dissection. JAMA. 1990;264:2537–2541.

78. Crowley JJ, Kenny A, Dardas P, et al. Identification of right atrial thrombi using transesophageal echocardiography. Eur Heart J. 1995;16:708–710.

79. Cujec B, Polasek P, Voll C, et al. Transesophageal echocardiography in the detection of potential cardiac source of embolism in stroke patients. Stroke. 1991;22:727–733.

80. Cunha CLP, Giuliani ER, Callahan JA, et al. Echocardiographic findings in patients with prosthetic heart valve malfunction. Mayo Clin Proc. 1980;55: 231–242.

81. Cyran SE. Coarctation of the aorta in the adolescent and adult: Echocardiographic evaluation prior to and following surgical repair. Echocardiography. 1993;10:553–563.

82. Daily PO, Trueblood HW, Stinson EB, et al. Management of acute aortic dissections. Ann Thorac Surg. 1970;10:237–247.

83. Dajani AS, Bisno AL, Chung KJ, et al. Prevention of bacterial endocarditis. Recommendations by the American Heart Association. JAMA. 1990;22:2919–2933.

84. Daniel WG, Angermann C, Engberding R, et al. Transesophageal echocardiography in patients with cerebral ischemic events and arterial embolism—a European multicenter study (abstract). Circulation. 1989;80(Suppl II):473.

85. Daniel WG, Erbel R, Kasper W, et al. Safety of transesophageal echocardiography: A multicenter survey of 10,419 examinations. Circulation. 1991;83:817–821.

86. Daniel WG, Freeberg RS, Grote J, et al. Incidence of left atrial thrombi in patients with non-valvular atrial fibrillation—a multicenter study using transesophageal echocardiography (abstract). Circulation. 1992;86(Suppl I):396.

87. Daniel WG, Mügge A. Transesophageal echocardiography. N Engl J Med. 1995;332(19):1268–1279.

88. Daniel WG, Nellessen U, Schröder E, et al. Left atrial spontaneous echo contrast in mitral valve disease: An indicator for an increased thromboembolic risk. J Am Coll Cardiol. 1988;11:1204–1211.

89. Davila-Roman V, Waggoner A, Hopkins W, et al. Right ventricular dysfunction in low output syndrome after cardiac operations: Assessment by transesophageal echocardiography. Ann Thorac Surg. 1995;60:1081–1086.

90. DeBakey ME, Henly WS, Cooley DA, et al. Surgical management of dissecting aneurysms of the aorta. J Thorac Cardiovasc Surg. 1965;49:130–149.

91. DeBelder MA, Lovat LB, Tourikis L, et al. Left atrial spontaneous contrast echoes—markers of thromboembolic risk in patients with atrial fibrillation. Eur Heart J. 1993;14:326–335.

92. Denning K, Dacian S, Hall D, et al. Doppler echocardiographic, 2-dimensional echocardiographic and invasive hemodynamic determination of valve orifice area in mitral stenosis: A comparative study. J Am Coll Cardiol. 1985;5:404.

93. Denning K, Rudolph W. Mitral valve apparatus. In Roelandt JRTC., Pandian NC (eds): Multiplane Transesophageal Echocardiography. New York, Churchill Livingstone; 1996:69–88.

94. Denning K, Wolfram D, Henneke KH, et al. Transesophageal Doppler echocardiographic assessment of flow velocity within pulmonary veins. Eur Heart J. 1988;9:I-379.

95. DeRook FA, Comess KA, Albers GW, et al. Transesophageal echocardiography in the evaluation of stroke. Ann Intern Med. 1992;117:922–932.

96. DeSanctis RW, Doroghazi RM, Austen WG, et al. Aortic dissection. N Engl J Med. 1987;317:1060–1067.

97. DeVille J, Corley D, Jin B, et al. Assessment of intracardiac masses by transesophageal echocardiography. Texas Heart Inst J. 1995;22:134–137.

98. Di Pasquale G, Andreoti A, Graxi P, et al. Cardioembolic stroke from atrial septal aneurysm. Stroke. 1988;19:640–643.

99. DiTullio M, Sacco RL, Gopal A, et al. Patent foramen ovale as a risk factor for cryptogenic stroke. Ann Intern Med. 1992;117:461–465.

100. Dodds GA III, Tice FD, Li J, et al. Aortic valve and thoracic aorta. In Roelandt JRTC, Pandian NG (eds): Multiplane Transesophageal Echocardiography. New York, Churchill Livingstone; 1996:89–116.

101. Dunker D, Stoddard M, Prince C, et al. Potential for contamination of transesophageal echocardiographic scopes by radionuclides from patients undergoing nuclear imaging studies. Am Heart J. 1995;130:397–398.

102. Dunn M, Alexander J, de Silva R, et al. Antithrombotic therapy in atrial fibrillation. Chest. 1989;95:118S–27S.

103. Duran CMG, Gometza B, Balasundaram A, et al. A feasibility study of valve repair in rheumatic mitral regurgitation. Eur Heart J. 1991;12(Suppl):34–38.

104. Eagle KA, De Sanctis RW. Aortic dissection. Curr Probl Cardiol. 1989;14:225–278.

105. Eagle KA, De Sanctis RW. Diseases of the aorta. In Braunwald E (ed): Heart Disease. Philadelphia, WB Saunders; 1992:1528–1557.

106. Elat Study Group: Embolism in left atrial thrombi: Baseline clinical and echocardiographic data. Cardiology. 1995;86:457–463.

107. Ellis CJ, Waite ST, Coverdale HA, et al. Transesophageal echocardiography in patients with prosthetic heart valves and systemic emboli: Is it a useful investigation? N Z Med J. 1995;108(1008):376–377.

108. Erbel R, Engberding R, Daniel W, et al. Echocardiography in diagnosis of aortic dissection. Lancet. 1989;1:457–461.

109. Erbel R, Mohr-Kahaly S, Oelert H, et al. Diagnostic strategies in suspected aortic dissection: Comparison

of computed tomography, aortography, and transesophageal echocardiography. Am J Cardiac Imaging. 1990;4:157–172.

110. Erbel R, Mohr-Kahaly S, Rennollet H, et al. Diagnosis of aortic dissection: The value of transesophageal echocardiography. Thorac Cardiovasc Surg. 1987; 35(Special Issue 1):126–133.

111. Erbel R, Rohmann S, Drexler M, et al. Improved diagnostic value of echocardiography in patients with infective endocarditis by transesophageal approach. A prospective study. Eur Heart J. 1988;9:43–53.

112. Essop R. Transesophageal echocardiography in infective endocarditis: The standard for the 1990s? Am Heart J. 1995;130:402–404.

113. Evangelista A, Carcia-del-Castillo H, Gonzalez-Alujas T, et al. Diagnosis of ascending aortic dissection by transesophageal echocardiography: Utility of M-mode in recognizing artifacts. J Am Coll Cardiol. 1996;27(1):102–107.

114. Eyre R, Hurley L, Burger A, et al. Use of dynamic two-dimensional transesophageal echocardiography for renal cell carcinoma with cavoatrial tumor thrombus. Urol Int. 1995;54:132–136.

115. Fatkin D, Herbert E, Feneley MP. Hematology correlates of spontaneous echo contrast in patients with atrial fibrillation and implications for thromboembolic risk. Am J Cardiol. 1994;73:672–676.

116. Feczko JD, Lynch L, Pless FE, et al. An autopsy case review of 142 non-penetrating (blunt) injuries of the aorta. J Trauma. 1992;33:846–849.

117. Fehske W, Omran H, Manz M, et al. Color coded Doppler imaging of the vena contracta as a basis for quantification of mitral regurgitation. Am J Cardiol. 1994;73:268–274.

118. Feigenbaum H (ed). Diseases of the Aorta in Echocardiography, 5th ed. Philadelphia, Lea & Febiger; 1994:632–633.

119. Feinberg M, Hopkins W, Davila-Roman V, et al. Multiplane transesophageal echocardiographic Doppler imaging accurately determines cardiac output measurements in critically ill patients. Chest. 1995;107(3):769–773.

120. Fenster PE, Comess KA, Marsh R, et al. Conversion of atrial fibrillation to sinus rhythm by acute intravenous procainamide infusion. Am Heart J. 1983;106: 501–504.

121. Fisher D, Fisher E, Budd J, et al. The incidence of patent foramen ovale in 1,000 consecutive patients: A contrast transesophageal echocardiography study. Chest. 1995;107(6):1504–1509.

122. Flachskampf FA, Weyman AE, Gillam L, et al. Aortic regurgitation shortens Doppler pressure half-time in mitral stenosis: Clinical evidence, in vitro simulation and theoretic analysis. J Am Coll Cardiol. 1990;16: 396–404.

123. Foster E, Schiller NB. The role of transesophageal echocardiography in critical care: UCSF experience. J Am Soc Echocardiogr. 1992;5:368–374.

124. Frazee RC, Mucha P, Farnell MB, et al. Objective evaluation of blunt cardiac trauma. J Trauma. 1986; 26:510–520.

125. Frazin L, Talano JV, Stephanides L, et al. Esophageal echocardiography. Circulation. 1976;54: 102–108.

126. Freedberg R, Goodkin G, Perez J, et al. Valve strands are strongly associated with systemic embolization: A transesophageal echocardiographic study. J Am Coll Cardiol. 1995;26(7):1709–1712.

127. Freeman W. Diseases of the thoracic aorta: Assessment by transesophageal echocardiography. *In* Freeman W, Seward JB, Khandheria BK, et al. (eds): Transesophageal Echocardiography. Boston, Little, Brown; 1994:425–467.

128. Freeman WK, Schaff HV, Khandheria BK, et al. Intraoperative evaluation of mitral regurgitation and repair by transesophageal echocardiography: Incidence and significance of systolic anterior motion. J Am Coll Cardiol. 1992;2:599–609.

129. Frohwein S, Klein L, Lane A, et al. Transesophageal dobutamine stress: echocardiography in the evaluation of coronary artery disease. J Am Coll Cardiol. 1995;25(4):823–829.

130. Fukuda N, Oki T, Luchi A, et al. Pulmonary and systemic venous flow patterns assessed by transesophageal Doppler echocardiography in congenital absence of the pericardium. Am J Cardiol. 1995;75: 1286–1288.

131. Gaither NS, Rogan KM, Stajduhar K, et al. Anomalous origin and course of coronary arteries in adults: Identification and improved imaging utilizing transesophageal echocardiography. Am Heart J. 1991; 122:69–75.

132. Gallet B, Malergue MC, Adam C, et al. Atrial septal aneurysm: A potential cause of systemic embolism. Br Heart J. 1985;53:310–312.

133. Galzerano D, Tuccillo B, Lama D, et al. Morphofunctional assessment of interatrial septum: A transesophageal echocardiographic study. Int J Cardiol. 1995;51:73–77.

134. Geibel A, Kasper W, Behroz A, et al. Risk of transesophageal echocardiography in awake patients with cardiac diseases. Am J Cardiol. 1988;62:337–339.

135. Gelernt MD, Mogtader A, Hahn RT. Transesophageal echocardiography to diagnose and demonstrate resolution of an acute massive pulmonary embolus. Chest. 1992;102:297–299.

136. Godwin JD, Breiman RS, Speckman JM. Problems and pitfalls in the evaluation of thoracic aortic dissection by computed tomography. J Comput Assist Tomogr. 1982;6:750–756.

137. Goldhaber SZ, Morpurgo M. Diagnosis, treatment and prevention of pulmonary embolism. Report of the WHO/International Society and Federation of Cardiology Task Force. JAMA. 1992;268:1727–1733.

138. Grayburn PA, Fehske W, Omran H, et al. Multiplane transesophageal echocardiographic assessment of mitral regurgitation by Doppler color flow mapping of the vena contracta. Am J Cardiol. 1994;74:912–916.

139. Grayburn PA, Smith MD, Gurley JC, et al. Effect of aortic regurgitation on the assessment of mitral valve orifice area by Doppler pressure half-time in mitral stenosis. Am J Cardiol. 1987;60:322–326.

140. Grimm R, Leung D, Black I, et al. Left atrial appendage "stunning" after spontaneous conversion of atrial fibrillation demonstrated by transesophageal Doppler echocardiography. Am Heart J. 1995;130:174–176.

141. Grogan M, Smith HCM, Gersh BJ, et al. Left ventricular dysfunction due to atrial fibrillation in patients initially believed to have idiopathic dilated cardiomyopathy. Am J Cardiol. 1992;69:1570–1573.

142. Grossman W. Profiles in valvular heart disease. *In* Grossman W (ed): Cardiac Catheterization and Angiography, 2nd ed. Philadelphia, Lea & Febiger; 1980:310–311.

143. Grote J, Mugge A, Schafers J, et al. Multiplane transesophageal echocardiography detection of a papillary fibroelastoma of the aortic valve causing myocardial infarction. Eur Heart J. 1995;16:426–429.

144. Gueret P, Vignon P, Fournier P, et al. Transesophageal echocardiography for the diagnosis and management of nonobstructive thrombosis of mechanical mitral valve prosthesis. Circulation. 1995;91(1):103–110.

145. Hàgen PT, Scholz DG, Edwards WD. Incidence and size of patent foramen ovale during the first 10 decades of life: An autopsy study of 965 normal hearts. Mayo Clin Proc. 1984;59:17–20.

146. Hanley PC, Tajik AJ, Hynes JK, et al. Diagnosis and classification of atrial septal aneurysm by two-dimensional echocardiography: Report of 80 consecutive cases. J Am Coll Cardiol. 1985;6:1370–1382.

147. Hausmann D, Mügge A, Daniel W. Identification of patent foramen ovale permitting paradoxic embolism. J Am Coll Cardiol. 1995;26(4):1030–1038.

148. Heidenreich P, Chou T, Smedira N, et al. Catheter fragmentation of massive pulmonary embolus: Guidance with transesophageal echocardiography. Am Heart J. 1995;130(6):1306–1308.

149. Heidenreich P, Stainback R, Redberg R, et al. Transesophageal echocardiography predicts mortality in critically ill patients with unexplained hypotension. J Am Coll Cardiol. 1995;26(1):152–158.

150. Helmcke F, Nanda N, Hsiung M, et al. Color Doppler assessment of mitral regurgitation with orthogonal planes. Circulation. 1987;75:175–183.

151. Himelman RB, Kusumoto F, Oken K, et al. The flail mitral valve: Echocardiographic findings by precordial and transesophageal imaging and Doppler color flow mapping. J Am Coll Cardiol. 1991;17:272–279.

152. Hoffman R, Flachskamp FA, Hanrath P. Planimetry of orifice area in aortic stenosis using multiplane transesophageal echocardiography. J Am Coll Cardiol. 1993;22:529–534.

153. Hoffman T, Kasper W, Meinertz T, et al. Determination of aortic valve orifice area in aortic valve stenosis by two-dimensional transesophageal echocardiography. Am J Cardiol. 1987;59:330–335.

154. Huei-ming Ma M, Hwang J-J, Lai L, et al. Transesophageal echocardiographic assessment of mitral valve position and pulmonary venous flow during cardiopulmonary resuscitation in humans. Circulation. 1995;92(4):854–861.

155. Hull RD, Hirsh J, Carter CJ, et al. Pulmonary angiography, ventilation lung scanning, and venography for clinically suspected pulmonary embolism with abnormal perfusion lung scan. Ann Intern Med. 1983;98:891–899.

156. Iliceto S, Papa A, Sorino M, et al. Combined atrial septal aneurysm and mitral valve prolapse: Detection by two-dimensional echocardiography. Am J Cardiol. 1986;54:1151–1154.

157. Isada L, Klein AL, Torelli J, et al. "Strands" on mitral valve prostheses by transesophageal echocardiography—another potential embolic source (abstract). J Am Coll Cardiol. 1992;19:32A.

158. Jain S, Helmcke F, Fan PH, et al. Limitation of pulmonary venous flow criteria in the assessment of mitral regurgitation severity by transesophageal echocardiography. Circulation. 1990;82:III-551.

159. Jones HR, Caplan LR, Come PC, et al. Cerebral emboli of paradoxical origin. Ann Neurol. 1983;13:314–9.

160. Kannel WB, Abbott RD, Savage DD, et al. Epidemiologic features of chronic atrial fibrillation: The Framingham Study. N Engl J Med. 1982;306:1018–1022.

161. Karalis DG, Chandrasekaran K, Victor MF, et al. Recognition and embolic potential of intraaortic atherosclerotic debris. J Am Coll Cardiol. 1991;17: 73–78.

162. Karp K, Teien D, Bjerle P, et al. Reassessment of valve area determinations in mitral stenosis by the pressure half-time method: Impact of left ventricular stiffness and peak diastolic pressure difference. J Am Coll Cardiol. 1989;13:594–599.

163. Kearney PA, Smith DW, Johnson SB, et al. Use of transesophageal echocardiography in the evaluation of traumatic aortic injury. J Trauma. 1993;3: 696–701.

164. Kennedy N, Ireland A, McConaghy PM. Transesophageal echocardiographic examination of a patient with venacaval and pericardial tears after blunt chest trauma. Br J Anesth. 1995;75:495–497.

165. Khandheria BK. Suspected bacterial endocarditis: To TEE or not to TEE. J Am Coll Cardiol. 1993;21: 222–224.

166. Khandheria BK, Freeman WK, Sinak LJ. Infective endocarditis: Evaluation by transesophageal echocardiography. *In* Freeman WK, Seward JB, Khandheria BK, et al (eds): Transesophageal Echocardiography. Boston, Little, Brown; 1994:307–337.

167. Khandheria BK, Oh J. Transesophageal echocardiography: State of the art and future directions. Am J Cardiol. 1992;69:61H–75H.

168. Khoury AF, Afridi I, Quinines MA, et al. Transesophageal echocardiography in critically ill patients: Feasibility, safety and impact on management. Am Heart J. 1994;127:1363–1371.

169. Kieny JR, Facelo A, Sacrez A, et al. Increase in radionuclide left ventricular ejection fraction after cardioversion of chronic atrial fibrillation in idiopathic dilated cardiomyopathy. Eur Heart J. 1992;13: 1290–1295.

170. Kissane RW. Traumatic heart disease: Nonpenetrating injuries. Circulation. 1953;6:421–425.

171. Kitchens JM, Flegel KM. Atrial fibrillation, stroke and anticoagulation: What is to be done? J Gen Intern Med. 1986;1:126–129.

172. Klein AL, Obarski TP, Stewart WJ, et al. Transesophageal Doppler echocardiography of pulmonary venous flow: A new marker of mitral regurgitation severity. J Am Coll Cardiol. 1991;18:518–526.

173. Kodali S, Jamieson WRE, Leia-Stephens M, et al. Traumatic rupture of the thoracic aorta: A twenty year review—1969–1989. Circulation. 1991; (Suppl III):33.

174. Konstadt S, Reich D, Kahn R, et al. Transesophageal echocardiography can be used to screen for ascending aortic atherosclerosis. Anesth Analg. 1995;81: 225–228.

175. Kopecky SL, Gersh BJ, McGoon MD, et al. The natural history of lone atrial fibrillation: A population based study over three decades. N Engl J Med. 1987; 317:669–674.

176. Kram HB, Wohlmuth DA, Appel PL, et al. Clinical and radiographic indications for aortography in blunt chest trauma. J Vasc Surg. 1987;6:168–176.

177. Kreis A, Lambertz H, Gerich N, et al. Value of the transesophageal echocardiographic pulmonary venous flow in classification of mitral insufficiency. Circulation. 1989;80:II-577.

178. Kronzon I, Winer HE, Cohen M. Noninvasive diagnosis of left coronary arteriovenous fistula communicating with the right ventricle. Am J Cardiol. 1982; 49:1811–1813.

179. Lagattolla N, Burnand G, Stewart A. Role of transesophageal echocardiography in determining the source of peripheral arterial embolism. Br J Surg. 1995;82:1651–1654.

180. Laissy J, Blanc F, Soyer P, et al. Thoracic aortic dissection: Diagnosis with transesophageal echocardiography versus MR imaging. Radiology. 1995; 194(2):331–336.

181. Lambertz H, Kreis A, Trümper H, et al. Simultaneous transesophageal atrial pacing and transesophageal two-dimensional echocardiography: A new method of stress echocardiography. J Am Coll Cardiol. 1990;16:1143–1153.

182. Larson EB, Stratton JR, Pearlman AS. Selective use of two-dimensional echocardiography in stroke syndromes (editorial). Ann Intern Med. 1981;95: 112–124.

183. Latham P, Hodgins L. A gastric laceration after transesophageal echocardiography in a patient undergoing aortic valve replacement. Anesth Analg. 1995;81:641–642.

184. Lattanzi F, Pcano E, Landini L, et al. In vivo identification of mitral valve fibrosis and calcium by real-time quantificative ultrasonic analysis. Am J Cardiol. 1990;65:355–359.

185. Laupacis A, Albers G, Dunn M, et al. Antithrombotic therapy in atrial fibrillation. Chest. 1992; 102(Suppl):426–433.

186. Lechet P, Mass JL, Lascault G, et al. Prevalence of patent foramen ovale in patients with stroke. N Engl J Med. 1988;3:1148–1152.

187. Lee RJ, Bartzokis T, Yeoh TK, et al. Enhanced detection of intracardiac sources of emboli by transesophageal echocardiography. Stroke. 1991;22:734–739.

188. Leibowitz G, Keller N, Daniel W, et al. Transesophageal versus transthoracic echocardiography in the evaluation of right atrial tumors. Am Heart J. 1995; 130(6):1224–1227.

189. Leung D, Black I, Cranney G, et al. Selection of patients for transesophageal echocardiography after stroke and systemic embolic events: Role of transthoracic echocardiography. Stroke. 1995;26(10): 1820–1824.

190. Levine DC, Fellows KE, Abrams HL. Hemodynamically significant primary anomalies of the coronary arteries. Circulation. 1978;58:25–34.

191. Liberthson RR, Sagar K, Berkoben JP, et al. Congenital coronary arteriovenous fistula: Report of 13 patients, review of the literature and delineation of management. Circulation. 1979;59:849–853.

192. Lin F, Chang H, Chern M, et al. Multiplane transesophageal echocardiography in the diagnosis of congenital coronary artery fistula. Am Heart J. 1995; 130(6):1236–1244.

193. Lown B, Perlroth MG, Kaidbey S, et al. "Cardioversion" of atrial fibrillation: A report on treatment of 65 episodes in 50 patients. N Engl J Med. 1963;269: 325–331.

194. Loyd D, Eng D, Ask P, et al. Pressure half-time does not always predict mitral valve area correctly. J Am Soc Echocardiogr. 1988;1:313–321.

195. Lynch M, Balk M, Lee R, et al. Role of transesophageal echocardiography in the management of patients with bronchogenic carcinoma invading the left atrium. Am J Cardiol. 1995;76:1101–1102.

196. Magarey FR. On the mode of formation of Lambl's excrescences and their relationship to chronic thickening of the mitral valve. J Pathol Bacteriol. 1949; 61:203–208.

197. Manning WJ, Leeman DE, Gotch PJ, et al. Pulsed Doppler evaluation of atrial mechanical function after electrical cardioversion of atrial fibrillation. J Am Coll Cardiol. 1989;13:617–623.

198. Manning WJ, Reis GJ, Douglas PS. Use of transesophageal echocardiography to detect left atrial thrombi before percutaneous balloon dilatation of mitral valve: A prospective study. Br Heart J. 1992; 67:170–173.

199. Manning WJ, Silverman DI, Gordon SPF, et al. Safety of cardioversion from atrial fibrillation using transesophageal echo to exclude atrial thrombi. N Engl J Med. 1993;328:750–755.

200. Manning WJ, Silverman DI, Katz SE, et al. Impaired left atrial mechanical function after cardioversion: Relationship to the duration of atrial fibrillation. J Am Coll Cardiol. 1994;23:1535–1540.

201. Manning W, Silverman D, Keighley C, et al. Transesophageal echocardiographically facilitated early cardioversion from atrial fibrillation using short-term anticoagulation: Final results of a prospective 4.5 year study. J Am Coll Cardiol. 1995;25(6): 1354–1361.

202. Marelli AJ, Child JS, Perloff JK. Transesophageal echocardiography in adult congenital heart disease. Cardiol Clin. 1993;11:505–520.

203. Marino P, Zanolla L, Perini GP, et al. Critical assessment of two-dimensional echocardiographic estimation of the mitral valve area in rheumatic mitral valve disease: Calcific deposits in the valve as a major determinant of the accuracy of the method. Eur Heart J. 1981;2:197–203.

204. Marwick TH, Torlli J, Obarski T, et al. Assessment of the mitral valve splitability score by transthoracic and transesophageal echocardiography. Am J Cardiol. 1991;68:1106–1107.

205. Matsumoto M, Hanrath P, Kremer P, et al. Evaluation of left ventricular performance during supine exercise by transesophageal M-mode echocardiography in normal subjects. Br Heart J. 1982;48:61–66.

206. Matsuzaki M, Shimizu M, Nomoto R, et al. Assessment of left ventricular anterior wall motion: A new application of esophageal echocardiography. J Cardiogr. 1978;8:113–124.

207. Melendez LJ, Chan KL, Cheung PK, et al. Incidence of bacteremia in transesophageal echocardiography: Prospective study of 140 consecutive patients. J Am Coll Cardiol. 1991;18:1650–1654.

208. Mentec H, Vignon P, Terre S, et al. Frequency of bacteremia associated with transesophageal echocardiography in intensive care unit patients: A prospective study of 139 patients. Crit Care Med. 1995; 23(7):1194–1199.

209. Mikell FL, Asinger RW, Elsperger KJ, et al. Regional stasis of blood in dysfunctional left ventricle: Echocardiographic detection and differentiation from early thrombosis. Circulation. 1982;66:755–763.

210. Miller FA, Khandheria BK, Tajik AJ. Echocardiographic assessment of prosthetic heart valves. *In* Freeman WK, Seward JB, Khandheria BK, et al (eds): Transesophageal Echocardiography. Boston, Little, Brown; 1994:243–306.

211. Mohr-Kahaly S, Erbel R, Puth M, et al. Aortic intraluminal hematoma visualized by transesophageal echocardiography (abstract). Circulation. 1991; 84(Suppl 2):II–128.

212. Mohr-Kahaly S, Puth M, Erbel R, et al. Intraluminal hematoma visualized by transesophageal echocardiography: An early sign of aortic dissection (abstract). J Am Coll Cardiol. 1991;17(Suppl A):20A.

213. Morris JJ Jr, Entman M, North WC, et al. The changes in cardiac output with reversion of atrial fibrillation to sinus rhythm. Circulation. 1965;31: 670–678.

214. Mügge A, Daniel W, Angermann C, et al. Atrial septal aneurysm in adult patients: A multicenter study using transthoracic and transesophageal echocardiography. Circulation. 1995;91(11): 2785–2792.

215. Mügge A, Daniel WG, Frank G, et al. Echocardiography in infective endocarditis: Reassessment of prognostic implications of vegetation size determined by the transthoracic and transesophageal approach. J Am Coll Cardiol. 1989;14:631–638.

216. Mügge A, Daniel WG, Hausmann D, et al. Diagnosis of left atrial appendage thrombi by transesophageal echocardiography: Clinical implications and follow-up. Am J Cardiac Imaging. 1990;4:173–179.

217. Murdoch I, Marsh MJ, Tibby SM, et al. Continuous hemodynamic monitoring in children: Use of transesophageal Doppler. Acta Pediatr. 1995;84: 761–764.

218. Nellesen U, Daniel WG, Matheis G, et al. Impending paradoxical embolism from atrial thrombus: Correct diagnosis by transesophageal echocardiography and prevention by surgery. J Am Coll Cardiol. 1985;5: 1002–1004.

219. Nellesen U, Schnittger I, Appleton CP, et al. Transesophageal two-dimensional echocardiographic and color Doppler flow velocity mapping in the evaluation of cardiac valve prosthesis. Circulation. 1988; 78:848–855.

220. Nienaber CA, van Kodolitsch Y, Nicolas V, et al. The diagnosis of thoracic aortic dissection by noninvasive imaging procedures. N Engl J Med. 1993;328:1–9.

221. Nikutta P, Mantey-Stiers F, Becht I, et al. Risk of bacteremia induced by transesophageal echocardiography: Analysis of 100 consecutive procedures. J Am Soc Echocardiogr. 1992;5:168–172.

222. Nishimura RA, Tajik AJ, Shub C, et al. Role of two-dimensional echocardiography in the prediction of in-hospital complications after acute myocardial infarction. J Am Coll Cardiol. 1984;4:1080–1087.

223. Oh JK, Click RL, Pellikka PA. Transesophageal echocardiography in ischemic heart disease. *In* Freeman WK, Seward JB, Khandheria BK, et al. (eds): Transesophageal Echocardiography. Boston, Little, Brown; 1994:167–185.

224. O'Leary P, Hagler D, Seward J, et al. Biplane intraoperative transesophageal echocardiography in congenital heart disease. Mayo Clin Proc. 1995;70: 317–326.

225. Olson LJ, Freeman WK, Enriquez-Sarano M, et al. Transesophageal echocardiographic evaluation of native valvular heart disease. *In* Freeman WK, Seward JB, Khandheria BK, et al (eds): Transesophageal Echocardiography. Boston, Little, Brown; 1994:187–242.

226. O'Murchu B, Seward J. Adult congenital heart disease: Obstructive and nonobstructive cor triatriatum. Circulation. 1995;92:3574.

227. Orsinelli D, Pearson A. Detection of prosthetic valve strands by transesophageal echocardiography: Clinical significance in patients with suspected cardiac source of embolism. J Am Coll Cardiol. 1995;26(7): 1713–1718.

228. Orsinelli D, Pearson AC. Usefulness of transesophageal echocardiography to screen for left atrial thrombus before elective cardioversion for atrial fibrillation. Am J Cardiol. 1993;72:1337–1339.

229. Oxorn D, Towers M. Traumatic aortic disruption: False positive diagnosis on transesophageal echocardiography. J Trauma. 1995;39(2):386–387.

230. Padayachee TS, Parsons S, Theobold R, et al. The detection of microbubbles in the middle cerebral artery during cardiopulmonary bypass: A transcranial Doppler ultrasound investigation using membrane and bubble oxygenators. Ann Thorac Surg. 1987; 44:298–302.

231. Pandian NG, Hsu T-L, Schwatz SL, et al. Multiplane transesophageal echocardiography: Imaging planes, echocardiographic anatomy, and clinical experience with a prototype phased array omniplane probe. Echocardiography. 1992;9:649–666.

232. Parmely L, Mattingly T, Manion W, et al. Non-penetrating traumatic injury of the aorta. Circulation. 1958;17:1086–1101.

233. Pearce FB, Sheikh KH, deBrujin NP, et al. Imaging of the coronary arteries by transesophageal echocardiography. J Am Soc Echocardiogr. 1989;2: 276–283.

234. Pearlman AS, Gardin JM, Martin RP, et al. Guidelines for physician training in transesophageal echocardiography: Recommendations of the American Society of Echocardiography Committee for physician training in echocardiography. J Am Soc Echocardiogr. 1992;5:187–194.

235. Pearson A. Noninvasive evaluation of the hemodynamically unstable patient: The advantages of seeing clearly. Mayo Clin Proc. 1995;70: 1012–1014.

236. Pearson A. Transesophageal echocardiographic screening for atrial thrombus before cardioversion of atrial fibrillation: When should we look before we leap? J Am Coll Cardiol. 1995;25(6):1362–1364.

237. Pearson AC, Castello R, Labovitz AJ. Safety and utilization of transesophageal in the critically ill patient. Am Heart J. 1990;119:1083–1089.

238. Pearson AC, Castello R, Wallace PM, et al. Effects of mitral regurgitation on pulmonary venous velocities

derived from transesophageal echocardiography. Circulation. 1989;80:II–571.

239. Pearson AC, Labovitz AJ, Tatineni S, et al. Superiority of transesophageal echocardiography in detecting cardiac source of embolism in patients with cerebral ischemia of uncertain etiology. J Am Coll Cardiol. 1991;17:66–72.

240. Pearson AC, Nagelhout D, Castello R, et al. Atrial septal aneurysm and stroke: A transesophageal echocardiographic study. J Am Coll Cardiol. 1991;18: 1223–1229.

241. Perloff JK, Child JS. Congenital Heart Disease in Adults. Philadelphia, WB Saunders; 1991.

242. Peterson J, Orsinelli D. Transesophageal echocardiography: When is it superior to standard imaging in clinical practice? Postgrad Med. 1995;97(3):47–61.

243. Peterson P, Godtfredsen J. Embolic complications in paroxysmal atrial fibrillation. Stroke. 1986;17: 622–626.

244. Pieper E, Hellemans I, Hamer H, et al. Additional value of biplane transesophageal echocardiography in assessing the genesis of mitral regurgitation and the feasibility of valve repair. Am J Cardiol. 1995;75: 489–493.

245. Poelaert J, Trouerbach J, DeBuyzere M, et al. Evaluation of transesophageal echocardiography as a diagnostic and therapeutic aid in a critical care setting. Chest. 1995;107(3):774–779.

246. Pop G, Sutherland GR, Koudstaal PJ, et al. Transesophageal echocardiography in the detection of intracardiac embolic sources in patients with transient ischemic attacks. Stroke. 1990;21:560–565.

247. Prevention of venous thrombosis and pulmonary embolism. NIH Consensus Development. JAMA. 1986;256:744–749.

248. Pritchett ELC. Management of atrial fibrillation. N Engl J Med. 1992;326:1264–1271.

249. Pu M, Vandervoort P, Griffin B, et al. Quantification of mitral regurgitation by the proximal convergence method using transesophageal echocardiography: Clinical validation of a geometric correction for proximal flow constraint. Circulation. 1995;92(8): 2169–2177.

250. Pugsley W, Klinger L, Paschalis C, et al. The impact of microemboli during cardiopulmonary bypass on neuropsychological functioning. Stroke. 1994;25: 1393–1399.

251. Redberg R, Sobol Y, Chou T, et al. Andenosin-induced coronary vasodilatation during transesophageal Doppler echocardiography. Circulation. 1995;92(2):190–196.

252. Resnekov L, McDonald L. Complications in 220 patients with cardiac dysrhythmia treated by phased direct current shock and indication for electric conversion. Br Heart J. 1967;29:926–936.

253. Rice M, Sahn D. Transesophageal echocardiography for congenital heart disease—who, what, and when. Mayo Clin Proc. 1995;70:401–402.

254. Roberts WC. Aneurysm (redundancy) of the atrial septum (fossa ovale membrane) and prolapse (redundancy) of the mitral valve. Am J Cardiol. 1984; 54:1153–1154.

255. Roberts WC, Buchbinder NA. Right-sided valvular infective endocarditis: A clinicopathologic study of twelve necropsy patients. Am J Med. 1972;53:7–19.

256. Robinson FJ. Lodging of an embolus in a patent foramen ovale. Circulation. 1950;2:304.

257. Rodriguez L, Thomas JD, Monterroso V, et al. Validation of the proximal flow convergence method; calculation of orifice area in patients with mitral stenosis. Circulation. 1993;88:1157–1165.

258. Rohmann S, Erbel R, Mohr-Kahaly S, et al. Use of transesophageal echocardiography in the diagnosis of abscess in infective endocarditis. Eur Heart J. 1995;16(Suppl B):54–62.

259. Saletta S, Lederman E, Fein S, et al. Transesophageal echocardiography for the initial evaluation of the widened mediastinum in trauma patients. J Trauma. 1995;39:137–142.

260. Samdarshi TE, Mahan EF, Nanda NC, et al. Transesophageal echocardiographic assessment of congenital coronary artery to coronary sinus fistulas in adults. Am J Cardiol. 1991;68:263–266.

261. Sanfilippo AJ, Picard MH, Newell JB, et al. Echocardiographic assessment of patients with infective endocarditis: Prediction of risk of complications. J Am Coll Cardiol. 1991;18:1191–1199.

262. Sansoy V, Abbott R, Jayaweera A, et al. Low yield of transthoracic echocardiography for cardiac source of embolism. Am J Cardiol. 1995;75:166–169.

263. Sawanda SG, Segar DS, Ryan T, et al. Echocardiographic detection of coronary artery disease during dobutamine infusion. Circulation. 1991;83: 1605–1614.

264. Schiller NB, Maurer G, Ritter SB, et al. Transesophageal echocardiography. J Am Soc Echocardiogr. 1989;2:354–357.

265. Schiller NB, Shah PM, Crawford M, et al. Recommendations for quantification of the left ventricle by two-dimensional echocardiography. J Am Soc Echocardiogr. 1989;2:358–367.

266. Schneider AT, Hsu TL, Schwartz SL, et al. Single, biplane, multiplane, and three-dimensional transesophageal echocardiography: Echocardiographic–anatomic correlations. Cardiol Clin. 1993;11: 361–387.

267. Schneider AT, Schwartz S, Pandian N, et al. Multiplane transesophageal echocardiography provides more precise echo-anatomic definition and functional assessment of the normal and pathologic mitral valve apparatus. J Am Coll Cardiol. 1993;21(2): 83A.

268. Schneider B, Hanrath P, Vogel P, et al. Improved morphologic characterization of atrial septal aneurysm by transesophageal echocardiography: Relation to cerebrovascular events. J Am Coll Cardiol. 1990;16:1000–1009.

269. Schnittger I. Value of transesophageal echocardiography before DC cardioversion in patients with atrial fibrillation: Assessment of embolic risk. Br Heart J. 1995;73:306–309.

270. Schweizer P, Bardos P, Erbel R, et al. Detection of left atrial thrombi by echocardiography. Br Heart J. 1981;45:148–156.

271. Schwartz SL, Vannan MA, Pandian NG. Evaluation of cardiac masses. *In* Roelandt JRTC, Pandian NG (eds): Transesophageal Echocardiography New York, Churchill Livingstone; 1996:199–211.

272. Seward JB. Congenital heart disease. *In* Freeman WK, Seward JB, Khandheria BK, et al (eds): Transesophageal Echocardiography. Boston, Little, Brown; 1994;385–423.

273. Seward JB. Ebstein's anomaly: Ultrasound imaging and hemodynamic evaluation. Echocardiography. 1993;10:641–664.

274. Seward JB, Khandheria BK, Edwards WB, et al. Biplanar transesophageal echocardiography: Anatomic correlations, image orientation, and clinical applications. Mayo Clin Proc. 1990;65: 1193–1213.

275. Seward JB, Khandheria BK, Freeman WK, et al. Multiplane transesophageal echocardiography: Image orientation, examination technique, anatomic correlation, and clinical applications. Mayo Clin Proc. 1993;68:523–551.

276. Seward JB, Khandheria BK, Oh JK, et al. Critical appraisal of transesophageal echocardiography: Limitations, pitfalls and complications. J Am Soc Echocardiogr. 1992;5:288–305.

277. Seward JB, Khandheria BK, Oh JK, et al. Transesophageal echocardiography: Technique, anatomic correlations, implementation, and clinical applications. Mayo Clin Proc. 1988;63:649–680.

278. Seward JB, Tajik AJ, Edwards WD, et al. Two-Dimensional Echocardiography Atlas, Vol 1: Congenital Heart Disease. New York, Springer-Verlag; 1987.

279. Shapiro W, Klein G. Alterations in cardiac function immediately following electrical conversion of atrial fibrillation to normal sinus rhythm. Circulation. 1968;38:1078–1084.

280. Sheikh WJ, DeBruijn NP, Rankin JS, et al. The utility of transesophageal echocardiography and Doppler color flow imaging in patients undergoing cardiac valve surgery. J Am Coll Cardiol. 1990;15: 363–372.

281. Sherman DG, Dyken ML, Fisher M, et al. Cerebral embolism. Chest. 1986;89(Suppl):82S–98S.

282. Shiina A, Seward JB, Edwards WD, et al. Two-dimensional echocardiographic spectrum of Ebstein's anomaly: Detailed anatomic assessment. J Am Coll Cardiol. 1984;3:356–370.

283. Shiina A, Tajik AJ, Smith HC, et al. Prognostic significance of regional wall motion abnormality in patients with prior myocardial infarction: A prospective correlative study of two-dimensional echocardiography and angiography. Mayo Clin Proc. 1986;61: 254–262.

284. Shively BK, Gurule FT, Roldan CA, et al. Diagnostic value of transesophageal compared with transthoracic echocardiography in infective endocarditis. J Am Coll Cardiol. 1991;18:391–397.

285. Shrestha NK, Moreno FL, Narcisco FV, et al. Two-dimensional echocardiographic diagnosis of left atrial thrombus in rheumatic heart disease: A clinicopathologic study. Circulation. 1983;67: 341–347.

286. Shyu KG, Lei MH, Hwang JJ, et al. Morphologic characterization and quantitative assessment of mitral regurgitation with ruptured chordae tendineae by transesophageal echocardiography. Am J Cardiol. 1992;70:1152–1156.

287. Silver MD, Dorsey JS. Aneurysm of the septum primum in adults. Arch Pathol Lab Med. 1978;102: 62–65.

288. Simon P, Owen AN, Moidl R, et al. Transesophageal echocardiographic follow-up of patients with surgically treated aortic aneurysms. Eur Heart J. 1995;16: 402–405.

289. Simpson IA, Sahn DJ, Valdes-Cruz LM, et al. Color flow mapping in patients with coarctation of the aorta: New observations and improved evaluation with color flow diameter and proximal acceleration as predictors of severity. Circulation. 1988;77: 7736–7744.

290. Singh A, Breisblatt W, Cutrone M, et al. Transesophageal echocardiography as an important tool in the diagnosis of postinfarction papillary muscle rupture. Cardiology. 1995;86:417–420.

291. Slater J, Lighty GW, Winer HE, et al. Doppler echocardiography and computed tomography in diagnosis of left coronary arteriovenous fistula. J Am Coll Cardiol. 1984;4:1290–1293.

292. Smith M, Cassidy M, Gurley J, et al. Echo Doppler evaluation of patients with acute mitral regurgita-

tion: Superiority of transesophageal echocardiography with color flow imaging. Am Heart J. 1995; 129(5):967–974.

293. Smith M, Cassidy J, Souther S, et al. Transesophageal echocardiography in the diagnosis of traumatic rupture of the aorta. N Engl J Med. 1995;332(6): 356–362.

294. Smith MD, Handshoe R, Handshoe S, et al. Comparative accuracy of two-dimensional echocardiography and Doppler pressure half-time methods in assessing severity of mitral stenosis in patients with and without commissurotomy. Circulation. 1986;73: 100–107.

295. Smith MD, Harrison MR, Pinton R, et al. Regurgitant jet size by transesophageal compared with transthoracic Doppler color flow imaging. Circulation. 1991;83:79–86.

296. Sohn D, Shin G, Oh J, et al. Role of transesophageal echocardiography in hemodynamically unstable patients. Mayo Clin Proc. 1995;70:925–931.

297. Solomon SL, Brown JJ, Glazer HS, et al. Thoracic aortic dissection: Pitfalls and artifacts in MR imaging. Radiology. 1990;177:223–228.

298. Spain MG, Smith MD, Grayburn PA, et al. Quantitative assessment of mitral regurgitation by color Doppler flow imaging: Angiographic and hemodynamic correlations. J Am Coll Cardiol. 1989;13: 585–590.

299. Stekelberg JM, Khandheria BK, Anhalt JP, et al. Prospective evaluation of the risk of bacteremia associated with transesophageal echocardiography. Circulation. 1991;84:177–180.

300. Stewart WJ, Currie PJ, Salcedo EE, et al. Evaluation of mitral leaflet motion by echocardiography and jet direction by Doppler color flow mapping to determine the mechanism of mitral regurgitation. J Am Coll Cardiol. 1992;20:1353–1361.

301. Stoddard MF, Arce J, Liddell NE, et al. Two-dimensional transesophageal echocardiographic determination of aortic valve area in adults with aortic stenosis. Am Heart J. 1991;122:1415–1422.

302. Stoddard MF, Dawkins PR, Longaker RA. Mobile strands are frequently attached to the St Jude Medical mitral valve prosthesis as assessed by two-dimensional transesophageal echocardiography. Am Heart J. 1992;124:671–678.

303. Stoddard MF, Dawkins PR, Prince C, et al. Left atrial appendage thrombus is not uncommon in patients with acute atrial fibrillation and a recent embolic event: A transesophageal echocardiographic study. J Am Coll Cardiol. 1995;25(2):452–459.

304. Stoddard MF, Longaker RA. Role of transesophageal echo prior to cardioversion in patients with atrial fibrillation (abstract). J Am Coll Cardiol. 1993; 21(Suppl A):28A.

305. Stoddard MF, Prince C, Ammash NM, et al. Two-dimensional transesophageal echocardiographic determination of mitral valve area in adults with mitral stenosis. Am Heart J. 1994;127:1348–1353.

306. Stoddard MF, Prince C, Morris G. Coronary flow reserve assessment by dobutamine transesophageal Doppler echocardiography. J Am Coll Cardiol. 1995;25(2):325–332.

307. Stoddard MF, Prince C, Tuman WL, et al. Angle of incidence does not affect accuracy of mitral stenosis area calculation by pressure half-time: Application to Doppler transesophageal echocardiography. Am Heart J. 1994;127:1562–1572.

308. Stöllberger C, Brainin M, Abzieher F, et al. Embolic stroke and transesophageal echocardiography: Can clinical parameters predict the diagnostic yield? J Neurol. 1995;242:437–442.

309. Stone D, Godard J, Corretti M, et al. Patent foramen ovale: Association between the degree of shunt by contrast transesophageal echocardiography and the risk of future ischemic neurologic events. Am Heart J. 1996;131:158–161.

310. Stone D, Hawke M, LaMonte M, et al. Ulcerated atherosclerotic plaques in the thoracic aorta are associated with cryptogenic stroke: A multiplane transesophageal echocardiographic study. Am Heart J. 1995;130:105–108.

311. Strauer B. The significance of coronary reserve in clinical heart disease. J Am Coll Cardiol. 1990;15: 775–783.

312. Streifler JY, Furlan AJ, Barnett HJM. Cardiogenic brain embolism: Incidence, variants, and treatment. *In* Barnett HJM, Mohr JP, Stein BM, (eds): Stroke Pathophysiology, Diagnosis, and Management. New York, Churchill Livingstone; 1992:967–994.

313. Sutton DC, Cahalan MK. Intraoperative assessment of left ventricular function with transesophageal echocardiography. Cardiol Clin. 1993; 11:399–408.

314. Tardif J, Miller D, Pandian N, et al. Effects of variations in flow on aortic valve area in aortic stenosis based on in vivo planimetry of aortic valve area by multiplane transesophageal echocardiography. Am J Cardiol. 1995;76:193–198.

315. The Stroke Prevention in Atrial Fibrillation Investigators. Predictors of thromboembolism in atrial fibrillation: I. Clinical features of patients at risk. Ann Intern Med. 1992;116:1–5.

316. Thomas JD, Wilkins GT, Choong CY, et al. Inaccuracy of mitral pressure half-time immediately after percutaneous mitral valvotomy. Dependence on transmitral gradient and left atrial and ventricular compliance. Circulation. 1988;78:980–993.

317. Tice F, Harrison JK, Heame SE, et al. Can transthoracic or transesophageal echocardiography predict successful Inoue balloon mitral commissurotomy? Am Coll Cardiol. 1994;22:194A.

318. Tice F, Heinle S, Harrison J, et al. Transesophageal echocardiographic assessment of reversal of systolic pulmonary venous flow in mitral stenosis. Am J Cardiol. 1995;75:58–60.

319. Tingleff J, Joyce F, Petterson G. Intraoperative echocardiographic study of air embolism during cardiac operations. Ann Thorac Surg. 1995;60:673–677.

320. Tribouilloy C, Shen WF, Quere JP, et al. Assessment of severity of mitral regurgitation by measuring regurgitant jet width at its origin with transesophageal Doppler color flow imaging. Circulation. 1992;85:1248–1253.

321. Tsai LM, Chen JH, Fang CJ, et al. Clinical implications of left atrial spontaneous echo contrast in nonrheumatic atrial fibrillation. Am J Cardiol. 1992;70:327–331.

322. Tsai LM, Chen JH, Ten JK, et al. Right coronary artery-to-left ventricle fistula identified by transesophageal echocardiography. Am Heart J. 1992;124:1106–1109.

323. Tunick PA, Perez JL, Kronzon I. Protruding atheromas in the thoracic aorta and systemic embolization. Ann Intern Med. 1991;115:423–427.

324. Urbanowicz JH, Kernoff RS, Oppenhiem G, et al. Transesophageal echocardiography and its potential for esophageal damage. Anesthesiology. 1990;72:40–43.

325. Van Reet RE, Quinones MA, Poliner LR, et al. Comparison of two-dimensional echocardiography with gated radionuclide ventriculography in the evaluation of global and regional left ventricular function in acute myocardial infarction. J Am Coll Cardiol. 1984;3:243–252.

326. Van Son JA, Vander Woude JC, Cheng W, et al. Surgical closed atrial septotomy under transesophageal guidance. Ann Thorac Surg 1995;60(5):1403–1404.

327. Velvis H, Schmidt KG, Silverman NH, et al. Diagnosis of coronary artery fistulas by two-dimensional echocardiography, pulsed Doppler ultrasound and color flow imaging. J Am Coll Cardiol. 1989;14:968–976.

328. Venkatesh B, Vannan MA, Roelandt JRTC, et al. Laboratory setup, patient preparation and procedure. In Roelandt JRTC, Pandian NG (eds): Multiplane Transesophageal Echocardiography. New York, Churchill Livingstone; 1996:15–16.

329. Vered Z, Mossinson D, Peleg E, et al. Echocardiographic assessment of prosthetic valve endocarditis. Eur Heart J. 1995;16(Suppl B):63–67.

330. Verhorst PM, Kamp O, Visser CA, et al. Left atrial appendage flow velocity assessment using transesophageal echocardiography in nonrheumatic atrial fibrillation and systemic embolism. Am J Cardiol. 1993;71:192–196.

331. Vignon P, Gueret P, Vedrinne J, et al. Role of transesophageal echocardiography in the diagnosis and management of traumatic aortic disruption. Circulation. 1995;92:(10):2959–2968.

332. Vilacosta I, Castillo JA, San Roman JA, et al. New echo–anatomical correlations in aortic dissection. Eur Heart J. 1995;16:126–128.

333. Vlahakes G, Warren R. Traumatic rupture of the aorta. N Engl J Med. 1995;332(6):389–390.

334. Walker WA, Pate FW. Medical management of acute traumatic rupture of the aorta. Ann Thorac Surg. 1990;50:965–967.

335. Wareing TH, Davila-Roman VG, Brazilai B, et al. Strategy for reduction of stroke in cardiac surgical patients. Ann Thorac Surg. 1993;55:1400–1408.

336. Webster MW, Chancellor AM, Smith JH, et al. Patent foramen ovale in young stroke patients. Lancet. 1988;2:11–12.

337. Weinberg DM, Mancini GBJ. Anticoagulation for cardioversion of atrial fibrillation. Am J Cardiol. 1989;63:745–746.

338. Weiss R, Brier J, O'Connor W, et al. The usefulness of transesophageal echocardiography in diagnosing cardiac contusions. Chest. 1996;109:73–77.

339. Wheat MW Jr. Current status of medical therapy of acute dissecting aneurysms of the aorta. World J Surg. 1980;4:563–569.

340. Winniford MD, Rossen JD, Marcus ML. Clinical importance of coronary flow reserve measurements. Mod Concepts Cardiovasc Dis. 1989;58:31–35.

341. Wong M, Tei C, Shah PM. Sensitivity and specificity of two-dimensional echocardiography in the determination of valvular calcification. Chest. 1983;84:423–427.

342. Yasick A, Samra S. An unusual complication of transesophageal echocardiography. Anesth Analg. 1995;81:654–661.

343. Yoshida K, Yoshikawa J, Hozumi T, et al. Detection of left main coronary artery stenosis by transesophageal color Doppler and two-dimensional echocardiography. Circulation. 1990;81:1271–1276.

344. Zabalgoitia M, Gandhi DK, Abi-Mansour P, et al. Transesophageal stress echocardiography: Detection of coronary artery disease in patients with normal resting left ventricular contractility. Am Heart J. 1991;122:1456–1463.

345. Zabalgoitia M, Gandhi DK, Evans J, et al. Transesophageal echocardiography in the awake elderly

patient: Its role in the clinical decision-making process. Am Heart J. 1990;120:1147–1153.

346. Zabalgoitia-Reyes M, Herrera C, Ghandi DK, et al. A possible mechanism for neurologic ischemic events in patients with atrial septal aneurysm. Am J Cardiol. 1990;66:761–764.

347. Zanolla L, Marino P, Nicolosi GL, et al. Two-dimensional echocardiographic evaluation of mitral valve calcification. Sensitivity and specificity. Chest. 1982;82:154–157.

348. Zehetgruber M, Mundigler G, Christ G, et al. Estimation of coronary flow reserve by transesophageal coronary sinus Doppler measurements in patients with syndrome X and patients with significant left coronary artery disease. J Am Coll Cardiol. 1995; 25(5):1039–1045.

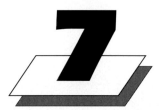

Exercise and Pharmacologic Echocardiography

DONNA EHLER and LINDA J. CROUSE

Before the mid-1980s, noninvasive evaluation of patients with known or suspected coronary artery disease (CAD) consisted predominantly of exercise electrocardiography (ECG) performed alone or in conjunction with thallium scintigraphy or gated blood pool radioventriculography. However, exercise ECG is unreliable in many subgroups of patients, including those who have had a myocardial infarction or undergone angioplasty or coronary bypass surgery; those taking medications, such as digoxin or antiarrhythmic, diuretic, and antidepressant agents, which can affect the ECG; those with bundle branch block or other resting repolarization abnormalities; those with valvular heart disease, including mitral valve prolapse; and women.[6] Stress radioventriculography and nuclear perfusion imaging may overcome many of these limitations, but they are relatively expensive, must be scheduled in advance, and for perfusion studies require repeated imaging after a delay of several hours. Furthermore, their clinical utility is confined to the assessment of CAD, and radionuclide techniques carry the risk of radiation exposure.

Exercise echocardiography avoids the disadvantages of other techniques, and over the past decade it has evolved as a test ideally suited for evaluating patients with known or suspected CAD or valvular heart disease. It is now accepted as a cost-effective and reliable tool for detecting the presence, extent, and distribution of coronary stenosis in a variety of patient groups, including those undergoing initial or preoperative screening, those who have had surgical or percutaneous revascularization, and those who have previously suffered a myocardial infarction. Widely available and relatively inexpensive, echocardiography is a high-resolution technique that can rapidly depict regional wall motion both at rest and after exercise. Regional wall motion analysis of echocardiograms obtained before and immediately after exercise allows highly accurate prediction of the extent and distribution of CAD, as demonstrated by the correlation with angiography.[11] In addition, stress echocardiography can be used to assess left ventricular size and ejection fraction. Consequences of previous myocardial infarction, such as thrombus or aneurysm formation, can be detected. Cardiac echocardiography can also identify causes of chest pain unrelated to vascular obstruction, including hypertrophic cardiomyopathy, aortic dissection, and pericardial disease, and with Doppler flow recording can be used to evaluate the severity and hemodynamic significance of valvular heart lesions. Finally, exercise echocardiography has unsurpassed sensitivity, specificity, and predictive value in evaluating the effect of treatment, which will be increasingly important as scrutiny of

135

diagnostic procedures for cost-containment purposes become more prevalent.

Basic Physiologic Principles of Cardiac Stress

MYOCARDIAL FUNCTION

The physiologic effects of stress on myocardial contractility are complex. In this text, we will present only the basic concepts pertinent to echocardiographic evaluation. Myocardial ischemia occurs when the global or regional oxygen supply is insufficient to meet the body's demand. An existing coronary artery occlusion may be clinically silent if it does not create a disparity between oxygen demand and oxygen supply to the corresponding myocardial region. When the myocardial blood flow reserve becomes inadequate, as is the case during exercise or inotropic stimulation, an insufficient oxygen supply will result in ischemia and impaired myocardial function. Because significant coronary artery stenoses often have little or no effect in the resting state, the evaluation of patients during or immediately after exercise has become standard. It is important to emphasize that exercise echocardiography predicts regional coronary insufficiency by detecting exertional changes in regional wall motion due to myocardial ischemia. Except in patients with cardiomyopathy, such changes will not occur in the absence of ischemia even if coronary narrowing is present. Therefore, patients must be encouraged to exercise as vigorously and as long as possible so as to evoke an ischemic episode.

An ischemic episode consists of a sequence of several underlying pathophysiologic events. First, myocardial perfusion becomes nonhomogeneous, decreasing in myocardium, which is supplied by the obstructed vessel. Next, ischemic myocardium undergoes a change in diastolic function, resulting in slowed relaxation, increased stiffness, and increasing end-diastolic pressure. Progressive contractile failure ensues, producing segmental hypokinesis, akinesis, and even dyskinesis. Significant shifts of the ST segment (depression or elevation) may appear on the ECG and, finally, the patient may experience symptoms such as chest pain[25] (Fig. 7-1). Because systolic contractile failure is one of the earliest detectable consequences of myocardial ischemia, preceding ECG changes and chest pain, the addition of imaging modalities to ECG stress testing increases the diagnostic accuracy of noninvasive testing.

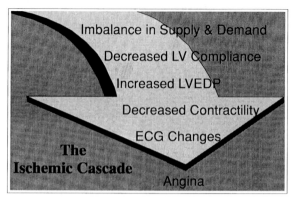

Figure 7-1. The ischemic cascade. Systolic contractile failure occurs as one of the earliest consequences of myocardial ischemia.

Radionuclide techniques are useful adjuncts to the stress ECG, and their ability to predict the presence or absence of CAD and to assess regional myocardial viability is widely accepted. Exercise echocardiography has several advantages over radionuclide techniques. In addition to those mentioned above, echocardiography is based on a segmental approach, which affords a more complete assessment of left ventricular wall motion. Real-time echocardiographic imaging permits instantaneous recording of beat-to-beat information rather than relying on averaged data obtained over several minutes. Also of importance, echocardiographic methods are considerably less expensive and are more convenient for the patient.

Historical Perspective

EARLY INVESTIGATORS

A correlation between CAD and exercise-induced regional wall motion abnormalities detected by two-dimensional echocardiography was first reported in 1979 by Wann et al.[42] Echocardiograms were recorded in 28 patients before and during supine bicycle exercise. Because of technical limitations due to respiratory interference, however, only 71% of the images could be interpreted. Subsequently, Limacher et al.[17] used two-dimensional echocardiography before and after a maximal treadmill exercise to evaluate 73 patients for CAD. Based on detection of wall motion abnormalities or decreased left ventricular ejection fraction, a sensitivity of 91% and a specificity of 88% were reported. The echocardiographic images were recorded on videotape, requiring the interpreter to shuttle back and forth through the videotape to compare resting and postexercise images. Robertson et al.[33] obtained echocardiograms before and immediately after treadmill exercise in 30 patients referred for cardiac catheterization. Successful postexercise images were recorded in 92% of these patients. This study demonstrated a correlation between a provoked regional wall motion abnormality and the specific artery that was constricted. The persistence of segmental abnormalities for as long as 30 min after exercise was also noted and was found to correspond to the severity of disease.

These and other investigators validated the usefulness of echocardiography in evaluating regional myocardial function in patients with known or suspected CAD. However, technical difficulties in recording and interpreting the images limited its clinical application. In particular, exertional hyperventilation produced exaggerated movement of the heart across the imaging window and interposed lung tissue between the chest wall and the heart during much of the respiratory cycle. These respiratory effects made it difficult for the interpreter to assess individual myocardial segments. Further uncertainty resulted from the need to shuttle the videotape back and forth from rest to exercise images, making simultaneous side-by-side comparison impossible. These problems led to limited correlation with angiographic findings.[9,10,22,24,33,42]

DIGITAL TECHNOLOGY

Although digital computer technology had been used for some time in other areas of cardiology, for example in nuclear medicine and to some extent in angiography, it was not until the mid-1980s that digital technology began to be applied to cardiac ultrasonography.[2,3,26,31,36,40] Digital image acquisition has largely overcome the technical obstacles described above. The ability to acquire, store, and replay a single cardiac cycle in cine-loop format and to compare rest and exercise images side by side has increased the accuracy of the test and has made it easier to perform. A sequence of images confined to systole can be acquired, digitized, stored, and replayed. Resting images are acquired in multiple views so that each myocardial segment can be evaluated. After exercise or pharmacologic challenge to provoke ischemia, images are acquired in each view and digitized. The software allows a sequence of systolic images from a single cycle to be continuously replayed. A cycle in which cardiac excursion and lung interpolation do not interfere can be selected, providing a steady image for analysis. The rest and exercise images can be displayed side by side, allowing the interpreter to analyze each myocardial segment and identify even subtle exercise-induced abnormalities (Fig. 7-2).

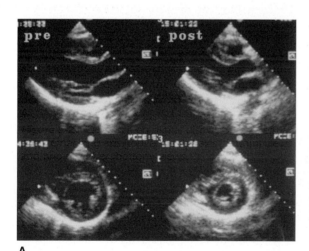
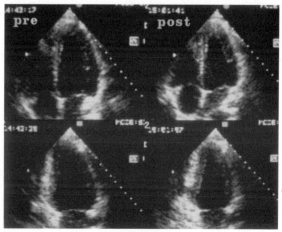

A **B**

Figure 7-2. Quad screen digital display of rest (left) and postexercise (right) images (**A**) in the parasternal long axis (top) and short axis (bottom) views and (**B**) in the apical four-chamber (top) and two-chamber (bottom) views.

Indications for Stress Echocardiography

According to currently accepted practice, any patient who will undergo both echocardiography and treadmill testing is a candidate for exercise echocardiography. Most often, the test is used (1) to screen new patients for CAD; (2) to assess the status before or after an intervention, for example, to detect restenosis after angioplasty or to evaluate graft patency after coronary bypass surgery; (3) to determine the prognosis after myocardial infarction; and (4) to evaluate the hemodynamic significance of valvular heart disease.

As a initial screening test for CAD, exercise echocardiography is especially useful in patients who have a high likelihood of a false-positive treadmill test, such as women, those with conduction or resting repolarization abnormalities, and those taking antihypertensive or antiarrhythmic medications, digoxin, and diuretics. It is also useful for assessing the effectiveness of initial medical therapy.

Exercise echocardiography is also useful before and after interventions. Before angioplasty, it can be used to assess the physiologic significance of a lesion. Angiographically detected lesions that are mild or even mild to moderate but do not induce significant wall motion abnormality may not require angioplasty. Angioplasty should not be undertaken unless physiologic abnormalities are present, as restenosis occurs in 35% of cases.[14] To avoid this risk, patients without exercise-induced wall motion abnormalities can be followed with serial exercise echocardiography to determine when intervention will be required. After angioplasty, it can demonstrate early improvement of resting wall motion abnormalities or an inadequate result and can detect restenosis or new disease. After bypass grafting, it can also be performed at 6 weeks to obtain a baseline for comparison with routine follow-up exams, as well as to detect inadequate revascularization or new disease. Annual follow-up exercise echocardiography can detect new abnormalities with a sensitivity of greater than 90%.

Echocardiography has proven valuable for rapidly and accurately assessing the effects of reperfusion therapy during myocardial infarction.[27] Dobutamine stress echocardiography is now commonly used to determine the extent of myocardial damage and to assess myocardial viability after myocardial infarction. Exercise echocardiography after myocar-

dial infarction can be used to determine the left ventricular ejection fraction and, most important, to determine the extent and distribution of existing CAD, which allows the most appropriate therapy (i.e., medical or interventional) to be selected. Consequences of previous myocardial infarction, such as thrombus or aneurysm formation, can also be detected.

Echocardiography is also well suited for screening patients for other causes of cardiac morbidity and mortality, such as pericardial disease, cardiomyopathy, aortic dissection, and valvular heart disease. Like CAD, a latent or known valvular abnormality may cause significant hemodynamic changes with stress. Stress Doppler echocardiography to evaluate changes in valve gradient and pulmonary artery pressure is especially useful in patients with mitral valve disease.[13,38] Patients undergo resting echocardiography and Doppler evaluation and then perform either bicycle or treadmill exercise. Bicycle ergonometry is preferred for Doppler studies of valvular disease because it allows recording during peak exertion. Doppler recording immediately after treadmill exercise can also be performed successfully. Exercise or postexercise Doppler recordings are then compared with those obtained at rest.

Contraindications for Exercise Echocardiography

Contraindications for performing exercise echocardiography are the same as those for treadmill exercise testing. They include very recent myocardial infarction, unstable angina, potentially life-threatening cardiac dysrhythmias, acute pericarditis, severe hypertension, and acute pulmonary embolism. Occasionally unexpected findings that would be contraindications to stress echocardiography are detected on the resting echocardiogram. These include significant left ventricular outflow tract obstruction or aortic stenosis, apical thrombus, cardiac masses or tumors, congenital anomalies, significant pericardial effusion or tamponade, and severe left ventricular dysfunction.

Recording and Display of Images

In our laboratory, echocardiography is performed with the patient in the left lateral decubitus position on a custom examination bed that has a dropout leaf. The patient is positioned with the apex of the heart over this leaf, which can then be lowered to make the lateral precordium accessible to the image transducer. The arrangement provides comfortable support for the patient and gives the sonographer ample access to the apical imaging windows. Image quality is greatly improved with this technique. Imaging is performed from the patient's left side rather than from the right side to avoid the necessity of reaching around the patient, especially when acquiring apical views (Fig. 7-3).

Resting (baseline) images are acquired with a 2.5- or 3.5-MHz transducer in the parasternal long and short axis and the apical four- and two-chamber views. The images in each view are recorded on videotape, and are simultaneously digitized and stored with a computerized system that converts the ultrasound images to a digital format. By convention, the sequence of digitized images, or cine-loop, consists of eight frames. The goal is to record systolic wall motion during a representative cardiac cycle. The interim delay setting, or time between successive frames, can be varied, but in the majority of adult patients the standard setting is 50 msec. The first frame is acquired at the onset of systole and the last is acquired 350 msec later. Image acquisition is triggered by the ECG (Fig. 7-4).

After the resting images have been obtained, the patient performs maximal, symptom-limited ex-

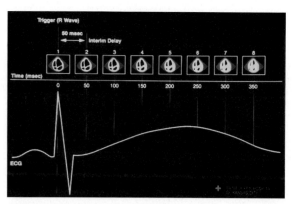

Figure 7-4. Eight-frame cine-loop. Eight consecutive frames are acquired at intervals of 50 msec during the systolic portion of a single cardiac cycle and are replayed as a continuous cine-loop.

ercise. Although upright or supine bicycle exercise is used successfully in many centers, this requires imaging during exercise, which we have found is very technically challenging. We therefore use treadmill exercise, performed according to the Bruce or modified Bruce protocol, with conventional monitoring of symptoms, blood pressure, and ECG. After exercise, no cool-down period is allowed. Instead, immediately after the test is stopped, the patient is repositioned on the examination table, and imaging is repeated in all four views as rapidly as possible and over multiple cardiac cycles. The sonographer can later select which eight-frame cine-loop is optimal and most representative for each view. The images selected are those acquired within 1 min after the end of exercise. Echocardiographic monitoring and videotape recording are continued for the next 2 to 3 min of recovery. Often, recovery-phase imaging shows gradually improving contractile function, which confirms the interpreter's assessment of stress-induced wall motion abnormality, making the diagnosis of coronary insufficiency more secure.

The digitized images are then reformatted so that rest and stress images for a particular view are displayed side by side. Usually, two views (both parasternal or both apical views) are displayed simultaneously in a "quad-screen" format to facilitate the assessment of exercise-induced changes in regional and global contractility. The standard playback setting displays each frame for 100 msec, for a total

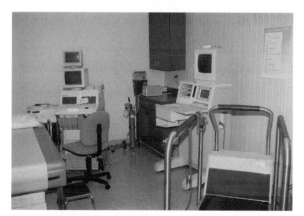

Figure 7-3. The setup for exercise echocardiography. Echocardiograms are obtained with the patient in the left lateral decubitus position on an examination bed specifically designed for cardiac sonography. Close proximity of the treadmill and the examination bed facilitates rapid acquisition of postexercise images.

display length of 800 msec. Regional wall motion is described at rest, and exercise-induced abnormalities are assessed. The extent and distribution of coronary stenoses are predicted based on the distribution of provoked wall motion abnormalities. The interpretation of the echocardiograms is described below.

Pharmacologic Stress Echocardiography

A sizable minority of patients are unable to perform an adequate exercise test because of peripheral vascular disease, musculoskeletal or neurologic disorders, pulmonary disease, or obesity. To evaluate such patients, pharmacologic agents may be used instead of exercise to provoke ischemia. In the past, such agents were used with radioactive tracers to delineate myocardial perfusion and viability. The use of pharmacologic stress in conjunction with echocardiography was an important advance in the noninvasive evaluation of cardiovascular disease.[18,21,28] Coronary vasodilators, such as dipyridamole and adenosine, have been used primarily with thallium scanning. Because they do not increase the metabolic demands on the heart to a significant degree or provoke ischemia, they are less suitable for echocardiographic studies than is dobutamine.[20]

DOBUTAMINE

Dobutamine is a synthetic sympathomimetic amine that has favorable pharmacologic properties for clinical use.[15] As commercially formulated, it possesses alpha-2 as well as beta-1 and beta-2 adrenergic stimulating properties, which provide a potent inotropic (muscular) response with a relatively blunted chronotropic (blood pressure) response. Dobutamine has a rapid onset of action, generally within 2 min, and reaches peak activity within 10 min. Its plasma half-life, even in patients with congestive heart failure, is approximately 2.5 min. It has proven to be safe and well tolerated in conjunction with echocardiographic imaging,[5,34] and its usefulness as an alternative to exercise testing to detect CAD and to diagnose multivessel disease after myocardial infarction has been well established.[5,8,18,34]

Certain exclusion criteria should be followed, as with any test involving stress or pharmacologic agents. These include class III or IV New York Heart Association heart failure, high-grade atrioventricular block, angina at rest, significant ventricular arrhythmias, severe systemic hypertension, acute myocardial infarction within the past 5 days, hypertrophic cardiomyopathy, atrial fibrillation with an uncontrolled ventricular response, critical aortic stenosis, and hypersensitivity to dobutamine. In some centers, patients with inadequate resting echocardiograms are excluded; however, we do not use this criterion. Beta blockers may be discontinued 48 hr before the test, if possible, and oral intake should be restricted to clear liquids for at least 6 hr before the test.

Dobutamine is infused with a calibrated infusion pump. During the infusion, a single-channel ECG is monitored continuously, and multichannel ECGs, blood pressure, and heart rate are recorded every 3 min. Hemodynamic variables, dosages, and symptoms are recorded on a flow sheet as well. Dobutamine can be infused rapidly or gradually, depending on the nature of the test, in dosage increments of 5 to 10 μg/kg/min up to a peak rate of 40 μg/kg/min. Rapid infusion reduces the duration of the test without compromising its safety or diagnostic utility and may be preferred. For determination of myocardial viability, a peak dose of 10 μg/kg/min appears to be optimal, as demonstration of dobutamine-enhanced contractility is good evidence of underlying myocardial viability, and higher doses may result in subsequent ischemia and lack of sensitivity in defining viability.[29]

Echocardiographic images are obtained at rest, at each infusion level, and during recovery. As described above, the images are recorded on videotape and acquired digitally in each of the four standard echocardiographic views. Unless symptoms occur, dobutamine stress is terminated after the target heart rate has been obtained or after regional wall motion abnormalities have been demonstrated unequivocally. The infusion is stopped for angina requiring sublingual nitroglycerin, significant arrhythmias, severe systolic hypertension, significant dobutamine-induced hypotension (systolic blood pressure less than 100 mm Hg), or significant regional wall motion abnormalities or symptoms.

In patients who do not achieve 85% of the predicted maximal heart rate during the dobutamine infusion, the addition of atropine increases the sensitivity of the test for the detection of coronary artery disease.[4] Atropine, 0.25 mg, is administered intravenously 1 min into the peak dobutamine infusion rate (40 μg/kg/min) and is repeated to a maximum dose of 1.0 mg if necessary to achieve 85% of the predicted maximal heart rate. Dobutamine-atropine stress echocardiography is a relatively safe test with few adverse effects that greatly improves the predictive value of dobutamine stress echocardiography.[23,30]

Interpretation of the dobutamine stress echocardiograms is similar to that of exercise echocardiograms, which is described below. In patients being screened for CAD, the only normal response is a hypercontractile one. After revascularization or myocardial infarction, improved regional wall motion induced by dobutamine is normal even if the response is not hypercontractile. Improved contraction of an akinetic segment at a low dose followed by deterioration at higher doses indicates a viable myocardial segment with a severely restricted vascular supply.

Dobutamine stress echocardiography has high sensitivity, specificity, and predictive accuracy for detecting CAD and predicting future cardiac events.[1,19,37] In the detection of CAD, we have achieved sensitivity of 90%, specificity of 81%, and positive predictive accuracy of 88%. Among our patients undergoing preoperative assessment of the risk of perioperative cardiac events, sensitivity was 86%, specificity was 100%, and overall accuracy was 95%.[34,35]

Evaluation of Valvular Heart Disease

Echocardiographic evaluation of patients with valvular heart disease is typically performed at rest. However, symptoms of valve disease frequently occur only during exertion. Therefore, exercise Doppler echocardiography permits a more complete assessment of the physiologic significance of valvular heart lesions.[39] Correlation of symptoms with hemodynamic measurements during exercise may also help determine the significance of a specific valvular pathology. Exercise Doppler echocardiography is useful for evaluating patients with exertional dyspnea or fatigue who have mild to moderate hypertension, prosthetic valves, or mild to moderate mitral valve disease at rest. Several studies have demonstrated a significant increase in mean transmitral gradient with exercise in a significant number of patients with mild mitral stenosis or a prosthetic mitral valve.[7,12,16,32,41,43] Doppler evaluation of pulmonary artery pressure allows further assessment of the hemodynamic consequences of exercise in these groups. In patients with mild rheumatic mitral valve disease, it may also be important to look for severe exercise-induced mitral regurgitation.[38] Exercise Doppler echocardiography can play an important role in differentiating the underlying cause of symptoms in patients with valvular heart disease.

Interpretation of Exercise Echocardiograms

To some extent, the interpretation of exercise echocardiograms depends on the type of patient being evaluated. In the absence of previous myocardial infarction, coronary artery bypass grafting, or angioplasty, the normal response to stress is hypercontractile function regardless of function at baseline, increased left ventricular ejection fraction, and decreased left ventricular volume. Any other response is abnormal, indicating coronary insufficiency. After bypass grafting or angioplasty, a normal response consists of improved but not necessarily hypercontractile segmental performance on postexercise compared with resting images. After myocardial infarction, failure of an akinetic segment on the baseline images to improve after exercise could indicate either nonviable tissue or viable tissue with a compromised vascular supply. Exercise echocardiography cannot distinguish between these two possibilities. (In such cases, however, dobutamine stress echocardiography could be used to assess viability.)

Interpretation of the test includes evaluation of the blood pressure, ECG, and symptomatic and echocardiographic responses to exercise. Resting cine-loops are displayed adjacent to postexercise cine-loops in each of the four standard views (Fig. 7-5). With the quad screen format, two views can be displayed simultaneously. Each segment in each view is interpreted as normal, hyperkinetic, hypokinetic, akinetic, or dyskinetic, and each segment's response to stress is described. The status of coronary arteries or bypass grafts is predicted by consolidating the myocardial segments into three perfusion zones (Fig. 7-6). Anterior, septal, and apical segments are perfused by the left anterior descending coronary artery; posterolateral segments by the left

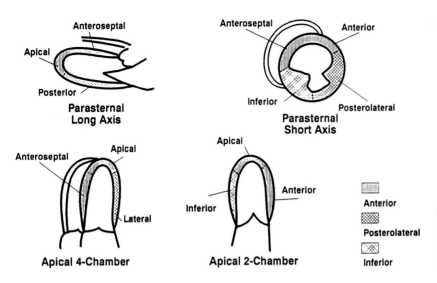

Figure 7-5. The myocardial segments in each of the four standard echocardiographic views. Each segment can be seen in more than one view.

circumflex coronary artery; and inferior segments by the right coronary artery and/or left circumflex artery, depending on dominance. Each myocardial segment is seen in more than one echocardiographic view. Because each major coronary distribution is represented in at least two views, coronary insufficiency in a specific perfusion zone can be predicted in the majority of patients. It is important to examine all segments in each coronary distribution systematically.

The ability to detect provoked wall motion abnormalities requires skill in the analysis and description of segmental contractile function. To obtain a close correlation between the echocardiographic and angiographic findings demands meticulous attention to the subtleties and nuances of localized, transient changes in wall motion. It is important to remember that wall motion abnormalities resulting from provoked myocardial ischemia can be quite transient, often resolving by 60 or 90 sec after exercise termination.

An exercise echocardiogram is interpreted as positive if any of three findings are present: (1) an exercise-induced wall motion abnormality; (2) an increase in left ventricular volume; or (3) a decrease in global ejection fraction. An exercise-induced wall

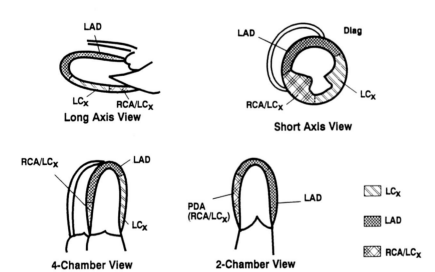

Figure 7-6. The correlation between myocardial segments and the perfusion zones of the three major coronary vessels: left anterior descending artery, left circumflex artery, and right coronary artery. The distributions of the left circumflex and right coronary arteries may overlap.

motion abnormality is the most sensitive indicator of the presence of CAD. The greater the wall motion abnormality, the more severe the stenosis. Increased left ventricular volume is a sensitive indicator of double- or triple-vessel disease. Decreased ejection fraction indicates significant CAD but is the least sensitive indicator. In general, the more severe the abnormalities, the more likely they are to represent severe stenoses. For example, a wall that is akinetic after exercise is much more likely to represent a 90% or greater lesion, whereas a mildly hypokinetic wall that reperfuses within 1 min may indicate a 60% lesion. Also, the longer the abnormality persists into the recovery period, the more abnormal the coronary artery is.

Many factors affect wall motion abnormalities. The duration of exercise is important because without adequate exercise, wall motion will not become hyperkinetic. Patients should exercise until symptoms appear because the longer the duration of ischemia during exercise, the longer wall motion abnormalities will persist into the recovery period and the easier it will be to perform and interpret the exercise echocardiograms. Lack of hyperkinetic wall motion causes the greatest difficulty in interpreting the test. It can also occur because of hypertension, mild cardiomyopathy, a hyper- or hypothyroid condition, or alcohol use. In these cases, it is necessary to review the treadmill flow sheet and make sure that the stress was adequate before the test can be interpreted as abnormal.

FALSE-NEGATIVE EXAMINATIONS

False-negative results are uncommon. They may be caused by mild coronary artery disease, inability to reach the maximal heart rate, or the presence of extensive collateral vessels. Because of the high sensitivity of the test, even lesions causing 50% stenosis can be readily identified, so there is little risk of missing a significant lesion. Inadequate exercise is a greater problem because if the patient does not exercise enough to induce ischemia, the test will not be positive. In such cases, dobutamine stress echocardiography may be appropriate. Rapid reperfusion as a result of extensive collaterals may cause a false-negative result. In such cases, the wall motion abnormality will disappear during acquisition of the digital images. Rapid resolution of wall motion abnormalities can also indicate limited ischemia or rapidly changing loading conditions.

FALSE-POSITIVE EXAMINATIONS

False-positive results, although not common, do occur more frequently than false-negative results. Cardiomyopathy, by definition, will give a false-positive exercise echocardiography test. Inadequate exercise can also cause a false-positive result, especially in elderly patients. If wall motion is not uniformly hyperdynamic, this may be attributed to inadequate exercise. In very elderly patients, false-positive tests may be due to early myocardial dysfunction, left ventricular hypertrophy, left ventricular fibrosis, and aging of the heart. High blood pressure, in the range of 220/110 mm Hg, is another source of false-positive results. Severe hypertension may cause endocardial underperfusion and diffuse, patchy abnormalities. In such cases, the hypertension can be managed more aggressively and exercise echocardiography can be repeated.

PITFALLS AND ARTIFACTS

Care should be taken to carefully evaluate resting wall motion abnormalities. They may represent a prior infarction, but they are present 50% of the time in patients with greater than 70% stenosis. After angioplasty, resting function will recover within 48 hr in about 50% of patients.

Left bundle branch block causes abnormal septal motion, but septal thickening is normal. Cardiomyopathies are more common in patients with left bundle branch block. Because abnormal septal motion may make it difficult to assess the anteroseptal wall, the two-chamber view must be used to analyze wall motion in the distribution of the left anterior descending artery (Fig. 7-7).

In patients with left ventricular hypertrophy, it is necessary to examine the inferior basal segments carefully. In some cases, right coronary artery disease cannot be excluded on rest or postexercise images. To minimize this possibility, we angle the transducer below the mitral valve plane on the four-chamber view to obtain a more complete view of the inferobasal wall.

It is not always necessary to see the endocardium in its entirety. Sometimes ischemia can be detected by a change in the shape of the ventricle even though the endocardium is not well seen. Technically poor-quality studies should not be interpreted as showing ischemia simply because the endocardium is not visible. However, on a good-quality study, the endocardium may be difficult to see because of ischemia-induced thinning. It is also important to separate endocardium from other structures, such as chordae and apical trabeculation, which may mimic the endocardial border.

Atypical acoustic windows may cause problems when interpreting stress echocardiograms. Use of a low parasternal window may create the appearance of anteroseptal hypokinesis and left anterior descending disease. Sometimes, to see the apex clearly, it is necessary to obtain the apical views from a higher intercostal space, which will foreshorten the image and give the appearance of right ventricular dilatation (Fig. 7-8). Obtaining a subcostal view is the best way to show the right ventricular size clearly. It is important to evaluate for right ventricular dilatation, which may be caused by right coronary artery ischemia or pulmonary hypertension and severe lung disease. If right ventricular dilatation is present, the inferior basal region must be carefully inspected for regional wall motion abnormalities.

Another phenomenon that may indicate ischemia is endocardial brightening. Using this indicator when only subtle wall motion abnormalities are present helps secure a diagnosis of ischemia. For this reason, we recommend keeping the ultrasound gain setting constant for rest and exercise imaging.

The interpretation of dobutamine studies is

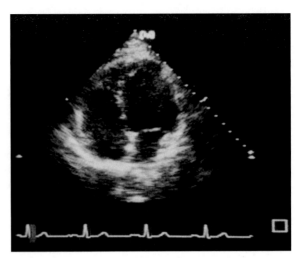

Figure 7-8. Echocardiogram in the apical four-chamber view recorded from an intercostal space that is too high. Note the foreshortening of the ventricles, which gives the false appearance of right ventricular dilatation. Apical images should be acquired from the lowest imaging window to avoid this pitfall.

complicated by the reduction in left ventricular size that occurs with decreased systemic vascular resistance due to vasodilation. It is a good idea to allow patients to drink clear fluids rather than restrict intake altogether before the test so that they will not become volume depleted. With dobutamine, endocardial visualization may be impaired by hyperpnea and cardiac translation. The increased inotropic response may cause difficulty with interpretation because uniform thickening is not always present.

Conclusion

CAD is the leading cause of death among adults in the United States. Reliable diagnosis is the first step toward reducing the morbidity and mortality that result from coronary insufficiency. Exercise echocardiography has emerged as a far superior alternative to standard stress electrocardiography, not only in detecting the presence or absence of CAD but also in delineating the extent and distribution of disease. In each of the three major patient groups in whom reliable prediction of the status of coronary vascular anatomy is most important and most frequent—patients being screened for CAD, those who have undergone angioplasty, and those who

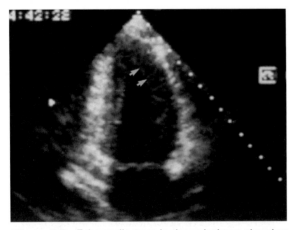

Figure 7-7. Echocardiogram in the apical two-chamber view. This view is best for evaluating perfusion in the distribution of the left anterior descending coronary artery (anterior wall, arrow) in patients with left bundle branch block.

TABLE 7-1. Comparison of Sensitivity, Secificity, and Predictive Accuracy of Electrocardiography (ECG) and Exercise Echocardiography as an Initial Screening Test for Coronary Artery Disease, After Coronary Artery Bypass Grafting (CABG), and After Percutaneous Transluminal Coronary Angioplasty (PTCA)

| | Sensitivity | | Specificity | | Predictive Accuracy | | | |
| | | | | | Positive | | Negative | |
Group	ECG	Echo	ECG	Echo	ECG	Echo	ECG	Echo
Initial screening (*n* = 228)	51%	97%	62%	64%	82%	90%	28%	87%
After CABG (*n* = 125)	41%	98%	67%	92%	91%	99%	16%	86%
After PTCA (*n* = 185)	51%	95%	73%	82%	88%	95%	28%	82%

Data are from reference 12. All patients underwent coronary angiography after noninvasive testing.

have had coronary artery bypass grafting—exercise echocardiography is more sensitive, specific, and accurate than stress electrocardiography[12] (Table 7-1). It also permits a more comprehensive assessment of other causes of cardiac morbidity and mortality, including thrombus, aneurysm formation, valvular heart disease, occult congenital heart disease, cardiomyopathy, cardiac masses and tumors, and pericardial disease. As experience with the technique grows and as methods are developed to overcome imaging difficulties in some patients, exercise echocardiography will evolve into a uniquely informative, noninvasive technique that can be applied to a variety of patient groups in whom exercise electrocardiography has serious limitations. Increased image storage capacity, greater network capabilities, advances in imaging techniques such as the use of echocardiographic contrast agents, and automated wall motion analysis and other quantitative methods hold great promise for the future development of exercise echocardiography.

REFERENCES

1. Afridi I, Quinones MA, Zoghbi WA, et al. Dobutamine stress echocardiography: Sensitivity, specificity, and predictive value for future cardiac events. Am Heart J. 1994;127:1510–1515.
2. Armstrong WF, O'Donnell J, Dillon JC, et al. Complementary value of two-dimensional exercise echocardiography to routine treadmill exercise testing. Ann Intern Med. 1986;105:829–835.
3. Armstrong WF, O'Donnell J, Ryan T, et al. Effect of prior myocardial infarction and extent and location of coronary disease on accuracy of exercise echocardiography. J Am Coll Cardiol. 1987;10:531–538.
4. Baptista J, Arnese M, Roelandt JR, et al. Quantitative coronary angiography in the estimation of the functional significance of coronary stenosis: Correlations with dobutamine-atropine stress test. J Am Coll Cardiol. 1994;23:1434–1439.
5. Berthe C, Pierard LA, Hiernaux M, et al. Predicting the extent and location of coronary artery disease in acute myocardial infarction by echocardiography during dobutamine infusion. Am J Cardiol. 1986; 58:1167–1172.
6. Borer JS, Brensike JF, Redwood DR, et al. Limitations of the electrocardiographic response to exercise in predicting coronary artery disease. N Engl J Med. 1975;293:367–371.
7. Braverman AC, Thomas JD, Lee RT. Doppler echocardiographic estimation of mitral valve area during changing hemodynamic conditions. Am J Cardiol. 1991;78:1485–1490.
8. Coma-Canella I. Sensitivity and specificity of dobutamine-electrocardiography test to detect multivessel disease after acute myocardial infarction. Eur Heart J. 1990;11:249–257.
9. Crawford MH, Among KW, Vance WS. Exercise 2-dimensional echocardiography. Am J Cardiol. 1983; 51:1–6.
10. Crawford MH, Petru MA, Amon KW, et al. Comparative value of 2-dimensional echocardiography and radionuclide angiography for quantitating changes in left ventricular performance during exercise limited by angina pectoris. Am J Cardiol. 1984;53: 42–46.
11. Crouse LJ, Harbrecht JJ, Vacek JL, et al. Exercise echocardiography as a screening test for coronary artery disease and correlation with coronary arteriography. Am J Cardiol. 1991;67:1213–1218.
12. Crouse LJ, Kramer PH. Clinical applicability of echocardiographically detected regional wall-motion

abnormalities provoked by upright treadmill exercise. Echocardiography. 1992;9:97–106.

13. Dahan M, Paillole C, Martin D. Determinants of stroke volume response to exercise in patients with mitral stenosis: A Doppler echocardiographic study. J Am Coll Cardiol. 1993;21:384–389.

14. Holmes DR, Vlietstra RE, Smith HC, et al. Restenosis after percutaneous transluminal coronary angioplasty. A report from the PTCA Registry of the National Heart, Lung and Blood Institute. Am J Cardiol. 1984;53:77C–81C.

15. Lawless CE, Loeb HS. Pharmacokinetics and pharmacodynamics of dobutamine. *In* Chatterjee K (ed): Dobutamine—A Ten-Year Review. Part 1. New York, NCM Publishers; 1989:33–47.

16. Leavitt JI, Coats MH, Falk RH. Effects of exercise on transmitral gradient and pulmonary artery pressure in patients with mitral stenosis or a prosthetic mitral valve: A Doppler echocardiographic study. J Am Coll Cardiol. 1991;17:1520–1526.

17. Limacher MC, Quinones MA, Poliner LR, et al. Detection of coronary artery disease with exercise two-dimensional echocardiography. Circulation. 1983; 67:1211–1218.

18. Mannering D. The dobutamine stress test as an alternative to exercise testing for acute myocardial infarction. Br Heart J. 1988;59:521–526.

19. Marcovitz PA, Armstrong WF. Accuracy of dobutamine stress echocardiography in detecting coronary artery disease. Am J Cardiol. 1992;69: 1269–1273.

20. Marwick T, D'Hondt A, Baudguin T, et al. Optimal use of dobutamine stress for the detection and evaluation of coronary artery disease: Combination with echocardiography or scintigraphy, or both? J Am Coll Cardiol. 1993;22:159–167.

21. Marwick T, Willemaart B, D'Hondt AM, et al. Selection of the optimal nonexercise stress for the evaluation of ischemic regional myocardial dysfunction and malperfusion. Circulation. 1993;87:345–354.

22. Mason SJ, Weiss JL, Weisfeldt JL, et al. Exercise echocardiography: Detection of wall motion abnormalities during ischemia. Circulation. 1979;59:1.

23. McNeill AJ, Fioretti PM, El-Said E-SM, et al. Enhanced sensitivity for detection of coronary artery disease by addition of atropine to dobutamine stress echocardiography. Am J Cardiol. 1992;70:41–46.

24. Morganroth J, Chen CC, David D. Exercise cross-sectional echocardiographic diagnosis of coronary artery disease. Am J Cardiol. 1981;47:20–26.

25. Nestro RW, Kowalchuk GJ. The ischemic cascade: Temporal sequence of hemodynamic, electrocardiographic, and symptomatic expressions of ischemia. Am J Cardiol. 1987;59:23C–30C.

26. Oberman A, Fan PH, Nanda NC, et al. Reproducibility of two-dimensional exercise echocardiography. J Am Coll Cardiol. 1989;14:923–928.

27. Oh JK, Gersh BJ, Nassed LA Jr, et al. Effects of acute reperfusion on regional myocardial function: Serial two-dimensional echocardiography assessment. Int J Cardiol. 1989;22:161–168.

28. Pierard LA, Berthe C, Carlier AA, et al. Hemodynamic alterations during ischemia induced by dobutamine stress testing. Eur Heart J. 1989;10: 783–790.

29. Pierard LA, De Landsheere CM, Berthe C, et al. Identification of viable myocardium by echocardiography during dobutamine infusion in patients with myocardial infarction after thrombolytic therapy: Comparison with positron emission tomography. J Am Coll Cardiol. 1989;15:1021–1031.

30. Poldermans D, Fioretti PM, Boersma E, et al. Safety of dobutamine-atropine stress echocardiography in patients with suspected or proven coronary artery disease. Am J Cardiol. 1994;73:456–459.

31. Presti CF, Armstrong WF, Feigenbaum H. Comparison of echocardiography at peak exercise and after bicycle exercise in evaluation of patients with known or suspected coronary artery disease. J Am Soc Echocardiogr. 1988;1:119–126.

32. Reisner SA, Lichtenberg GS, Shapiro JR, et al. Exercise Doppler echocardiography in patients with mitral prosthetic valves. Am Heart J. 1989;118: 755–759.

33. Robertson SW, Feigenbaum H, Armstrong WF, et al. Exercise echocardiography: A clinically practical addition in the evaluation of coronary artery disease. J Am Coll Cardiol. 1983;2:1085–1091.

34. Rosamond TL, Rowland AJ, Harbrecht JJ, et al. Outpatient dobutamine echocardiography: Safety and clinical utility (abstract). Circulation. 1990; 83(suppl III):

35. Rosamond TL, Rowland AJ, Willhoite DJ, et al. Hypotension during dobutamine stress echocardiography: Significance of the absence of regional hypokinesis. J Am Coll Cardiol. 1991;17:193A.

36. Ryan T, Vasey CG, Presti CF, et al. Exercise echocardiography: Detection of coronary artery disease in patients with normal left ventricular wall motion at rest. J Am Coll Cardiol. 1988;11:993–999.

37. Segar DS, Brown SE, Swada SG, et al. Dobutamine stress echocardiography: Correlation with coronary lesion severity as determined by quantitative angiography. J Am Coll Cardiol. 1992;19:1197–1202.

38. Tischler M, Battle RW, Saha M, et al. Observations suggesting a high incidence of exercise-induced severe mitral regurgitation in patients with mild rheumatic mitral valve disease at rest. J Am Coll Cardiol. 1995;25:128–133.

39. Tischler MD, Plehn JF. Applications of stress echocardiography: Beyond coronary disease. J Am Soc Echocardiogr. 1995;8:185–197.

40. Vasey CG, Armstrong WF, Ryan T, et al. Prediction of the presence and location of coronary artery disease by digital exercise echocardiography. J Am Coll Cardiol. 1986;7:15A.

41. Voelker W, Jacksch R, Dittmann H, et al. Validation of continuous-wave Doppler measurements of mitral valve gradients during exercise: A simultaneous Doppler-catheter study. Eur Heart J. 1989;10: 737–746.

42. Wann LS, Faris JV, Childress RH, et al. Exercise cross-sectional echocardiography in ischemic heart disease. Circulation. 1979;60:1300–1308.

43. Weiss P, Hoffman A, Burckhardt D. Doppler sonographic evaluation of mechanical and bioprosthetic mitral valve prostheses during exercise with a rate corrected pressure half time. Br Heart J. 1992;67: 466–469.

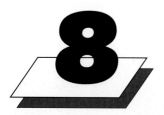

8

Contrast Echocardiography

MARK N. ALLEN

Introduction

The use of contrast to help visualize cardiac structures was reported as early as 1968.[52,53] Since the time of its initial uses, contrast echocardiography has gained great attention because of the development of newer contrast agents, advances in technology, and increased safety. Today contrast agents are used to enhance the visualization of cardiac structures and Doppler signals. They are used in the evaluation of left and right heart structures,[74,159,178] pulmonary artery pressures,[73] degree of mitral regurgitation,[132,168] aortic stenosis,[42] left ventricular function with and without stress echocardiography,[2,14,18,23,28,29,41,54,179] presence and degree of patent foramen and other shunts,[39,60,69,72,121,153,154,155] and coronary artery visualization, stenosis, and perfusion.[5,17,63,88]

Spontaneous Contrast

The term *contrast* is used to describe the enhancement of ultrasound images or Doppler signals. The appearance of these highly reflective entities can result from internal or intrinsic properties or from introduced agents containing highly reflective microbubbles that enhance the ultrasound signal. The former is frequently called *spontaneous contrast (SEC)*, a term used to describe the appearance of discrete reflections in the blood inside cardiac chambers, cavities, or vessels without previous injection of echocontrast medium or fluids containing microbubbles.[4] There are many explanations for SEC.[101,102,106,107,112,144,161] These range from the formation of blood aggregates *(rouleaux)*,[161] bubbles produced from gas absorbed from the intestines and transported to the heart via porta-systemic shunting,[107] the persistence of microbubbles in the circulation from recent or remote intravenous injections,[144] erythrocytes and platelet formations in low-flow regions,[101,102] and shear forces or shear rate of the blood.[146,147]

SEC is typically observed when blood becomes echogenic in a particular region of decreased flow.[4] Shear rate, particle size, and particle frequency appear to be important factors in the observation of SEC.[146,147] SEC is not seen with shear rates greater than 40 sec. Only in low-flow states do shear rates below 40 sec permit SEC observation.[7] The ratio of blood particle size and wavelength also plays a critical role in SEC observation. The larger the particle size, the more likely SEC will be seen. Higher-frequency (decreased-wavelength) transducers permit higher resolution and enhanced backscattering, ultimately allowing increased sensitivity to SEC.[4]

The appearance of SEC is typically noted in regions with abnormal flow states. However, SEC can also be seen in patients with no significant abnormalities.[20,108] Any of the cardiac chambers or vessels may demonstrate SEC in the presence of the above-mentioned conditions. SEC is commonly noted in the left atrium in association with mitral stenosis,[25,89] atrial fibrillation,[12,19,74] or impaired left ventricular diastolic function.[124] SEC can be found in the left atrium in the presence of these conditions. In any of these states, common findings include left atrial size greater than 2.4 cm (corrected base index and measured from the anteroposterior dimension), mitral velocity time integral (corrected for heart rate) of less than 10 cm, and mean peak velocity in the left atrial appendage of .12 m/sec.[124]

SEC is also noted in the left ventricle when systolic function is impaired, and in patients with coronary artery disease and regional wall motion abnormalities,[42] dilated cardiomyopathies,[37] and left ventricular (LV) aneurysms or pseudoaneurysms. When LV function improves, SEC usually disappears. A dilated or dissected thoracic aorta is another site for SEC (Fig. 8-1). In dilated aortas, cardiac output is decreased, setting the stage for a low-flow state. In aortic dissections, SEC is seen in the false lumen. The presence of SEC can indicate the flow status and therefore the size of the tear. If no SEC is seen, this suggests a higher flow state and a larger tear.[40,147] Smaller tears typically demonstrate SEC. With higher-frequency transesophageal echocardiography (TEE) transducers and excellent image quality, SEC can be seen in normal aortas.[4]

SEC of the RV occurs when there is significant RV dysfunction.[30] SEC of the right atrium (RA) is seen in RA enlargement, atrial fibrillation or flutter, elevated RV pressure, moderate or severe mitral valve disease, or right-to-left interatrial shunts.[20] SEC is seen in the inferior vena cava (IVC) from a subcostal echocardiographic view in patients with

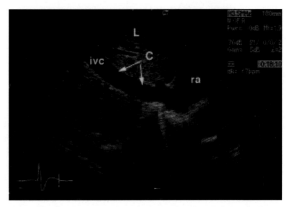

Figure 8-2. Subcostal transthoracic view of the IVC with spontaneous contrast noted (arrow). IVC, inferior vena cava; ra, right atrium; c, spontaneous contrast; l, liver.

constrictive pericarditis[65] and in patients with no cardiac abnormalities (Fig. 8-2).[108]

SEC has the potential to induce embolic events due to thrombus formation.[24,55,95,163,182] It is important to document the presence of SEC in the left atrium (LA). In studies comparing groups of patients with and without documented systemic embolism, the presence of SEC was high in the group with embolic events.[163] SEC can be used as a predictor of embolic events in patients at high risk. Careful evaluation of cardiac chambers with proper transducer frequency may help identify SEC. TEE is a reliable tool since its probes typically use higher transmit frequencies and offer better unobscured views of the cardiac chambers.

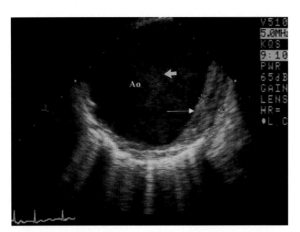

Figure 8-1. Cross-sectional transesophageal view of the aorta with spontaneous contrast within the lumen (short arrow). A mural thrombus is also noted (long arrow).

Contrast Agents

Visualization of cardiac structures can be enhanced with the use of contrast agents. Microbubbles are very efficient reflectors of ultrasound.[142] However, although the process appears relatively simple, the concept of using microbubbles as reflectors to enhance cardiac images poses several challenges. The microbubbles of contrast used must be small to avoid causing potentially harmful effects, must remain tiny after injection, must stay in the circulation and remain stable long enough to be detected by ultrasound, must be tolerated by patients, and must be the proper size.

Initially, contrast agents were as simple as agitated saline solution or agents with surfactant properties such as renografin or cardiogreen, which with vigorous shaking produced small bubbles. These agents could be used only to enhance right-sided chambers and were used to identify intracardiac shunts, septal defects, and right-sided valvular insufficiency. In order to be useful in the left heart, contrast agents had to become small enough to pass and survive the pulmonary circulation. Today typical contrast agents are injected into a peripheral vein, where they enter the right heart and pass through the pulmonary vasculature into the left heart. The diameter of the capillaries within the pulmonary vasculature is roughly 8 μm.[170] Therefore, in order for these contrast agents to be useful, their suspensions or mixtures must possess microbubbles with a diameter of 8 μm or less to pass through these tiny vessels. The bubble size of most contrast agents ranges from 0.1 to 8 μm. One agent, Quantison, possesses particles with a mean diameter of 12 μm and must be injected intra-arterially since its bubbles are too large to pass through the pulmonary capillaries.[10]

There are numerous agents commercially available and in developmental stages today. Table 8-1 identifies some of the current agents. The materials that are used to help produce or carry the microbubbles vary from product to product (see Table 8-1). The reflective property of the microbubbles comes from the material within the microbubbles or spheres, which in most agents consists of gas or air. The acoustic impedance of these gas or air bodies differs from that of blood and accounts for the

TABLE 8-1. CONTRAST AGENTS

Agent	Manufacturer	Composition
CURRENTLY AVAILABLE AGENTS		
SHU 454 (Echovist)	Echovist Schering AG Berlin	Galatose base
SHU 508A (Levovist)	Levovist Shering AG, Berlin	Galatose base
Albunex	Mallinckrodt Medical, Inc., St. Louis, MO	Human albumin
Optison™	Mallinckrodt Medical, Inc., St. Louis, MO	Human albumin with octafluoropropane gas
LATE DEVELOPMENTAL STAGE		
Echogen	Sonus Pharmaceutical, Bothell, WA	Dodecafluoropentane
BY 963		Air-containing microbubbles in suspension of soya-based phospholipid
FSO 69	Molecular Biosystems, Inc., San Diego, CA	Proteinaceous gas-filled microspheres
EARLY DEVELOPMENTAL STAGE		
Imagent (AFO145)	Alliance Pharmaceutical Corp., San Diego, CA	Unspecified components, surfactants, sodium chloride, phosphate buffers, gaseous perfluorohexane
BR1	Bracco Research SA, Carouge-Geneva	Suspension of microbubbles filled with dense gas and sulfur hexafluoride
SHU 563A		Air-filled microspheres with a thin layer of a biodegradable cyanacrylate polymer
Quantison and Quantison Depot	Andaris, Nottingham, United Kingdom	Resembles human albumin microcapsules
Perflurocarbons— exposed sonicated dextrose albumin (RESDA)		Sonicated solutions of glucose and human albumin
Aersomes	Imarex, Tucson, AZ	Lipid bilayers of dipalmitoylphosphatidylcholine filled with gas rather than liquid

Source: Ref. 142.

strong signals, which can be 4×10^5 stronger than that of red blood cells.[99] Other factors affecting the reflective properties of microbubbles include transmit frequency, microbubble diameter, microbubble concentration, and microbubble survival rate.

Smaller-diameter bubbles reflect more strongly. Ideally, contrast agents that can hold their bubble size relatively constant would be ideal. However, bubble diameter varies due to resonant frequency and internal and external pressures exerted on the bubble. An increase in microbubble concentration may also help increase the contrast effect.[172] The survival rates of microbubbles depend on the properties of the solutions used to carry them, the amount of gas in the surrounding medium, the interaction of the microbubbles in concentrated solution, and the encapsulation of the bubbles.[172]

Bubble life can be prolonged by decreasing the surface tension and other pressures surrounding the bubbles. Surfactants help to reduce the surface tension of bubbles and therefore are used in many of the materials in contrast agents. The use of strong encapsulating materials also helps to prolong bubble life. Materials such as gelatins and saccharides help to stabilize the bubbles. The old adage of "safety in numbers" also applies to bubbles. Larger concentrations of bubbles help prolong bubble life. In a bolus with a large concentration of bubbles, the bubbles located toward the outside tend to protect those on the inside, slowing the dissolution process.[142,172]

Eventually, these microbubbles disappear, resolve, or dissolve. The process by which microbubbles disappear depends largely on the contrast material. Galactose- and albumin-based agents dissolve in the bloodstream and are removed by the liver or kidneys. Other agents, such as Echogen, become dissolved in the blood and are eventually excreted in expired air.[142]

Safety Considerations

Naturally of concern is the safety of these products, both the microbubbles and the contrast agent used to store them. The toxicity of microbubbles is related to bubble size, stability, and uniformity. Large microbubbles pose a potential risk of gas embolism by becoming trapped within smaller blood vessels.[86] Studies have concluded that the diameter of air microbubbles size must be less than 10 μm in order

for the bubbles to pass safely through the capillary vasculature.[33,177] The most serious side effects from peripherally injected contrast agents such as agitated saline are transient cerebrovascular defects, presumably from gas embolization in patients with right-to-left shunts.[15,92] These complications resolve within several minutes, with no long-lasting residual effects. The safety of more recent contrast agents continues to be studied.

Most contrast agents use a particular material to suspend or help create the microbubbles. The safety of these materials has been the focus of recent studies. The toxicity of these carrier materials is related to their osmolarity, viscosity, and surfactant properties. Carrier agents are composed of gelatin, ionic, nonionic albumin, saccharide, or fluorocarbons.[118]

Gelatin-based contrast agents are no longer available in the United States due to an occasional allergic reaction, although they are still used in Europe. Other side effects include transient T-wave changes, transient second degree atrioventricular (AV) block, and QRS axis deviation.[140] However, the majority of patients in the study experienced no side effects. Newer gelatin-based products are being developed and tested; few side effects have been reported.[11]

The osmolality of a material is related to its concentration. A highly concentrated material may draw fluids from other sources in order to equalize the amounts of solids and liquid within the material. A carrier agent with a high osmolality or hyperosmolality may lead to a drop in coronary flow, creating cardiodepressive effects.[57,118] The viscosity of a material is related to its frictional property. The viscosity of a carrier material influences the size and stability of the microbubbles and appears to have an inverse effect on microbubble size and stability.[85,118] Highly viscous contrast agents are associated with transient changes in coronary flow and left ventricular function. Surfactant is a material that reduces surface tension. Contrast agents with good surfactant properties increase the stability of microbubbles.

Right Heart Applications

Contrast echocardiography in the evaluation of the right heart has many uses, including enhancing RV endocardial borders,[159] determining cardiac output,[32,47] and enhancing Doppler spectral displays of tricuspid and pulmonary regurgitation, which in turn helps to determine pulmonary artery systolic and diastolic pressures, respectively.[78,96,157] Agitated saline is most widely used for these applications; however, other contrast agents can also be used.

SYSTOLIC PULMONARY ARTERY PRESSURES

Systolic pulmonary artery pressures can be determined by transthoracic echocardiography if a high-quality tricuspid regurgitant signal is present on a spectral Doppler display. Using the modified Bernoulli equation, $P = 4\ V^2$, systolic pulmonary artery pressures can be calculated by adding the estimated central venous pressure.[9,58,87,169] However, a significant number of patients have only trivial tricuspid regurgitation or suboptimal or incomplete signals with poorly developed envelopes and peak velocities. In patients with possible pulmonary hypertension, the ability to quantify pulmonary artery pressures is crucial. Contrast agents can aid in the detection and display of tricuspid regurgitant signals. Usually agitated saline is sufficient to help identify the presence of tricuspid regurgitation; however, this effect can be short-lived, making it difficult to obtain an adequate signal.[78] Albunex has also been used to enhance the regurgitant signal, reportedly with better results than those obtained with simple agitated saline[8,16,78] (Fig. 8-3).

The severity of tricuspid regurgitation can also be determined by the use of contrast echocardiography. Detection and clearance time of injected contrast within the IVC can indicate the severity of tricuspid regurgitation.[32,73,110] Clearance time of more than 20 cardiac cycles is consistent with severe tricuspid regurgitation.[110]

PULMONARY DIASTOLIC PRESSURES

Diastolic pulmonary artery pressures can be estimated from a Doppler spectral display of a pulmonic valve regurgitant signal by measuring the end-diastolic velocity.[58,93,103,105] However, like Doppler signals of tricuspid regurgitation, distinct pulmonary regurgitation signals are not always clearly seen. Contrast on the right side of the heart can

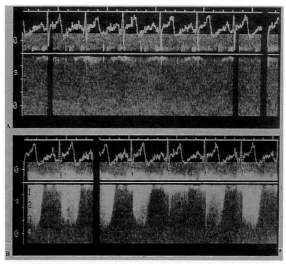

Figure 8-3. (**A**) Spectral Doppler display from across the tricuspid valve; notice the absence of flow below the baseline. (**B**) Doppler display from the same patient following intravenous injection of Albunex. The resulting signal allows visualization of the spectral envelope and peak velocity measurements (3.7 m/sec). (From Nanda NC, Schlief R, Goldberg BB [eds]: Advances in Echo Imaging Using Contrast Enhancement, 2nd ed. Dordrecht, the Netherlands, Kluwer; 1993:230. Reprinted with permission.)

reliably and accurately enhance pulmonic valve regurgitant Doppler signals.[157]

CARDIAC OUTPUT

The presence of contrast in the RV can help delineate endocardial borders. The shape of the RV and the orientation of the RV to the sound waves in most views do not always allow a clear view of all wall segments. Contrast echocardiography is useful in helping to define the endocardial borders of the RV, allowing for a more accurate assessment of ejection fraction.[159] Additionally, changes in the intensity of the contrast within a chamber can be used to measure cardiac output.[77] It has been observed that the contrast effect lasts longer in patients with congestive heart failure than in patients with normal systolic function.[32] With contrast echocardiography, cardiac output can be calculated using indicator dilution curves that measure the quantity of the injected indicator, the mean concentration of the indicator, and the total duration of the curve.[77] However, many factors can affect these measurements, and further work is being done to determine absolute flows.

Valvular Applications

MITRAL VALVE

The accurate assessment and quantification of mitral regurgitation (MR) remains an echocardiographic challenge. Many techniques are used to provide some quantifiable data on the volume and severity of MR. Color flow Doppler is currently one of the more common methods used. MR jets using this method, although widely accepted, may not always be reproducible or reliable since improper color or image gain settings, image dropout, poor images, masking from calcification, and eccentric jets can make visualization and therefore assessment of MR severity difficult.

The use of contrast agents to enhance Doppler signals in the left heart increases the sensitivity of MR signals.[132,158,167,168] The tiny bubbles contained or suspended in contrast agents reflect sound waves with a higher intensity than red blood cells.[45,109] TEE has proven to be better than transthoracic echocardiography (TTE) in detecting and displaying MR in technically difficult studies. Contrast agents such as SHU 508A and sonicated albumin enhance Doppler signals and increase the visualization of MR jets when used in conjunction with color Doppler exams[132,158,167,168] (Fig. 8-4). The bubbles contained in these agents are small enough to pass through the pulmonary vascular bed, enabling them to be seen in the left heart. Studies comparing TEE and contrast-enhanced color and continuous wave Doppler TTE evaluation of MR have correlated very well.[168] The signal-to-noise ratio improves with the use of contrast agents, so that peak velocities can be confidently measured.

The dose of these agents is critical in defining a clear signal. If the contrast agent is too concentrated, artifact will be seen; if the concentration is insufficient, the effect will be less dramatic or inadequate. For SHU 508A the recommended dose is 200 to 400 mg/ml in an amount of 8 to 16 ml. The duration of a signal of significant intensity is 100 to 140 sec.[168]

PULMONARY VEIN FLOW

Doppler signals obtained from the pulmonary veins have been used to provide information on diastolic LV function (dysfunction), as well as to determine the severity of MR and LA pressures.[79,80,82,83,90,91,104,133] Pulmonary venous flow is typically obtained from apical windows, where depth can make visualization and placement of the pulsed Doppler range gate difficult. Pulmonary venous flow patterns are inadequate in as many as 27% of patients using TTE,[81] but they improve significantly with the use of TEE.[21] TTE with intravenously injected SHU 508A and sonicated albumin improves the quality of the pulmonary venous Doppler signal. The biphasic and peak flow velocities after contrast injection compare well with those obtained with TEE, with no alteration in velocity[168,174] (Fig. 8-5).

AORTIC STENOSIS

Doppler TTE remains one of the best methods to evaluate and quantify aortic stenosis.[148,180] The peak velocity and gradients can be obtained from a number of different acoustic windows with relative ease and accuracy. However, these measurements can be difficult to obtain in some patients because the required velocity envelopes are not always clearly delineated. Contrast agents may be used to enhance these signals[116,168] (Fig. 8-6). Agents capable of passing through the pulmonary vascular bed can be used to enhance aortic stenosis signals. With the use of sonicated human albumin in this clinical setting, the duration of the contrast effect is influenced by LV systolic pressure.[117] The higher the systolic pressure, the shorter the duration of contrast. This may be explained by the observation that

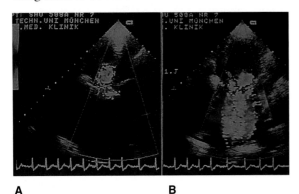

A   **B**

Figure 8-4. (**A**) Transthoracic four-chamber view with a color Doppler display of the mitral valve. The small size of the jet suggests minimal or mild MR. (**B**) Intravenous injection of SHU 508A dramatically reveals the MR using color Doppler. (From Nanda NC, Schlief R, Goldberg BB (eds): Advances in Echo Imaging Using Contrast Enhancement, 2nd ed. Dordrecht, the Netherlands, Kluwer; 1993: 245. Reprinted with permission.) (See also Color Plate 23.)

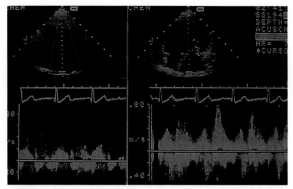

Figure 8-5. (A) Pulsed wave recordings of the right upper pulmonary vein from an apical four-chamber view in a patient with MR. The spectral display is not well appreciated. **(B)** The same view with contrast enhancement demonstrating systolic reversal. (From Nanda NC, Schlief R, Goldberg BB (eds): Advances in Echo Imaging Using Contrast Enhancement, 2nd ed. Dordrecht, the Netherlands, Kluwer; 1993:249. Reprinted with permission.)

sonicated human albumin is sensitive to high pressures.[51,145] It also seems reasonable that in the presence of aortic insufficiency, the duration of contrast would also be prolonged.

Intravenous administration of contrast agents has proven to be useful in enhancing aortic, MR,

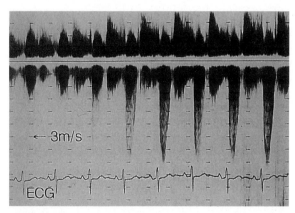

Figure 8-6. Continuous Doppler recording across an aortic valve in a patient with aortic stenosis. The signals to the left of the image are indistinct and cannot be measured. Following contrast injection (right side of the image), the aortic signals are clearly delineated and can be measured. (From Nanda NC, Schief R, Goldberg BB (eds): Advances in Echo Imaging Using Contrast Enhancement, 2nd ed. Dordrecht, the Netherlands, Kluwer; 1993:256. (Reprinted with permission.)

and pulmonary venous flow signals in patients. This technique offers a noninvasive alternative to TEE in these clinical settings.

Stress Echocardiography

Stress echocardiography has emerged as an accurate and safe method of evaluating known or suspected coronary artery disease. Using two-dimensional echocardiography, baseline and postexercise images of the heart in numerous tomographic planes can be obtained and compared, allowing a detailed assessment of regional wall motion and wall thickening. However, detailed images of the endocardial borders are not always possible in roughly 10–20% of patients.[46] Identification of the endocardial walls in the lateral, inferior basal, and apical regions is particularly problematic in patients with poor acoustic windows. Peripheral injection of contrast agents capable of passing through the pulmonary vascular bed enhances endocardial borders by opacifying the LV, improving the interpretation of regional wall motion and therefore of ejection fraction during exercise and pharmacologic stress echocardiography.[2,23,27,34,41,78,94,166,179] Studies have demonstrated that endocardial border delineation improves with contrast injection in 83% of patients and that confidence in assessing regional wall motion improves 77% in patients in whom confidence was low before contrast injection.[27,28]

Myocardial Perfusion

Injection of echocontrast agents directly into the coronary arteries enhances visualization of the myocardium. The resultant increase in reflectivity of the myocardium provides information regarding the distribution of myocardial perfusion and allows assessment of coronary flow.[3,5,14,18,29,54,62,63,64,66,67,75,76,97,98,111,122,126,127,128,130,131,134,135,136,138,139,165] Enhancement of the myocardium by contrast agents can be achieved by injecting the agent directly into the coronary arteries[1,11,122,126,134,138] or by injecting it intravenously.[76,166] Both methods have advantages and disadvantages. Direct injection of contrast agents into the coronary circulation provides sufficient contrast to perfuse the myocardium. However, due to the highly reflective properties of the contrast material, images in the near field may effectively obscure images in the far field by masking. This technique is also invasive since it needs to be done in conjunction with coronary angiography or angioplasty and therefore must be performed in a cardiac catheterization lab or another highly controlled environment.

Contrast agents capable of reaching the coronary arteries and hence the myocardium from a venous site would hold great promise since only access to a peripheral vein is required. However, there are several problems that must be solved for this technique to be useful. Roughly 5–10% of cardiac output contributes to the coronary blood supply. Resting blood flow through the coronary arteries ranges from 250 to 500 ml/min. The coronary arteries begin as two large branches that gradually branch into smaller and smaller vessels, eventually terminating in capillaries no larger than the diameter of a single red blood cell.[150] With this in mind, several problems may arise that may limit the ability of contrast agents to "illuminate" the myocardium.

In order for a contrast agent injected from a venous site to reach the coronary arteries, the number of microbubbles in the agent must be sufficient to be detected in the myocardium. Further, the microbubbles must be stable enough to survive the pulmonary circulation since only about 5–10 of every 100 microbubbles will reach the coronary circulation. Another problem with this approach is that the concentration of microbubbles within a given area will be less in the myocardium due to the size of the vessel relative to the concentration in the same area of a blood pool.[137] To overcome these problems, a number of changes have been proposed, including agents with a high and longer persistence once injected.[137] These newer agents are being investigated, and it seems reasonable that within a relatively short period of time, these problems will be overcome.

Shunts

PATENT FORAMEN OVALE

Contrast echocardiography is valuable in identifying right-to-left shunts such as patent foramen ovale,[6,26,60,69,72,153,154,155] interatrial defects,[121] and pulmonary arteriovenous malformations.[39,50]

Paradoxic embolus from patent foramen ovale (PFO) may cause stroke in patients even in the absence of clinically demonstrable venous thrombosis or pulmonary hypertension.[6] Identification of PFO by a reliable method is therefore important. The use of hand-agitated saline solution injected into a peripheral vein is the usual procedure in attempting to assess PFO. In the presence of a PFO, the contrast will appear dramatically in the right heart, while just a few bubbles may be observed in the left heart immediately (usually within the first or second cardiac cycle) after opacification of the right heart.[26] Although pressures within the left heart are normally higher than those within the right side, transient reversal of the usual left-to-right pressure gradient during any phase of the cardiac cycle results in some reversal or bidirectional occurrence of microbubbles. Contrast can occasionally be seen in the left heart in the absence of a PFO, but it will not be observed until after several complete cardiac cycles or until some small microbubbles have passed through the pulmonary vasculature.

Contrast echocardiography can be used to identify this lesion in conjunction with TTE or TEE. TEE and contrast injection is more accurate and is considered to be the gold standard in this clinical setting[6] (Fig. 8-7). The accuracy of contrast with TTE to detect PFO depends on the type of contrast material, the site of the injection, and the respiratory maneuvers or provocations performed during the injections.[61] In patients without suspected paradoxic embolus, PFO can be detected by contrast TTE in only 5–13% of patients during normal respiration and in 7–24% of those with Valsalva respiration, compared to 3–39% using contrast TEE.[61] The incidence of PFO found at autopsy is 24–36%.[56] Increasing right-sided pressures by performing the Valsalva maneuver or by coughing greatly increases the sensitivity of the contrast in PFO.[38,105] Color Doppler and TTE are not helpful in detecting PFO.[59,176]

Transcranial Doppler (TCD) scanning of the middle cerebral artery during intravenous injection of contrast can diagnose intracardiac right-to-left shunting.[69,72] The diagnosis of PFO by TCD is considered positive when a spike appears on the Doppler display 4–25 sec following an intravenous injection of a contrast agent.[69,72] The sensitivity of TCD

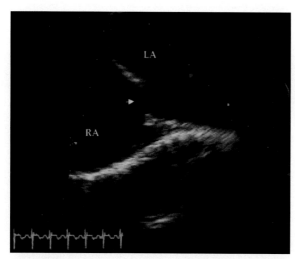

Figure 8-7. TEE demonstrating a PFO. Note the contrast crossing between the left atrium (LA) and right atrium (RA) (arrow).

compared to contrast TEE ranges from 68% to 93% in several studies, with a specificity of 94%–100%.[36,69,84] Passage of the bubbles through the pulmonary vasculature may produce false-positive results using this technique, but a strict time limit of 4 to 15 seconds between completion of the injection and observation of the Doppler signals may reduce this problem.[72]

ATRIAL SEPTAL DEFECTS AND OTHER SHUNTS

The use of contrast during TTE and TEE is helpful in the evaluation of atrial septal defects[121] and pulmonary AV fistulas.[39] The patterns of contrast in patients with PFO are similar to those in patients with atrial septal defects. This procedure is particularly valuable in patients with atrial septal defect repairs when the integrity of the patch must be examined.[160] Pulmonary AV shunts may be diagnosed with contrast echocardiography by timing the visualization of bubbles in the right heart versus the left heart. In pulmonary AV fistulas, a communication exists between the right pulmonary artery and the left heart (LA or pulmonary veins). Normally, contrast agents that are incapable of crossing the pulmonary vasculature will be filtered out and will not appear in the left heart in the absence of a communication. In pulmonary AV fistulas, the contrast will

first appear in the right heart and after several cardiac cycles will appear in the left heart. This late appearance of contrast in the left heart differentiates pulmonary AV fistulas from right-to-left atrial shunts.[149] The use of contrast agents in visualizing ventricular septal defects is seldom helpful unless the defect is large.

Summary

Contrast echocardiography will have an increasingly important role in the echocardiography lab in the near future. Technological advances in equipment and in contrast agents will enable relatively easy applications in most clinical settings. Some of the most interesting and exciting echocardiography research is being performed in this area.

REFERENCES

1. Abrams G, Jaffe C, Hoffer P, et al. Diagnostic utility of contrast echocardiography and lung perfusion scan in patients with hepatopulmonary syndrome. Gastroenterolgy. 1995;109:1283–1288.
2. Agati L, Voci P, Autore C, et al. Combined use of dobutamine echocardiography and myocardial contrast echocardiography in predicting regional dysfunction recovery after coronary revascularization in patients with recent myocardial infarction. Eur Heart J. 1997;18:771–779.
3. Agati L, Voci P, Bilotta F, et al. Dipyridamole myocardial contrast echocardiography in patients with single vessel coronary artery disease: Perfusion, anatomic, and functional correlates. Am Heart J. 1994;128:28–35.
4. Aiazian AA, Taams MA, Ten Cate FJ, et al. Spontaneous echocontrast: Etiology, technology dependence and clinical implications. *In* Nanda NC, Schlief R, Goldberg BB (eds): Advances in Echo Imaging using Contrast Enhancement. Dordrecht, the Netherlands, Kluwer; 1997:65–83.
5. Bach D, Muller D, Cheirif J, et al. Regional heterogeneity on myocardial contrast echocardiography without severe obstructive coronary artery disease. Am J Cardiol. 1995;75:982–986.
6. Belkin R, Pollack B, Ruggiero M, et al. Comparison of transesophageal and transthoracic echocardiography with contrast and color flow Doppler in the detection of patent foramen ovale. Am Heart J. 1994;128:520–525.
7. Beppu S, Nimura Y, Sakakibara H, et al. Smoke-

like echo in the left atrial cavity in mitral valve disease: Its features and significance. J Am Coll Cardiol. 1985;6:744–749.

8. Beppu S, Shimizu TK, Ishikura F, et al. Contrast enhancement of Doppler signals by sonicated albumin for estimating right ventricular systolic pressure. Am J Cardiol. 1991;67:1148–1149.

9. Berger M, Haimowitz A, Van Tosh A, et al. Quantitative assessment of pulmonary hypertension in patients with tricuspid regurgitation using continuous wave Doppler ultrasound. J Am Coll Cardiol. 1985;6:359–365.

10. Berwing K, Schlepper M. Kontrast-Echokardiographische Darstellungdes linken ventrikels bei peripher venoser Kontrastmittelingiektion bie patienten. Z Kariol. 1985;74(suppl 5):15.

11. Berwing K, Schlepper M. Echocardiographic imaging of the left ventricle by peripheral intravenous injection of echo-contrast agent in patients. Am Heart J. 1988;115:399.

12. Black IW, Hopkins AP, Lee LCL, et al. Left atrial spontaneous echo contrast: A clinical and echocardiographical analysis. J Am Coll Cardiol. 1991;18:398–404.

13. Block R, Brodsky L, Ostoic T, et al. Optimizing albunex in the left ventricle: An analysis of the technical parameters of four ultrasound systems in canines and humans. J Am Soc Echocardiogr. 1996;9:787–794.

14. Bolognese L, Antoniucci D, Rovai D, et al. Myocardial contrast echocardiography versus dobutamine echocardiography for predicting functional recovery after acute myocardial infarction treated with primary coronary angioplasty. J Am Coll Cardiol. 1996;28:1677–1683.

15. Bommer WJ, Shah PM, Allen H, et al. The safety of contrast echocardiography. J Clin Ultrasound. 1983;11:292–294.

16. Byrd BF, O'Kelly BF, Schiller NB. Contrast echocardiography enhances tricuspid but not mitral regurgitation. Clin Cardiol. 1991;14(suppl 5): V-10–V-14.

17. Caiati C, Aragona P, Iliceto S, et al. Improved Doppler detection of proximal left anterior descending coronary artery stenosis after intravenous injection of a lung crossing contrast agent: A transesophageal Doppler echocardiographic study. J Am Coll Cardiol. 1996;27:1413–1421.

18. Camarano G, Ragosta M, Gimple L, et al. Identification of viable myocardium with contrast echocardiography in patients with poor left ventricular systolic function caused by recent or remote myocardial infarction. Am J Cardiol. 1995;75:215–219.

19. Castello R, Pearson AC, Labovitz AJ, et al. Prevalence and clinical implications of atrial spontaneous contrast in patients undergoing transesophageal echocardiography. Am J Cardiol. 1990;65:1149–1153.

20. Castello R, Pearson AC, Fagan L, et al. Spontaneous echocardiographic contrast in the descending aorta. Am Heart J. 1990;120:915–919.

21. Castello R, Pearson AC, Lenzen P, et al. Evaluation of pulmonary venous flow by transesophageal echocardiography in subjects with a normal heart: Comparison with transthoracic echocardiography. J Am Coll Cardiol. 199;18:65–71.

22. Chandwaney R, Zajac E, Salvidar J, et al. Contrast echocardiography displays increased subendocardial perfusion after nitroglycerin administration. J Am Soc Echocardiogr. 1997;10:210–214.

23. Cheirif J, Meza M, Murgo J, et al. Dobutamine echocardiography and myocardial contrast echocardiography. Two new techniques for the assessment of myocardial viability. Texas Heart Instit J. 1995;22:33–39.

24. Chimowitz MI, De Geaorgia MA, Poole RM, et al. Left atrial spontaneous echo contrast is highly associated with previous stroke in patients with atrial fibrillation or mitral stenosis. Stroke. 1994;25:1295–1305.

25. Corimer B, Vahanian A, Lung B, et al. Influence of percutaneous mitral comissurotomy on left atrial spontaneous contrast of mitral stenosis. Am J Cardiol. 1993;71:842–847.

26. Cross S, Thomson L, Evans S, et al. Inter- and intra-observer variability in detection of patent foramen ovale with contrast echocardiography. Eur Heart J. 1993;12:388–390.

27. Crouse L. Sonicated serum albumin in contrast echocardiography: Improved segmental wall motion depiction and implications for stress echocardiography. Am J Cardiol. 1992;69:42H–45H.

28. Crouse L, Cheirif J, Hanly D, et al. Opacification and border delineation improvement in patients with suboptimal endocardial border definition in routine echocardiography: Results of the Phase III Albunex Multicenter Trial. J Am Coll Cardiol. 1993;22:1494–1500.

29. De Filippi C, Willett D, Irani W, et al. Comparison of myocardial contrast echocardiography and low dose dobutamine stress echocardiography in predicting recovery of left ventricular function after coronary revascularization in chronic ischemic heart disease. Circulation. 1995;92:2863–2868.

30. De Georgia MA, Chimowitz MI, Hepner A, et al. Right atrial spontaneous contrast echocardiographic and clinical features. Int J Cardiac Imaging. 1994;10:227–232.

31. De Jong N, Ten Cate F, Vletter W, et al. Quantification of transpulmonary echocontrast effects. Ultrasound Med Biol. 1993;19:279–288.

32. DeMaria AN, Bommer W, George L, et al. Combined peripheral venous injection and cross-sectional echocardiography in the evaluation of cardiac disease. Am J Cardiol. 1978;41:370.

33. Dick CD, Feinstein SR, Peterson EM, et al. Biodistribution of transpulmonary echocardiographic contrast agents. Circulation. 1987;76(suppl IV): 506.

34. Distante A, Rovai D. Stress echocardiography and myocardial contrast echocardiography in visibility assessment. Eur Heart J. 1997;18:771–779.

35. Dittrich H. Transient ischemic attack after air contrast echocardiography. Ann Intern Med. 1995; 123:731–732.

36. DiTullo M, Sacco RL, Venketasubramanian N, et al. Comparison of diagnostic techniques for the detection of a patent foramen ovale in stroke patients. Stroke. 1993;24:1020–1024.

37. Doud DN, Jacobs WR, Moran JF, et al. The natural history of left ventricular spontaneous contrast. J Am Soc Echocardiogr. 1990;3:465–470.

38. Dubourg O, Bourdarias JP, Farcot JC, et al. Contrast echocardiographic visualization of cough induced right-to-left shunt through a patent foramen ovale. J Am Coll Cardiol. 1984;4:587–594.

39. Duch P, Chandrasekaran K, Mulhern, et al. Transesophageal echocardiographic diagnosis of pulmonary arteriovenous malformation. Role of contrast and pulsed Doppler echocardiography. Chest. 1994;105:1604–1605.

40. Erbel R, Mohr-Kahaly S, Oelert H, et al. Diagnostic strategies in suspected aortic dissection: Comparison of computed tomography, aortography and transesophageal echocardiography. Am J Cardiac Imaging. 1990;4:157–172.

41. Falcone R, Marcovitz P, Perez J, et al. Intravenous albunex during dobutamine stress echocardiography: Enhanced localization of left ventricular endocardial borders. Am Heart J. 1995;130:254–258.

42. Fan PH, Kapur KK, Nanda NC. Color guided Doppler echocardiographic assessment of aortic valve stenosis. J Am Coll Cardiol. 1988;12: 441–449.

43. Feigenbaum H. Echocardiography, 2nd ed. Philadelphia, Lea & Febiger; 1976:350.

44. Feinstein S. Advances in contrast echocardiography. Invest Radiol. 1993;28(suppl 4):S26–S31.

45. Feinstein S, Ten Cate FJ, Zwehl W, et al. Two-dimensional contrast echocardiography. I. In vitro development and quantitative analysis of echocontrast agents. J Am Coll Cardiol. 1984;3:14–20.

46. Freeman AP, Giles RW, Walsh WF, et al. Regional left ventricular wall motion assessment: Comparison of two-dimensional echocardiography and radionuclide angiography with contrast angiography in healed myocardial infarction. Am J Cardiol. 1985;56:8–12.

47. Galanti G, Jayaweera AR, Villanueva FS, et al. Transpulmonary transit of microbubbles during contrast echocardiography: Implications for estimating cardiac output and pulmonary blood volume. J Am Soc Echocardiogr. 1993;6:272–278.

48. Gandhok N, Block R, Ostoic T, et al. Reduced output states affect the left ventricular opacification of intravenously administered Albunex. J Am Soc Echocardiogr. 1997;10:25–30.

49. Geny B, Mettauer B, Muan B, et al. Safety and efficacy of a new transpulmonary echo contrast agent in echocardiographic studies in patients. J Am Coll Cardiol. 1993;22:1193–1198.

50. Gin K, Fenwick J, Pollick C, et al. The diagnostic utility of contrast echocardiography in patients with refractory hypoxemia. Am Heart J. 1993;125: 1136–1141.

51. Gottlieb S, Ernst A, Litt L, et al. Effect of pressure on echocardiographic videodensity from sonicated albumin: An in-vitro model. J Am Soc Echocardiogr. 1990;3:238.

52. Gramiak R, Shah P. Echocardiography of the aortic root. Invest Radiol. 1968;3:356–388.

53. Gramiak R, Shah P, Kramer D. Ultrasound cardiography: Contrast study in anatomy and function. Radiology. 1969;92:939–948.

54. Groundstroem K, Tarkka M, Kirklin J, et al. Single right coronary artery assessed by contrast angiography and transesophageal echocardiography. Eur Heart J. 1995;16:1739–1741.

55. Gueret P, Vignon P, Fournier P, et al. Transesophageal echocardiography for the diagnosis and management of nonobstructive thrombosis of mechanical mitral valve prosthesis. Circulation. 1995;91: 103–110.

56. Hagen PT, Scholz DG, Edwards WD. Incidence and size of patent foramen ovale during the first 10 decades of life: an autopsy study of 965 normal hearts. Mayo Clin Proc. 1984;59:17–20.

57. Hajduczki I, Rajagopalam RE, Meerbaum S, et al. Effects of intracoronary administered echocontrast agents on epicardial coronary flow, ECG and global and regional hemodynamics. J Cardiovasc Ultrasonogr. 1987;6:85–93.

58. Hatle L, Angelsen B. Doppler Ultrasound in Cardiology: Physical Principles and Clinical Applications, 2nd ed. Philadelphia, Lea & Febiger; 1985.

59. Hausmann D, Mügge A, Becht I, et al. Diagnosis of patent foramen ovale by transesophageal echocardiography and association with cerebral and peripheral embolic events. Am J Cardiol. 1992;70: 668–672.

60. Hausmann D, Mügge A, Daniel W. Identification of patent foramen ovale permitting paradoxic embolism. J Am Coll Cardiol. 1995;26:1030–1038.

61. Hausmann D, Mügge A, Kühn H, et al. Contrast echo-enhancement during transesophageal echocardiography: Indications and clinical benefits. *In* Nanda NC, Schlief R, Goldberg B, (eds): Advances in Echo Imaging Using Contrast Enhancement, 2nd ed. Dordrecht, the Netherlands, Kluwer; 1997: 289–308.

62. Himbert D, Seknadji P, Karila-Cohen D, et al. Myocardial contrast echocardiography to assess spontaneous reperfusion during myocardial infarction. Lancet. 1997;349:617–619.

63. Hirata N, Nakano S, Sakai K, et al. Extent and distribution of the perfusion areas of the coronary artery selected for bypass grafting: Assessment by intraoperative myocardial contrast echocardiography. J Thorac Cardiovasc Surg. 1994;107:323–325.

64. Hirata N, Shimazaki Y, Nakano S, et al. Evaluation of regional myocardial perfusion in areas of old myocardial infarction after revascularization by means of intraoperative myocardial contrast echocardiography. J Thorac Cardiovasc Surg. 1994;108: 1119–1124.

65. Hjemdahl-Monsen CE, Daniels J, Kaufman D, et al. Spontaneous contrast in the inferior vena cava in a patient with constrictive pericarditis. J Am Coll Cardiol. 1984;4:165–167.

66. Iliceto S, Marangelli V, Marchese A, et al. Myocardial contrast echocardiography in acute myocardial infarction. Pathophysiological background and clinical applications. Eur Heart J. 1996;17: 344–353.

67. Iliceto S, Galiuto L, Marchese A, et al. Analysis of microvascular integrity, contractile reserve, and myocardial visibility after acute myocardial infarction by dobutamine echocardiography and myocardial contrast echocardiography. Am J Cardiol. 1996;77:441–445.

68. Iliceto S, Caiati C, Argona P, et al. Improved Doppler signal intensity in coronary arteries after intravenous peripheral injection of a lung crossing contrast. J Am Coll Cardiol. 1994;23:191–193.

69. Jauss M, Kaps M, Kerberle M, et al. A comparison of transesophageal echocardiography and transcranial Doppler sonography with contrast medium for detection of patent foramen ovale. Stroke. 1994; 25:1265–1267.

70. Jayaweera A, Skyba D, Kaul S, et al. Technical factors that influence the determination of microbubble transit rate during contrast echocardiography. J Am Soc Echocardiogr. 1995;8:198–206.

71. Jayaweera A, Ismail S, Kaul S. Attenuation deforms time intensity curves during contrast echocardiography: Implications for assessment of mean transit rates. J Am Soc Echocardiogr. 1994;7:590–597.

72. Job F, Ringelstein E, Grafen Y, et al. Comparison of transcranial contrast Doppler sonography and transesophageal contrast echocardiography for the detection of patent foramen ovale in young stroke patients. Am J Cardiol. 1994;74:381–384.

73. Jullien T, Valtier B, Hongnat J, et al. Incidence of tricuspid regurgitation and vena caval backward flow in mechanically ventilated patients. A color Doppler and contrast echocardiographic study. Chest. 1995;107:488–493.

74. Kato H, Nakanishi M, Maekawa N, et al. Evaluation of left atrial appendage stasis in patients with atrial fibrillation using transesophageal echocardiography with an intravenous albumin-contrast agent. Am J Cardiol. 1996;78:365–369.

75. Kaul S, Jayaweera A. Myocardial contrast echocardiography has the potential for the assessment of coronary microvascular reserve. J Am Coll Cardiol. 1993;21:356–358.

76. Kaul S. Myocardial contrast echocardiography in coronary artery disease: Potential applications using venous injections of contrast. Am J Cardiol. 1995; 71:61D–68D.

77. Kemp W, Byrd BJ III. Right heart echo-enhancement in the assessment of pulmonary artery pressures and right ventricular function. *In* Nanda NC, Schlief R, Goldberg BB (eds): Advances in Echo Imaging using Contrast Enhancement, 2nd ed. Dordrecht, the Netherlands, Kluwer; 1997:233.

78. Kemp W, Kerins D, Syr Y, et al. Optimal Albunex dosing for enhancement of Doppler tricuspid regurgitation spectra. Am J Cardiol. 1997;79:232–234.

79. Keren G, Sherez J, Megidish R, et al. Pulmonary venous flow pattern—its relationship to cardiac dynamics. A pulsed Doppler echocardiographic study. Circulation. 1985;71:1105–1112.

80. Klein AL, Bailey AS, Cohen GI, et al. Effects of mitral stenosis on pulmonary venous flow as measured by Doppler transesophageal echocardiography. Am J Cardiol. 1993;72:66–72.

81. Klein AL, Burstow DJ, Tajik AJ, et al. Effects of age on left ventricular dimensions and filling dy-

namics in 117 normal persons. Mayo Clin Proc. 1994;69:212–224.

82. Klein AL, Hatle LK, Burstow DJ, et al. Doppler characterization of left ventricular diastolic function in cardiac amyloidosis. J Am Coll Cardiol. 1989; 13:1017–1026.

83. Klein AL, Stewart WJ, Bartlett J, et al. Effects of mitral regurgitation of pulmonary venous flow and left atrial pressure: An intraoperative transesophageal echocardiographic study. J Am Coll Cardiol. 1992;20:1345–1352.

84. Klotzsch C, Janssen G, Berlit P. Transesophageal echocardiography and contrast TCD in the detection of patent foramen ovale: Experience with 111 patients. Neurology. 1994;44:1603–1606.

85. Koenig K, Meltzer RS. Effect of viscosity on the size of microbubbles generated for use as echocardiographic contrast agents. J Cardiovasc Ultrasonogr. 1986;5:3–4.

86. Kort A, Krougon I. Microbubble formation: In vitro and in vivo observations. J Clin Ultrasound. 1982;10:117–120.

87. Kostucki W, Vandenbossche H, Friart A, et al. Pulsed Doppler regurgitant flow patterns of normal valves. Am J Cardiol. 1986;58:309–313.

88. Kozakova M, Palombo C, Zanchi M, et al. Increased sensitivity of flow in the left coronary artery by transesophageal echocardiography after intravenous administration of transpulmonary stable echocontrast agent. J Am Soc Echocardiogr. 1994;7: 327–336.

89. Kronzon I, Tunick PA, Colossman E, et al. Transesophageal echocardiography to detect atrial clots in candidates for percutaneous transseptal mitral balloon valvuloplasty. J Am Coll Cardiol. 1990;16: 1320–1322.

90. Kuecherer HF, Kusumoto F, Muhiudeen IA, et al. Pulmonary venous flow patterns by transesophageal pulsed Doppler echocardiography: Relation to parameters of left ventricular systolic and diastolic function. Am Heart J. 1991;122:1683–1693.

91. Kuecherer HF, Muhiudeen IA, Kusumoto FM, et al. Estimation of mean left atrial pressure from transesophageal pulsed Doppler echocardiography of pulmonary venous flow. Circulation. 1990;82: 1127–1139.

92. Lee F, Ginzton L. A central complication of contrast echocardiography. J Clin Ultrasound. 1983; 11:292–294.

93. Lee RT, Lord CP, Plappert T, et al. Prospective Doppler echocardiographic evaluation of pulmonary artery diastolic pressure in the medical intensive care unit. Am J Cardiol. 1989;64:1366–1370.

94. Leischik R, Bartel T, Mohelkamp S, et al. Stress echocardiography: New techniques. Eur Heart J. 1997;18(suppl D):D49–D56.

95. Leung DY, Black IW, Cranney GB, et al. Prognostic implications of left atrial spontaneous echo contrast in nonvalvular atrial fibrillation. J Am Coll Cardiol. 1994;24:755–762.

96. Lieppe W, Behar VS, Scallion R, et al. Detection of tricuspid regurgitation with two-dimensional echocardiography and peripheral vein injections. Circulation. 1978;57:128–132.

97. Lim Y, Nanto S, Masuyama T, et al. Myocardial salvage: Its assessment and prediction by the analysis of serial myocardial contrast echocardiograms in patients with acute myocardial infarction. Am Heart J. 1994;128:649–656.

98. Lim Y, Masuyama T, Nanto S, et al. Left ventricular papillary muscle perfusion assessed with myocardial contrast echocardiography. Am J Cardiol. 196;78: 955–958.

99. Lubbers J, Van den Berg JW. An ultrasonic detector for microgas emboli in a blood line. Ultrasound Med Biol. 1976;2:301–310.

100. Lynch JJ, Schuchard GH, Gross CM, et al. Prevalence of right-to-left shunting in a healthy population: Detection by Valsalva maneuver contrast echocardiography. Am J Cardiol. 1984;53: 1478–1480.

101. Mahony C, Ferguson J. The effect of heparin versus citrate on blood echogenicity in vitro: The role of platelet and platelet-neutrophil aggregates. Ultrasound Med Biol. 1992;18:851–859.

102. Mahony C, Ferguson J, Fischer PL. Red cell aggregates and the echogenicity of whole blood. Ultrasound Med Biol. 1992;18:579–586.

103. Masuyama T, Kodama K, Kitabatake A, et al. Continuous-wave Doppler echocardiographic detection of pulmonary regurgitation and its application to noninvasive estimation of pulmonary artery pressure. Circulation. 1986;74:484–492.

104. Masuyama T, Lee J-M, Nagano R, et al. Doppler echocardiographic pulmonary venous flow-velocity pattern for assessment of the hemodynamic profile in acute congestive heart failure. Am Heart J. 1995; 129:107–113.

105. Masuyama T, Uematsu M, Nakatani S, et al. Doppler echocardiographic assessment of changes in pulmonary artery pressure associated with vasodilating therapy in patients with congestive heart failure. J Am Soc Echocardiogr. 1991;4:35–42.

106. Merino A, Hauptman P, Badimon L, et al. Echocardiographic "smoke" is produced by an interaction of erythrocytes and plasma proteins modulated by

shear forces. J Am Coll Cardiol. 1992;20: 1661–1668.

107. Meltzer RS, Lancess CT, Stewart GR, et al. Spontaneous echocardiographic contrast on the right side of the heart. J Clin Ultrasound. 1982;10:240–242.

108. Meltzer RS, Klig V, Visser CA, et al. Spontaneous echographic contrast in the inferior vena cava. Am Heart J. 1985;110:826.

109. Meltzer RS, Tickner EG, Sahines TP, et al. The source of ultrasound contrast effect. J Clin Ultrasound. 1980;8:121–127.

110. Meltzer RS, Vered Z, Roelandt J, et al. Systematic analysis of contrast echocardiograms. Am J Cardiol. 1983;52:375–380.

111. Meza M, Mobarek S, Sonnemaker R, et al. Myocardial contrast echocardiography in human beings: Correlation of resting perfusion defects to sestamibi single photon emission computed tomography. Am Heart J. 1996;132:528–535.

112. Mitusch R, Lange V, Stierle U, et al. Transesophageal echocardiographic determinants of embolism in nonrheumatic atrial fibrillation. Int J Cardiac Imaging. 1995;11:27–34.

113. Mizushige K, DeMaria A, Toyama Y, et al. Contrast echocardiography for evaluation of left ventricular flow dynamics using densitometric analysis. Circulation. 1993;88:588–595.

114. Mor-Avi V, Akselrod S, David D, et al. Myocardial transit time of the echocardiographic contrast media. Ultrasound Med Biol. 1993;19:625–648.

115. Nageuh S, Vaduganathan P, Ali N, et al. Identification of hibernating myocardium: Comparative accuracy of myocardial contrast echocardiography, rest-redistribution thallium-201 tomography and dobutamine echocardiography. J Am Coll Cardiol. 1997;29:985–993.

116. Nakatani S, Imanishi T, Terasawa A, et al. Clinical application of transpulmonary contrast-enhanced Doppler technique in the assessment of severity of aortic stenosis. J Am Coll Cardiol. 1992;20: 973–978.

117. Nakatani S, Miyatake K. Contrast-enhanced Doppler in the assessment of aortic stenosis. *In* Nanda NC, Schlief R, Goldberg BB (eds): Advances in Echo Imaging Using Contrast Enhancement, 2nd ed. Dordrecht, the Netherlands, Kluwer; 1997: 253–263.

118. Nanda NC, Cartensen EL. Echo-enhancing agents: Safety. *In* Nanda NC, Schlief R, Goldberg BB (eds): Advances in Echo Imaging Using Contrast Enhancement, 2nd ed. Dordrecht, the Netherlands, Kluwer; 1997:115–131.

119. Nanto S, Masuyama T, Lim Y, et al. Demonstration of functional border zone with myocardial contrast echocardiography in human hearts: Simultaneous analysis of myocardial perfusion and wall motion abnormalities. Circulation. 1993;88:447–453.

120. Nihoyannopoulos P. Contrast echocardiography. Clin Radiol. 1996;(suppl 1):28–30.

121. Okura H, Yoshikawa J, Yoshida K, et al. Quantification of left to right shunts in secundum atrial septal defect by two dimensional contrast echocardiography with use of Albunex. Am J Cardiol. 1995;75: 639–642.

122. Perchet H, Dupouy P, Duval-Moulin A, et al. Improvement of subendocardial myocardial perfusion after percutaneous transluminal coronary angioplasty. A myocardial contrast echocardiography study with correlations between myocardial contrast reserve and Doppler coronary reserve. Circulation. 1995;91:1419–1426.

123. Perkins A, Frier M, Hindle A, et al. Human biodistribution of an ultrasound contrast agent (Quantison) by radiolabeling and gamma scintigraphy. Br J Radiol. 1997;70:603–611.

124. Pop GAM, Meeder HJ, Roelandt JRTC, et al. Transthoracic echo/Doppler in the identification of patients with chronic non-valvular atrial fibrillation at risk for thromboembolic events. Eur Heart J. 1994;15:1545–1551.

125. Porter T, Xie F, Anderson J, et al. Multifold sonicated dilutions of albumin with fifty percent dextrose improves left ventricular contrast videointensity after intravenous injection in human beings. J Am Soc Echocardiogr. 1994;7:465–471.

126. Porter T, D'Sa A, Turner C, et al. Myocardial contrast echocardiography for the assessment of coronary blood flow reserve: Validation in humans. J Am Coll Cardiol. 1993;21:349–355.

127. Porter T, Li S, Kricsfeld D, et al. Detection of myocardial perfusion in multiple echocardiographic windows with one intravenous injection of microbubbles using transient response second harmonic imaging. J Am Coll Cardiol. 1997;29:791–799.

128. Porter T, Xie F, Kricsfeld D, et al. Improved myocardial contrast with second harmonic transient ultrasound response imaging in humans using intravenous perfluorocarbon-exposed sonicated dextrose albumin. J Am Coll Cardiol. 1996;27: 1479–1501.

129. Porter T, Xie F, Kricsfeld D, et al. Improved endocardial border resolution during dobutamine stress echocardiography with intravenous sonicated dextrose albumin. J Am Coll Cardiol. 1994;23: 1440–1443.

130. Porter T, D'sa A, Pesko L, et al. Usefulness of myocardial contrast echocardiography in detecting the

immediate changes in antegrade blood flow reserve after coronary angioplasty. Am J Cardiol. 1993;71: 893–896.

131. Redberg RF. Coronary flow by transesophageal Doppler echocardiography: Do saccharide-based contrast agents sweeten the pot? J Am Coll Cardiol. 1994;23:191–193.

132. Rodriguez A, Tardif J, Dominguez M, et al. Transthoracic echocardiographic assessment of periprosthetic mitral regurgitation using intravenous injection of sonicated albumin. Am J Cardiol. 1997;79: 829–834.

133. Rossvoll O, Hatle LK. Pulmonary venous flow velocities recorded by transthoracic Doppler ultrasound: Relation to left ventricular diastolic pressures. J Am Coll Cardiol. 1993;21:1687–1696.

134. Rovai D, Ferdeghini E, Mazzarisi A, et al. Quantitative aspects in myocardial contrast echocardiography. Eur Heart J. 1995;16(suppl J):42–45.

135. Rovai D, Zanchi M, Lombardi M, et al. Residual myocardial perfusion in reversibly damaged myocardium by dipyridamole contrast echocardiography. Eur Heart J. 1996;17:296–301.

136. Rovai D, DeMaria A, L'Abbate A. Myocardial contrast echo effect: The dilemma of coronary blood flow and volume. J Am Coll Cardiol. 1995;26: 12–17.

137. Rovai D, DeMaria A, Lombardi M, et al. Assessment of myocardial perfusion with various intravenous echo-contrast agents: *In* Nanda NC, Schlief R, Goldberg BB (eds): Advances in Echo Imaging Using Contrast Enhancement, 2nd ed. Dordrecht, the Netherlands, Kluwer; 1997:371–385.

138. Sakata Y, Kodama K, Adachi T, et al. Comparison of myocardial contrast echocardiography and coronary angiography for assessing the acute protective effects of collaterals recruitment during occlusion of the left anterior descending coronary artery at the time of elective angioplasty. Am J Cardiol. 1997;79: 1329–1333.

139. Sakuma T, Hayashi Y, Shimohara A, et al. Usefulness of myocardial contrast echocardiography for the assessment of serial changes in risk areas in patients with acute myocardial infarction. Am J Cardiol. 1996;78:1273–1277.

140. Sanatoso T, Roelandt J, Mansyoer H, et al. Myocardial perfusion imaging in humans by contrast echocardiography using polygelin colloid solution. J Am Coll Cardiol. 1985;6:612–620.

141. Sapin P, Salley R. Atrial desaturation and orthodeoxia after atrial septal defect repair: Demonstration of the mechanism by transesophageal and contrast echocardiography. J Am Soc Echocardiogr. 1997;10:588–592.

142. Schlief R. Echo-enhancing agents: Their physics and pharmacology. *In* Nanda NC, Schlief R, Goldberg BB (eds): Advances in Echo Imaging Using Contrast Enhancement, 2nd ed. Dordrecht, the Netherlands, Kluwer; 1997:85–113.

143. Schwarz K, Bezante G, Chen X, et al. Quantitative echo contrast concentration measurements by Doppler sonography. Ultrasound Med Biol. 1993; 19:289–297.

144. Segal R, Baltazar RF, Mower MM, et al. Spontaneous contrast visualization on the right side of the heart during echocardiography. Am J Med Sci. 1986;292:363–366.

145. Shapiro JR, Reisner SA, Lichtenberg GS, et al. Intravenous contrast echocardiography in humans: Systolic disappearance of left ventricular contrast after transpulmonary transmission. J Am Coll Cardiol. 1990;16:1603–1607.

146. Sigel B, Coelho JCH, Spidos DG, et al. Ultrasound of blood during stasis and coagulation. Invest Radiol. 1981;16:71–76.

147. Sigel B, Maci J, Beirler JC, et al. Variable ultrasound echogenicity in flowing blood. Science. 1982;218: 1321–1323.

148. Skjaerpe T, Hegrenaes L, Hatle L. Noninvasive estimation of valve area in patients with aortic stenosis by Doppler ultrasound and two-dimensional echocardiography. Circulation. 1985;72:810–818.

149. Snider RA, Serwer GA. Abnormal vascular connections and structures. *In:* Echocardiography in Pediatric Heart Disease. Chicago, Year Book; 1990; 273–274.

150. Spaan JAE. Basic coronary physiology. Heart function and coronary flow. *In* Spaan JAE (ed): Coronary Blood Flow. Mechanics, Distribution and Control. Dordrecht, the Netherlands, Kluwer; 1991:1–4.

151. Srivastava T, Undesser E. Transient ischemic attack after air contrast echocardiography in patients with septal aneurysm. Ann Intern Med. 1995;122:396.

152. Stewart D, Sobczyyk W, Bond S, et al. Use of two dimensional and contrast echocardiography for venous cannula placement in venovenous extracorporeal life support. ASAIO J. 1996;42:604–606.

153. Stollberger C, Schneider B, Abzieher F, et al. Diagnosis of patent foramen ovale by transesophageal contrast echocardiography. Am J Cardiol. 1993;71: 604–606.

154. Stone D, Godard J, Corretti M, et al. Patent foramen ovale association between the degree of shunt by contrast transesophageal echocardiography and

the risk of future ischemic neurologic events. Am Heart J. 1996;131:158–161.

155. Sun J, Stewart W, Hanna J, et al. Diagnosis of patent foramen ovale by contrast versus color Doppler by transesophageal echocardiography: Relation to atrial size. Am Heart J. 1996;131:239–244.

156. Sutherland G, Stewart M, Groundstroem K. Color Doppler myocardial imaging: A new technique for the assessment of myocardial function. J Am Soc Echocardiogr. 1994;7:441–458.

157. Tanabe K, Asanuma T, Yoshitomi H, et al. Doppler estimation of pulmonary artery end diastolic pressure using contrast enhancement of pulmonary regurgitant signals. Am J Cardiol. 1996;78:1145–1148.

158. Terasawa A, Mikatake K, Nakatani S, et al. Enhancement of Doppler flow signals in the left heart chambers by intravenous injection of sonicated albumin. J Am Coll Cardiol. 1993;21:737–742.

159. Tokgozoglu S, Caner B, Kabaki G, et al. Measurement of right ventricular ejection fraction by contrast echocardiography. Int J Cardiol. 1997;59:71–74.

160. Valdes-Cruz LM, Pieroni DR, Rowland JM, et al. Recognition of residual post-operative shunts by contrast echocardiographic techniques. Circulation. 1977;55:148.

161. Van Camp G, Cosyns B, Vandenbossche JL. Nonsmoke spontaneous contrast in left atrium intensified by respiratory maneuvers: A new transesophageal echocardiographic observation. Br Heart J. 1994;72:446–451.

162. Vedrinne J, Duperret S, Bizollon T, et al. Comparison of transesophageal and transthoracic contrast echocardiography for detection of an intrapulmonary shunt in liver disease. Chest. 1997;111:1236–1240.

163. Verhorst PM, Kamp O, Visser CA, et al. Left atrial appendage flow velocity assessment using transesophageal echocardiography in nonrheumatic atrial fibrillation and systemic embolism. Am J Cardiol. 1993;71:192–196.

164. Vernon S, Camarano G, Kaul S, et al. Myocardial contrast echocardiography demonstrates that collateral flow can preserve myocardial function beyond a chronically occluded coronary artery. Am J Cardiol. 1996;78:958–960.

165. Villaneuva F, Jankowski R, Manaugh C, et al. Albumin microbubble adherence to human coronary endothelium: Implications for assessment of endothelial function using myocardial contrast echocardiography. J Am Coll Cardiol. 1997;30:689–693.

166. Voci P, Bilotta F, Merialdo P, et al. Myocardial contrast enhancement after intravenous injection of sonicated albumin microbubbles: A transesophageal echocardiography dipyridamole study. J Am Soc Echocardiogr. 1994;7:337–346.

167. Von Bibra H, Becher H, Firschke C, et al. Enhancement of mitral regurgitation and normal left atrial color Doppler flow signals with peripheral venous injection of a saccharide-based contrast agent. J Am Coll Cardiol. 1993;22:521–528.

168. Von Bibra H, Sutherland G, Becher H, et al. Clinical evaluation of left heart Doppler contrast enhancement by a saccharide-based transpulmonary contrast agent. J Am Coll Cardiol. 1995;25:500–508.

169. Waggoner A, Quinones M, Young JB, et al. Pulsed Doppler echocardiographic detection of right-sided valve regurgitation. Am J Cardiol. 1981;47:279–286.

170. Weibel ER. Morphometry of the Human Lung. New York, Academic Press; 1975:78.

171. Weisse A, Desai R, Rajihah G, et al. Contrast echocardiography as an adjunct in hemorrhagic or complicated pericardiocentesis. Am Heart J. 1996;131:822–825.

172. Weyman A. Miscellaneous Echocardiographic techniques I: Contrast echocardiography. *In* Weymen A (ed): Principles and Practice of Echocardiography. Philadelphia, Lea & Febiger; 1994:302–326.

173. Wiencek J, Feinstein S, Rajihah G, et al. Pitfalls in quantitative contrast echocardiography: The steps to quantitation of perfusion. J Am Soc Echocardiogr. 1993;6:395–416.

174. Williams M, McClements B, Picard M, et al. Improvement of transthoracic pulmonary venous flow Doppler signal with intravenous injection of sonicated albumin. J Am Coll Cardiol. 1995;16:1741–1746.

175. Winkelmann J, Kenner M, Dave, R, et al. Contrast echocardiography. Ultrasound Med Biol. 1994;20:506–515.

176. Wu CC, Chen WJ, Chen MF, et al. Left-to-right shunt through patent foramen ovale in adult patients with left sided cardiac lesions: A transesophageal echocardiographic study. Am Heart J. 1993;125:1369–1374.

177. Xie F, Shapir J, Meltzer R. Toxicity of intracoronary microbubbles in contrast echo. Circulation. 1987;76(suppl IV):505.

178. Yao S, Ilercil A, Meisner J, et al. Improved Doppler echocardiographic assessment of the left atrial appendage by peripheral vein injection of sonicated albumin microbubbles. Am Heart J. 1997;133:400–405.

179. Yvorchuk K, Sochowski R, Chan K, et al. Sonicated albumin in exercise echocardiography: Technique

and feasibility to enhance endocardial visualization. J Am Soc Echocardiogr. 1996;9:462–469.

180. Zoghbi WA, Farmer KL, Soto JG, et al. Accurate noninvasive quantification of stenotic aortic valve area by Doppler echocardiography. Circulation. 1986;73:452–459.

181. Zotz, R, Geneth S, Waaler A, et al. Left ventricular volume determination using Albunex. J Am Soc Echocardiogr. 1996;9:1–8.

182. Zotz RJ, Pinnau U, Genth S, et al. Left atrial thrombi despite anticoagulant and antiplatelet therapy. Clin Cardiol. 1994;17:375–382.

9

Three-Dimensional Echocardiography

JIEFEN YAO, LISSA SUGENG, GERALD MARX, and NATESA G. PANDIAN

Two-dimensional echocardiography is very useful in providing cardiologists with information about cardiac structures and function with multiple tomographic views of the heart. Spectral Doppler and color Doppler scans provide us with qualitative and quantitative information on normal and abnormal blood flows and pressures within the heart and great vessels. These two-dimensional approaches have been playing an important role in diagnostic cardiology over the past two decades. Nevertheless, the heart is a three-dimensional organ with complex geometry and intricate spatial relationships in terms of structure, function, and flow. Therefore, for assessment of cardiac disorders, physicians often mentally reconstruct three-dimensional images of the pathology from a limited number of cross-sectional views of the heart while employing two-dimensional ultrasound examinations. Accurate evaluation of cardiac abnormalities requires sophisticated knowledge of the anatomy, geometry, and hemodynamics of the heart and considerable experience. Not surprisingly, intraobserver and interobserver variability is sometimes significant both in qualitative appraisal and in quantitative assessment of various cardiac disorders.[9,13,32] It has been realized for years that a technique with the ability to display the heart in multiple dimensions would be very helpful in the evaluation of various cardiovascular disorders. The earliest attempt to develop three-dimensional echocardiography was made in the 1970s, and great progress has been made since then.[5,12,23,26] Initially three-dimensional echocardiography was used to explore means of accurately measuring ventricular volumes and myocardial masses without the need for geometric assumptions.[1,38] These approaches, which yielded only static, wire-frame images, required tedious manual tracing of numerous two-dimensional echocardiographic images. Recently, dynamic volume-rendered, three-dimensional echocardiography, a technique that yields both tissue depiction images and accurate quantitative information, has emerged as a very promising tool.[27] In this chapter, we will discuss the methodology, instrumentation, current clinical experience with, and future directions of clinically relevant three-dimensional echocardiographic techniques, with a major focus on dynamic volume-rendered, three-dimensional echocardiography.

Methodology for Three-Dimensional Echocardiography

The ideal method to examine the heart in multiple dimensions easily and rapidly would be one that directly visualizes it on line in three dimensions as imaging is performed. This would require receiving signals from all parts of the organ and instantly performing signal processing as data are being collected. This concept is being explored with a prototype transducer that yields a pyramidal volume of ultrasound signals. On-line three-dimensional echocardiography, however, has not yet become a clinical tool. There are viable alternative approaches which utilize a plethora of two-dimensional images and perform three-dimensional reconstructions. Systematic acquisition of two-dimensional images encompassing the whole heart, or a given region, provides a cubic data set. Generally, a two-dimensional ultrasound unit and a computer dedicated to three-dimensional data processing are needed for this purpose. The acquired images are then processed and transformed into a three-dimensional data set which can be reconstructed into three-dimensional displays. Although there are different techniques for three dimensional echocardiography, the following procedures are essential: (1) two-dimensional echocardiographic image acquisition; (2) data processing; (3) two-dimensional multiplanar review; (4) three-dimensional image reconstruction and display; and (5) quantitative data analysis.

Data Acquisition

Multiple two-dimensional image samples are necessary for three-dimensional reconstruction. These samples need to be collected throughout the whole cardiac cycle for dynamic three-dimensional display of the cardiac structures. Furthermore, the images have to be acquired with electrocardiographic and respiratory gaiting for optimal spatial and temporal registration. There are two major modes of two-dimensional image acquisition for three-dimensional echocardiography: random data acquisition and sequential data acquisition. The latter is the most often used method in volume-rendered, three-dimensional echocardiography.

RANDOM DATA ACQUISITION

In random mode data acquisition, also referred to as *free-hand imaging*, two-dimensional images of the heart are collected either with the transducer at one acoustic window, tilted in different directions, or with the transducer at multiple windows.[17,31] The position and orientation of the transducer, and thus of the image plane, are detected and registered by sensor devices such as magnetic sensors, acoustic sensors, and goniometry. An image, or a line computed from one image, is usually taken as a reference to align other images acquired in a random fashion in their actual anatomic order. The advantage of this mode of data acquisition is the flexibility of using different acoustic windows. The disadvantage, on the other hand, is that big gaps may result between scanned images, and inaccuracy may arise from computer interpolation during data processing. While accurate results have been demonstrated for volume and mass measurements, this approach has not yet yielded good-quality tissue-depiction images so far.

SEQUENTIAL DATA ACQUISITION

In sequential data acquisition, two-dimensional images are collected in a predetermined step. Different algorithms have been applied to develop three-dimensional reconstructions with sequential scanning. Polygon cavity reconstruction has been used for the left ventricle in the form of wire-frame formation or surface rendering. For volume-rendered, three-dimensional reconstruction, the following modes of data acquisition have been employed: parallel slicing, rotational scanning, and fan-like imaging (Fig. 9-1).

Polygon Imaging

The method referred to as *polygon reconstruction* for left ventricular cavity analysis uses three apical views (four-chamber, two-chamber, and long axis views) which are 60 degrees apart from each other and are acquired either manually or with computer-controlled automatic rotation of the probe or transducer.[14] The endocardial border of the left ventricle can be traced manually or detected automatically. The borders between these views are extrapolated by the computer according to geometric assumptions of the left ventricle. The reconstructed images

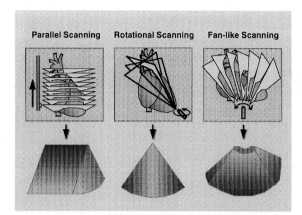

Figure 9-1. *Schematics showing different modes of sequential data acquisition for three-dimensional echocardiography and the shape of the resultant three-dimensional data set. Left: parallel scanning. Middle: rotational scanning. Right: fan-like scanning.*

of the left ventricular cavity are wire framed or surface rendered and can be viewed in a dynamic mode from different directions (Fig. 9-2). The biggest and smallest volumes during one cardiac cycle are computed automatically, and the ejection fraction is given as well. Accurate results have been achieved for left ventricular volume and function assessment using this method.

Parallel Slicing

In this mode of data acquisition, two-dimensional images are acquired in equidistant steps with the transducer moved in a linear direction. The total distance between the first and last images and the intervals between slices can be predefined by the computer. This mode of image acquisition yields a prism-shaped three-dimensional data set. Parallel scanning has been used with both transthoracic and transesophageal approaches.[10,18,26,36] With transthoracic echocardiography, a monitoring device controlled by the computer is mounted on the probe. With transesophageal echocardiography (TEE), a special TEE probe is attached to a sliding device controlled by the computer. The distal portion of the probe is enclosed in a casing carriage which is straightened after the probe is introduced into the esophagus. The transducer is moved linearly in equal steps, and tomographic images of the heart for one cardiac cycle are collected.[26] This transesophageal probe has also been used successfully for transthoracic data acquisition in infants and

children.[10] Besides its application in various cardiac disorders, this device is especially useful in viewing longitudinal structures such as the descending thoracic aorta. It has also been employed for three-dimensional data acquisition with intravascular ultrasound.[29] This mode of acquisition may result in good image quality, and higher resolution can be obtained with a smaller volume of the data set, but the need for a relatively bigger acoustic window limits its application.

Rotational Scanning

During rotational data acquisition, two-dimensional images are collected while the probe or the transducer within the probe is rotated around an axis in equal steps from 0 through 180 degrees. Such an acquisition yields a cone-shaped three-dimensional data set. This mode of image acquisition can be applied in any acoustic window and, therefore, is most frequently employed in clinical studies, both transthoracically and transesophageally.[11,21,28] In transthoracic data acquisition, the probe stays at a vantage acoustic window and the rotation of the probe is achieved with a computer-controlled steering logic device adapted to the probe. A multiplane surface probe is also being evaluated and has been used for transthoracic three-

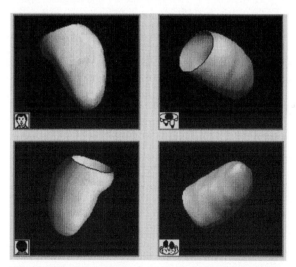

Figure 9-2. *Three-dimensional images of the left ventricular cavity acquired with polygon reconstruction from three apical views of the left ventricle. Changes in left ventricular shape and size can be appreciated in dynamic mode viewed from multiple directions. Orientation of the image is shown with an icon in the lower left corner of each picture. Only diastolic images are shown here.*

dimensional data acquisition. The transducer within the probe can be rotated through 180 degrees in equal steps during data acquisition, obviating the need for an external carriage device. The collected images can be stored directly on an optical drive incorporated into the ultrasound unit. Similarly, with a transesophageal approach, two-dimensional images are collected with a multiplane TEE probe when the transducer is rotated in predefined steps.

Fan-Like Imaging

With fan-like data acquisition, the probe is tilted in an arc in equal steps, with the imaging plane distributed in a fan-shaped pyramidal data set. This method has been employed at parasternal and subcostal windows.[7] The advantage of this mode of data acquisition is that an adequate data set can be achieved from a relatively smaller acoustic window. It can be used for acquisition of both small and large structures such as the entire heart or a pericardial effusion.

ARTIFACTS AND TEMPORAL GATING

The heart is a highly dynamic organ. Artifacts in three-dimensional data sets can be caused by many factors such as patient movement, respiratory interference, or irregular heartbeats. To diminish the artifacts which evolve mainly from malalignment of the images due to unexpected movement of the patient or of the ultrasound probe during data acquisition, the patient is usually asked to stay motionless and is encouraged to breathe smoothly in a comfortable and relaxed position which should allow optimal imaging of the heart. Gain settings need to be optimized and caution taken to avoid dropout of important structures.

Appropriate gating to an electrocardiogram (EKG) is necessary for synchronized registration of the images in different phases of one cardiac cycle and to avoid malalignment of images caused by irregular heartbeats. Distances between R waves of the EKG (R-R intervals) can be detected and a range set for the gating. This facilitates well-triggered image acquisition with a stable heart rate and, at the same time, data can be acquired in an acceptable period of time. Usually, the maximum R-R interval for the gating should not exceed 20% of the minimum or less than 150 msec.

The heart shifts in the chest cavity during respiration and may cause moving artifacts in the three-dimensional image. Such artifacts can be minimized by proper respiratory gating. Recording of thoracic impedance is most often used for this purpose. The increase in thoracic impedance during inspiration and the decrease during expiration can be recorded using EKG electrode leads. Nasal thermometers, which detect temperature changes in the nasal cavity during respiration, can also be used for this purpose. The respiratory gating can be set to either the inspiration or expiration phase.

DATA PROCESSING

For volume-rendered, three-dimensional echocardiography, the data set needs to be postprocessed by the computer before it can be reviewed or further analyzed. Calibration is performed first for later quantitative measurement. The images are realigned according to their spatial and temporal orders and reformatted into a matrix of rectangular pixels. Gaps between the adjacent images are filled automatically by the computer through an interpolation algorithm, and two-dimensional pixels are turned into volume-rendered cubic voxels while the three-dimensional data are transformed into a Cartesian coordinate system.

Various filters can be used to diminish the artifacts from ultrasonic noise or small movement by removing low-level noises, smoothing the images, and preserving the edges of the structure. Moving artifacts caused by patient or probe movement are difficult to eliminate later and therefore should be avoided during data acquisition.

THREE-DIMENSIONAL MULTIPLANAR IMAGE REVIEW

The postprocessed three-dimensional data set can be reviewed in numerous two-dimensional imaging planes in any arbitrary direction. The two-dimensional cutting planes can be ordered by the Cartesian coordinate system with three axes perpendicular to each other. Several methods are available for multiplanar image reconstruction from the three-dimensional data set. With the anyplane method, arbitrary placement and orientation of the images can be realized by manipulating cutting angles. The paraplane method produces a group of parallel equidistant cutting planes which can be used to review the continuity of a complex pathology and for volume or mass measurement. An arbitrary long axis can be decided by choosing two points in the three-dimensional data set. A group of cutting planes around this axis (long axis views) or perpendicular to the axis (short axis views) is formed. Another method generates three cutting planes perpendicular to each other, providing information on the spatial extension of the studied structure.

THREE-DIMENSIONAL IMAGE RECONSTRUCTION AND DISPLAY

For viewing three-dimensional objects on a two-dimensional screen of the computer monitor, several forms of three-dimensional image reconstruction and display techniques have been developed, as described below.

1. *Wire-frame formation.* When contours of two-dimensional echocardiographic images are connected with traced lines, a cage-like frame is formed to display the cardiac structures. It has been used mainly in assessment of chamber volume, myocardial mass, and geometry of the ventricles.[1,15,16,25,31,38] Although a surface can be applied to the wire frame, the lack of tissue depiction and the need for tedious manual tracings or semiautomatic border detection of the two-dimensional echocardiographic images have limited its use in many clinical settings.
2. *Surface-rendering technique.* With this technique, a surface is applied to a three-dimensional structure and a solid appearance is produced. Structures underneath the surface are not visible.

The distance and depth of three-dimensional objects can be shown if shading and lighting techniques are combined.

3. *Volume-rendering technique.* This recent development in three-dimensional echocardiography provides better appreciation of cardiac structures with a more detailed anatomic description. The use of different shading techniques enhances its tissue-depicting ability.[4,7,33] With distance coding, the distance of an object is converted into a gray scale. The points which are more distant from the observer are shaded with color darker than those that are closer to the observer. With texture-coding techniques, the gray scale level of the superficial cardiac tissue is generated according to its appearance on two-dimensional images representing the texture of the tissue. With the technique of gray scale gradient shading, the surface of the three-dimensional object is illuminated as if a light is shed on it from the observer. Usually all these shading techniques are mixed together to create a realistic three-dimensional echocardiographic image. The most updated computer for three-dimensional echocardiography has the ability to reconstruct the dynamic images of the heart in any desired projection. Three-dimensional echocardiography provides us with many novel viewing projections of the cardiac structures and pathologies. Surgical views can be generated so that the surgeon can study the pathologic anatomy before the heart is open.[33] For example, the mitral valve can be viewed from above by removing the left atrium, imitating an atriotomy. The thickness,

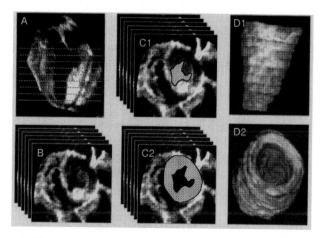

Figure 9-3. Schematic depicting the method of quantifying left ventricular volume and myocardial mass using three-dimensional echocardiography. With an appropriate reference image (**A**), the three-dimensional data set is electronically dissected into multiple parallel, equidistant transverse slices (**B**). The myocardium and the cavity are traced separately (**C1** and **C2**). The area and volume of the traced region on each slice, as well as the total volume on all slices, are calculated automatically by the computer. The traced region, which can be labeled specifically, can be extracted later from the rest of the data set and reconstructed into three-dimensional images (**D1** and **D2**).

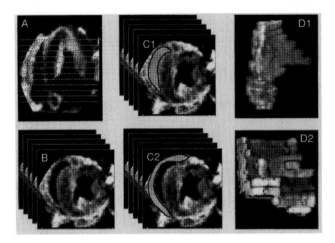

Figure 9-4. Schematic showing the method of quantifying the right ventricular volume and myocardial mass using a three-dimensional data set. After an appropriate reference image (**A**) is chosen, the three-dimensional data set of the right ventricle is sectioned into parallel, equidistant transverse slices (**B**). The myocardium or the cavity of the right ventricle is traced (**C1** and **C2**). The area and volume of the traced region on each slice, as well as the total volume of all traced slices, are automatically calculated by the computer. The traced region, when labeled specifically, can be extracted from the rest of the data set and reconstructed into three-dimensional images (**D1** and **D2**).

mobility, and coaptation of the valvular leaflets can be appreciated in detail. Abnormalities such as an interatrial septal defect can be viewed *en face* from the left or right atrium. With current instrumentation, it takes less than 60 sec for the reconstruction of a dynamic three-dimensional image.

QUANTITATIVE ANALYSIS OF THREE-DIMENSIONAL ECHOCARDIOGRAPHY

The advantage of three-dimensional echocardiography in yielding accurate quantitative data adds to its strength in many clinical and investigational applications. Its reliability in measuring chamber volume, myocardial mass, and cardiac function without the use of geometric assumptions has been well validated.[1,16,20,31,34,38] With volume-rendered, three-dimensional echocardiography, the data set of the heart is dissected into parallel, equidistant slices (usually short axis slices) and is viewed on a two-dimensional image. The slice thickness can be adjusted. The chamber, or myocardium, that one is interested in can be contoured manually or with an automatic/semiautomatic border detection algorithm. The volume of this region on each side is the product of its area and slice thickness. Summation of the volume of each slice yields the total volume (Figs. 9-3, 9-4). This measurement can also be applied to assess the volume of intracardiac masses, pericardial effusion, or aneurysms.[18] Another quantitative ability of three-dimensional echocardiography is the facility to measure distances, areas, and circumferences using two-dimensional cutting planes. The area of the valvular orifice, atrial or ventricular septal defects, and cross-sectional area of great vessels can be obtained. Distance can also be measured directly on three-dimensional images. Accurate assessment of the diameters of irregularly shaped structures has become possible.

Current Clinical Experience with Three-Dimensional Echocardiography

Initial experience with three-dimensional echocardiography has demonstrated its feasibility in various cardiovascular settings, including the echocardiographic laboratory, the patient's bedside, the operating room, and the emergency room, in both pediatric and adult patients. It can be performed with either transthoracic or transesophageal approaches. In addition to its quantitative ability, three-dimensional echocardiography generates dynamic multidimensional images that portray the cardiac anatomy, pathology, and regional wall motion of the ventricles in a realistic manner.

CONGENITAL CARDIOVASCULAR DISEASES

The complexities of the pathologic anatomy in congenital heart defects could be challenging to the cardiologist when only two-dimensional imaging capability is available. Several studies with three-dimensional echocardiography have indicated the potential strength of this technique in a better appraisal of congenital cardiac disorders.[3,10,22,29,30,36]

In patients with atrial septal defects, the *en face* view of the atrial septum, from either the left or the right side, gives direct visualization of the site and size of the defect (Fig. 9-5). The major and minor diameters of the defect measured directly on three-dimensional images are more reliable than those measured on two-dimensional images. Other information, such as the size of the limbus of the defect, can also be obtained from direct measurement on the three-dimensional images. The information on the distances between the defect and the other nearby structures such as the aorta, superior vena cava, inferior vena cava, and tricuspid valve is useful in planning how an atrial septal defect should be closed, i.e., by a transcatheter closure device (which needs adequate tissue surrounding the defect) or by surgery. The dynamic geometry of the defect in diastole and systole, the mobility of the septum, and the presence of an aneurysm can also be appreciated with three-dimensional echocardiography.[3,22] Similarly, in patients with ventricular septal defects, the site, size, and number of defect(s) can be evaluated from either the right or the left side of the septum or from any vantage projection. In patients with tetralogy of Fallot, the relationship between the ventricular septum, the defect, and the aorta can be appreciated in various views.[30]

Three-dimensional echocardiography is also helpful in a variety of congenital heart diseases. For example, it can disclose the site and shape or subaortic fibromuscular obstruction by viewing the three-dimensional projections of the lesion from above or below or from longitudinal views of the left ventric-

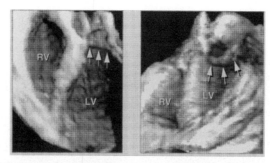

Figure 9-6. Three-dimensional echocardiographic images in a patient with a subaortic membrane (arrows) viewed from two different projections. RV = right ventricle; LV = left ventricle.

ular outflow tract (Fig. 9-6). In patients with complex anomalies, three-dimensional echocardiography may help to provide information on spatial relationships of the malpositioned cardiac structures. Three-dimensional echocardiography is helpful in evaluating abnormalities such as atrioventricular canal, single ventricle, aortic coarctation, pulmonary stenosis, cor triatriatum, tricuspid atresia, double outlet right ventricle, and so on.[2,10,21,30]

VALVULAR HEART DISEASES

One of the most common applications of three-dimensional echocardiography is the evaluation of valvular diseases. Both atrioventricular and semilunar valves can be viewed from above, from below, or from longitudinal projections with three-dimensional echocardiography. As the most frequently affected valve, the mitral valve and its apparatus have been the focus of investigation in a number of studies. The physiologic shape of the mitral valve and annulus has been studied with wire-framed, three-dimensional echocardiography.[19] In patients with mitral valve prolapse, the prolapsing part of the mitral valve is shown crisply as a portion of the leaflet bulging into the left atrium in a more precise manner than depicted by two-dimensional echocardiography (Fig. 9-7). In cases of rheumatic mitral stenosis, thickening and restrictive motion of the leaflets or the subvalvular structures are delineated clearly[27,33] (Fig. 9-8). The mitral valve area can be measured accurately in appropriate two-dimensional sections derived from a three-dimensional data set, obviating the difficulty of im-

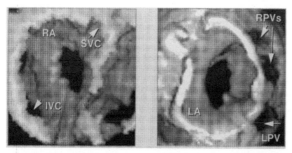

Figure 9-5. Three-dimensional images of an atrial septal defect viewed en face from the right atrium (RA) (left) and left atrium (LA) (right). SVC = superior vena cava; IVC = inferior vena cava; RPVs = right pulmonary veins; LPV = left pulmonary vein.

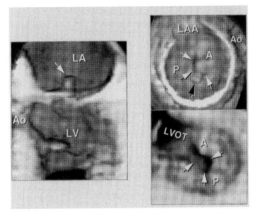

Figure 9-7. Images of a flail mitral valve viewed in a longitudinal projection (left) and transverse projections (right). The flail portion of the anterior mitral leaflet is clearly seen (arrow). In the view from the left atrium (top right), the prolapsing portion of the anterior mitral leaflet is seen doming into the left atrium (white arrows), along with a discrete flail portion (black arrow). When viewed from below, the prolapsing portion is shown as an indentation (arrows) in systole (bottom right). LA = left atrium; LV = left ventricle; Ao = aorta; LAA = left atrial appendage; A = anterior mitral leaflet; P = posterior mitral leaflet; LVOT = left ventricular outflow tract.

aging at the true tips of the leaflets with conventional two-dimensional echocardiography (Fig. 9-9). The aortic valve can also be examined from above (as if looking down from the ascending aorta), from below (looking up from the left ventricle), or from longitudinal views.[24,26] The number of cusps, which is sometimes difficult to decide by the two-dimensional approach, is clearly shown by

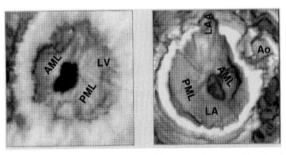

Figure 9-8. Three-dimensional images of a stenotic mitral valve viewed from below (left panel) and from above (right panel). The thickened leaflets and restricted opening of the valve are well depicted. LV = left ventricle; AML = anterior mitral leaflet; PML = posterior mitral leaflet; LA = left atrium; LAA = left atrial appendage; Ao = aorta.

three-dimensional echocardiography (Fig. 9-10). The excursion and flexibility of the leaflets can also be portrayed crisply.

EVALUATION OF INTRACARDIAC FLOW JETS

Three-dimensional reconstruction techniques can be applied to color Doppler data as well. Two-dimensional color Doppler signals are acquired and transferred to gray scale volumetric signals to create three-dimensional images of abnormal flow jets or intracardiac shunts (Fig. 9-11). The dynamic display of three-dimensional images appears to be helpful in the appraisal of the origin, direction, surface geometry, and spatial distribution of the flow jets, as well as the size and shape of the proximal flow convergence zone.[8]

ISCHEMIC CARDIAC DISEASES

In patients with coronary artery disease, regional wall motion abnormalities can be visualized easily by dynamic three-dimensional echocardiography in different orientations and projections. The size and extent of left ventricular aneurysm or mural clot is well depicted by a three-dimensional display (Fig. 9-12). The ischemic or infarcted myocardial mass can be assessed by measuring the absolute volume or weight of the dysfunctional regions or by calculating the percentage of left ventricle involved in regional dysfunction.[37] With the utilization of myocardial contrast agents, the myocardial area at risk can be quantified by defining the regions of perfusion detected.[6]

AORTIC DISORDERS

Images of the ascending aorta can be obtained from parasternal or suprasternal windows via transthoracic scanning for three-dimensional reconstruction. The descending aorta can be imaged by transesophageal scanning. Aortic lesions can be viewed from above, as if an aortotomy is performed, from below, or in longitudinal cuts. Three-dimensional images readily demonstrate the site and extent of aortic coarctation, aneurysm, or thrombus. Short- and long axis images of the aorta help reveal the true and false lumens of the dissected aorta, the flap of the ruptured intima, and the inlet and outlet of the dissection.

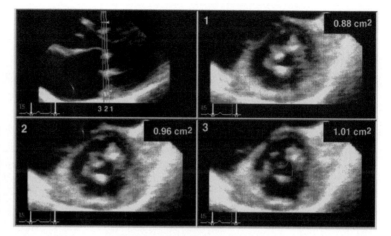

Figure 9-9. Measurement of the mitral valve area at the tip of the valve on two-dimensional cutting planes which have been extracted from a three-dimensional data set. Parallel images derived by free direction of the cutting plane assure the measurement at the smallest valve opening (measurement 1).

MISCELLANEOUS CARDIOVASCULAR DISEASES

In patients with left or right ventricular outflow tract obstruction, the site and severity of the involvement are easily demonstrated in dynamic three-dimensional images. Three-dimensional mass measurements can be used in patients with hypertrophic cardiomyopathy for defining septal and mitral valve abnormalities. The shape and site of attachment of intracardiac masses (including tumors, vegetations, and thrombus) can be well delineated by three-dimensional echocardiography and their volume quantified (Fig. 9-13). The distribution of

pericardial effusion can be demonstrated and the quantity measured.

Future Direction

Three-dimensional echocardiography has proven useful in the assessment of many cardiovascular disorders. Work is in progress to facilitate the process of data acquisition. The availability of a multiplane transthoracic probe may avoid the need for an external carriage device and free-hand imaging. Echocardiographic machines with three-dimensional data-

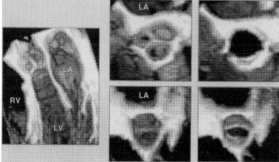

Figure 9-10. Three-dimensional images of the aortic valve. The image on the left shows the longitudinal view of the heart, which displays the left ventricle (LV), right ventricle (RV), interventricular septum, left atrium (LA), ascending aorta, left ventricular outflow tract, and aortic valve in diastole. The upper right images demonstrate a normal aortic valve in diastole and systole viewed from above, as if an aortotomy has been performed. The lower right images show a bicuspid aortic valve.

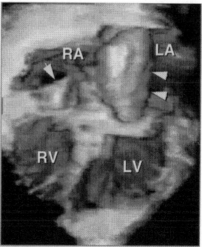

Figure 9-11. Three-dimensional display of mitral regurgitation jet (double arrows) in a four-chamber format. A jet of tricuspid valve regurgitation is also seen (single arrow) in the right atrium (RA). RV = right ventricle; LA = left atrium; LV = left ventricle.

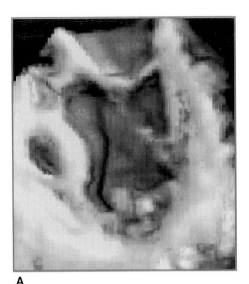
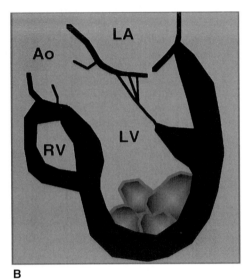

A   **B**

Figure 9-12. (**A,B**) Three-dimensional display of an infarcted left ventricle (LV) acquired from a transesophageal approach. An irregularly shaped clot is noted at the apex. Ao = aorta; LA = left atrium; RV = right ventricle.

acquisition systems for on-line image collection and storage are on their way toward clinical use. Data processing for three-dimensional echocardiography has been refined and made more automated. It can be expected that the data processing will be on line along with two-dimensional data acquisition. Color encoding of three-dimensional images is being developed; this could facilitate understanding of cardiac lesions. Holography is able to give unique three-dimensional views of the heart; further inves-

tigation is needed to assess its clinical utility.[35] Developments in quantification algorithms could allow faster volume or mass computations using automatic or semiautomatic border detection methods. Three-dimensional surface area measurement will provide useful information not obtainable with other techniques. In the future, physical models derived from three-dimensional echocardiography might be used for teaching demonstrations, preoperative rehearsals, or experimental investigations.

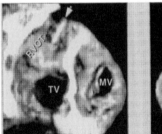
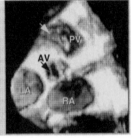

Figure 9-13. A pulmonary valve (PV) vegetation (white arrow) in a patient with endocarditis is demonstrated by three-dimensional echocardiography. Its size, shape, attachment, and mobility are well appreciated. Left: right ventricular outflow tract (RVOT) view. Right: short axis view from above at the level of the base of the heart. TV = tricuspid valve; MV = mitral valve; AV = aortic valve; LA = left atrium; RA = right atrium.

REFERENCES

1. Ariet M, Geiser EA, Lupkiewicz SM, et al. Evaluation of a three-dimensional reconstruction to compute left ventricular volume and mass. Am J Cardiol. 1984;54:415–420.
2. Bartel T, Muller S, Geibel A. Preoperative assessment of cor triatriatum in an adult by dynamic three dimensional echocardiography was more informative than transesophageal echocardiography or magnetic resonance imaging. Br Heart J. 1994;72:498–499.
3. Belohlavek M, Foley DA, Gerber TC, et al. Three-dimensional ultrasound imaging of the atrial septum: Normal and pathologic anatomy. J Am Coll Cardiol. 1993;22:1673–1678.
4. Cao QL, Pandian NG, Azevedo J, et al. Enhanced comprehension of dynamic cardiovascular anatomy by three-dimensional echocardiography with the use

of mixed shading techniques. Echocardiography. 1994;11:627–633.

5. Dekker DL, Piziali R, Dong E. A system for ultrasonically imaging the human heart in three dimensions. Comput Biomed Res. 1974;7:544–553.

6. Delabays A, Cao QL, Yao J, et al. Contrast three-dimensional echocardiography in acute myocardial infarction: 3-D reconstruction of perfusion defects yields accurate estimate of infarct mass and extent (abstract 718-4). J Am Coll Cardiol. 1996; 27(2)(suppl A):63A.

7. Delabays A, Pandian NG, Cao QL, et al. Transthoracic real-time three-dimensional echocardiography using a fan-like scanning approach for data acquisition: Methods, strength, problems, and initial clinical experience. Echocardiography. 1995;12:49–59.

8. Delabays A, Sugeng L, Pandian NG, et al. Dynamic three-dimensional echocardiographic assessment of intracardiac blood flow jets. Am J Cardiol. 1995;76: 1053–1058.

9. Folland ED, Parisi A, Moynihan PF, et al. Assessment of left ventricular ejection fraction and volume by real-time two-dimensional echocardiography. Circulation. 1979;60:760–766.

10. Fulton DR, Marx GR, Pandian NG, et al. Dynamic three-dimensional echocardiographic imaging of congenital heart defects in infants and children by computer-controlled tomographic parallel slicing using a single integrated ultrasound instrument. Echocardiography. 1994;11:155–164.

11. Fyfe DA, Ludomirsky A, Sandhu S, et al. Left ventricular outflow tract obstruction defined by active three-dimensional echocardiography using rotational transthoracic acquisition. Echocardiography. 1994;11:607–615.

12. Ghosh A, Nanda NC, Maurer G. Three-dimensional reconstruction of echocardiographic images using the rotation method. Ultrasound Med Biol. 1982; 6:655–661.

13. Gueret P, Meerbaum S, Wyatt HL, et al. Two-dimensional echocardiographic quantification of left ventricular volumes and ejection fraction. Circulation. 1980;62:1308–1318.

14. Gustavsson T, Pascher R, Caidahl K. Model based dynamic 3D reconstruction and display of the left ventricle from 2D cross-sectional echocardiograms. Comput Med Imaging Graphics. 1993;17:273–278.

15. Handschumacher MD, Lethor JP, Siu SC, et al. A new integrated system for three-dimensional echocardiographic reconstruction: Development and validation for ventricular volume with application in human subjects. J Am Coll Cardiol. 1993;21: 743–753.

16. Jiang L, Siu SC, Handschumacher MD, et al. Three-dimensional echocardiography: In vivo validation for right ventricular volume and function. Circulation. 1994;89:2342–2350.

17. King DL, King DL Jr, Shao MY. Three-dimensional spatial registration and interactive display of position and orientation of realtime ultrasound images. Ultrasound Med. 1990;9:525–532.

18. Kupferwasser I, Mohr-Kahaly S, Erbel R, et al. Three-dimensional imaging of cardiac mass lesions by transesophageal echocardiographic computed tomography. J Am Soc Echocardiogr. 1994;7: 561–570.

19. Levine RA, Handschumacher MD, Sanfilippo AJ, et al. Three-dimensional echocardiographic reconstruction of the mitral valve, with implications for the diagnosis of mitral valve prolapse. Circulation. 1989;80:589–598.

20. Linker DT, Mortiz WE, Pearlman AS. A new three-dimensional echocardiographic method of right ventricular volume measurement: In vitro validation. J Am Coll Cardiol. 1986;8:101–106.

21. Ludomirsky A, Vermilion R, Nesser J, et al. Transthoracic real-time three-dimensional echocardiography using the rotational scanning approach for data acquisition. Echocardiography. 1994;11:599–606.

22. Marx G, Fulton DR, Pandian NG, et al. Delineation of site, relative size and dynamic geometry of atrial septal defects by real-time three-dimensional echocardiography. J Am Coll Cardiol. 1995;25:482–490.

23. Matsumoto M, Matsuo H, Kitabatake A, et al. Three-dimensional echocardiograms and two-dimensional echocardiographic images at desired planes by a computerized system. Ultrasound Med Biol 1977;3:163–178.

24. Nanda NC, Roychoudhury D, Chung SM, et al. Quantitative assessment of normal and stenotic aortic valve using transesophageal three-dimensional echocardiography. Echocardiography. 1994;11: 617–625.

25. Nikravesh PE, Skorton DJ, Chandran KB, et al. Computerized three-dimensional finite element reconstruction of the left ventricle from cross-sectional echocardiograms. Ultrason Imaging. 1984;6:48–59.

26. Pandian NG, Nanda NC, Schwartz SL, et al. Three-dimensional and four-dimensional transesophageal echocardiographic imaging of the heart and aorta in humans using a computed tomographic imaging probe. Echocardiography. 1992;9:677–687.

27. Pandian NG, Roelandt J, Nanda NC, et al. Dynamic three-dimensional echocardiography: Methods and clinical potential. Echocardiography. 1994;11: 237–259.

28. Roelandt JRTC, Cate FJ, Vletter WB, et al. Ultrasonic dynamic three-dimensional visualization of the

heart with a multiplane transesophageal imaging transducer. J Am Soc Echocardiogr. 1994;7:217–229.

29. Roelandt JRTC, di Mario C, Pandian NG, et al. Three-dimensional reconstruction of intracoronary ultrasound images. Rationale, approaches, problems, and directions. Circulation. 1994;90:1044–1055.

30. Salustri A, Spitaels S, McGhie J, et al. Transthoracic three-dimensional echocardiography in adult patients with congenital heart disease. J Am Coll Cardiol. 1995;26:759–767.

31. Sapin PM, Schroedr KD, Smith MD, et al. Three-dimensional echocardiographic measurement of left ventricular volume in vitro: Comparison with two-dimensional echocardiography and cineventriculography. J Am Coll Cardiol. 1993;22:1530–1537.

32. Schiller NB, Acquatella H, Ports TA, et al. Left ventricular volume from paired biplane two-dimensional echocardiography. Circulation. 1979;60:547–555.

33. Schwartz SL, Cao QL, Azevedo J, et al. Simulation of intraoperative visualization of cardiac structures and study of dynamic surgical anatomy with real-time three-dimensional echocardiography. Am J Cardiol. 1994;73:501–507.

34. Siu SC, Rivera JM, Guerrero JL, et al. Three-dimensional echocardiography: In vivo validation for left ventricular volume and function. Circulation. 1993;88(part 1):1715–1723.

35. Vannan MA, Cao QL, Pandian NG, et al. Volumetric multiplexed transmission holography of the heart with echocardiographic data. J Am Soc Echocardiogr. 1995;8:567–575.

36. Vogel M, Lösch S. Dynamic three-dimensional echocardiography with a computed tomography imaging probe: Initial clinical experience with transthoracic application in infants and children with congenital heart defects. Br Heart J. 1994;71:462–467.

37. Yao J, Cao QL, Delabays A, et al. How well does three-dimensional echocardiographic quantification of dysfunctional left ventricular mass reflect actual anatomic infarct mass? Experimental studies (abstract 708-4). J Am Coll Cardiol. 1996;27(2)(suppl A):49A.

38. Zoghbi WA, Buckey JC, Massey MA, et al. Determination of left ventricular volumes with use of a new nongeometric echocardiographic method: Clinical validation and potential application. J Am Coll Cardiol. 1990;15:610–617.

PART III

The Complete Exam

10

The Transthoracic Exam

MARK N. ALLEN

Introduction

This chapter explains the sequence of a typical echocardiographic exam from the time the patient enters the echocardiography lab until he or she departs. The steps and sequences outlined here are meant to serve as guidelines and variations may be necessary depending on the specific lab. It is always important for everyone in the lab to follow a similar protocol. As accreditation of cardiac labs becomes an issue, having established protocols will become even more important.

Patients should be greeted kindly and compassionately. This statement may seem simple, but in today's fast-paced, hectic workplace, it becomes easy to lose focus. Health care employees must always remember that the patient may be apprehensive about coming to the hospital, doctor's office, or clinic. What is routine to us may be frightening to individuals unaccustomed to a health care environment. Hospital settings in particular may cause some individuals a great deal of apprehension. The overall "tone" of the exam can be determined from the moment you greet the patient. Attempts to place the patient at ease should always be given priority.

Before scanning begins, a complete medical history should be taken. The sonographer should have a clear understanding of the reason for the exam. Inpatient charts should be reviewed for any pertinent information that would be useful for the exam, including a description of any cardiac condition(s).

The patient's height, weight, heart rate, and blood pressure should be recorded. Accurate height and weight determinations are necessary in the event that a measurement needs to be corrected for body surface area or height, as is the case for left ventricular mass determinations.

Patient Preparation

After the appropriate introduction and initial medical history, the sonographer should explain the procedure and the steps that will be taken. Patients should be given an opportunity to ask questions about the procedure. They are then provided with a gown and asked to remove their clothing from the waist up. Placing the gown with the opening to the back provides greater privacy for patients. The sleeve can be removed from the left arm and draped loosely across the chest and over the sonographer's hand and transducer. This provides the patient with privacy and warmth and does not interfere with the exam.

The patient is then positioned on the bed and made as comfortable as possible; a fidgeting patient makes a poor target. The patient should be kept warm and comfortable, with attention to privacy. The patient is first placed in a supine position. Special beds with a drop section located at chest level or a mattress with a cut section in the same position are available and can make a significant difference in the success of the exam. A three-lead electrocardiogram (EKG) is placed on the patient's chest. The EKG signal provides timing for electrical events, which is helpful in making measurements and calculations. Once the EKG is placed, the patient is asked to turn onto the left side, assuming a left lateral decubitus position (Fig. 10-1). This position facilitates imaging of the heart by stretching the intercostal spaces and positioning the heart closer to the chest wall. The exam can then be performed from the left or right side of the patient. If scanning from the right, the operator and system are positioned to the right of the patient. The patient turns to the left and away from the sonographer. The sonographer then reaches around the patient to scan.

If scanning from the left, the sonographer and system are positioned to the left of the patient, and the patient turns toward the sonographer (Fig. 10-2). Scanning the patient from the left is preferable for several reasons. First, it allows the sonographer to have eye contact with the patient. Second, the patient is able to watch the video monitor, which can help keep the patient occupied; the sonographer can explain or point out various structures without providing any diagnostic information. Third, the sonographer can see if the patient is experiencing any distress during the exam. Fourth, it reduces the chance of back injury for the sonographer. When scanning from the right, the sonographer needs to reach around the patient, potentially overextending back muscles. Fifth, the sonographer is able to see where the transducer is being placed and avoids fumbling around for the proper windows. It is important for the sonographer to be able to scan with the left as well as the right hand, since many in-patient hospital situations may dictate the scanning side. Occasionally, creative scanning tech-

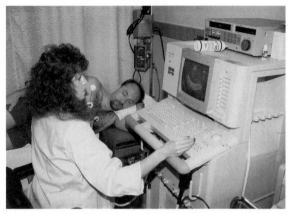

Figure 10-2. Demonstration of left-sided scanning. The machine and the sonographer are to the patient's left. The patient is able to watch the screen, and the sonographer can maintain eye contact with the patient.

niques are required in order to obtain the images. The sonographer should make every attempt to achieve a comfortable position in order to help reduce fatigue and injury.

Views

The American Society of Echocardiography has developed guidelines for two-dimensional and Doppler echocardiography.[10] These guidelines can be used as reference points in developing protocols. Unlike the planes described by anatomists, the echocardiography planes are described with respect to the positions in which the sound waves transect the heart.[11] A complete exam includes imaging as well as conventional (pulsed and continuous wave) and color Doppler components. Some sonographers prefer to obtain all images and follow with a complete Doppler study, while others prefer to perform the Doppler exam along with the imaging. Whatever the preference, all sonographers in a particular lab should follow the same procedure. For simplicity, the following section uses an integrated approach to scanning.

There are only a few acoustic windows from which numerous planes and views of cardiac structures can be obtained.[1,6] These include the left parasternal, apical, subcostal, suprasternal, and right parasternal views. Once there is an understanding of these fundamental windows, all necessary views can be obtained by fine-tuning the transducer's po-

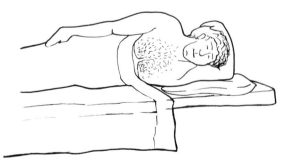

Figure 10-1. Drawing of a patient in the left lateral decubitus position, with the left arm extended over the head.

Display 10-1   Structures Viewed from the Various Transducer Positions

LEFT PARASTERNAL LONG-AXIS VIEW

Anterior right ventricular free wall
Right ventricular cavity
Interventricular septum, including membranous
   portion
Left ventricle
Left ventricular posterior wall
Mitral valve and apparatus
Left ventricular outflow tract
Aortic valve—left and noncoronary cusps
Aortic root
Left atrium
Descending thoracic aorta
Coronary sinus
Pericardium

PARASTERNAL SHORT-AXIS VIEW

Left ventricle—all wall segments
Aortic valve—all three cusps
Pulmonic valve
Tricuspid valve
Right atrium
Right ventricle
Main pulmonary artery
   Left and right branches
Interatrial septum
Pericardium
Left atrium

APICAL FOUR-CHAMBER VIEW

Left ventricle
   Septal wall
   Apex
   Lateral wall
Right ventricle
Left atrium
Right atrium
Mitral valve—anterior and posterior leaflets
Tricuspid valve

APICAL TWO-CHAMBER VIEW

Left ventricle
   Anterior wall
   Inferior wall
   Apex
Left atrium
   Left atrial appendage
Coronary sinus
Mitral valve

APICAL LONG-AXIS VIEW

Left ventricle
   Septum

Posterior wall
   Apex
Left atrium
Aortic valve
Ascending aorta
Mitral valve
   Both leaflets
Right ventricle (small portion)

APICAL FOUR-CHAMBER VIEW WITH AORTA

Left ventricle
   Septal wall
   Apex
   Lateral wall
Right ventricle
Left atrium
Right atrium
Atrioventricular valves
Aortic valve
Ascending aorta/left ventricular outflow tract

SUBCOSTAL FOUR-CHAMBER VIEW

Left ventricle
   Septal wall
   Lateral wall
Right ventricle
Left atrium
Right atrium
Atrioventricular valves

SUBCOSTAL SHORT-AXIS VIEW

Left ventricle—short axis
Right ventricle
Tricuspid valve
Pulmonic valve
Right ventricular outflow tract
Main pulmonary artery

SUBCOSTAL INFERIOR VENA CAVA VIEW

Inferior vena cava
Hepatic veins
Right atrium

SUPRASTERNAL VIEW

Ascending aorta
Aortic arch
Descending aorta
Left common carotid artery
Left subclavian artery
Innominate artery
Right pulmonary artery

sition. This last point is important because once an image is located, even a poor-quality image, it can be improved by fine manipulations of the transducer. Larger movements of the probe can lead to frustration as suboptimal images continuously come in and out of view. Display 10-1 summarizes the various views and the structures seen in each.

Left Parasternal Views

Before the discussion on scanning technique begins, it should be reiterated that M-mode or two-dimensional images will be best if the sound wave is positioned perpendicular or at 90 degrees to the structures. Doppler, on the other hand, will yield the best result if the angle between the Doppler sample and blood flow is parallel or 0 or near 0 degrees. With this in mind, a poor image will not necessarily mean a poor Doppler signal. The operator should therefore not struggle to obtain an ideal two-dimensional image before beginning a Doppler interrogation.

LEFT PARASTERNAL LONG-AXIS VIEW

The echocardiographic exam usually begins with a left parasternal long-axis view. Figures 10-3 through 10-6 illustrate the proper transducer position and the various images obtained from this position. The transducer is placed at the third, fourth, or fifth interscostal space, depending on the patient's chest configuration. Patients with pectus excavatum may have a lower left parasternal window. The transducer is placed in such a manner that the sound waves transect the heart in the longitudinal axis. With most transducers, the index marker is positioned toward the patient's right shoulder (Fig. 10-3*A*). A depth of at least 20 cm is initially used to

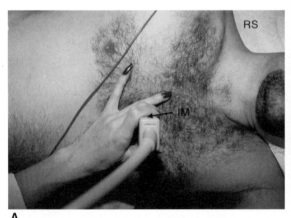

A

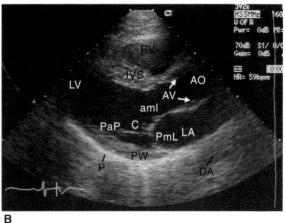

B

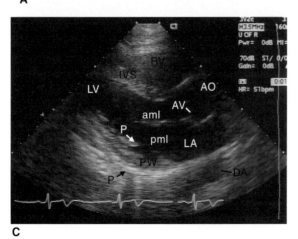

C

Figure 10-3. (**A**) Left parasternal long-axis view with the transducer positioned to the left of the sternum and the index marker (IM) pointed toward the right shoulder (RS). (**B**) Left parasternal long-axis image in systole. Most of the left-sided structures are noted. LA, left atrium; LV, left ventricle; AML, anterior mitral valve leaflet; PML, posterior mitral valve leaflet; IVS, interventricular septum; PW, posterior left ventricular wall; RV, right ventricular wall; Ao, aorta; AV, aortic valve; PAP, papillary muscle; C, chordae tendinae; DA, descending thoracic aorta; P, pericardium. (**C**) Left parasternal long-axis view in diastole. Most of the left-sided structures are noted. LA, left atrium; LV, left ventricle; AML, anterior mitral valve leaflet; PML, posterior mitral valve leaflet; IVS, interventricular septum; PW, posterior left ventricular wall; RV, right ventricular wall; Ao, aorta; AV, aortic valve; PAP, papillary muscle; C, chordae tendinae; DA, descending thoracic aorta; P, pericardium.

rule out obvious pericardiac pathology such as peri-cardial or pleural effusions. The depth is then re-duced for maximal cardiac resolution. Once a stan-dard parasternal long-axis view is obtained, at least 10 cardiac cycles are recorded. Some systems have a two-dimensional colorization feature that enables the operator to view the image in a variety of colors rather than just gray. Some systems can capture a series of frames or a loop whereby a particular car-diac cycle is continuously played back. Colorization is helpful in visualizing detail since the human eye can discern more color hues than grays. The loop function is helpful in patients with irregular cardiac rhythms. From this view many of the left-sided structures are seen, including the left atrium and the basal parts of the left ventricle with the posterior and septal walls. In addition, the anterior and posterior leaflets of the mitral valve and their chordae tendi-nae and the posterolateral papillary muscle are visu-alized; the left ventricular outflow tract, the right and noncoronary cusps of the aortic valve, and a proximal section of the ascending thoracic aorta, including the coronary sinus and descending tho-racic aorta, are all seen (Fig. 10-3*B*). From this posi-tion an M-mode scan can be done across the aortic valve and left atrium, and measurements of the aor-tic cusps' excursion, aortic root, and left atrial diam-eter can be made. These measurements can and should be made from the two-dimensional images as well. If M-mode is still used in your lab, the cursor can be moved toward the left ventricular apex through the mitral valve apparatus to the left ventri-cle. Once the cursor is at the tips of the mitral valve leaflets, measurements of the left ventricle are made. Great care should be taken to ensure that the M-mode cursor is perpendicular to the structures being measured.

M-mode is used to make the following standard measurements: aortic root at the aortic valve com-missure level, left atrial diameter (end systole), left ventricular cavity internal dimension (end diastole and end systole), left ventricular septum, and poste-rior wall thickness at end diastole. These same mea-surements are made in two-dimensional imaging. A loop or cine review feature found on most systems is used to obtain freeze-frames at the proper point in the cardiac cycle. An apical long-axis view may be used if the parasternal long axis is suboptimal. The most accurate measurements are reported and should fit the clinical impression. Left ventricular

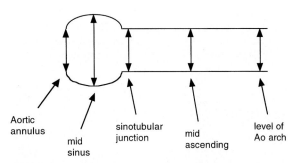

Schematic of Aortic root and ascending aorta

Figure 10-4. *Ascending aorta from the parasternal long-axis view. Measurements can be made along the length of the aorta as far as the image can be seen.*

mass calculations should be made only if there are no left ventricular diastolic shape deformities. The diameter of the ascending thoracic aorta is measured at the following levels: annulus, midsinus, sinotubu-lar junction, midtubular, middescending, and arch (Fig. 10-4).

TRICUSPID INFLOW VIEW

From this transducer position a number of non-standard imaging planes can be obtained. Tricuspid inflow images are obtained by moving the trans-ducer laterally and inferiorly while maintaining a parasternal long-axis image and rotating the probe approximately 15 to 30 degrees[1] (Fig. 10-5*A*). In addition to visualizing the tricuspid valve, the right atrium and right ventricle can be seen. From this view, the sonographer can get a good appreciation of valvular structure and function. Conditions such as tricuspid stenosis, prolapse, and vegetations can be detected. This view is perhaps most helpful in detecting the presence of tricuspid regurgitation (Fig. 10-5*B*). Due to the parallel placement of the continuous wave cursor to tricuspid valve flow from this view, it is possible to measure tricuspid valve gradients and to estimate pulmonary artery pres-sures. Color Doppler can be used to identify the presence and extent of regurgitation as well.

The ascending aorta can also be imaged in most patients by sliding the transducer along the left ster-nal border toward the neck, enabling measurements to be made along the course of the aorta. In a stan-dard parasternal long-axis view the proximal por-

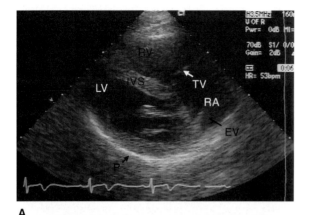

A

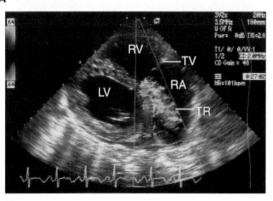

B

Figure 10-5. (**A**) Modified parasternal long-axis view of the right ventricular inflow tract and tricuspid valve. RA, right atrium; RV, right ventricle; TV, tricuspid valve; LA, left atrium; LV, left ventricle; IVS, interventricular septum; PW, posterior left ventricular wall; P, pericardium; EV, eustachian valve. (**B**) Modified parasternal long-axis view of the right ventricular inflow of tricuspid valve with color flow Doppler. Tricuspid regurgitation is noted as a blue-mosaic signal noted in systole. RA, right atrium; RV, right ventricle; TV, tricuspid valve; LV, left ventricle; TR, tricuspid regurgitation. (See also Color Plate 24.)

tion of the aorta can be visualized well; however, more distal regions of the ascending aorta are frequently cut out of the sector. To visualize more distal regions of the ascending aorta, quality images of the left ventricle must be sacrificed.

DOPPLER IN THE PARASTERNAL LONG-AXIS VIEW

Color Doppler is used in this view to evaluate the mitral and aortic valves for regurgitation (Fig. 10-6A,B). The membranous portion of the interventricular septum is interrogated with color Doppler for ventricular septal defect (VSD). If a VSD is

found, continuous wave Doppler (CW) is used to measure the peak trans-ventricular gradients.

In order to best visualize the mitral valve, aortic valve, and outflow tract, the "res" or "zoom" function can be used. These functions allow a magnified view of these structures without jeopardizing the resolution because, in most ultrasound systems, the line density is preserved within the magnified region.

PARASTERNAL SHORT-AXIS VIEWS

From a parasternal long-axis view, the transducer is rotated 90 degrees (Fig. 10-7) clockwise to reveal the heart in the cross-sectional orientation. Figures 10-7 through 10-15 illustrate the proper transducer position and the various images obtained from this position. The transducer index marker is positioned toward the patient's head. Interrogation of the heart from a parasternal short-axis view begins at the base of the heart. The transducer is angled anteriorly toward the patient's right shoulder to reveal the aorta in cross section. The aorta should be in the center of the image (Fig. 10-8A,B). Toward the left of the screen are the right atrium, tricuspid valve, and part of the right ventricle. The right ventricle is also noted at the top of the screen and continues to the left of the screen to turn into the right ventricular outflow tract. To image these structures more clearly, the transducer is angled toward the patient's left shoulder. This angulation reveals the pulmonic valve, the main pulmonary artery, and the bifurcation of the left and right pulmonary arteries[6,9] (Fig. 10-9A,B).

The transducer is then angled posteriorly toward the cardiac apex. Recordings should be made along each plane, starting at the base and traveling down through the mitral valve (Fig. 10-10A) and the papillary muscles (Fig. 10-10B) to the apex and then back toward the base. At least 10 cardiac cycles should be recorded at each level. The image colorization and/or cine loop function can be used in these views when there are irregular cardiac rhythms or in patients with limited image quality.

DOPPLER IN PARASTERNAL SHORT-AXIS VIEWS

Following a complete exam by two-dimensional echocardiography, a color Doppler exam is performed across all valves. From a short-axis view at

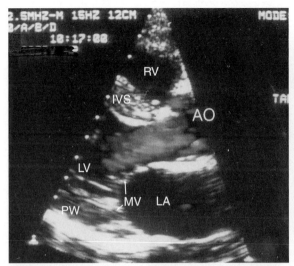

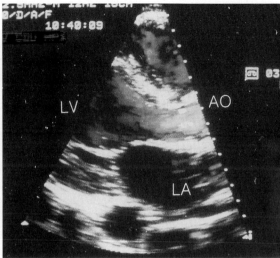

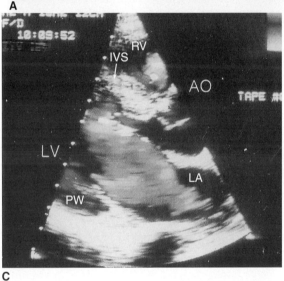

Figure 10-6. (**A**) Left parasternal long-axis view in systole with color Doppler demonstrating flow through the left ventricular outflow tract. The flow is coded red because the angle of flow is directed toward the transducer. (**B**) In this frame the flow is blue because the angle of flow is directed away from the transducer. LA, left atrium; LV, left ventricle; MV, mitral valve; IVS, interventricular septum; PW, posterior left ventricular wall; RV, right ventricular wall; Ao, aorta. (From Kisslo J, et al. Doppler Color Flow Imaging. New York, Churchill Livingstone; 1988: Figs. 3-18 (**A**) and 6-1 (**B**). Reprinted with permission.) (**C**) Left parasternal long-axis view in diastole demonstrating normal color flow patterns across the mitral valve. The flow is coded red because the angle of flow is directed more toward the transducer than away. LA, left atrium; LV, left ventricle; IVS, interventricular septum; PW, posterior left ventricular wall; RV, right ventricular wall; Ao, aorta. (From Kisslo J, et al. Doppler Color Flow Imaging. New York, Churchill Livingstone; 1988:74–75. Reprinted with permission.) (See also Color Plates 25, 26, and 27.)

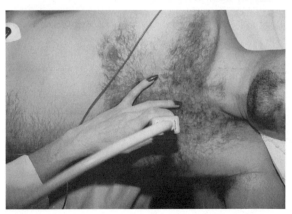

Figure 10-7. Transducer position for obtaining left parasternal short-axis views. The index marker is directed toward the patient's head.

the base of the heart, color Doppler is used to evaluate the pulmonic, tricuspid, and aortic valves. The interatrial septum and portions of the interventricular septum can be seen.[4] Color Doppler is helpful in identifying septal defects. Once the shunt is identified by color Doppler echocardiography, CW Doppler is used to quantitative degrees of the shunt and to measure velocities and gradients.

The parasternal short-axis view of the pulmonic and tricuspid valves is well suited for a Doppler exam since flow across these valves is nearly parallel to the orientation of the sound beam and Doppler cursor. Slight angulation of the transducer toward the patient's right shoulder may be necessary in order to see the pulmonic valve clearly (Fig. 10-11) and to-

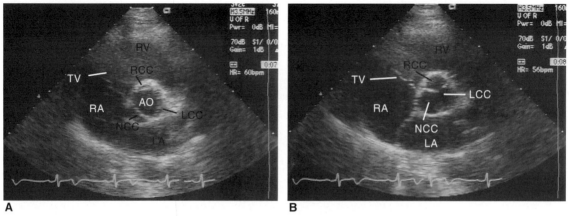

Figure 10-8. (**A**) A left parasternal short-axis view in systole with the transducer angled toward the base of the heart. (**B**) The same view seen in diastole; note that the aortic valve is closed. Ao, aorta; LA, left atrium; RA, right atrium; RV, right ventricle; TV, tricuspid valve; LCC, left coronary cusp; RCC, right coronary cusp; NCC, noncoronary cusp.

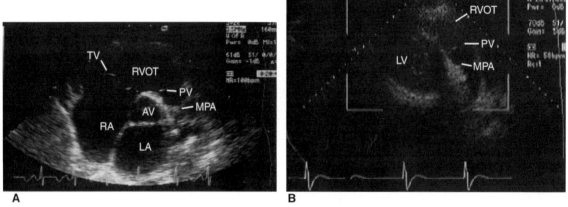

Figure 10-9. (**A**) Left parasternal short-axis view with the transducer angled toward the patient's right side to reveal the tricuspid valve. (**B**) With a more leftward angulation, the pulmonic valve can be visualized. AV, aortic valve; LA, left atrium; RA, right atrium; RVOT, right ventricular outflow tract; TV, tricuspid valve; MPA, main pulmonary artery; PV, pulmonic valve.

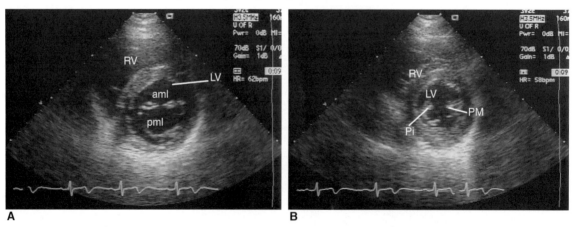

Figure 10-10. (**A**) Left parasternal short-axis view at the level of the mitral valve. LV, left ventricle; RV, right ventricle; aml, anterior mitral valve leaflet; pml, posterior mitral valve leaflet. (**B**) Left parasternal short-axis view at the level of the papillary muscles. LV, left ventricle; RV, right ventricle; P, papillary muscle.

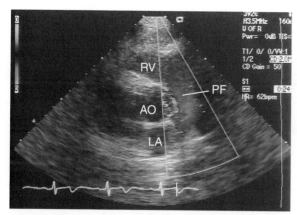

Figure 10-11. A left parasternal short-axis view at the base of the heart and at the level of the pulmonic valve. A blue jet is noted in this systolic frame because flow across the pulmonic valve in this imaging plane is away from the transducer. LA, left atrium; RA, right atrium; RV, right ventricle; Ao, aorta; MPA, main pulmonary artery; PF, pulmonic valve flow; PI, pulmonic valve insufficiency. (See also Color Plate 28.)

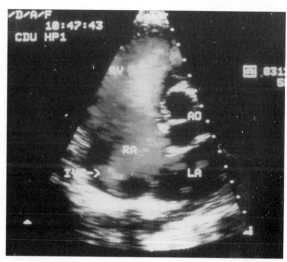

Figure 10-12. Color flow Doppler in a left parasternal short-axis view angled toward the tricuspid valve. The jet is red since flow is toward the transducer. Color flow is noted originating from the inferior vena cava (IVC) as it enters the right atrium. LA, left atrium; RA, right atrium; RV, right ventricle; Ao, aorta. (From Kisslo J, et al. Doppler Color Flow Imaging. New York, Churchill Livingstone; 1988:83. Reprinted with permission.) (See also Color Plate 29.)

ward the left shoulder to see the tricuspid valve (Fig. 10-12).

The Doppler cursor can be placed across the pulmonic valve to measure pulmonic valve gradients and the presence of pulmonary insufficiency (Fig. 10-13). Moving the cursor to the left of the screen allows Doppler interrogation of the tricuspid valve (Figure 10-14). In patients with aortic insufficiency, the short-axis view can be used to evaluate the regurgitant lesion (Fig. 10-15). Since the aortic valve is in the cross section, the precise location of the jet can be seen from this view. This is helpful, in distinguishing between valvular and perivalvular lesions.

Apical Views

To obtain adequate apical views, the sonographer should first feel for the point of maximal impulse (PMI). Using two fingers positioned just below the left breast, a small focal pulse can be palpated. Once this pulse is located, the transducer is positioned directly over it to obtain apical views. Figures 10-16 through 10-22 illustrate the proper transducer position and the various images obtained from this position. The transducer is placed with the index marker positioned toward the patient's left shoulder (Fig. 10-16). The apex of the left ventricle and the

mitral valve should be centered in the imaging sector. At least 10 cardiac cycles of the left ventricular walls are taken in this position. Endocardial borders should be optimized by appropriately adjusting gain, time gain compensation, or other system functions.

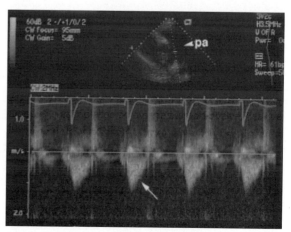

Figure 10-13. Left parasternal short-axis view with CW Doppler cursor placed across the pulmonic valve. Peak velocities can be measured.

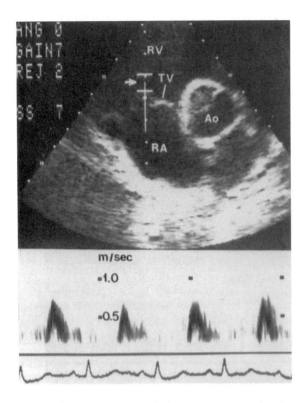

Figure 10-14. Left parasternal short-axis view with the PW Doppler cursor placed across the tricuspid valve. The typical spectral display of tricuspid flow is noted. E, E wave; A, A wave; LA, left atrium; RV, right ventricle. (From Berger M. Doppler Echocardiography in Heart Disease. New York: Marcel Dekker, Inc.)

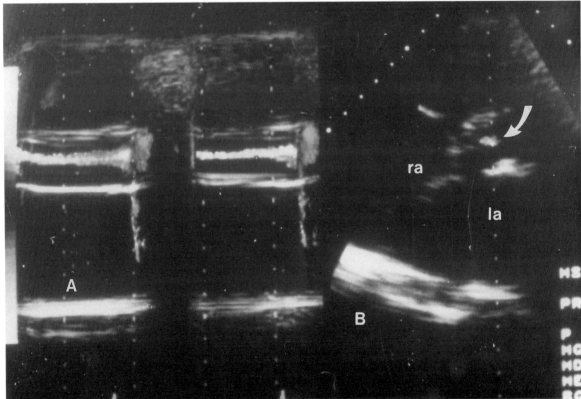

Figure 10-15. Left parasternal short-axis view at the level of the aorta. This is a color Doppler frame demonstrating a central diastolic color jet identifying a mild degree of aortic insufficiency (arrow). (See also Color Plate 30.)

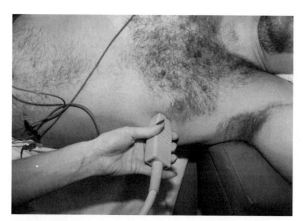

Figure 10-16. Patient and transducer position for an apical four-chamber view.

The apical views allow the sonographer to visualize many structures of the heart. Assessment of wall motion, as well as Doppler interrogation of valves and cardiac chamber size, can all be performed from these views. Four standard views can be obtained from this position: apical four-chamber view, apical two-chamber view, apical four-chamber view with aorta (commonly referred to as the *apical five-chamber view*), and apical long-axis view. All these views can be obtained by maintaining the transducer's face in the same position. The various views can then be obtained by merely rotating the transducer around a focal point.[9]

APICAL FOUR-CHAMBER VIEW

The sound beam is directed superiorly and toward the right shoulder.[6,11] This view allows visualization of all four cardiac chambers (left atrium, right atrium, right ventricle, and left ventricle). The septal wall, lateral free wall, and apex of the left ventricle are seen in this view. Both atrioventricular valves are also seen: the mitral and tricuspid valves. The interventricular and interatrial septa can also be visualized from this view and should be seen in the middle of the sector. An apical four-chamber view can be obtained by placing the transducer properly over the true cardiac apex. The apex of the left ventricle should be at the center of the sector where the septum and lateral wall meet, almost creating a point[7] (Fig. 10-17*A,B*). A rounded apex typically means that the image is foreshortened and does not represent a true apical four-chamber view (Fig. 10-18). The mitral and tricuspid valves should be seen

swinging open widely (in patients with no pathology). The walls of the left and right atria should be clearly seen, and pulmonary veins should be seen entering the left atrium. The right ventricle, located to the left of the screen, should appear as a triangular shape. Once these characteristic features are noted, the operator is assured of a true apical four-chamber view.

Like the other apical views, this view is particularly important in evaluating the size and function of the ventricles and atria, as well as valvular structure and function.[5] Because this view allows simul-

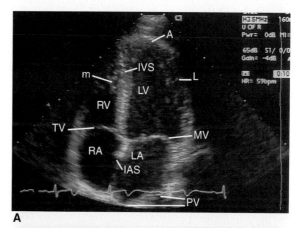

A

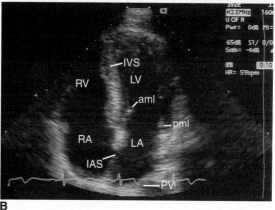

B

Figure 10-17. (**A**) Apical four-chamber view in systole; notice the closure of the mitral and tricuspid valves, as well as the more apical displacement of the tricuspid valve—an anatomic distinction from the mitral valve. (**B**) Apical four-chamber view in diastole; notice the normally wide separation of the atrioventricular valves. LA, left atrium; RA, right atrium; LV, left ventricle; RV, right ventricle; IVS, interventricular septum; L, lateral wall; A, apex; IAS, interatrial septum; PV, pulmonary veins; TV, tricuspid valve; MV, mitral valve; aml, anterior mitral valve leaflet; pml, posterior mitral valve leaflet; m, moderator band.

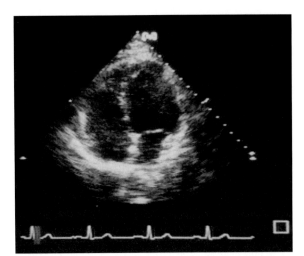

Figure 10-18. Foreshortened apical four-chamber view. Note the rounded appearance of the apex. Such views distort normal anatomic structures and lead to misinterpretations of function.

taneous visualization of all four cardiac chambers, their relative sizes, orientation, and function can be assessed. The apical four-chamber view is important in the evaluation of left ventricular function because the septal wall, lateral wall, and apex can be visualized. Wall motion abnormalities, ventricular aneurysms, and clot can all be seen from this view.[8] Ventricular size can be measured; however, one must keep in mind that the sound beam runs parallel to the lateral and septal walls using the system's lateral resolution, which can create side lobe and reverberation artifacts. As a result, there may be dropout of endocardial echoes or artifacts masking true endocardial borders. Therefore, caution should be exercised in making the measurements and in reporting any data.

The presence of right ventricular involvement in myocardial infarction can also be determined from this view since the right ventricular septum and lateral free wall can be seen. Dilatation of the right ventricle can be assessed by comparing its size with that of the left ventricle or by making actual measurements. The presence of thrombus or masses within the right ventricle can be noted. The moderator band is frequently seen in this view and should not be confused with the abnormalities. Knowledge of the moderator band's location and position will avoid this problem. Remember from Chapter 1 that the moderator band is located apically and runs

from the septum to the lateral wall. In clinical situations of anterior myocardial infarction or left ventricular apical aneurysms, the right ventricular apex should be closely scanned for the presence of a VSD.[7]

Left and right atrial size can be appreciated from the apical four-chamber view, allowing a good comparison. Superior-inferior and lateral-medial measurements and areas of both atria can be obtained from a four-chamber view. However, resolution errors that affect the ventricles also apply to the atria. The lateral free walls and septum are parallel to the sound beam, potentially creating artifacts. The presence of left or right atrial masses can be documented. The site of attachment, if seen, can help determine the nature of the mass. A number of normal variants can also be seen, particularly of the right atrium. A large series of trabeculations called the *Chiari network* are very prominent in some patients. In addition, the eustachian valve, a fetal remnant, can be seen in many patients (Fig. 10-19). Knowledge of their presence and location can help avoid misdiagnoses.

All four pulmonary veins can be seen entering the left atrium. Proper depth and gain settings will reveal both left and right veins. The absence of

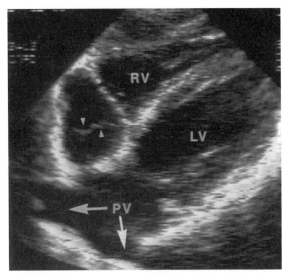

Figure 10-19. A prominent eustachian valve, as seen in this subcostal view, is commonly noted in the right atrium in some patients and should not be confused with a clot or tumor. These structures can be noted in apical views as well. LA, left atrium; RA, right atrium; LV, left ventricle; RV, right ventricle. (From Feigenbaum H. Echocardiography, 5th ed. Baltimore: Lea & Febiger, 1994.)

veins, abnormal insertion sites, and vein diameter can be appreciated. Careful attention to the pulmonary veins is important for anatomic identification, as well as for Doppler interrogation (Fig. 10-20).

Diastolic and systolic motion of the mitral and tricuspid valve are seen from this view. Abnormal valve motion, vegetations, torn chordae, and ruptured papillary muscles can all be seen. The anterior mitral valve leaflet arises from its medial attachment at the ventricular septum. The posterior leaflet arises from the lateral wall. The septal tricuspid leaflet is identified by its attachment of the ventricular septum. The large anterior tricuspid valve leaflet inserts on the lateral wall. The posterior tricuspid leaflet is not seen in this view. An important physical distinction between the mitral and tricuspid valves is made here. The attachment of the septal leaflet of the tricuspid valve occurs at the midportion of the membranous septum and is positioned 5 to 10 mm more apically relative to the mitral valve.[11] This distinction is important in identifying the mitral and tricuspid valves, as well as in identifying the ventricles. In congenital defects, knowledge of this difference is extremely helpful in correctly identifying chambers and valves.

DOPPLER IN THE APICAL FOUR-CHAMBER VIEW

The apical four-chamber view is excellent for Doppler interrogation of the mitral and tricuspid valves due to the parallel flow of the mitral valve and the nearly parallel flow of the tricuspid valve to the Doppler sound beam. The Doppler exam frequently begins with color Doppler in order to evaluate the flow patterns of the mitral and tricuspid valves (Fig.

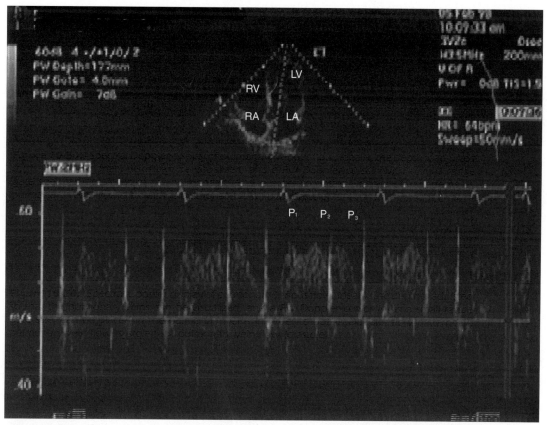

Figure 10-20. Spectral Doppler display of pulmonary venous flow. Ideally, the depth is adjusted so that the pulmonary veins can be visualized, and a PW Doppler cursor (with a small range gate size) can be placed in the pulmonary veins in order to obtain Doppler flow patterns. P, pulmonary vein flow (systole); P_d, pulmonary vein flow (diastole).

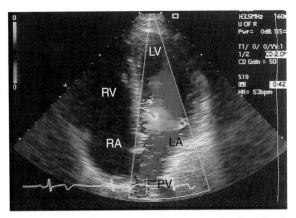

Figure 10-21. Apical four-chamber view in diastole. A red color flow Doppler pattern is noted because flow across the valve is toward the transducer. Flow from the pulmonary veins can be appreciated in this view. LA, left atrium; RA, right atrium; LV, left ventricle; RV, right ventricle; PV, pulmonary veins. (See also Color Plate 31.)

10-21) and for the presence of regurgitation. Once the flow patterns are identified, the pulsed or continuous wave Doppler cursor can be aligned parallel with the color jet to provide a Doppler flow signal (Fig. 10-22*A,B*). Velocities and pressure gradients can then be obtained. The use of color Doppler to identify flow patterns helps reduce scanning time and aids in identifying variations in flow, such as those seen in prosthetic valves.

In patients with regurgitation, the peak velocities can be obtained more quickly and accurately by using color Doppler to guide the pulsed wave (PW) Doppler or continuous wave (CW) Doppler cursor to the lesion. To measure maximum velocities and peak gradients, Doppler CW is typically used because of its ability to record velocities above the Nyquist limit. By contrast, if range resolution is the objective and precise location of flow is needed, pulsed Doppler (PW) is used. Doppler CW is used if systolic pulmonary artery pressures have to be calculated from tricuspid regurgitation gradients or the if PISA calculations have to be performed on either valve to determine regurgitant fraction and effective regurgitant orifice area. In the latter case, the maximum tricuspid regurgitation or mitral regurgitation velocities are needed for the calculation.

APICAL TWO-CHAMBER VIEW

By rotating the transducer roughly 30–45 degrees counterclockwise (Fig. 10-23), an apical two-cham-

ber view of the left ventricle is obtained. Figures 10-23 and 10-24 illustrate the proper transducer position and the various images obtained from this position. The plane of the sound wave is anterior-posterior and angled toward the right shoulder. This view allows visualization of the anterior and inferior walls of the left ventricle. A true apical two-chamber view is obtained when no right-sided structures are seen. To the left of the image at the atrioventricular junction, a small circular structure is also noted. This landmark is the coronary sinus. The left atrial appendage noted to the right of the screen at the level of the left atrium is also frequently seen and can be used as a landmark for positioning the transducer as well. The left ventricular apex and mitral valve should be centered in the sector (Fig. 10-24).

This view allows left ventricular size and function to be evaluated. To the right of the screen, the anterior wall of the left ventricle is seen. To the left of the screen, the inferior wall of the left ventricle is noted. The anterior leaflet of the mitral valve is to the right of the screen, and the posterior leaflet is to the left. The size of the coronary sinus, located near the posterior leaflet at the atrioventricular junction, can be appreciated in this view. A dilated coronary sinus can indicate cardiac abnormalities such as abnormal attachment of the pulmonary veins, as well as other abnormalities. The left atrial appendage can be seen to the right of the screen as a triangular structure angled toward the ventricle. Its opening is noted just below the anterior mitral valve leaflet attachment. Although this structure can be seen, transthoracic imaging is typically limited in evaluating it for clot. The left atrial appendage is not always seen, and the tip is frequently obscured by the lung. Transesophageal echocardiography is ideally suited for evaluating this region.

In addition to chamber size, area, and function, a number of pathologic processes can be seen. As with the apical four-chamber view, the presence of wall motion abnormalities of either the anterior or inferior walls can be appreciated. The presence of left ventricular thrombus can be documented. If thrombus is suspected in the apical four-chamber view, its presence should be confirmed in the two-chamber view as well as in the apical long-axis view before making a definitive diagnosis. The presence of left atrial masses, as well as chamber size and left atrial areas, can be calculated from this view.

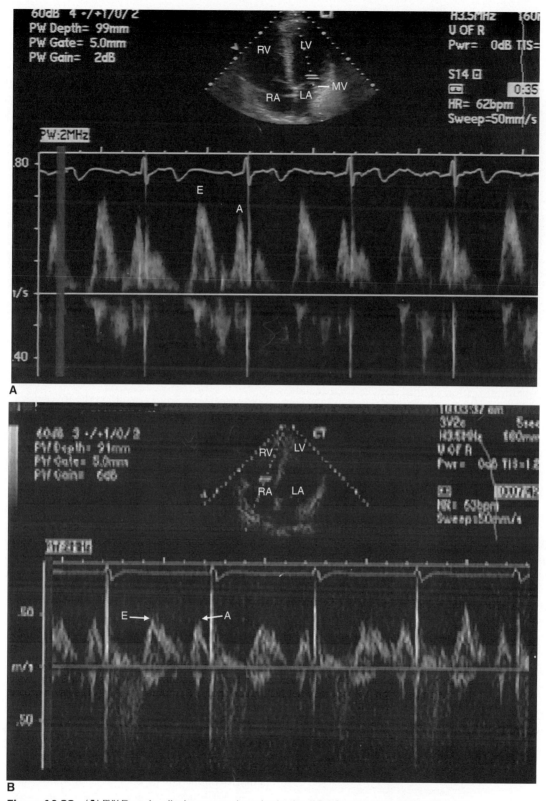

Figure 10-22. (**A**) PW Doppler display across the mitral valve (MV) from an apical four-chamber view. The E wave and A wave are appreciated in this view. (**B**) PW Doppler display across the tricuspid valve (TV). LA, left atrium; RA, right atrium; LV, left ventricle; RV, right ventricle.

195

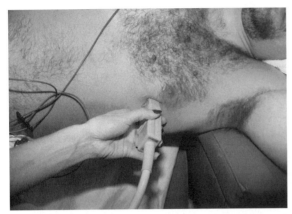

Figure 10-23.   Patient and transducer position for an apical two-chamber view. The transducer is oriented in such a way that the sound beam transects the chest (heart) from right shoulder to left hip.

DOPPLER IN THE APICAL TWO-CHAMBER VIEW

Doppler interrogation in this view is done mainly to evaluate flow across the mitral valve. In a patient with no cardiac disease, the flow pattern across the mitral valve appears as two peaks. An E wave that occurs in early diastole represents the rapid filling phase of diastole. The second wave, the A wave, is seen as a result of atrial contraction. The E wave is normally larger than the A wave, but age, pressure differences, and pathology may cause a variety of patterns. Color Doppler is frequently performed first in order to appreciate flow direction. The Doppler cursor can then be aligned with the color jet in order to obtain spectral Doppler displays for velocity and pressure measurements.

APICAL LONG-AXIS VIEWS

Apical long-axis views can be obtained by further rotation of the transducer counterclockwise approximately 30–45 degrees from the apical two-chamber view while maintaining the head of the transducer at the same location as for the apical four-chamber view (Fig. 10-25). Figures 10-25 through 10-28 illustrate the proper transducer position and the various images obtained from this position. As with all the apical views, one merely rotates the transducer around a stationary point. The posterior apex can be best appreciated from this view. The apical long-axis view allows the following structures to be seen: left atrium, mitral valve (anterior and posterior leaflets), left ventricle (including the septum and posterior walls, as well as portions of the apex), left ventricular outflow tract, aortic valve, and ascending aorta (Fig. 10-26). This view is frequently referred to as the *apical three-chamber view*, but since only two chambers are visualized, the more appropriate name is the *apical long-axis view*.

This view is identical to the left parasternal long-axis view, except that the transducer is positioned over the cardiac apex. In fact, this view can be used in stress echocardiography when parasternal windows are suboptimal.

Wall motion abnormalities, aneurysms, and the presence of clot can all be evaluated from this image. Mitral valve structure and integrity can be appreciated since both the anterior and posterior leaflets are observed. The left atrium is seen clearly, allowing complete evaluation of its contents, size, and area. The left ventricular outflow tract, aortic valve, and ascending aorta can also be seen toward the right of the screen. This view is particularly useful for evaluating the left ventricular outflow tract for the presence of subaortic obstruction or membranes. A small portion of the right ventricle is also noted in this view, but little diagnostic information can be obtained from the right ventricle.

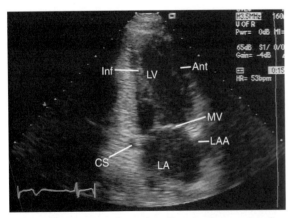

Figure 10-24.   Two-dimensional image of a two-chamber view. Only the left atrium (LA) and left ventricle (LV) are seen in this view. Proper transducer placement will reveal the coronary sinus (cs) and left atrial appendage (LAA). No right heart structures should be noted in this view. Inf, inferior wall of the left ventricle; Ant, anterior wall of the left ventricle.

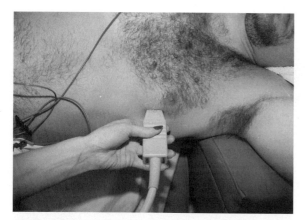

Figure 10-25. *Patient and transducer position for apical long-axis views. The transducer is rotated approximately 30 to 45 degrees from an apical two-chamber position.*

DOPPLER IN THE APICAL LONG-AXIS VIEWS

Similar to the apical two-chamber view, Doppler interrogation of the mitral valve can be done in color (Fig. 10-27), PW and CW Doppler (Fig. 10-28). Blood flow velocities, the presence of regurgitation, and stenosis can all be ascertained. The orientation of the outflow tract is ideally suited for Doppler since flow is parallel to the Doppler sound beam. Maximum velocities across the outflow tract and aortic valve can be obtained. In aortic stenosis,

it is possible to measure valvular and outflow tract velocities with CW and PW Doppler, respectively. The diameter of the left ventricular outflow tract can also be measured from this view.

In subaortic stenosis, the apical long-axis image may help identify the site of obstruction. Subaortic membranes can be difficult to visualize, but they may be seen from these views. By mapping the left ventricular outflow tract with PW Doppler, the site of obstruction can be located. The pulsed wave cursor is "walked" up the outflow tract toward the aortic valve, and the maximum velocity is recorded at each level. Normally, velocities in the outflow tract do not exceed 1 m/sec. If obstruction is present, the velocities will typically exceed the Nyquist limit, alerting the sonographer to the presence of subaortic obstruction.

Due to the anatomic orientation of the left ventricular outflow tract, color Doppler is ideal for evaluating the aortic valve for the presence of insufficiency. In the presence of aortic insufficiency, a red mosaic jet is typically observed in diastole. Color

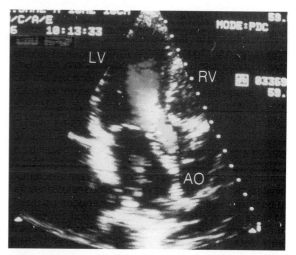

Figure 10-27. *Apical long-axis view with color flow Doppler. Flow in the outflow tract is normally blue since it is directed away from the transducer; however, red flow is also noted. This red flow is due to aliasing, which is common in this view since the velocity of blood in a normal left ventricular outflow tract can exceed the Nyquist limit. This is an important point since some may be inclined to call the red flow aortic insufficiency (AI). AI can easily be ruled out since the aliased flow occurs in systole. (From Kisslo J, et al. Doppler Color Flow Imaging. New York, Churchill Livingstone; 1988:79. Reprinted with permission.) (See also Color Plate 32.)*

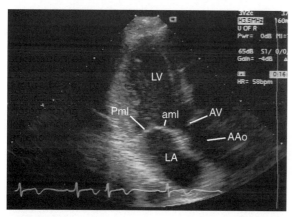

Figure 10-26. *Two-dimensional image of an apical long-axis image. Note that both the mitral and aortic valves are closed during isovolumic relaxation. LA, left atrium; LV, left ventricle; AV, aortic valve; Aao, ascending aorta; aml, anterior mitral valve leaflet; pml, posterior mitral valve leaflet.*

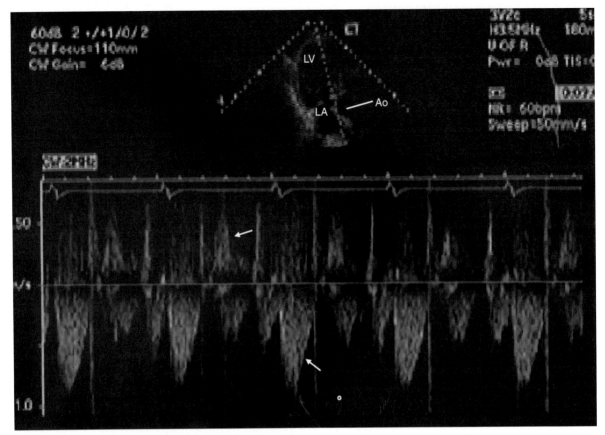

Figure 10-28. Spectral Doppler tracings across the apical long-axis view. LA, left atrium; LV, left ventricle; Ao, aorta; aortic valve flow (arrow); mitral valve flow (open arrow).

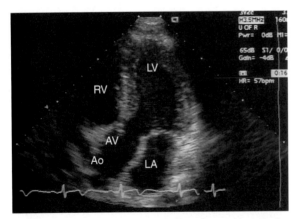

Figure 10-29. Apical four-chamber view with anterior angulation in order to visualize the aortic valve (AV) and aorta (Ao). LA, left atrium; LV, left ventricle; RV, right ventricle.

helps to define the direction of the jet. Aortic insufficiency can be directed straight into the left ventricle, toward the interventricular septum, or toward the anterior mitral valve leaflet. Identifying the direction of the jet is helpful in placing the CW or PW Doppler cursor.

APICAL FOUR-CHAMBER VIEW WITH AORTA

Returning to an apical four-chamber view, the transducer is angled anteriorly toward the chest wall (Fig. 10-29). This brings the left ventricular outflow tract, the aortic valve, and portions of the ascending aorta into view. Figures 10-29, 10-30, and 10-31 illustrate the proper transducer position and the various images obtained from this posi-

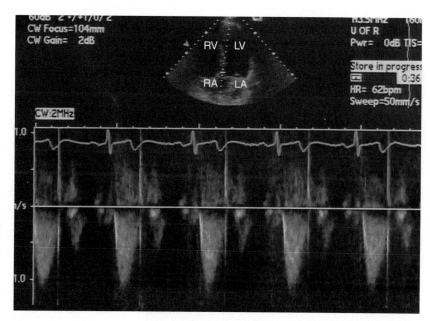

Figure 10-30. Spectral display across the left ventricular outflow tract in an apical four-chamber view with anterior angulation. LA, left atrium; LV, left ventricle; RV, right ventricle; RA, right atrium.

tion. This view adds little information to the imaging portion of the exam other than aortic valve motion. However, it is critical in evaluating the aortic valve and left ventricular outflow tract by Doppler. Doppler measurements can be made from this view in both stenosis and regurgitation because the Doppler cursor can be aligned parallel to the left ventricular outflow tract and valve (Fig. 10-30). Subaortic obstructions can also be as-

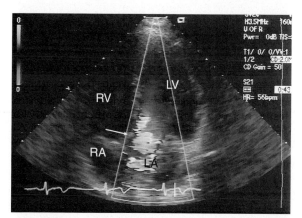

Figure 10-31. Color flow Doppler from an apical four-chamber view and anterior angulation. Color flow is typically blue, but due to aliasing red may also be seen (arrow). LA, left atrium; RA, right atrium; LV, left ventricle; RV, right ventricle. (See also Color Plate 33.)

sessed. The presence of systolic anterior motion of the mitral valve, subaortic membranes, and interventricular septal thickening can be seen and their consequence appreciated by Doppler interrogation. Color flow Doppler in this view demonstrates a blue jet with some red aliasing due to the Nyquist limit (Fig. 10-31).

MODIFIED APICAL VIEWS

At times it becomes necessary to modify standard views in order to obtain structural or functional information. Figures 10-32 and 10-33 illustrate the images obtained from such a position. In an apical four-chamber view the tricuspid valve will be angled slightly toward the left, so that flow across the valve is moving at a 25 to 30 degree angle to the peak of the sector. The Doppler angle is therefore greater than 0, making alignment and accurate Doppler assessment of the tricuspid valve difficult. This problem can be corrected by sliding the transducer medially and up one interspace (Fig. 10-32*A,B*). Tricuspid flow will then be parallel to the Doppler beam. The view resembles a cross between an apical four-chamber view and a short-axis view. Color Doppler can then be used to identify regurgitant jets and guide the CW Doppler cursor to record the peak trans tricuspid gradients (Fig. 10-33).

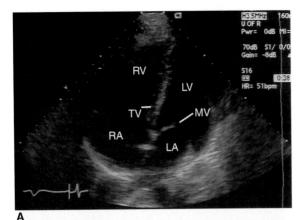

A

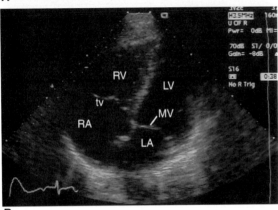

B

Figure 10-32. Modified apical four-chamber view with emphasis on the tricuspid valve. From this view, tricuspid flow is more parallel to the sound beam, allowing a clear Doppler signal. (**A**) Diastolic frame with atrioventricular valves open. (**B**) Systolic frame with atrioventricular valves closed. LA, left atrium; RA, right atrium; LV, left ventricle; RV, right ventricle; TV, tricuspid valves; MV, mitral valve.

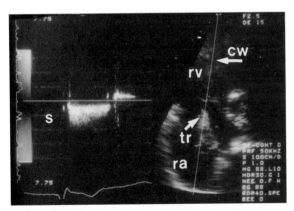

Figure 10-33. Modified four-chamber view with spectral Doppler. The angle of tricuspid flow is nearly parallel to the sound beam, allowing better Doppler interrogation of the tricuspid flow. (See also Color Plate 34.)

Subcostal Views

The subcostal view is considered a standard view and should be performed on all patients (Fig. 10-34). It is an ideal view to image the heart in patients with chronic obstructive pulmonary disease (COPD). Images of the heart from this view can be obtained in the majority of adults. Figures 10-34 through 10-39 illustrate the proper transducer position and the various images obtained from this position. Three subcostal views can be obtained from the subcostal transducer position: the subcostal four-chamber view (Fig. 10-35), the subcostal short-axis views (Fig. 10-36A,B), and the inferior vena cava/hepatic vein view[2,3] (Fig. 10-37). For all these views the patient is asked to lie supine, with the knees bent and the feet flat on the bed. The transducer is placed just below the xyphoid process. The left lobe of the liver, which runs from right to left, serves as an excellent acoustic window. In the

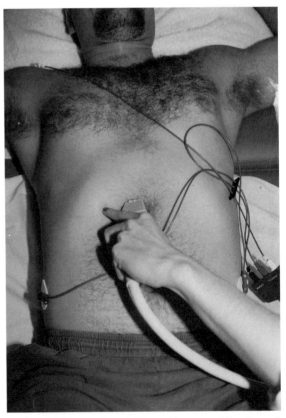

Figure 10-34. Patient and transducer position for subcostal views. The patient is supine, with the knees bent. A deep inspiration is held to help bring in the image.

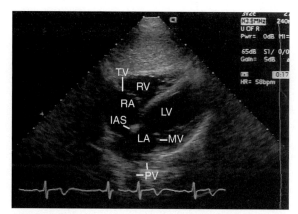

Figure 10-35. Subcostal four-chamber view. This view allows all four chambers to be seen with the right ventricle closest to the transducer. This view facilitates the evaluation of right ventricular systolic function. The interatrial septum can also be interrogated for evidence of atrial septal defects or patent foramen ovale. LA, left atrium; RA, right atrium; LV, left ventricle; RV, right ventricle; TV, tricuspid valves; MV, mitral valve; IAS, interatrial septum; pv, pulmonary veins.

subcostal four-chamber and short-axis views, the patient is usually asked to take a deep breath and maintain it as long as possible. This decreases intrathoracic pressures and causes the diaphragm to expand, pushing abdominal organs down while expanding the thoracic cage and pulling the heart down. This facilitates visualization of the heart from this position.

SUBCOSTAL FOUR-CHAMBER VIEW

The subcostal four-chamber view is obtained by placing the transducer such that the sound beam transects the body into ventral (top) and dorsal (bottom) halves. The transducer is angled toward the patient's left shoulder. This view is comparable to the apical four-chamber view demonstrating all four cardiac chambers. The right heart is positioned closest to the transducer and is therefore displayed at the top of the sector, with the right atrium to the left and the right ventricle to the right. In fact, this is one of the best views for evaluating right ventricular function and size and for making a right ventricular free wall measurement. This is one of the few views that allows a large part of the right ventricle to be seen. Since the right ventricle lies perpendicular to the sound beam, artifacts such as reverberation commonly seen in the right ventricle from an apical

position are not a problem in this view. In addition, in patients in cardiac tamponade where there is cardiac compromise, the presence of right ventricular free wall diastolic invagination or collapse can best be appreciated.

In addition to the right ventricle, the left atrium is seen toward the lower right region of the sector and the left ventricle toward the upper right side of the sector. Maximum excursion of both mitral and tricuspid valves can be appreciated. The interatrial and interventricular septa can be seen. From these

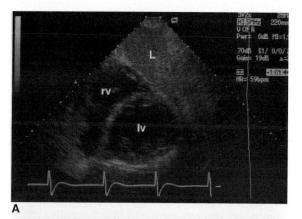

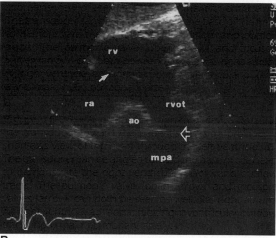

Figure 10-36. (**A**) Subcostal short-axis views. Rotating the transducer toward the patient's left side provides a short-axis view of the heart through the left ventricle. (**B**) The transducer can be angled toward the base of the heart to demonstrate the right ventricular inflow and outflow tracts. The pulmonic valve (open arrow) and tricuspid valves (arrow) can both be seen as well. Ra, right atrium; rv, right ventricle; ao, aorta; rvot, right ventricular outflow tract; mpa, main pulmonary artery.

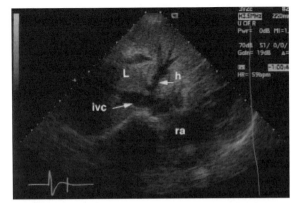

Figure 10-37. Subcostal view with the transducer angled toward the patient's right side. The inferior vena cava (IVC) and hepatic veins (hv) can be seen entering the right atrium. In this subcostal view the patient is asked to breathe normally so that normal respiratory variations of the IVC can be observed. RA, right atrium; L, liver.

views, the motion of the septa, the presence of interatrial septal aneurysm, or lipomatous hypertrophy of the interatrial septum can be visualized. Atrioventricular relationships can also be studied and should demonstrate a more apically positioned tricuspid valve. Slight anterior angulation of the transducer will align the sound beam with the aorta and the aortic valve. The left atrium and mitral valve will no longer be seen clearly.

DOPPLER IN THE SUBCOSTAL FOUR-CHAMBER VIEW

The long axis of the heart is close to 45 degrees from the point of the imaging sector. This large angle makes Doppler interrogation difficult. Aligning CW or PW Doppler cursors across the valve yields little success. Color Doppler, being less dependent on angle, can be used to evaluate the septa for evidence of atrial septal defects (Fig. 10-38), patent foramen ovale, and VSD. Identification of these lesions is possible, but further quantification is limited.

SUBCOSTAL SHORT-AXIS VIEW

This view is obtained by beginning with a subcostal four-chamber view and rotating the transducer 90 degrees clockwise so that it is pointed farther left toward the patient's left arm. This view resembles

the parasternal short-axis view (Fig. 10-36*A*). By angling the transducer slightly anteriorly toward the base of the heart, the right ventricular outflow tract, pulmonic valve, and main pulmonary artery with bifurcation can be seen (Fig. 10-36*B*). The tricuspid valve and right atrium are seen to the left of the screen. Toward the top of the screen, the right ventricle is noted. The left atrium is toward the bottom of the screen and slightly to the left. The aorta and aortic valve are typically in the center of the sector.

If the transducer is rotated counterclockwise toward the patient's right shoulder while maintaining a short-axis view, an inferior vena cava/hepatic view is obtained (Fig. 10-37). To obtain optimal subcostal views, the patient is usually asked to inhale and hold the breath. This maneuver is typically not performed in this view since it is important to evaluate the normal respiratory variation of the inferior vena cava. In patients with elevated right heart pressures, the inferior vena cava may be dilated and will remain fixed throughout the respiratory cycle. Evidence of metastatic masses can also be seen in this view. Some of the hepatic veins are seen emptying into the right atrium. Color Doppler is useful for examining flow in the inferior vena cava and hepatic veins (Fig. 10-39).

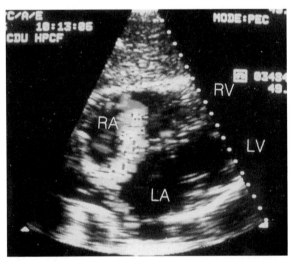

Figure 10-38. Subcostal four-chamber view with color Doppler. Flow is noted crossing the interatrial septum via a large interatrial septal defect (ASD). RA, right atrium; RV, right ventricle; LA, left atrium; LV, left ventricle. (From Kisslo J, et al. Doppler Color Flow Imaging. New York, Churchill Livingstone; 1988:144. Reprinted with permission.) (See also Color Plate 35.)

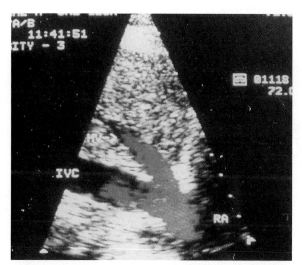

Figure 10-39. *Subcostal inferior vena cava image with color flow Doppler. The jet is blue because flow in this view is normally moving away from the transducer. Red flow would indicate significant tricuspid regurgitation. IVC, inferior vena cava; RA, right atrium; HV, hepatic veins. (See also Color Plate 36.)*

Suprasternal Views

Suprasternal views should be a routine part of adult echocardiograms. The suprasternal long-axis view is obtained with the patient supine and the head extended backward. Figures 10-40 through 10-43 illustrate the proper transducer position and the various images obtained from this position. The transducer is placed in the suprasternal notch, with the index marker pointed up toward the patient's head (Fig. 10-40). This view allows visualization of the ascending thoracic aorta, aortic arch, and descending thoracic aorta (Fig. 10-41 A,B). In addition, the left common carotid and left subclavian arteries can be seen. The scan plane is directed in an inferior and posterior plane. This view is used to evaluate for coarctation of the aorta and to help identify significant aortic insufficiency.

In adults, the suprasternal views are not always clear. In other patients, it is not possible to image the ascending and descending aortas in the same plane, so the transducer is angled toward the right to see the ascending aorta (Fig. 10-42, *top*) and toward the left to see the descending aorta (Fig. 10-43, *top*).

The suprasternal short-axis view is obtained by rotating the transducer 90 degrees clockwise from its long-axis orientation. This view reveals the aorta

in the short-axis view and aligns the right pulmonary artery in the long-axis view (Fig. 10-41B).

Nonimaging Views

In order to obtain adequate Doppler information across the valves, images are usually helpful in aiding the proper alignment of the cursors with blood flow. However, Doppler interrogation can be performed without images, and in some cases this is preferable. In aortic stenosis, it is important to confirm the peak pressure gradient from several different views. In fact, apical standard imaging windows are not always available, so information must be obtained elsewhere.

SUPRASTERNAL VIEW

The suprasternal notch is ideal for Doppler interrogation of the aorta due to the relatively superficial nature of the aorta in this region. Using a CW

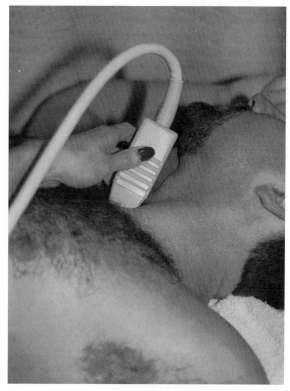

Figure 10-40. *Patient and transducer positions for a suprasternal view. The patient is asked to lie supine, with the head extended (chin up). The transducer is placed in the suprasternal notch.*

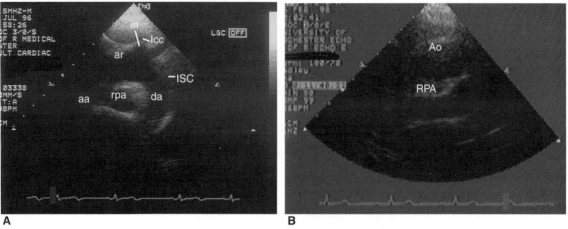

Figure 10-41. **(A)** Suprasternal long-axis view of the ascending aorta (aa), aortic arch (ar), and descending aorta (da). The right pulmonary artery (rpa) lies in the center of the sector, just below the arch. The innominate (in), left common carotid (lcc), and left subclavian (lsc) arteries can be seen from this image. **(B)** Suprasternal short-axis view at the arch demonstrating the aorta in cross section (Ao) and the right pulmonary artery (rpa) in long axis.

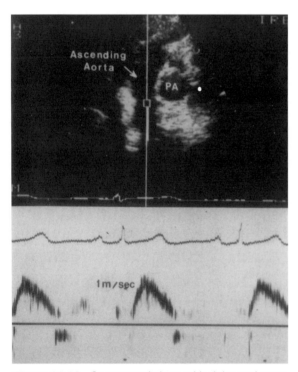

Figure 10-42. Suprasternal views with rightward angulation of the transducer to evaluate the ascending aorta (*top*).PW Doppler reveals normal velocities and flow patterns (*bottom*). PA, right pulmonary artery. (From Berger M. Doppler Echo in Heart Disease. Dekker; 1987:79, Fig. 23. Reprinted with permission.)

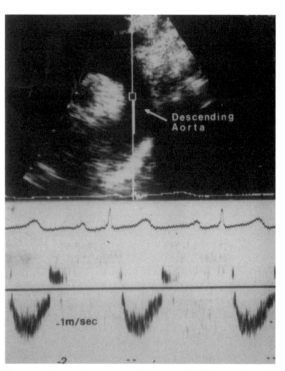

Figure 10-43. Suprasternal views with leftward angulation of the transducer to evaluate the descending aorta (*top*). PW Doppler reveals normal velocities and flow patterns (*bottom*). (From Berger M. Doppler Echo in Heart Disease. Dekker; 1987:81, Fig. 30. Reprinted with permission.)

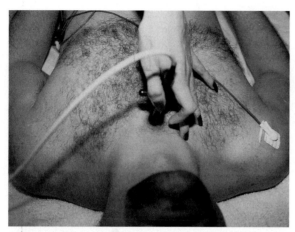

Figure 10-44. Patient and transducer positions for an independent Doppler exam of the aorta. The probe is angled in a posterior-inferior fashion and is then angled toward the left for interrogation of the descending aorta or toward the right for interrogation of the ascending and aortic valves.

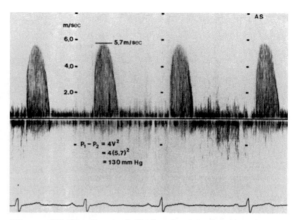

Figure 10-46. Spectral display from a right parasternal location using a nonimaging Doppler transducer. Note the display above the baseline because flow is toward the transducer. (From Berger M. Doppler Echocardiography in Heart Disease. New York: Marcel Dekker; 1987.

Doppler probe, velocities from the ascending as well as the descending aorta can be obtained. The probe is first positioned in the suprasternal notch, much the same way as the imaging probe (Fig. 10-44). To obtain Doppler signals from the descending aorta, the probe is angled toward the patient's left side and angled posteriorly (Fig. 10-43, *bottom*). To obtain Doppler recordings from the ascending aorta, the probe is angled toward the patient's right side (Fig. 10-42, *bottom*).

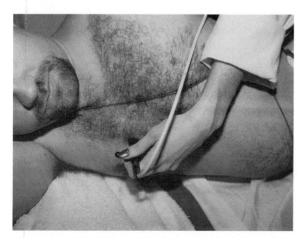

Figure 10-45. Patient and transducer position for obtaining Doppler signals across the aortic valve from a right parasternal location. The patient lies in a right lateral decubitus position with the right arm extended over the head. The probe is angled around the chest until a clear, well-defined signal is appreciated.

RIGHT PARASTERNAL VIEW

The right parasternal window is perhaps one of the better positions to obtain peak aortic velocities. In this view, the patient is asked to turn onto the right side and to extend the right arm over the head (Fig. 10-45). The probe is placed anywhere from the second through the fifth intercostal space near the right sternal border. If no signal is detected at one intercostal space, another position is used. If a faint signal or click is heard, the probe should be stationed in this area and fine manipulations used to tune into the central jet. The correct position will reveal a well-defined spectral display (Fig. 10-46) with a crisp audio signal. This position is challenging for most sonographers new to the profession. This technique should be practiced on patients with no aortic stenosis so that it is less intimidating when it becomes necessary to obtain signals in patients with aortic stenosis.

Summary

This chapter has presented a step-by-step protocol for a routine echocardiogram. Each situation will be different, and modifications may be required. However, it is important to have a thorough understanding of the basic concepts and views since nonstandard images can be confusing and lead to misdiagnosis. It takes years to learn the many facets of echocardiography, and only continuous scanning and careful attention to detail will enable the sonographer to feel comfortable performing the more difficult exams.

REFERENCES

1. Bansal RC, Tujik AS, Seward JB, Offord KP. Feasibility of detailed two-dimensional echocardiographic examination in adults. Prospective study of 200 patients. Mayo Clin Proc. 1980;55:291–308.
2. Bierman FZ, Williams RG. Subxyphoid two-dimensional imaging of the interatrial septum in infants and neonates with congenital heart disease. Circulation. 1979;60:80–90.
3. Chang S, Feigenbaum H, Dillon J. Subxyphoid echocardiography. Chest. 1975;68:233–235.
4. Dillon JC, Weyman AE, Feigenbaum H, et al. Cross-sectional echocardiographic examination of the interatrial septum. Circulation. 1977;55:115–120.
5. Eggleton RC, et al. Visualization of cardiac dynamics with real-time B-mode ultrasonic scanners. *In* White D (ed): Ultrasound Medicine. New York, Plenum; 1975.
6. Griffith JM, Henry WL. A sector scanner for real-time two-dimensional echocardiography. Circulation. 1974;49:1147–1152.
7. Hickman HO, et al. Cross-sectional echocardiography of the apex. Circulation. 1977;56:589.
8. Kisslo J, VonRamm OT, Thurstone FL. Cardiac imaging using a phased array ultrasound system: Clinical technique and application. Circulation. 1976;53:262–267.
9. Kloster FE, Roelandt J, Cate FJ, et al. Multiscan echocardiography II: Technique and initial clinical results. Circulation. 1973;48:1075–1084.
10. Report of the American Society of Echocardiography Committee on Nomenclature and Standards in two-dimensional imaging. Circulation. 1980;62:212.
11. Tajik AJ, Seward JB, Hagler DJ, et al. Two-dimensional real-time ultrasonic imaging of the heart and great vessels. Technique image orientation structure, and validation. Mayo Clin Proc. 1978;53:271–303.

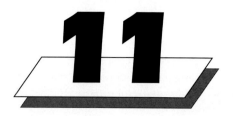

How to Perform a Transesophageal Exam

KARL SCHWARZ and MARK N. ALLEN

Introduction

Transesophageal echocardiography (TEE) shares many of the strengths and weaknesses of transthoracic echocardiography (TTE). The greatest strength that all ultrasound imaging modalities share is their inherently high spatial and temporal resolution. Spatial resolution is determined primarily by imaging frequency, ultrasound pulse duration, and the ability of the ultrasound scanner to focus and orient the ultrasound beam. Modern scanners use innovative crystal designs combined with phased array and computer technology to focus the ultrasound beam, not just in the two-dimensional imaging plane but also in the plane perpendicular to the imaging plane (referred to as *dynamic elevation beam forming* by some manufacturers). The result is a two-dimensional image that represents the structure contained in a very thin slice of tissue. Herein also lies the greatest weakness of two-dimensional ultrasound. The high spatial and temporal resolution of ultrasound may result in missed diagnoses if the structure in question does not happen to be in the two-dimensional plane at the time the image is created. A good example is a mobile valvular vegetation located in a position not included in a standard imaging plane. If the operator fails to pan through the valve in a stepwise fash-

ion, stopping and waiting in each position for many cardiac cycles to pass, the mobile vegetation may never come into view and may be missed.

TEE differs from TTE mainly in the resolution of the images obtained and in the additional structures that may be viewed routinely. The higher resolution of TEE is due to the higher frequencies used for imaging, made possible by the less attenuating transesophageal window. In most adult cases, 5.0 or 7.0 MHz can be used for imaging from the TEE window, where 5.0 MHz or less would be required for the TTE window. The simple change in frequency can double or more than double image resolution. The other advantage of TEE over TTE is its ability to image the posterior cardiac structures in the optimal midfield ultrasound beam (aorta, atria, and cardiac valves). These structures are seen less well in the TTE approach due to attenuation at maximum imaging depth or due to absence of an acoustic window for the structure in question. The more posterior the structure is from the TTE window, the lower the image resolution due to divergence and attenuation of the ultrasound beam, resulting in a reduced signal-to-noise ratio.

The other significant area where TEE differs from TTE is in the use of many different ultrasound imaging planes, including many "off-axis" planes,

207

depending on the type of TEE probe used (mono-plane vs. biplane vs. multiplane). Image data need to be interpreted in the context of the imaging plane. For example, an apparent perforation in a cardiac valve may just be an off-axis view of an otherwise normal commissure line. Likewise, two-dimensional and M-mode measurements made from the TEE window need to be interpreted based on the imaging plane used.

In general, a TEE exam should be even more complete than a TTE exam. This is due to higher resolution imaging and the greater number of structures that can be viewed from the TEE window. If the patient is properly prepared, a standard TEE exam takes 12 to 20 min to complete. Complex cases, such as a difficult aortic valve case or a difficult congenital case, may take 5 min more to complete. Most patients should be comfortable during this period if properly prepared. A "goal-directed" exam is indicated only when a patient cannot tolerate a complete study, due either to uncontrollable discomfort with the probe or to a medical condition that requires urgent treatment.

What follows is a protocol established at our institution. It is included here to serve as a guide. There are numerous protocols, many dependent on the type of probe used. Regardless of the protocol used, TEE should be performed by an experienced echocardiographer with the appropriate training and skills.

Room Setup

When considering performing TEE for the first time, it is important to consider where the exam will take place. Additional equipment will be required, so an appropriate amount of space needs to be available. A good starting point would be to plan on at least 250 square feet. In addition to the exam room, there should be a separate location for the disinfection or sterilization of the TEE probe. This is usually a secure equipment room or utility room.

The necessary equipment for the performance of TEE exams includes an ultrasound system with TEE capabilities, a TEE probe, a comfortable exam table, patient monitoring equipment such as an oximeter, suction (wall or portable), a small work table, blood pressure devices, a lock box for required medications, and advanced cardiac life support emergency equipment. Table 11-1 list the necessary equipment.[18] The bulk of the equipment is positioned toward the patient's head. This allows easy access to necessary and emergency equipment.

Appropriate personnel also need to be considered. Minimally, this includes the physician who will pass the probe and an echocardiographic assistant, usually a nurse. A cardiac sonographer may also be present to assist with system controls and patient support duties. Once prepared, the patient is placed in a left lateral decubitus position. Pillows are used to help support the patient. Figure 11-1 demon-

TABLE 11-1. Suggested Materials Necessary for TEE

IV normal saline solution, 500 cc	Necessary medications (see text)
Venoset tubing	Two bath towels
Two three-way stopcocks	Four pairs of latex or latex-free gloves
Extension set	30 cc of Surgilube
Yankauer suction tube	Two yellow gowns (one for the operator, one for the assistant)
Suction device with Yankauer bulbous tip	30 cc (vial) bacteriostatic normal saline
Two connecting tubes	Two 20-cc Luer lock syringes
One 4 × 4	One bite block (padded)
Tubex connector	One medicine cup
3-cc syringe with needle	One cannula for Lidocaine spray
1.5-in. needle	One large absorbent pad (pink)
One tongue depressor	Echocardiogram machine
Videotape	TEE probe

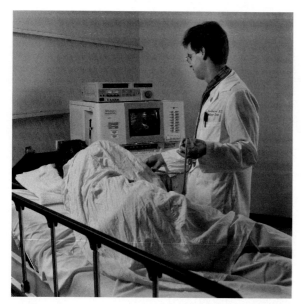

Figure 11-1. Room setup for TEE imaging. The physician is to the left of the patient, as is the ultrasound system. A nurse stays to the right of the patient and monitors the patient.

strates the general position of the patient and physician for TEE.

Preparation of the Patient

Patients scheduled for TEE need to fast for a minimum of 4 hr, except for medications. Outpatients should be accompanied by a relative or friend since sedation may be required. Patients are instructed not to operate a motor vehicle for up to 12 hr following the procedure. A medical history and informed consent are obtained. The procedure should be thoroughly explained, with time allotted for any questions the patient may have.

An automated blood pressure device and pulse oximeter are connected to the patient. An electrocardiogram is continuously displayed, using a separate system or the ultrasound system. A peripheral intravenous line is also established according to institutional guidelines. Ideally, this line is begun in the right arm since the patient will be in the left lateral decubitus position, potentially obstructing venous flow.

Personnel performing the procedure should wear appropriate protection, including protective eyewear or shields, latex-free gloves, gowns, and masks. Special precautions should be taken when performing TEE on patients suspected of having contagious or infectious diseases in accordance with institutional infection control policies and procedures.

The echocardiographer is responsible for the safety of the patient and the diagnostic power of the TEE exam. TEE is almost always performed by the attending echocardiographer; only advanced and specially selected fellows should be allowed to pass or manipulate the TEE probe. Table 11-2 lists the necessary training components for developing skills in TEE.[13] The physician performing the TEE exam needs to have extensive experience with echocardiography, a knowledge of cardiac disease and hemodynamic changes that occur with acquired as well as congenital disorders, an understanding of diagnostic differentials for various pathologic conditions, and a knowledge of basic ultrasound image formation and Doppler assessment. The American Society of Echocardiography has established the necessary skills needed by physicians in performing

TABLE 11-2. **Recommended Training Components for Developing and Maintaining Skills in TEE**

Component	Objective	Duration	No. of Cases (Approx.)
General echocardiography, Level II	Background needed for performance and interpretation	6 months or equivalent	300
Esophageal intubation	TEE probe introduction	Variable	25
TEE examination	Skills in TEE performance and interpretation	Variable	50
Ongoing education	Maintenance of competence	Annual	50 to 75

Source: Pearlman AS et al. Guidelines for physician training in transesophageal echocardiography. J Am Soc Echocardiogr (March/April) 1992; 5:188–189.

◤◤◤ **TABLE 11-3. Skills Needed to Perform TEE**

Cognitive Skills

Knowledge of appropriate indications, contraindications, and risks of TEE

Understanding of differential diagnostic considerations in each clinical case

Knowledge of physical principles of echocardiographic image formation and blood flow velocity measurement

Familiarity with the operation of the ultrasonographic instrument, including the function of all controls affecting the quality of the data displayed

Knowledge of normal cardiovascular anatomy, as visualized tomographically

Knowledge of alterations in cardiovascular anatomy resulting from acquired and congenital heart diseases

Knowledge of normal cardiovascular hemodynamics and fluid dynamics

Knowledge of alterations in cardiovascular hemodynamics and blood flow resulting from acquired and congenital heart diseases

Understanding of component techniques for general echocardiography and TEE, including when to use these methods to investigate specific clinical questions

Ability to distinguish adequate from inadequate echocardiographic data, and to distinguish an adequate from an inadequate TEE examination

Knowledge of other cardiovascular diagnostic methods for correlation with TEE findings

Ability to communicate examination results to patient, other health care professionals, and medical record

Technical Skills

Proficiency in performing a complete standard echocardiographic examination, using all echocardiographic modalities relevant to the case

Proficiency in safely passing the TEE transducer into the esophagus and stomach, and in adjusting probe position to obtain the necessary tomographic images and Doppler data

Proficiency in operating correctly the ultrasonographic instrument, including all controls affecting the quality of the data displayed

Proficiency in recognizing abnormalities of cardiac structure and function as detected from the transesophageal and transgastric windows, in distinguishing normal from abnormal findings, and in recognizing artifacts

Proficiency in performing qualitative and quantitative analysis of the echocardiographic data

Proficiency in producing a cogent written report of the echocardiographic findings and their clinical implications

Source: Pearlman AS et al. Guidelines for physician training in transesophageal echocardiography. J Am Soc Echocardiogr (March/April) 1992; 5:188–189.

TEE exams[13] (Table 11-3). TEE should not be used as a general screening technique, but should be performed when clinically relevant questions cannot be answered transthoracically.

Preparation of the patient for the TEE exam starts with an evaluation of the clinical history to determine the goal of the exam and potential areas where complications may develop. All TEE exams should be complete studies, but identification of exam goals may alert the operator to special circumstances that might require nonstandard imaging or the need to review prior studies for comparison. The most common complications that can be avoided by a good history are drug reactions (see below), bleeding (history of esophageal varices,

bleeding diathesis, anticoagulant usage, etc.), emesis/aspiration (recent ingestion of food and tube feeding in the debilitated patient), and esophageal perforation (Zenker's diverticulum, severe dysphagia, esophageal radiation or tumor). If any are identified, the echocardiographer must clear the TEE with the patient's primary care physician or cardiologist. The patient is then instructed on the procedure used to pass the probe and on maneuvers that the patient can use to reduce the gag sensation (relaxation, slow and shallow breathing, thinking of other things).

Almost all patients require a topical anesthetic to lessen the gag sensation. A variety of topical agents can be used, but Lidocaine is generally regarded as having the lowest risk-to-benefit ratio. A metered dose delivery system is recommended to allow for accurate dosing. Lidocaine is available in a 10% solution in which 10 mg is delivered with each metered puff. The four quadrants of the oral pharynx are anesthetized with a single puff each, and the patient is asked to swallow. Administration of Lidocaine may be associated with mild coughing if some of the atomized spray is inhaled. The same four-spray protocol is repeated in 1 to 2 min for a total dose of 80 mg. Suppression of the gag reflex is tested with a tongue blade, and additional Lidocaine is given if needed. The typical patient requires between 80 and 160 mg of Lidocaine for effective suppression of the oral pharyngeal component of the gag reflex. Lidocaine should be used with caution in patients with known sensitivity to the drug (rare), and the total dose should not exceed 4.5 mg/kg (or 160 mg in adults). When used in children, a more dilute formulation (0.5% or 1.0%) is recommended to avoid overdosage. High plasma concentrations of Lidocaine are manifested by the drug's central nervous system stimulatory effects (anxiety, restlessness, confusion, blurred vision, dizziness, tremulousness, and, in higher concentrations, unconsciousness and seizures). The most dangerous complications with overdosage are cardiovascular collapse, cardiac arrhythmias, and death.

In many centers, no general sedation is given prior to the insertion of the probe. While it is certainly possible to intubate and fully scan the majority of patients without generalized sedation, it is common practice to use low-dose IV sedation prior to probe insertion. The most common agents used for this purpose are midazolam (Versed) and meperidine (Demerol), either alone or in combination. Midazolam is a benzodiazepine that has an onset of action within 1 to 5 min following IV administration and produces amnesia of the procedure in many patients in addition to sedation. The drug is administered by IV bolus in aliquots of 0.5 to 1.0 mg. Following each dose, the patient is observed for 3 to 5 min to determine the level of sedation and to monitor for hypotension or respiratory depression. It is common practice to use an automatic blood pressure device and a fingertip pulse oximeter for these purposes. The desired result is an awake but comfortable patient, and this is usually achieved with a total dose of less than 5.0 mg in the adult. If the desired effect has not been achieved, the addition of low-dose meperidine is usually very effective (25 to 100 mg). Midazolam and meperidine both have a two-phase elimination pattern, with the first phase lasting for 5 to 20 min and the second phase lasting for 4 to 12 hr. The duration of the first phase is ideal for the TEE procedure, and the patient is usually awake enough within 15 min to be moved out of the exam room and into a less extensive observation area. If the effects of midazolam need to be reversed quickly, that can be achieved with the use of flumazenil (Romazicon, 0.2 mg IV), and meperidine can be reversed with naloxone (Narcan, 0.1 to 0.2 mg). Both midazolam and meperidine are metabolized first in the liver, followed by excretion in the urine; therefore, the dosage of either drug may need to be reduced. The elimination time may be prolonged in patients with hepatic and/or renal insufficiency. The TEE room should be equipped with a lock box to secure all medications.

Passage of the Probe

The most important factor in successful intubation is correct positioning of the patient relative to the ultrasound probe. The correct position is one in which the oral cavity, posterior pharynx, esophagus, and eventually the ultrasound probe are all in the same two-dimensional plane.[16] If there are twists in the probe or if the neck is rotated, it will be very difficult to pass the probe. The left lateral decubitus position is the preferred position for achieving this alignment among ambulatory patients and those who can be moved in bed (including most intubated patients). This position promotes clearance of oral secretions, with or without the aid of suction; and this effect can be augmented with the use of the head-up or reverse Trendelenburg position.[10–20] The patient's knees and neck are flexed toward the chest (fetal position). A doubled-over pillow under the head (not shoulders) can be used to keep the neck midline. Patients who cannot roll onto the side and must remain supine for the TEE exam should be intubated and mechanically ventilated. This is required to protect the airway, as oral secretions will likely pass into the trachea as they collect in the posterior pharynx during the TEE exam. The supine patient should have the midline and face forward. To the extent possible, the oral cavity should be clear of other lines and hoses.

A bite guard with a foam rim to protect the teeth is placed in the mouth and held in position by an assistant (edentulous patients require no bite guard). The occasional intubated and mechanically ventilated patient will require systemic paralysis to place the guard. This can be achieved with a variety of nondepolarizing neuromuscular blocking agents. Examples include Atracurium Besylate (dose: 0.5 mg/kg), Pancuronium Bromide (dose: 0.06 to 0.1 mg/kg), and Vecuronium Bromide (dose: 0.08 to 0.1 mg/kg). These drugs have an onset of action in 3 to 5 min and a duration of effect of 20 to 60 min.

Several methods can be used to pass the ultrasound probe, but by far the easiest way is to have the patient swallow the probe[11] (Fig. 11-2). This is achieved by having the operator steer the well-lubricated ultrasound probe into the posterior pharynx using anteflexion on the movable tip. There may be a small amount of resistance as the probe passes around the back of the tongue, but any significant resistance should be investigated. In this position, the tip of the probe is angled directly toward the trachea. To avoid tracheal intubation, the operator must counterrotate the probe by exerting *mild*

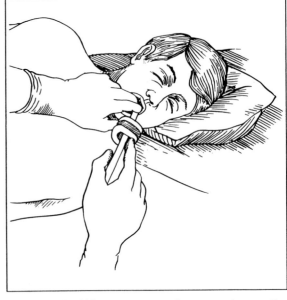

Figure 11-3. Using one or two fingers to depress the tongue, the probe is advanced to the posterior oropharynx. Then the patient is asked to swallow, facilitating further advancement of the probe.

extension pressure (posterior rotation). The patient is asked to swallow, and the probe passes into the esophagus in the terminal phase of the swallow as the tip gently presses against the posterior pharynx.

Another way of passing the probe involves using one or two fingers to depress the tongue. The transducer is then passed under the fingers and advanced to the oropharynx. The patient is asked to swallow, and the probe passes into the esophagus in the terminal phase of the swallow as the tip gently presses against the posterior pharynx[11] (Fig. 11-3).

IMAGING VIEW AND FLOW OF THE EXAM

The goal of TEE is to provide complete imaging of the cardiac and pericardial structures. A disciplined approach to the sequence of the exam is the best method of achieving that goal. Exam sequencing may be view-based or structure-based; described below is a combination of both approaches. Figure 11-4 demonstrates the basic views and the transducer orientation necessary to achieve them.[14]

The TEE standard procedure is an example of how the TEE exam may be sequenced, starting from

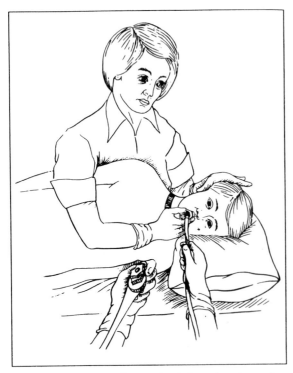

Figure 11-2. Swallowing method of passing the probe. The well-lubricated ultrasound probe is inserted into the posterior pharynx using anteflexion on the movable tip.

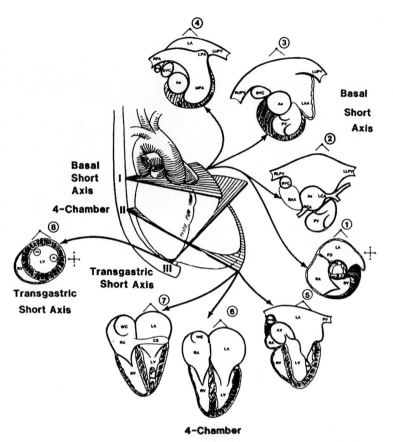

Figure 11-4. Diagram of common scan planes: basal short-axis (I), four-chamber (frontal long-axis (II), and transgastric short-axis (III), resultant tomographic planes of section (1 through 8). Basal short-axis sections: aortic root (1), coronary arteries (2), left atrial appendage (3), and pulmonary artery bifurcation (4). Four-chamber sections: left ventricular outflow view (5), four-chamber view (6), and coronary sinus view (7). Transgastric short-axis section; ventricular short-axis view (8). AL, anterolateral papillary muscle; Ao, aorta; Av, aortic valve; Cs, coronary sinus; FO, fossa ovalis; IVC, inferior vena cava; L, left coronary cusp; LA, left atrium; LAA, left atrial appendage; LCA, left coronary artery; LLPV, left lower pulmonary vein; LPA, left pulmonary artery; LUPV, left upper pulmonary vein; LV, left ventricle; MPA, main pulmonary artery; N, noncoronary cusp; PM, posteromedial papillary muscles; PV, pulmonary valve or pulmonary vein; R, right coronary cusp; RA, right atrium; RAA, right atrial appendage; RCA, right coronary artery; RLPV, right lower pulmonary vein; RPA, right pulmonary artery; RUPV, right upper pulmonary vein; RV, right ventricle; SVC, superior vena cava. Directional axes: A, anterior; L, left; P, posterior; R, right. (From Seward JB, Khandheria BK, Oh JK, et al. Transesophageal echocardiography: Technique, anatomic correlations, implementation, and clinical applications. Mayo Clin Proc. 1988;63: 649–680. Reprinted with permission.)

the point at which the probe is inserted. If intubation was accomplished without a great deal of swallowed air in the esophagus, then the first structure imaged should be the left ventricle from the four-chamber view. Otherwise, the probe should be advanced directly to the stomach for the transgastric views (see "Transgastric and Lower Esophageal Views" below), after which time the esophagus should have cleared the trapped air and the probe can be withdrawn to the four-chamber view.

Transesophageal Standard Imaging Procedure

LOWER AND MIDESOPHAGEAL VIEWS

The TEE probe is positioned in the four-chamber view, ensuring that the axial alignment of the image centerline passes through the mitral valve and left ventricular apex. This is done by advancing the probe to the 20-cm marker. At least 10 cardiac cycles should be observed in each plane. To obtain a four-chamber view using a biplane TEE probe, the transducer is fixed in a longitudinal position (Fig. 11-5). The transverse position provides a short-axis image of the left ventricle (Fig. 11-6). Using the system's "zoom" or "res" function may also aid in improving resolution. If imaging is difficult, the

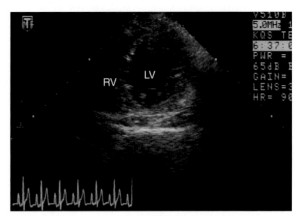

Figure 11-6. Cross-sectional view of the left ventricle (LV) from a transverse plane. RV, right ventricle.

transmit frequency of the probe is changed from 5.0 to 3.5 MHz.

For assessment of regional or global left ventricular dysfunction, minimal depth settings are required and the area of interest should be magnified. Close attention to the affected endocardium will help to rule out mural thrombus. Off-axis imaging views may be necessary.

In order to interrogate the valves, a frequency of 5.0 or 7.0 MHz is used. Using a biplane probe, the transverse plane with slight rotation will allow visualization of the mitral valve (Fig. 11-7). In order

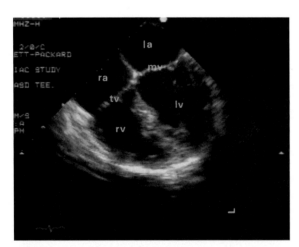

Figure 11-5. TEE four-chamber view. la, left atrium; ra, right atrium; rv, right ventricle; lv, left ventricle; mv, mitral valve; tv, tricuspid valve.

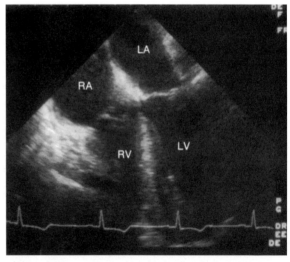

Figure 11-7. TEE four-chamber view with emphasis on the mitral valve. LA, left atrium; LV, left ventricle; RA, right atrium; RV, right ventricle.

to best delineate the anatomy, the valve is "zoomed" or "res'd." The image is aligned at the center of the valve for at least five cardiac cycles while the ultrasound probe is held steady. Using a slow, stepwise, sweeping motion, the valve is interrogated. The tip of the ultrasound transducer is flexed or extended in order to see as much of the valve as possible. This step is repeated in the longitudinal plane with similar stepwise panning by rotating the shaft of the probe while keeping the tip's angulation fixed.

This procedure is repeated with color Doppler, making sure that the entire commissure line from annulus to annulus is imaged. If mitral regurgitation has been detected, the lesion site is again interrogated with two-dimensional imaging to investigate the origin of the jet and the extent of regurgitation[8,12] (confirm all findings in the transverse plane). If a regurgitant fraction is to be calculated, the size of the mitral annulus is measured in two dimensions, the velocity time integral by pulsed wave Doppler is obtained at the mitral annulus, and the velocity time integral of the mitral regurgitation jet and the maximum velocity of the mitral regurgitation jet are all obtained from this view. In addition, the degree of mitral regurgitation can be obtained using the proximal isovelocity surface area (PISA) method (these measurements are discussed in subsequent chapters). If mitral stenosis has been detected, continuous wave Doppler is used to measure the mean gradient, velocity time integral, and pressure half-time.

From a midesophageal position, the aortic valve can be seen using the T plane at 5.0 or 7.0 MHz. Visualization of the aortic valve is accomplished by rotating the probe clockwise, withdrawing it slightly, and flexing the head slightly (Fig. 11-8). The ventricular and aortic sides of the valve should be evaluated by slowly panning through the valve. The operator should observe this area along the commissure line for several beats to evaluate for mobile masses. The transducer is rotated to the leftmost position in order to image all three leaflets in the short-axis view (Fig. 11-9). The transducer is rotated all the way to the rightmost position so that the aortic valve can be imaged in a true long axis (Fig. 11-10). At least five cycles at each level of panning should be performed throughout the valve

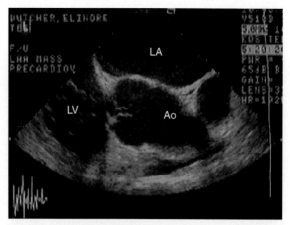

Figure 11-8. Longitudinal view of the aortic valve. LA, left atrium; LV, left ventricle; Ao, aorta.

image. Color Doppler is used at this level to investigate aortic insufficiency in the transverse plane. If the jet appears to be more than mild, the extent of the jet in the left ventricular outflow tract and left ventricular cavity should be investigated. If there is a question of aortic valve stenosis, the left ventricular outflow tract is measured in systole (T plane). The velocity time integral across both the left ventricular outflow tract using pulsed wave Doppler and across the aortic valve using continuous wave Doppler can be obtained from the subcostal view. The measurements should be confirmed by transthoracic imaging and Doppler after the TEE exam is complete.

To image the left atrium, the image is returned to the four-chamber view and the depth is reduced so that only the atria and atrioventricular valves are seen. The left atrial appendage can be imaged using the L plane with a frequency of 5.0 MHz (Fig. 11-11). The left atrial appendage should be magnified in order to rule out the presence of thrombus

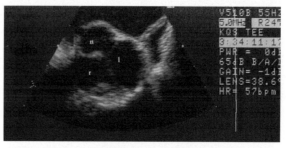

Figure 11-9. Transverse plane at the level of the aortic valve. All three cusps can be visualized. l, left coronary cusp; r, right coronary cusp; n, noncoronary cusp.

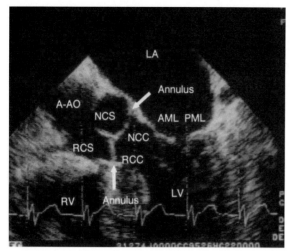

Figure 11-10. Longitudinal view of the aortic valve. LA, left atrium; LV, left ventricle; RV, right ventricle; AAo, ascending aorta; aml, anterior mitral valve leaflet; pml, posterior mitral valve leaflet; ncc, noncoronary cusp; rcc, right coronary cusp.

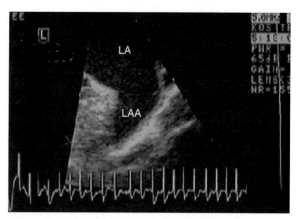

Figure 11-12. Magnified view of the left atrial appendage (LAA). Close interrogation of the appendage is important to rule out the presence of clot. LA, left atrium.

(Fig. 11-12). With slight rotation of the shaft of the probe, the left atrial appendage can be interrogated. The appendage should be imaged with color Doppler (Fig. 11-13). To obtain the best color images, the Nyquist limit should be lowered to approximately 25 cm/sec to confirm flow through the structure (this can help to rule out hypoechoic thrombi). Since flow in the left atrial appendage tends to be lower in rate, it is important to lower the Nyquist limits so that flow can be seen. If the left atrial ap-

pendage appears enlarged or if the cardiac rhythm is something other than sinus, check the peak flow velocity in the main body of the appendage using pulsed wave Doppler. The remainder of the left atrium is scanned for thrombi by rotating the shaft of the transducer while in the L plane, making sure to image all of the structure from pulmonary vein to pulmonary vein.

Ascending Aorta Imaging

While still in the L plane, the shaft of the transducer is rotated so that the ascending thoracic aorta is in view. The diameter of the vessel is measured at the

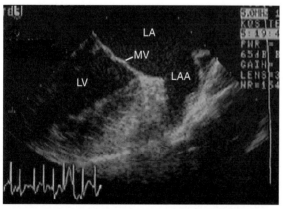

Figure 11-11. Longitudinal two-chamber view of the left atrium (LA) and ventricle (LV). The left atrial appendage (LAA) is seen from this view. MV, mitral valve.

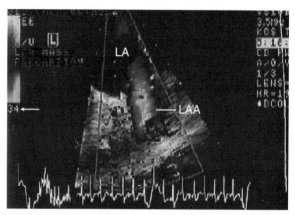

Figure 11-13. Magnified view of the left atrial appendage (LAA) with color flow Doppler. Doppler scanning is performed to identify the presence of a low-flow state, which could help predict clot formation. The color scale is usually adjusted downward so that low flow can be identified. LA, left atrium. (See also Color Plate 37.)

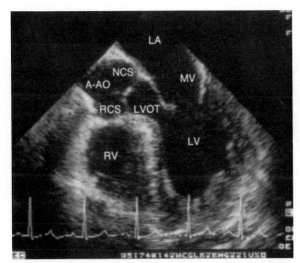

Figure 11-14. Longitudinal view of the ascending aorta. LA, left atrium; LV, left ventricle; MV, mitral value; RV, right ventricle; LVOT, left ventricular outflow tract; AAo, ascending aorta; NCS, noncoronary cusp; RCS, right coronary cusp.

aortic valve annulus, sinotubular junction, and upper extent of the image plane. This view is essential in identifying aortic plaques, aneurysms, and dissections. Color flow Doppler is used to evaluate flow in this region. From this view, the right and noncoronary cusps of the aortic valve and ascending aorta are seen. (Fig. 11-14).

Pulmonary Valve Imaging

The shaft of the probe is rotated slightly while still in the L plane. The valve is imaged in a slow, stepwise fashion, and color Doppler is used as necessary to evaluate flow. The pulmonary vessels can be seen from this view. The left upper pulmonary vein is seen entering the left atrium above the left atrial appendage. A ridge of tissue is often seen separating these two structures.

Tricuspid Valve Imaging

The T plane of the multiplane device is used to image the tricuspid valve, with the head of the TEE probe just above the gastroesophageal junction (Fig. 11-15). Using anterior-posterior flexion of the TEE probe head, the valve can be interrogated. Color Doppler is used to check for regurgitation. If tricuspid regurgitation is detected, the continuous wave beam is aligned with the tricuspid regurgitant jet and the gradient measured. If the jet is poorly

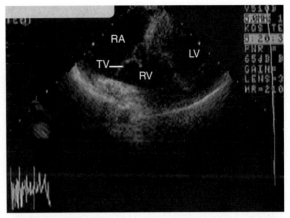

Figure 11-15. Transverse plane with imaging of the tricuspid valve (TV). RA, right atrium; RV, right ventricle; LV, left ventricle.

defined, a small quantity of agitated saline can be injected to enhance the signal.

Returning the probe to the four-chamber position, the right atrium and ventricle are imaged in the T plane. At least five cardiac cycles should be allowed to assess right ventricular systolic function. The shaft is rotated, and the depth is adjusted appropriately for right atrial inferior vena cava imaging. The image is centered on the fossa ovalis portion of the interatrial septum and switched to the L plane. The septum is examined in detail, as well as the inferior vena cava and the superior vena cava (Fig. 11-16). If there is a catheter or pacer wire in

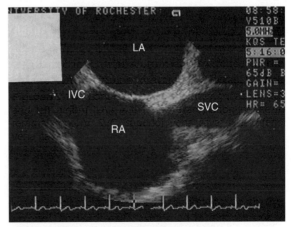

Figure 11-16. Longitudinal plane of the right atrium (RA) and left atrium (LA), with close examination of the interatrial septum. SVC, superior vena cava; IVC, inferior vena cava.

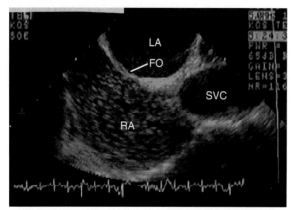

Figure 11-17. Longitudinal plane of the right atrium (RA) and left atrium (LA), with close examination of the interatrial septum in the region of the foramen ovale (FO). Injection of contrast material helps to identify the presence of a patent foramen ovale. SVC, superior vena cava.

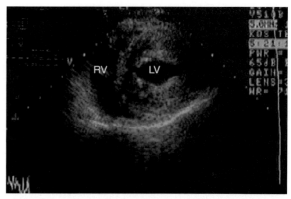

Figure 11-18. Transgastric view of the left ventricle (LV) in a transverse plane, demonstrating the left ventricle in cross section. RV, right ventricle.

the right heart, follow its course from the superior vena cava on down (the superior vena cava may also be imaged in the short-axis view by withdrawing the probe in the T plane). While the probe is centered on the fossa ovalis portion of the interatrial septum, evidence of transseptal shunting can be seen by activating the color Doppler and lowering the Nyquist limit to 20–30 cm/sec. Evidence of right-to-left shunting across the interatrial septum is found by two-dimensional imaging of the fossa ovalis in the L plane and with an injection of 10–20 cc of hand-agitated saline while the patient coughs (Fig. 11-17). If an obvious atrial septal defect is present, check for the proper anatomic location of all four pulmonary veins.

TRANSGASTRIC AND LOWER ESOPHAGEAL VIEWS

Transgastric views are obtained by advancing the probe farther into the esophagus. The left ventricle is imaged in the short-axis orientation using the T plane (Fig. 11-18), and a two-chamber view of the left ventricle is obtained from the L plane (Fig. 11-19). From this view, it may be necessary to use a lower frequency, such as 3.5 MHz, in order to optimize the image. The left ventricle should be panned through in a short-axis view from apex to base. If there is a wall motion abnormality, this view is used to assess for mural thrombus. If there is a

suspicious mitral or aortic stenosis or subaortic stenosis, the L plane with lateral angulation is used to measure velocities across the aortic valve with continuous wave Doppler, as well as across the left ventricular outflow tract with pulsed wave Doppler. Rotating the shaft of the probe to the right will provide short-axis and long-axis images of the right ventricle using the T and L planes, respectively. The transgastric view can be used to rule out pericardial effusions.

While in the transverse plane, the shaft of the probe is rotated counterclockwise and withdrawn slightly to image the descending thoracic aorta (Fig. 11-20). Imaging depth, gain, and frequency (use 7

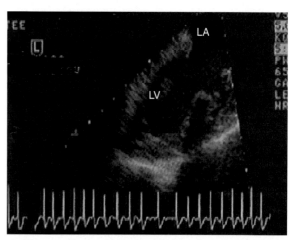

Figure 11-19. Transgastric view of the left ventricle (LV) in a longitudinal view demonstrating a two-chamber view. LA, left atrium.

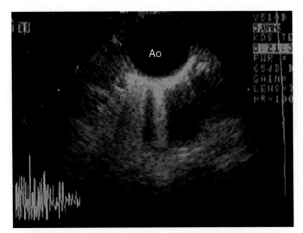

Figure 11-20. Descending thoracic aorta (Ao) in a transverse plane.

MHz) are all adjusted in order to optimize the image. Slow withdrawal of the probe will allow imaging of the length of the descending thoracic aorta, stopping at several levels to image in the L plane (Fig. 11-21). If plaque or other pathology is detected, documentation of mobile components, dissection, and intramural hemorrhage (low-velocity scale color Doppler) should be done. Once the top of the descending thoracic aorta is reached, anterior flexion of the probe head and clockwise rotation of the shaft of the probe will provide images of the arch and great vessels in both planes. These structures are

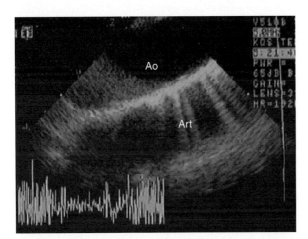

Figure 11-21. Descending thoracic aorta (Ao) in a longitudinal plane. The apparent second aorta running posterior to the true aorta is an artifact (Art), a frequent finding in this view.

fully evaluated for any periaortic or visible pleural pathology.

Interpreting the Transesophageal Data

The TEE report contains both descriptive and quantitative data. In many cases, the improved image definition is the reason the attending echocardiographer chose to order a TEE exam rather than a TTE exam. To achieve this goal, the attending echocardiographer must thoroughly image and describe all pathology found. This often requires a review of the videotaped images after image acquisition to confirm, describe, and quantify the findings. Attention to detail is the responsibility of the attending echocardiographer. For example, to simply report a valvular mass without describing its mobility, leaflet location, size, echocardiographic character, differential diagnosis, pertinent negative findings, and underlying leaflet pathology is inadequate.

In all cases, the findings of the TEE exam should be correlated as much as possible with the patient's history and clinical findings.

TEE Reporting

The complete TEE report should contain the following elements:

1. A clinical history that explains the purpose of the examination.
2. A description of the procedure, including who provided consent, premedications used, and documentation of any complications.
3. A list of standard cardiac measurements that were made (e.g., size of the left atrium).
4. A description of the left atrium, including chamber size (normal or enlarged), presence of masses/thrombi, presence of echo "smoke," a description of the interatrial septum, and the results of IV contrast injection. If indicated, the anatomy of the pulmonary veins should be described.
5. Left ventricular wall motion scores should be obtained. A detailed description of global and regional left ventricular function should be provided, including documentation of hemodynamic state (heart rate, rhythm, blood pressure).

Left ventricular wall motion should be described in regional terms (anterior, inferoposterior, etc.) and using a vascular model of regional left ventricular function (i.e., left anterior descending distribution). An explanation must be provided when there is a wide discrepancy between regional function and global left ventricular function (left ventricular ejection fraction). Any pathology (echo "smoke," masses/thrombi, etc.) should be described in detail.

6. The right atrium and right ventricle are described at least in terms of size and function. All right heart catheters and wires should be described in terms of position and associated pathology.

7. Each of the cardiac valves should be described separately on the echocardiographic report. In all cases, there should be a detailed description of valvular structure and function. When pathology is identified, associated findings and secondary signs should be completely documented (e.g., flow reversal in pulmonary veins for mitral regurgitation or the aorta for aortic insufficiency). This includes a full Doppler assessment of stenosis, of regurgitation with calculation of the valve area, and/or of the regurgitant orifice area.

8. The pericardium and any pleural pathology (or lack of pathology) should be described.

9. The aorta from the aortic valve to the diaphragm should be described in detail. This includes documentation of the vessel size and any pathology (plaques, thrombi, dissection, intramural hemorrhage, anterior displacement, etc.).

Summary

TEE is a valuable tool in the assessment of many cardiac abnormalities. The ability to image the heart with minimal attenuation effects lends itself to accurate assessment of valves and chambers. It is not completely noninvasive, however, and requires skill in performance as well as in interpretation. Training and commitment to continuous development of skills are necessary to prevent potential problems.

This technique has changed considerably over the years, and the number of potential views seem endless. A critical and academic approach to this technique is essential. Unfamiliar views of normal and abnormal cardiac structures can easily lead to confusion and misinterpretation.[15] A thorough understanding of cardiac anatomy and TEE is essential.

REFERENCES

1. Abel M, Nishimura R, Callahan M, et al. Evaluation of intraoperative transesophageal two-dimensional echocardiography. Anesthesiology. 1987;66:64–68.

2. Cahalan MK, Litt L, Botvinick EH, et al. Advances in noninvasive cardiovascular imaging: Implications for the anesthesiologist. Anesthesiology. 1987;66:356–372.

3. Daniel WG, Schroder E, Mugge A, et al. Transesophageal echocardiography in infective endocarditis. Am J Cardiac Imaging. 1988;2:78–85.

4. De Bruijn NP, Clements FM, Kisslo J. Transesophageal applications in color flow imaging. Echocardiography. 1987;4:557–567.

5. Erbel R. Transesophageal echocardiography. Echocardiography. 1986;3:287–291.

6. Erbel R, Borner N, Steller D, et al. Detection of aortic dissection by transesophageal echocardiography. Br Heart J. 1987;58:45–51.

7. Geibel A, Caspar W, Betroz A, et al. Risk of transesophageal echocardiography in awake patients with cardiac diseases. Am J Cardiol. 1988;62:337–339.

8. Goldman M, Fuster V, Guardino T, et al. Intraoperative echocardiography for the evaluation of valvular regurgitation: Experience in 263 patients. Circulation. 1986;74:143–149.

9. Gussenhoven E, Taams M, Roelandt J, et al. Transesophageal two-dimensional echocardiography: Its role in solving clinical problems. J Am Coll Cardiol. 1986;8:975–979.

10. Gussenhoven E, Van Herwerden L, Roelandt J, et al. Intraoperative two-dimensional echocardiography in congenital heart disease. J Am Coll Cardiol. 1987;9:565–572.

11. Khandheria BK, Tajik AJ, Freeman WK. Transesophageal echocardiographic examination: Technique, training and safety. *In* Freeman WK, Seward JB, Khandheria BK, et al (eds): Transesophageal Echocardiography. Boston, Little, Brown; 1994:9–54.

12. Maurer G, Lawrence SC, Chaux A, et al. Intraoperative Doppler color flow mapping for assessment of valve repair for mitral regurgitation. Am J Cardiol. 1987;60:333–337.

13. Pearlman AS, Gardin JM, Martin RP, et al. Guidelines for physician training in transesophageal echocardiography: Recommendations of the American Society of Echocardiography Committee for Physician Training in Echocardiography. J Am Soc Echocardiogr. 1992;5:187–194.

14. Schiller NB, Maurer G, Ritter SB, et al. Transesophageal echocardiography. 1989;2:354–357.

15. Schnittger I. Transesophageal Doppler echocardiography (editorial). Mayo Clin Proc. 1988;63: 726–728.

16. Seward JB, Khandheria BK, Oh JK, et al. Transesophageal echocardiography: Technique, anatomic correlations, implementation and clinical applications. Mayo Clin Proc. 1988;63:649–680.

17. Shively BK, Schiller NB. Transesophageal echocardiography in the intraoperative detection of myocardial ischemia and infarction. Echocardiography. 1986;3: 433–443.

18. Venkatesh B, Vannan M, Roelandt J, et al. Laboratory setup, patient preparation, and procedure. *In* Roelandt JRTC, Pandian NG (eds): Multiplane Transesophageal Echocardiography. New York, Churchill Livingstone; 1996:15–24.

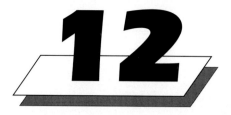

The Stress Echocardiographic Exam

DONNA EHLER

The sonographer's role in echocardiography is vital to the overall accuracy and acceptance of the technique. The ability of the sonographer to record high-quality echocardiographic images which represent the anatomy and physiology of the heart has earned the specialty of cardiac sonography its well-deserved respect. The past 25 years have brought numerous technological advances in ultrasound. The addition of each new modality has always heightened the challenge for the sonographer. Stress echocardiography is no exception. Because of computer image technology, the ability to incorporate the evaluation of provokable myocardial ischemia into the echocardiographic exam is possible. This technique does, however, introduce new challenges to the sonographer performing the exam. The sonographer must be persistent in attaining the highest-quality images possible. Acquisition of images quickly, during the time period immediately after exercise makes this especially challenging for the sonographer.

Two-dimensional echocardiography is extremely well suited for evaluation of myocardial wall motion because it is tomographic and has high spatial resolution. When performing exercise echocardiography for evaluation of known or suspected coronary artery disease, the ability to visualize each myocardial segment optimally becomes paramount.

The sonographer's focus changes from recording the whole-heart "snapshot" to specific visualization of each coronary artery perfusion region. Stress echocardiography takes time to perfect; a sonographer can expect to feel comfortable performing this technique after 50–60 exams on patients with varying levels of technical difficulty. Performing exercise echo exams on patients already undergoing treadmill electrocardiography may provide beginning stress echo sonographers an opportunity to improve their technique without negative consequence to the patient. The additional time is minimal, and the patients are not billed for the echocardiogram. The stress ECG information is unaltered.

Setting Up a Stress Echo Lab: Equipment

With the exception of the digital acquisition computer, equipment necessary for performing stress echocardiography is frequently already in place in a cardiology department (Fig. 12-1). The ultrasound system used for routine physiologic echocardiography is ideally suited for use in stress echo. The system must have high-quality image resolution and good depth penetration and meet criteria similar to those used for routine echocardiography. The transducer options should allow the sonographer to

Equipment	Personnel
Ultrasound system	Cardiac sonographer
Digital image acquisition computer (frame grabber) - stand alone or integrated into the ultrasound system	Medical technician
Treadmill or bicycle ergometer	Nurse
12-lead electrocardiograph - monitor/recorder	Cardiologist
Echo examination bed	
Blood pressure cuffs / sphygmomanometer	
Emergency cart	

Figure 12-1. Equipment and personnel recommended for performing exercise echocardiography. The personnel and equipment recommended (with the exception of the frame grabber or other digital acquisition device or software) are frequently already in place in a cardiology department.

choose the highest possible frequency for any given patient. Each user/interpreter will have differing needs when selecting an ultrasound system to purchase.

Several methods of exercise have been used in conjunction with echocardiography. When evaluating for coronary artery disease (CAD), the exercise method employed must provide enough stress to induce myocardial ischemia. The resultant impaired myocardial function is then detected echocardiographically as a wall motion abnormality.

The use of bicycle ergometry has been validated as a technique which offers the ability to acquire images both during and immediately after exercise. Bicycle ergometry can be done with the patient upright or supine. These methods have the advantage of potentially detecting transient wall motion abnormalities at peak exercise which may otherwise go undetected if only postexercise imaging is done.[16] One possible disadvantage, though, is this method's dependence on patient cooperation to maintain a constant workload. Bicycle ergometry is, however, the method of choice when assessing hemodynamics in patients being evaluated for valvular heart disease. The ability to record valvular gradients, regurgitant lesions, and pulmonary artery pressure at peak exercise is advantageous.

Because treadmill testing is a widely available form of exercise in this country and because patients readily accept it, posttreadmill exercise echocardiography has become the desired choice for many cardiology laboratories.

Both treadmill and bicycle echocardiographic techniques have equivalent diagnostic accuracy.[8,16]

The type of echo exam bed used becomes very important when performing exercise echo. A bed specifically designed for use in echocardiography is optimal. Either a portion of the bed beneath the cardiac apex is cut away, or the section is hinged and drops down and out of the way. The patient can therefore be imaged in the full left lateral position, and the sonographer has quick, easy access to the apical imaging windows (Fig. 12-2).

Additional patient monitoring equipment necessary in the stress echo lab includes the electrocar-

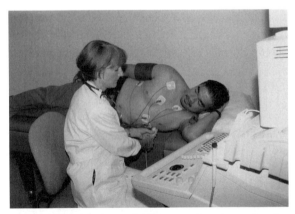

Figure 12-2. Photograph of an exercise echocardiogram being performed. The exam is performed with the patient in the left lateral decubitus position on a specially designed examination bed which gives the sonographer access to the apical imaging window.

diograph (12-lead) and a blood pressure monitoring system. The treadmill echocardiographic monitoring console is usually in place if treadmill testing is routinely done. Automated blood pressure monitoring equipment can be used, but it may be burdensome due to the additional cables and is often inaccurate when patients are exercising at high levels. Manual blood pressure monitoring is the preferred method, having blood pressure (BP) cuffs on both of the patient's arms and using a single, detachable sphygmomanometer. An emergency cart should be in the procedure room or in close enough proximity to access quickly if needed.

Probably the most important piece of equipment necessary for performing stress echocardiography is the digital image acquisition computer. Recording images on videotape has numerous drawbacks. The exaggerated cardiac motion that results from hyperventilation at peak exercise and immediately afterward produces discontinuous imaging from any fixed imaging window, making it difficult to focus detailed attention on each myocardial segment. Side-by-side image comparisons are also impossible, forcing the interpreter to shuttle back and forth through the videotape to compare rest to exercise wall motion. The ease with which exercise echocardiography is performed is greatly improved with the use of digital image acquisition. The acquisition device may be a stand-alone computer system or may be integrated into the ultrasound system. The recording of a single representa-

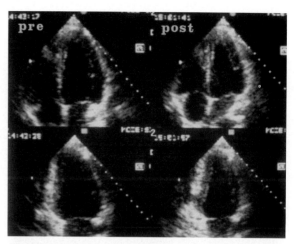

Figure 12-4. Quad screen digital display of the apical four-chamber (top) and apical two-chamber (bottom) views. Rest and postexercise images are displayed side by side for simultaneous analysis.

tive cardiac cycle from each of the imaging planes is all that is necessary. The display format allows the interpreter to view pre- and postexercise images simultaneously (Figs. 12-3, 12-4). The ability to assess regional wall motion abnormalities is thus enhanced, improving the reliability of this test.

Setting Up a Stress Echo Lab: Personnel

Ideally, four people work together to perform the typical stress echocardiogram. First, the medical technician prepares the patient for the procedure, including placement of the electrocardiogram (EKG) leads (Fig. 12-5), recording of baseline BP and EKG, obtains written consent from the patient, and, perhaps the most important aspect of the exam,

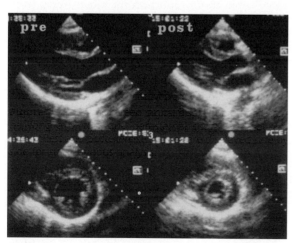

Figure 12-3. Quad screen digital display of the parasternal long axis (top) and parasternal short axis (bottom) views. Rest and postexercise images are displayed side by side for simultaneous analysis.

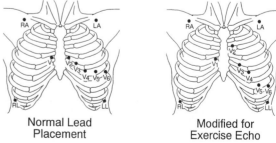

Normal Lead Placement   Modified for Exercise Echo

Figure 12-5. ECG lead placement for stress echocardiography. The standard lead placement is modified by moving V_2 up a rib interspace and moving V_5 and V_6 down an interspace.

instructs the patient. The person who completes this portion of the test is vital to its success and must explain the procedure thoroughly, emphasizing the importance of achieving maximal exertion and of returning quickly to the echo exam bed after exercise. Second, a qualified sonographer must perform the ultrasound imaging. Patient instruction should also be reiterated by this person. Third, a nurse should be present to monitor the patient during the treadmill test. The sonographer and the nurse work closely as a team to complete the treadmill test, monitoring the EKG and BP, and evaluating the patient's symptoms and perceived exertion level. Fourth, a physician must be available in case of an emergency. The physician does not need to be present in the procedure room for the entire exam, but must be near enough to respond quickly if needed.

The Room Setup: How Much Space Is Necessary?

Not much more space is necessary for stress echo than is used for standard treadmill testing. The configuration of the procedure room will vary somewhat, depending on the individual laboratory's preference. The equipment should be arranged with the end of the patient bed very close to the end of the treadmill. The shorter the distance the patient has to travel after exercise, the quicker the image acquisition can be started. The treadmill ECG console also needs to be close to the patient bed to ensure easy reach of the ECG cable. The room should be set up in such a manner that all of the personnel,

including the patient, are between the echo bed and the treadmill at all times. While monitoring the patient during exercise and while guiding the patient back to the echo bed, the ability to have immediate access to the patient in the event of an emergency is crucial. Additionally, the patient can maneuver easily onto the echo bed by simply sitting down, then reclining from the sitting position to the left lateral position and be immediately ready for imaging. This layout assumes that the imaging is being done left-handed and can be varied to accommodate the right-handed sonographer. Exercise echo is more efficiently performed left-handed with this room configuration (Fig. 12-6), although many laboratories have had success with alternative approaches.

Digital Image Acquisition

The most important advantage of recording images in a digital format is the ability to display rest and stress images side-by-side. A single representative cardiac cycle is recorded and played in continuous loop format, or *cineloop*. If a digital signal is not generated directly from the ultrasound system, the analog signal must be converted to digital format using a separate acquisition computer, or frame grabber. Figure 12-7 represents a typical layout when converting an analog signal using a digital acquisition computer. The frame grabber computer receives the ultrasound image directly using a simple cable connection importing the video signal from the ultrasound system. The R wave of the ECG activates the image acquisition computer to begin its grab; therefore, a clean, stable signal is necessary. The signal directly from the stress equipment ECG recorder is ideally suited for this purpose. The ECG output, usually labeled the *ECG sync*, can be directly cabled to the acquisition computer. An alternative method for grabbing is to use the R-wave beep or audio signal directly from the ultrasound system. Most frame grabbers provide this method as an option. To view the ECG tracing on the ultrasound system, a separate adapter is connected directly to the patient cables from an ECG output channel of the stress equipment recorder. With the use of this adapter, attachment of an additional set of ECG leads to the patient is avoided. Finally, to ensure a clean, artifact-free signal, patient preparation must be adequate. The ECG lead attachments must be secure, the cable and lead wires must be in good

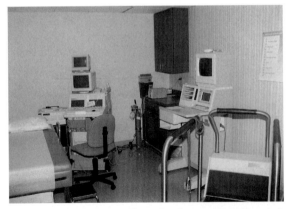

Figure 12-6. Room configuration for exercise echocardiography. The treadmill and examination bed are in close proximity to allow quick image acquisition after exercise.

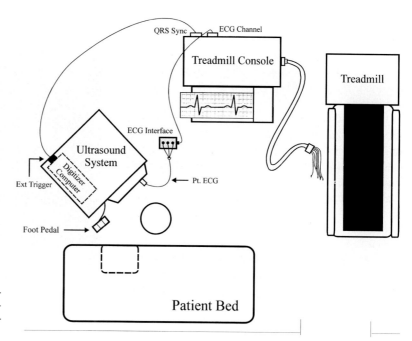

Figure 12-7. Diagram of connections between the ultrasound system, ECG recorder system, and digital acquisition computer.

repair, and the cable must be long enough to reach comfortably to the echo exam bed.

Acquisition Parameters

Direct digital image technology offers numerous advantages over analog format for stress echo use. The ultrasound signal is digital; therefore, no conversion is necessary, and the original quality of the image is preserved. The basic premise for cine-loop acquisition is the same, but higher image resolution and increased flexibility in recording and storage options are possible.

When an external digital acquisition system is used, eight frame cineloop recordings have been the convention for stress echocardiography. (Fig. 12-8) The first of these frames is acquired on the R wave of the ECG, and the subsequent seven are recorded at intervals that the user can vary. The interval setting is called the *interim delay*, and the standard setting used with the majority of adult patients is 50 msec. The length of the recording is therefore 350 msec, which ensures recording of all of systole and very little, if any, diastole. An interim delay setting of 33 msec can also be used if a rapid heart rate is anticipated. It is important to remem-

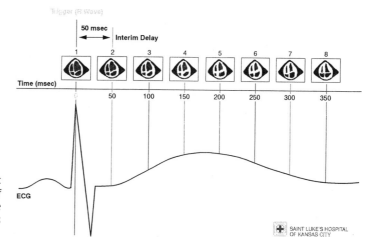

Figure 12-8. Eight-frame cine-loop. Eight consecutive frames are acquired at intervals of 50 msec during the systolic portion of a single cardiac cycle and are replayed as a continuous cine-loop.

ber, however, that the heart rate generally decreases rapidly after exercise. Too short an interim delay may result in failure to record systole in its entirety.

The digital computer allows acquisition of zoomed or windowed images for evaluation of segmental wall motion by capturing a specific region of interest from the ultrasound system. The use of this zoomed image in conjunction with the highest possible transducer frequency and a low depth setting will produce the best images for wall motion assessment. The sonographer must evaluate each patient for optimal settings to ensure the highest-quality recordings. Digital image resolution can also be adjusted. It is important to remember that higher-resolution settings utilize more computer memory. A low-resolution setting is adequate for stress echo use.

Display of the cine-loop is also variable. The standard playback setting displays each of the eight frames for 100 msec, providing a total display length of 800 msec. This allows one to view the images comfortably and assess regional wall motion accurately. The playback length can be adjusted easily by the viewer to speed up or slow down the cine-loop display. The viewer may also choose to edit the cine-loop. Frames can be trimmed from the beginning as well as the end, and a quick look at the first half of systole (the first four frames) can be selected on most digital image systems.

The screen format can be varied, from displaying a single cine-loop to a double, quad, or more if the viewer chooses. The quad screen format has become standard for most stress echocardiography use. The resting images are acquired and displayed as shown in Figure 12-9.

Standard Views

Digital images are acquired at rest in the four standard imaging planes: parasternal long axis, parasternal short axis, apical four-chamber and apical two-chamber views. Parasternal views should be recorded from the highest parasternal window possible. For the long axis view, the transducer should be angled to reflect maximum left ventricular endocardium visualization. This will decrease the amount of aortic root visualized. The short axis view is acquired at the level of the papillary muscles. A continuous line of LV endocardium should be seen in this view. The apical views are acquired from a low intercostal space displaying the ventricles maxi-

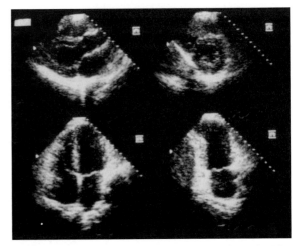

Figure 12-9. Quad screen digital display of standard images acquired at rest.

mally elongated. A foreshortened apical view has several associated pitfalls, such as false right ventricular dilatation, false anteroseptal wall motion abnormalities, and true apical abnormalities, which may be missed altogether. Additional views used for stress echo include the apical five-chamber view, the apical long axis view and a posterior angulation from the apical two-chamber view, which allows for increased visualization of the inferior wall. All of these additional views can be recorded and stored digitally.

Postexercise Image Acquisition

The goal of postexercise image recording is to acquire the highest-quality images in each of the standard views within a period of time in which ischemia, if provoked, is still present. Myocardial reperfusion may begin to occur as early as 1 min after the stress is terminated. Therefore, using 1 min after the treadmill is stopped as the interval in which to have all views recorded will ensure high diagnostic sensitivity of the technique.

When the patient has reached maximal exertion, the treadmill is stopped abruptly, and a timer is started immediately. The patient quickly returns to the echo exam table and resumes the left lateral position. Care must be taken to guide the patient to the correct position and at the same time guide the ECG cables so as not to disconnect them. Imaging is started from the parasternal window. A full disclosure acquisition method is used, which con-

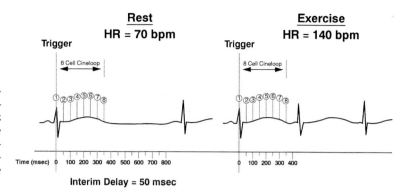

Figure 12-10. Diagram of synchronization of pre- and postexercise images. Standard acquisition parameters allow images to be recorded at a wide range of heart rates, to be synchronized, and to still display representative systolic cycles for comparative analysis.

tinually records cine-loops throughout the immediate post exercise period. Digital acquisition of all views is completed within the first minute following exercise. Imaging should be continued for 2–3 min to monitor reperfusion, if wall motion abnormalities have occurred.

The sonographer then views all of the digitized images, selecting representative cycles from each view. Several criteria must be considered when selecting postexercise images. The ideal selection is the image which has the best endocardial delineation, is recorded in the earliest postexercise time period, and best matches the resting image's tomographic plane. On occasion these criteria cannot all be met, and the sonographer must make choices. The "prettiest" image may not necessarily be the best selection. An image of lesser quality recorded early may be preferable to one of higher quality recorded later, possibly after myocardial reperfusion has started to occur. While other segments are not optimally seen, visualization of a specific myocardial segment may be necessary if the segment seen is supplied by an artery which has undergone intervention and restenosis or patency are in question. Sometimes trade-offs must be made, but carefully analyzing the selection process will maximize the technique's diagnostic utility. Upon completion of postexercise image selection, the pre- and postexercise images are synchronized (Fig. 12-10) and displayed side by side, with the resting images on the left upper and lower quadrants and the postexercise images in the corresponding right upper and lower quadrants (Figs. 12-11, 12-12). Additional digital images can be stored if desired.

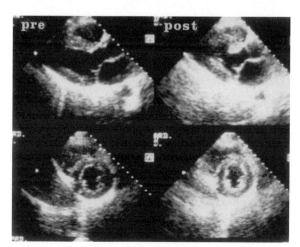

Figure 12-11. Pre- and postexercise quad screen digital display of parasternal long axis (top) and parasternal short axis (bottom) views of a patient with a subtotal left anterior descending (LAD) coronary artery stenosis.

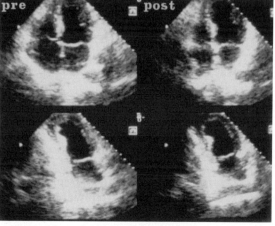

Figure 12-12. Pre- and postexercise quad screen digital display of apical four-chamber (top) and apical two-chamber (bottom) views of the same patient with a subtotal LAD coronary artery stenosis.

Standard Protocols

EXERCISE ECHO EXAM

1. Pre/posttreadmill protocol
   a. Resting, baseline images are acquired and recorded digitally and on videotape. Standard echocardiographic views are displayed in quad screen format.
   b. The patient performs maximal, symptom-limited treadmill exercise according to the Bruce or Modified Bruce protocol. ECG, BP, and patient symptoms are monitored continually throughout the test.
      (1) Upon completion of exercise, *a cooldown period is avoided*.
      (2) The patient is immediately assisted back to the echo exam bed.
   c. Postexercise images are acquired.
      (1) A timer is started *at the same time* that the treadmill belt is stopped.
      (2) Postexercise images are acquired digitally, using the full-disclosure method.
      (3) Digital acquisition is completed within *1 min* of exercise termination.
      (4) Videotape recording of images is continued for 2–3 min after exercise.
   d. Rest and exercise images are synchronized and displayed side by side on two quad screens.
   e. BP and ECG monitoring are continued for 6–10 min or until any induced changes return to baseline.
2. Upright bicycle protocol[10]
   a. Resting baseline images of the standard views are acquired and recorded digitally and on videotape.
   b. The patient is positioned on the bicycle, which is situated close to the ultrasound system, allowing the sonographer to access the apical imaging window.
   c. Baseline upright images are acquired from the apical window (apical four- and two-chamber views) and are stored digitally and on videotape.
   d. The bicycle stress test is performed according to a standard protocol which requires the patient to pedal at 60 revolutions per minute against 25 watts of resistance. The workload is increased by 25 watts every 2 min. ECG, BP, and patient symptoms are monitored continually throughout the test.
   e. Apical images are acquired at the end of each 2-min stage and are temporarily stored in digital memory. As each subsequent stage is completed, the temporarily stored images are replaced with the new images. The images acquired at the highest level of exercise are permanently stored digitally and are labeled as *peak*. All images are recorded on videotape.
   f. Once the patient reaches peak exertion, a cooldown period is avoided and the patient is immediately assisted back to the echo exam bed.
   g. Postexercise images are acquired.
      (1) A timer is started at the cessation of exercise.
      (2) Postexercise images are acquired using the full-disclosure method.
      (3) Video recording of images is continued for 2–3 min postexercise.
   h. Rest and postexercise images are synchronized and displayed side by side on two quad screens. Apical images are displayed using the quad screen format, but with each view using all four quadrants: rest—upper left, peak—upper right, immediate post—lower left, and post or baseline—lower right.
   i. BP and ECG monitoring are continued for 6–10 min or until any induced changes return to baseline.
3. Supine bicycle protocol: The following protocol is a synthesis of the protocol used by Dr. Thomas Ryan at Duke University in Durham, North Carolina, and the protocol used by Dr. William Zoghbi at the Baylor College of Medicine in Houston, Texas.
   a. The patient is placed on a specially designed supine ergometer bed (American Echo, Inc.), which is computer controlled. The bed is brought to a lateral tilt of 15–20 degrees to optimize imaging. Baseline images are acquired and recorded digitally and on videotape.
   b. The bed is returned to the horizontal supine position.
   c. The patient performs bicycle exercise while in the supine horizontal position, starting at a workload of 25 or 50 watts of resistance, and is encouraged to maintain a 60 revolutions per minute pedal rate.
      (1) Two- or 3-min stages may be used.

(2) The workload is increased at each stage by 25 watts of resistance.

d. Standard images are recorded on videotape for each stage.

e. ECG, BP, and patient symptoms are recorded continually throughout the test.

f. As the patient approaches maximal exertion, the bed is returned to the same degree of lateral tilt that was used during baseline image acquisition.

g. Peak images are obtained while the patient pedals and the peak heart rate is maintained. Images are recorded digitally and on videotape.

h. Video recording of images is continued for at least 2 min after exercise.

i. The patient is returned to the horizontal position, and BP and ECG monitoring are continued for 5 min, or until baseline conditions return.

j. Rest and exercise digital images are synchronized and displayed side by side in quad screen format.

4. Protocols vary for evaluation of hemodynamic function in valvular heart disease.[5,18,19]

All of the previously described protocols can be varied for use in evaluating valvular gradients, and regurgitant lesions and in estimating pulmonary artery pressure with exercise. The bicycle methods are better for this purpose because peak recordings can be obtained. The resting Doppler spectral tracing is recorded and measured for several cardiac cycles.

The patient exercises according to the desired protocol outlined, and spectral Doppler tracings are recorded at peak exercise or immediately afterward for comparison to rest measurements. Digital recording of the spectral tracing is not necessary, but simultaneous recording of regional wall motion can be done to evaluate for coronary artery disease if indicated.

For patients who are able, physical stress is the optimal method when evaluating for ischemia. For patients who are unable to exercise, pharmacologic stress is a satisfactory substitute.[1,3,6,12] Additionally, dobutamine echocardiography has proven to be a practical, safe, and accurate method for assessing the risk and the prognosis following acute myocardial infarction, and as an indicator of tissue viability in areas of resting myocardial dysfunction.[2,11,14]

5. Pharmacologic stress echo as a screening test for CAD: Dobutamine echocardiography can be performed safely and efficiently on an outpatient basis, as well as in the hospital setting (Fig. 12-13). Beta blockers should be discontinued (on the advice of the patient's physician) 48 hr before the test, and solid food intake should be restricted for 6 hr prior to the test.

6. Dobutamine echo protocol

a. After the procedure is reviewed with the patient, informed consent is obtained.

b. A saline lock is started, preferably in the patient's right hand.

c. Buretrol is inserted into a bag of D_5W and filled to a level of 115 cc.

Supplies	Medications
Infusion pump and tubing	Dobutamine
Normal saline (0.9 NaCl) or D5W	Sublingual nitroglycerin
IV access kit	Atropine (optional)
Continuous 12 lead ECG monitoring	Beta blocker for intravenous administration (optional)
Fully equipped crash cart with defibrillator	
Blood pressure cuff, stethoscope and sphygmomanometer or automatic blood pressure device	
Consent form	

Figure 12-13. Supplies necessary for performing dobutamine stress echocardiography.

d. Then 10 cc (125 mg) of dobutamine is injected into buretrol, bringing the total fluid volume to 125 cc.

e. After gentle shaking of buretrol to mix the fluids, tubing is connected to the delivery pump and the system is flushed.

f. Baseline ECG and BP are recorded.

g. Resting baseline echo images are acquired and recorded digitally and on videotape. The image acquisition protocol for use with dobutamine allows the display of each echo view in quad screen format, with each quadrant representing a different stage of pharmacologic stress. The baseline images are displayed in the upper left quadrant. The four standard views are acquired.

h. A dobutamine intravenous line is inserted into the saline lock, and infusion is started at a rate of 5 μg/kg/min. The dose rate is increased at 3-min intervals up to a maximal dose of 40 μg/kg/min. Incremental increases are 5, 10, 20, 30, and 40 μg/kg/min. ECG, BP, and patient symptoms are monitored continually throughout the test.

i. Two minutes into each stage, the standard echo views are obtained, recorded on videotape, and acquired digitally as follows (Fig. 12-14):

  5 μg/kg/min: Record standard views on videotape.

  10 μg/kg/min: Acquire digital images and store in upper right quadrant.

  20 μg/kg/min: Record standard views on videotape.

  30 μg/kg/min: Acquire digital images and store in lower left quadrant.

  40 μg/kg/min, or peak dose: Dobutamine is infused for 3 min before echo images are recorded. Peak digital images are stored in the lower right quadrant.

j. Dobutamine infusion is stopped on completion of peak image acquisition.

k. BP and ECG monitoring are continued for 6–10 min or until any induced changes return to baseline. The half-life of dobutamine is approximately 2.5 min.

l. Once the patient returns to baseline, standard echo views are recorded and stored in the standard quad screen format.

ATROPINE

In patients who do not achieve 85% of the predicted maximal heart rate during dobutamine infusion, atropine may be added to further increase the heart rate response.[4,13,15] Atropine, 0.25 mg, is administered intravenously 1 min into the peak dobutamine infusion (40 μg/kg/min) and is repeated to a maximum dose of 1.0 mg if necessary to achieve 85% of the maximal predicted heart rate.

6. Pharmacologic stress echo is used to assess myocardial viability. Low doses of dobutamine have been shown to improve myocardial wall motion, which may represent contractile reserve. Dobutamine stress echocardiography can therefore be used as a measure of viable myocardial tissue in the setting of acute myocardial infarction and in patients who have undergone coronary revascu-

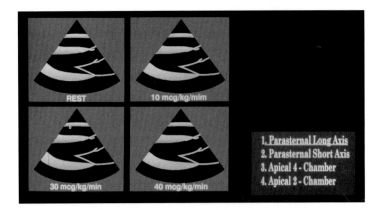

Figure 12-14. Diagram of a quad screen digital display of the parasternal long axis view images acquired during dobutamine stress echocardiography. An additional quad screen is used for each view imaged.

larization.[2,11,14] Described here is one protocol,[2] but many variations are being used successfully to evaluate myocardial viability.

  a. Dobutamine is prepared, and baseline ECG, BP, and echo images are recorded as described in the dobutamine echo protocol.

  b. Dobutamine infusion is started at a rate of 2.5 μg/kg/min and is increased at 3-min intervals. Incremental dose increases are 5, 7.5, 10, 20, 30, and 40 μg/kg/min.

  c. Two minutes into each infusion procedure, the standard echo images are obtained, recorded on videotape, and digitally acquired.

   (1) Two quad screens may be used to display images at baseline and for each of the seven infusion levels for each view.

   (2) A single quad screen display of resting, 5 μg/kg/min, 7.5 μg/kg/min, and recovery images may be used.

  d. Dobutamine infusion is stopped on completion of peak image acquisition, and patient monitoring is continued as described in the dobutamine echo protocol.

Technical Objectives in Performing Stress Echocardiography

The echocardiographically visualized myocardium is divided into segments. These segments are then consolidated into three perfusion zones (Fig. 12-15). Each zone correlates with the corresponding coronary artery. There are, of course, variations in the coronary distribution, with overlap most commonly seen in the area of the circumflex and right coronary artery distributions. The views recorded must represent each of the perfusion zones. If the four standard echo views are recorded—parasternal long and short axis, apical four- and two-chamber views—visualization of each of the coronary perfusion zones in two or more views is achieved. Additional views can and should be recorded to provide more information about each coronary distribution. This is important in areas where, in the standard views, the endocardial surface is not well visualized or in areas where other factors influence the ability to evaluate the contractile function of a segment. Important views to be recorded include the apical long axis, apical five-chamber, and apical four-chamber angle-down views. These additional views can be digitized and/or recorded on videotape as adjuncts to the standard views. The apical long axis view displays the posterior wall in its entirety, which is helpful if other views showing a circumflex coronary artery distribution are inadequate. In patients who have left ventricular hypertrophy, the inferior wall may appear thinned and hypokinetic. The four-chamber angle-down view helps visualize the inferior wall more extensively. This is a simple posterior angulation of the ultrasound beam to just below the mitral valve plane.

The gain, region of interest, and depth settings should remain constant for all stages of the stress

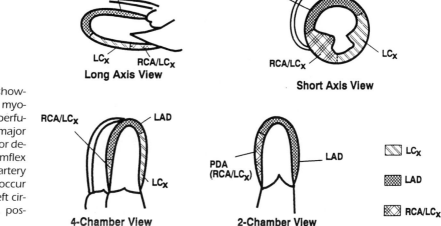

Figure 12-15. Diagram showing the correlation between myocardial segments and the perfusion zones of the three major coronary arteries: left anterior descending (LAD), left circumflex (Lc$_x$), and right coronary artery (RCA). Some overlap may occur in the right coronary and left circumflex distributions. PDA, posterior descending artery.

echo exam. The sonographer should set the gain so that it is adequate for all imaging planes. Occasionally, the gain will need to be adjusted somewhat at peak or postexercise, but this should be the exception, not the rule. The region of interest should also need to be adjusted only rarely. Depth settings should never be changed during the exercise echo exam, so a suitable depth for all windows needs to be selected.

Abnormal Rest Echo Findings

Occasionally, unexpected findings are discovered on the resting images. Patients are often referred to the echo laboratory with symptoms which may be caused by cardiac disorders other than coronary artery disease. If the resting echo reveals an unsuspected abnormality, it is important to notify the ordering physician of the findings. Abnormalities which may be contraindications for stress echo are as follows:

1. Unexpected resting wall motion abnormalities.
2. Significant left ventricular outflow tract obstruction or aortic valve stenosis.
3. Apical thrombus.
4. Cardiac masses or tumors.
5. Congenital anomalies.
6. Other unexpected finding which could be a non-CAD cause of symptoms.

Exercise echocardiography has evolved into a reliable, cost-effective tool for detecting and evaluating CAD and for assessing the functional significance of cardiac valvular lesions. As the future brings continued technological developments and as the use of this technique becomes more widespread, the challenges that occur today will undoubtedly be replaced by new ones. As diagnostic techniques come under increasing scrutiny as part of the broader cost-control environment, the sonographer's continued attention to providing the highest-quality exam will play a role in ensuring the value of stress echocardiography in the future.

REFERENCES

1. Afridi I, Quinones MA, Zoghbi WA, et al. Dobutamine stress echocardiography: Sensitivity, specificity, and predictive value for future cardiac events. Am Heart J. 1994;127:1510–1515.
2. Afridi I, Kleiman NS, Raizner AE, et al. Dobutamine echocardiography in myocardial hibernation. Circulation. 1995;91:663–670.
3. Bach DS, Armstrong WF. Dobutamine stress echocardiography. Am J Cardiol. 1992;69:90H–96H.
4. Baptista J, Arnese M, Roelandt JR, et al. Quantitative coronary angiography in the estimation of the functional significance of coronary stenosis: Correlations with dobutamine-atropine stress test. J Am Coll Cardiol. 1994;23:1434–1439.
5. Braverman AC, Thomas JD, Lee RT. Doppler echocardiographic estimation of mitral valve area during changing hemodynamic conditions. Am J Cardiol. 1991;68:1485–1489.
6. Cohen JL, Ottenweller JE, Achenkunju KG, et al. Comparison of dobutamine and exercise echocardiography for detecting coronary artery disease. Am J Cardiol. 1993;72:1226–1231.
7. Crouse LJ, Harbrecht JJ, Vacek JL, et al. Exercise echocardiography as a screening test for coronary artery disease and correlation with coronary arteriography. Am J Cardiol. 1991;67:1213–1218.
8. Crouse LJ, Kramer PH. Clinical applicability of echocardiographically detected regional wall-motion abnormalities provoked by upright treadmill exercise. Echocardiography. 1992;9:97–106.
9. Dahan M, Paillole C, Martin D, et al. Determinants of stroke volume response to exercise in patients with mitral stenosis: A Doppler echocardiographic study. J Am Coll Cardiol. 1993;21:384–389.
10. Davis C. Upright bicycle and treadmill stress echocardiography techniques and technical hints for the sonographer. J Am Soc Echocardiogr. 1994;7:194–200.
11. LaCanna G, Alfieri O, Giubbini R, et al. Echocardiography during infusion of dobutamine for identification of reversible dysfunction in patients with chronic coronary artery disease. J Am Coll Cardiol. 1994;23:617–626.
12. Marcovitz PA, Armstrong WF. Accuracy of dobutamine stress echocardiography in detecting coronary artery disease. Am J Cardiol. 1992;69:1269–1273.
13. McNeill AJ, Fioretti PM, El-Said E-SM, et al. Enhanced sensitivity for detection of coronary artery disease by addition of atropine to dobutamine stress echocardiography. Am J Cardiol. 1992;70:41–46.
14. Peirard LA, DeLandsheere CM, Berthe C, et al. Identification of viable myocardium by echocardiography during dobutamine infusion in patients with

myocardial infarction after thrombolytic therapy: Comparison with positron emission tomography. J Am Coll Cardiol. 1989;15:1021–1031.

15. Poldermans D, Fioretti PM, Boersma E, et al. Safety of dobutamine-atropine stress echocardiography in patients with suspected or proven coronary artery disease. Am J Cardiol. 1994;73:456–459.

16. Presti CF, Armstrong WF, Feigenbaum H. Comparison of echocardiography at peak exercise and after bicycle in evaluation of patients with known or suspected coronary artery disease. J Am Soc Echocardiogr. 1988;1:119–126.

17. Rosamond TL, Rowland AJ, Harbrecht JJ, et al. Outpatient dobutamine echocardiography: safety and clinical utility (abstract). Circulation. 1990; 82(suppl III):744.

18. Tischler M, Battle R, Madhumita S, et al. Observations suggesting a high incidence of exercise-induced severe mitral regurgitation in patients with mild rheumatic mitral valve disease at rest. J Am Coll Cardiol. 1995;25:128–133.

19. Tischler MD, Plehn JF. Applications of stress echocardiography: Beyond coronary disease-part II. J Am Soc Echocardiogr. 1995;8:185–197.

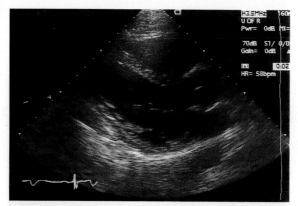

Color Plate 1. Two-dimensional colorized image of the left ventricle. Colorization can help to define endocardial borders and valvular detail (a) in technically difficult cases because the human eye is better able to detect shades of color than shades of gray. (See also Fig. 3-26.)

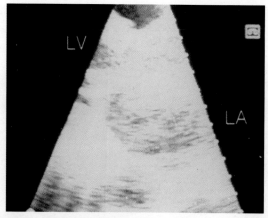

Color Plate 3. Overall gain set too high, masking the color jets. (From Kisslo J, Adams DB, Belkin RN. Doppler Color Flow Imaging. New York, Churchill Livingstone; 1988, Fig. 5-6b. Reprinted with permission) (See also Fig. 5-10.)

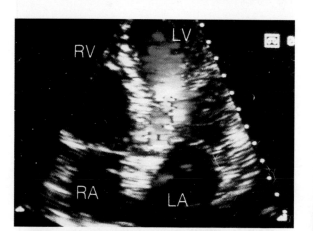

Color Plate 2. Effects of aliasing in color flow Doppler. Because color flow Doppler is a pulsed wave technique, velocities above the Nyquist limit will result in aliasing of the color display. In this example of normal flow across the aortic valve (blue is away from the transducer), a red jet is also noted. This jet denotes aliasing and should not be confused with aortic insufficiency. (From Kisslo J, Adams DB, Belkin RN. Doppler Color Flow Imaging. New York, Churchill Livingstone; 1988, Fig. 6-9b. Reprinted with permission.) (See also Fig. 5-9.)

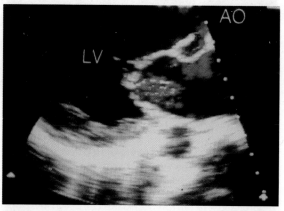

4

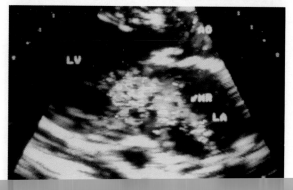

Color Plates 4 and 5. Parasternal long-axis view illustrating mitral regurgitation. The effects of color gain setting on the color display. A setting that is too low will not reveal the severity of the mitral regurgitation. In (**4**) the severity of the mitral regurgitation would be underestimated. (**5**) Demonstrated the proper gain settings and better defines the severity of the regurgitation. (From Kisslo J, Adams DB, Belkin RN. Doppler Color Flow Imaging. New York,

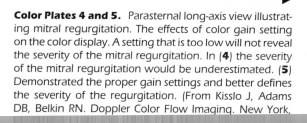

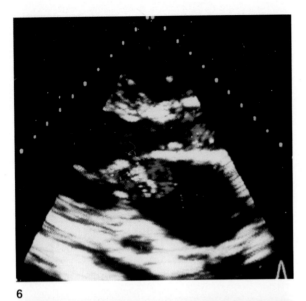

6

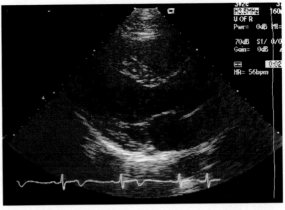

Color Plate 9. Colorization of the two-dimensional image can be helpful in identifying endocardial borders. This parasternal long-axis view demonstrates one of the many colors use to colorize the two-dimensional image. (See also Fig. 5-14.)

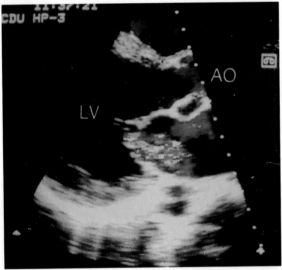

7

Color Plates 6 and 7. Reject or wall filters help eliminate background noise but can also eliminate "real" low flow states. A proper wall filter setting is needed to establish a balance between the two. (**6**) demonstrates a higher color reject, in turn eliminating some of the real signal. (**7**) demonstrates proper reject controls and best defines the mitral regurgitation. (From Kisslo J, Adams DB, Belkin RN. Doppler Color Flow Imaging. New York, Churchill Livingstone; 1988, Fig. 5-13a,b. Reprinted with permission) (See also Fig. 5-12A,B.)

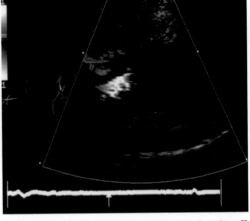

Color Plate 10. Tissue Doppler demonstrating the effects of color in identifying the amplitude or excursion of the endocardium. This technique may help to quantitate the severity of left ventricular dysfunction and to identify regional wall motion abnormalities. (From McDicken WN, Colour Doppler velocity imaging of the myocardium. Ultrasound Med Biol. 1992;18(6,7):653. Reprinted with permission.) (See also Fig. 5-15.)

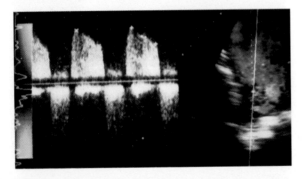

Color Plate 8. The use of color Doppler to guide the placement of a continuous wave Doppler cursor. By observing the direction of flow by color, the continuous wave the cursor can be placed nearly parallel to the direction of flow. This helps eliminate the need to optimize cursor placement. (See also Fig. 5-13.)

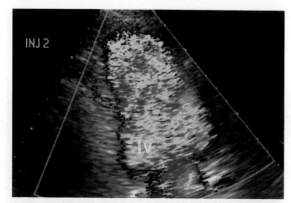

Color Plate 11. Color flow Doppler enhancement of contrast agents. This apical four-chamber view demonstrates fundamental imaging. With the addition of color flow the endocardial borders are better defined. (See also Fig. 5-16D.)

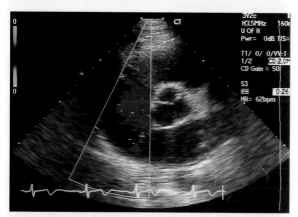

Color Plate 12. To improve the frame rate of color Doppler, a narrow sector is used to sample the area of interest. This parasternal short-axis view demonstrates normal flow across the tricuspid valve. (See also Fig. 5-17.)

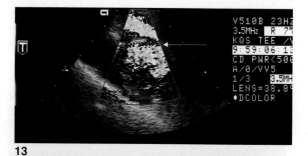

13

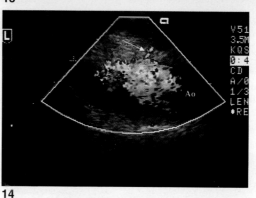

14

Color Plates 13 and 14. Cross-sectional view of a ruptured aorta. (**13**) Color Doppler demonstrates turbulent flow (arrow) outside the lumen of the ruptured descending thoracic aorta. (**14**) Long-axis view of an aorta tear. A small color jet (arrow) is noted crossing the aortic wall. Ao, aorta. (See also Fig. 6-9B, C.)

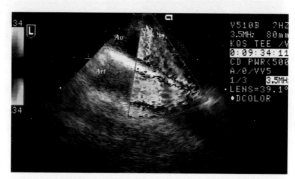

Color Plate 15. Artifact (Art) mimicking an aortic dissection. Note the poorly defined walls. In addition, artifacts such as these do not demonstrate the independent motion typical of a dissection. Ao, aorta. (See also Fig. 6-14.)

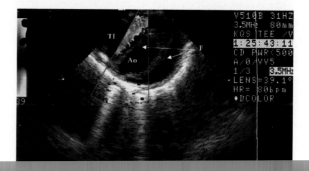

Color Plate 16. Cross-sectional view of the aorta (Ao) demonstrating two false lumens (F). Note the compression of the false lumens during systole. TL, true lumen. (See

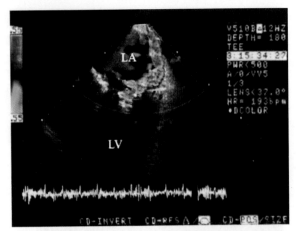

Color Plate 17. Color Doppler demonstration of an eccentric mitral regurgitant jet. TEE is helpful in identifying the pathology associated with eccentric jets. LA, left atrium; LV, left ventricle. (See also Fig. 6-27.)

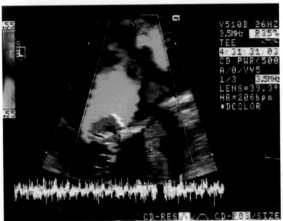

Color Plate 18. In moderate to severe cases of mitral stenosis an area of flow convergence can be seen on the atrial side of the valve. Flow convergence or PISA can be used to calculate mitral valve areas. Under the principles of flow, blood passing through any given hemisphere must also pass through the stenotic region. Using this principle, the instantaneous flow rate through the stenotic orifice can be calculated. The flow radius (r) is measured from the narrowest point of the convergence to the first aliased hemisphere. Since the mitral valve is domed, the angle of the convergence must be determined and corrected by dividing by 180 degrees. The velocity at which the first aliased hemisphere occurs ($V1$) is used in the calculation and can be obtained from the ultrasound system. The flow rate in cubic centimeters per second is calculated by multiplying $2\pi r^2 \times V1 \times$ the corrected angle. The flow rate is then divided by the peak mitral inflow velocity obtained by continuous Doppler to yield the mitral valve area. This calculation is covered in more detail in Chapter 13. (See also Fig. 6-29.)

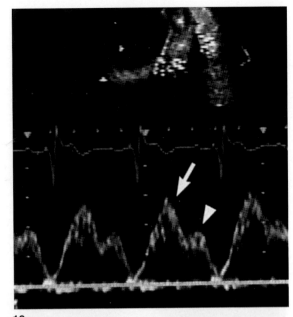

19

20

Color Plates 19 and 20. Pulsed wave spectral Doppler display of pulmonary venous flow in various degrees of mitral regurgitation. In moderate to severe mitral regurgitation (**19**), the systolic component is significantly reduced and the diastolic component is increased due to an increase in left atrial pressure. The low-velocity end-diastolic signal noted (small arrow) below the baseline is caused by atrial contraction. In severe mitral regurgitation (**20**), the systolic component is reversed (arrow) due to direct reflux of the mitral regurgitation into the pulmonary vein and an increase in atrial pressure. The increased diastolic component is due to the systolic regurgitation. (See also Fig. 6-31A, C.)

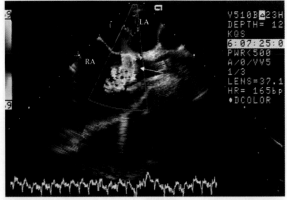

Color Plate 21. Secundum ASD (arrow) with color Doppler demonstration of a left-to-right shunt. Four-chamber view. LA, left atrium; RA, right atrium. (See also Fig. 6-40.)

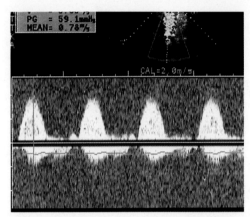

Color Plate 22. Longitudinal view of the right ventricular outflow tract demonstrating the pulmonic valve and narrowed main pulmonary artery. Color Doppler demonstrates turbulent flow, and conventional Doppler shows increased velocity across a stenotic pulmonic valve. (See also Fig. 6-43B.)

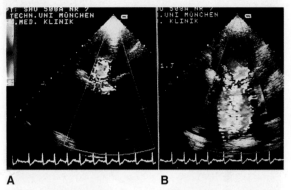

A   **B**

Color Plate 23. (**A**) Transthoracic four-chamber view with a color Doppler display of the mitral valve. The small size of the jet suggests minimal or mild MR. (**B**) Intravenous injection of SHU 508A dramatically reveals the MR using color Doppler. (From Nanda NC, Schlief R, Goldberg BB (eds): Advances in Echo Imaging Using Contrast Enhancement, 2nd ed. Dordrecht, the Netherlands, Kluwer; 1993: 245. Reprinted with permission.) (See also Fig. 8-4A, B.)

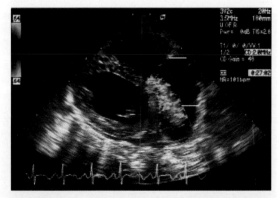

Color Plate 24. Modified parasternal long-axis view of the right ventricular inflow of tricuspid valve with color flow Doppler. Tricuspid regurgitation is noted as a blue-mosaic signal noted in systole. RA, right atrium; RV, right ventricle; TV, tricuspid valve; LV, left ventricle; TR, tricuspid regurgitation. (See also Fig. 10-5B.)

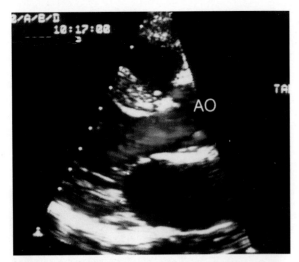

25

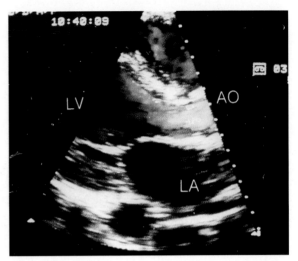

26

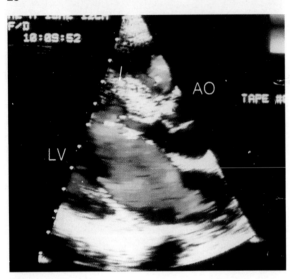

27

Color Plates 25, 26, 27. (**25**) Left parasternal long-axis view in systole with color Doppler demonstrating flow through the left ventricular outflow tract. The flow is coded red because the angle of flow is directed toward the transducer. (**26**) In this frame the flow is blue because the angle of flow is directed away from the transducer. LA, left atrium; LV, left ventricle; MV, mitral valve; IVS, interventricular septum; PW, posterior left ventricular wall; RV, right ventricular wall; Ao, aorta. (From Kisslo J, et al. Doppler Color Flow Imaging. New York, Churchill Livingstone; 1988:Fig. 3-18 (**25**) and 6-1 (**26**). Reprinted with permission.) (**27**) Left parasternal long-axis view in diastole demonstrating normal color flow patterns across the mitral valve. The flow is coded red because the angle of flow is directed more toward the transducer than away. LA, left atrium; LV, left ventricle; IVS, interventricular septum; PW, posterior left ventricular wall; RV, right ventricular wall; Ao, aorta. (From Kisslo J, et al. Doppler Color Flow Imaging. New York, Churchill Livingstone; 1988: Fig. 6-3. Reprinted with permission.) (See also Fig. 10-6A–C.)

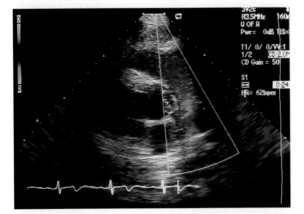

Color Plate 28. A left parasternal short-axis view at the base of the heart and at the level of the pulmonic valve. A blue jet is noted in this systolic frame because flow across the pulmonic valve in this imaging plane is away from the transducer. LA, left atrium; RA, right atrium; RV, right ventricle; Ao, aorta; MPA, main pulmonary artery; PF, pulmonic valve flow; PI, pulmonic valve insufficiency. (See also Fig. 10-11.)

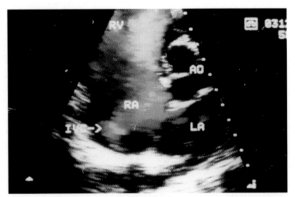

Color Plate 29. Color flow Doppler in a left parasternal short-axis view angled toward the tricuspid valve. The jet is red since flow is toward the transducer. Color flow is noted originating from the inferior vena cava (IVC) as it enters the right atrium. LA, left atrium; RA, right atrium; RV, right ventricle; Ao, aorta. (From Kisslo J, et al. Doppler Color Flow Imaging. New York, Churchill Livingstone; 1988: Fig. 6-14. Reprinted with permission.) (See also Fig. 10-12.)

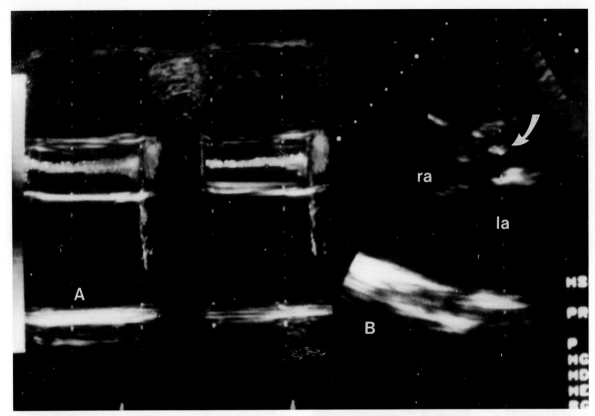

Color Plate 30. Left parasternal short-axis view at the level of the aorta. This is color Doppler frame demonstrating a central diastolic color jet identifying a mild degree of aortic insufficiency (arrow). (See also Fig. 10-15.)

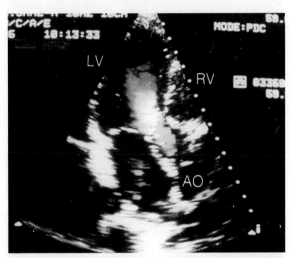

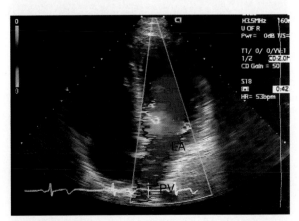

Color Plate 31. Apical four-chamber view in diastole. A red color flow Doppler pattern is noted because flow across the valve is toward the transducer. Flow from the pulmonary veins can be appreciated in this view. LA, left atrium; RA, right atrium; LV, left ventricle; RV, right ventricle; PV, pulmonary veins. (See also Fig. 10-21.)

Color Plate 32. Apical long-axis view with color flow Doppler. Flow in the outflow tract is normally blue since it is directed away from the transducer; however, red flow is also noted. This red flow is due to aliasing, which is common in this view since the velocity of blood in a normal left ventricular outflow tract can exceed the Nyquist limit. This is an important point since some may be inclined to call the red flow aortic insufficiency (AI). AI can easily be ruled out since the aliased flow occurs in systole. (From Kisslo J, et al. Doppler Color Flow Imaging. New York, Churchill Livingstone; 1988: Fig. 6-9A. Reprinted with permission.) (See also Fig. 10-27.)

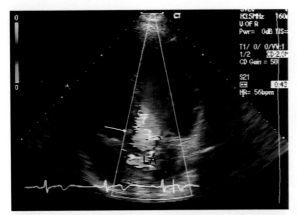

Color Plate 33. Color flow Doppler from an apical four-chamber view and anterior angulation. Color flow is typically blue, but due to aliasing red may also be seen (arrow). LA, left atrium; LV, left ventricle; RV, right ventricle. (See also Fig. 10-31.)

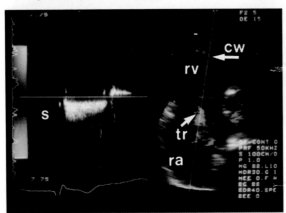

Color Plate 34. Modified four-chamber view with spectral Doppler. The angle of tricuspid flow is nearly parallel to the sound beam, allowing better Doppler interrogation of the tricuspid flow. LA, left atrium; LV, left ventricle; RV, right ventricle; TV, tricuspid valves; MV, mitral valve. (See also Fig. 10-33.)

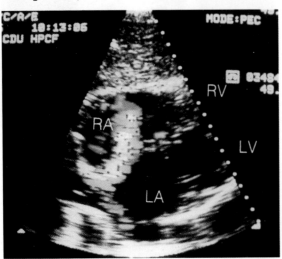

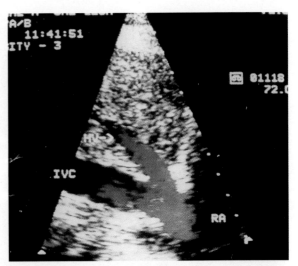

Color Plate 36. Subcostal inferior vena cava image with color flow Doppler. The jet is blue because flow in this view is normally moving away from the transducer. Red flow would indicate significant tricuspid regurgitation. IVC, inferior vena cava; RA, right atrium; HV, hepatic veins. (See also Fig. 10-39.)

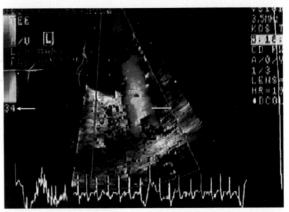

Color Plate 37. Magnified view of the left atrial appendage (LAA) with color flow Doppler. Doppler scanning is performed to identify the presence of a low-flow state, which could help predict clot formation. The color scale is usually adjusted downward so that low flow can be identified. LA, left atrium. (See also Fig. 11-13.)

Color Plate 35. Subcostal four-chamber view with color Doppler. Flow is noted crossing the interatrial septum via a large interatrial septal defect (ASD). RA, right atrium; RV, right ventricle; LA, left atrium; LV, left ventricle. (From Kisslo J, et al. Doppler Color Flow Imaging. New York, Churchill Livingstone; 1988: Fig. 10-1. Reprinted with permission.) (See also Fig. 10-38.)

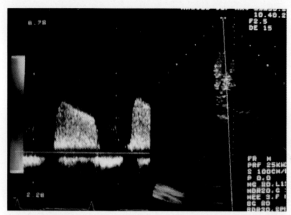

Color Plate 38. In mitral stenosis, pathology of the valve may result in an eccentric jet. The use of color flow Doppler echocardiography may help align the continuous wave (CW) Doppler cursor with the jet, allowing an adequate spectral display. (See also Fig. 13-10.)

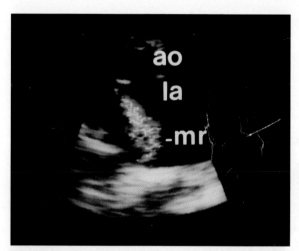

39

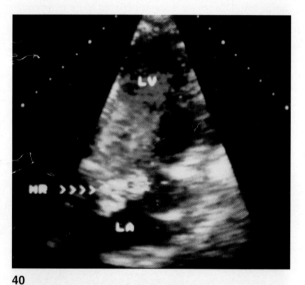

40

Color Plates 39 and 40. In assessing the degree of mitral regurgitation by color flow Doppler, a number of imaging planes should be used in order to get a better appreciation of the degree of regurgitation and the secondary findings associated with it. (**39**) Parasternal long-axis view of a patient with mild mitral regurgitation. (**40**) Apical four-chamber view of a patient who also has mild mitral regurgitation. (See also Fig. 13-20A, B.)

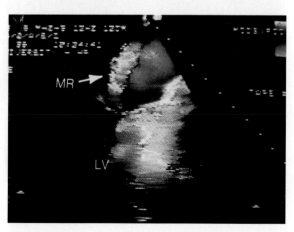

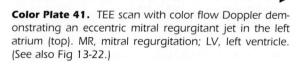

Color Plate 41. TEE scan with color flow Doppler demonstrating an eccentric mitral regurgitant jet in the left atrium (top). MR, mitral regurgitation; LV, left ventricle. (See also Fig 13-22.)

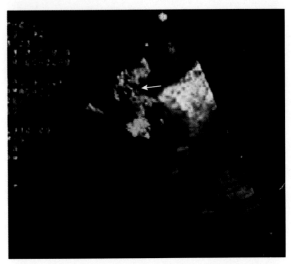

Color Plate 42. TEE scans of a patient with infective bacterial endocarditis that originated on the aortic valve. An aortic insufficiency jet lesion is believed to be responsible for the anterior mitral valve leaflet aneurysm (arrow). Color Doppler can be seen across the aneurysm. (See also Fig. 13-34 C.)

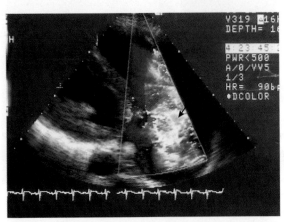

43

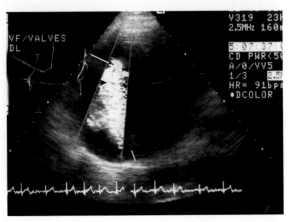

44

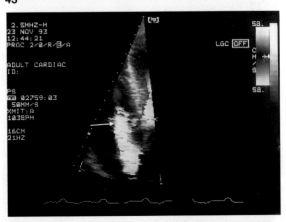

45

Color Plates 43, 44, and 45. (**43**) Modified left parasternal long-axis or right ventricular inflow view of a patient with significant tricuspid regurgitation (arrow). RA, right atrium; RV, right ventricle; LV, left ventricle; IVS, interventricular septum; PW, posterior wall; Ao, descending thoracic aorta; TR, tricuspid regurgitation. (**44**) Left parasternal short axis view of a patient with significant tricuspid regurgitation (TR) (arrow). Note the enlarged right and left atria. RA, right atrium; RV, right ventricle; LV, left ventricle; LA, left atrium; IAS, interatrial septum; TV, tricuspid valve. (**45**) Apical four-chamber view of a patient with tricuspid regurgitation (arrow). RA, right atrium; RV, right ventricle; LA, left atrium; LV, left ventricle; TV, tricuspid valve. (See also Fig. 15-8A–C.)

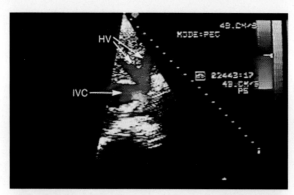

Color Plate 46. Subcostal view of hepatic veins and inferior vena cava (IVC) in a patient with significant tricuspid regurgitation. Note the systolic reflux flow in these vessels (red flow). HV, hepatic vein. (See also Fig. 15-10.)

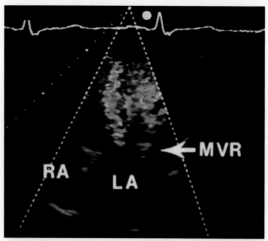

Color Plate 49. Apical four-chamber view from a patient with a porcine mitral valve replacement (MVR) showing color flow toward the apex along the septal wall and flow toward the base along the lateral wall. This pattern is the opposite of the color flow pattern through a normal native valve. RA, right atrium; LA, left atrium. (From Otto CM, Pearlman AS. *Textbook of Clinical Echocardiography.* Philadelphia, WB Saunders; 1995:18, Fig. 11-13. Reprinted with permission.) (See also Fig. 16-29.)

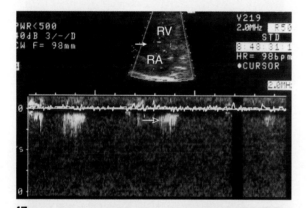

47

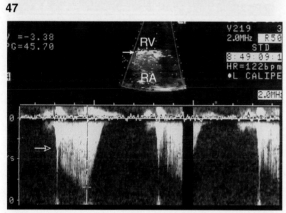

48

Color Plate 47 and 48. (**43**) A patient with trivial tricuspid regurgitation and a weak tricuspid regurgitation Doppler signal. With contrast enhancement (**48**) the tricuspid regurgitation is well demonstrated by color Doppler (open arrow) and the continuous wave Doppler signal is well demarcated (closed arrow). RA, right atrium; RV, right ventricle. (See also Fig. 15-12A,B.)

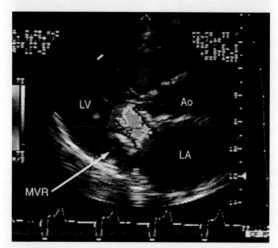

Color Plate 50. Parasternal long-axis image from a patient with a porcine mitral valve replacement (MVR) showing a normal left ventricular color flow pattern through the valve. LV, left ventricle; LA, left atrium; Ao, aorta. The jet (shown in blue due to aliasing) is directed toward the septum. (From Otto CM, Pearlman AS. *Textbook of Clinical Echocardiography.* Philadelphia, WB Saunders; 1995:19, Fig. 11-12. Reprinted with permission.) (See also Fig. 16-30.)

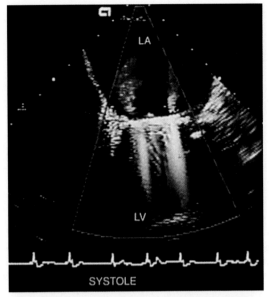

SYSTOLE

51

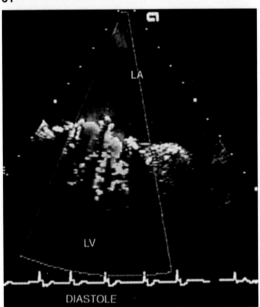

DIASTOLE

52

Color Plates 51 and 52. (**51**) Systolic color flow image of a bileaflet mitral valve prosthesis showing two normal jets of regurgitation. LA, left atrium; LV, left ventricle. (**52**) Diastolic color flow image of a bileaflet mitral valve prosthesis showing the three peaks that correspond to the two large lateral orifices and the smaller central slit-like orifice. LA, left atrium; LV, left ventricle. (From Otto CM, Pearlman AS. *Textbook of Clinical Echocardiography.* Philadelphia, WB Saunders; 1995, Fig. 11-5, top and bottom panels. Reprinted with permission.) (See also Fig. 16-31*A,B.*)

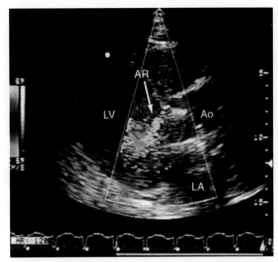

53

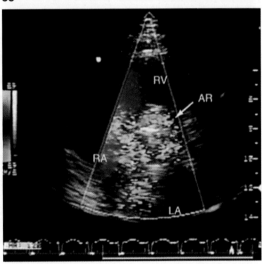

54

Color Plates 53 and 54. Color flow Doppler images in parasternal long-axis (top) and short-axis (bottom) views in a patient with aortic valve dehiscence due to endocarditis and paraprosthetic aortic regurgitation. Color flow imaging shows flow anterior to the prosthesis in a long-axis view with a circumferential pattern of regurgitation seen in the short-axis view. LV, left ventricle; LA, left atrium; RV, right ventricle; RA, right atrium, Ao, aorta; AR, aortic regurgitation. (From Otto CM, Pearlman AS. *Textbook of Clinical Echocardiography.* Philadelphia, WB Saunders; 1995:23, Fig. 11-18. Reprinted with permission.) (See also Fig. 16-38 [bottom].)

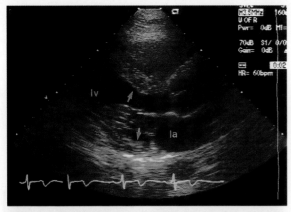

55

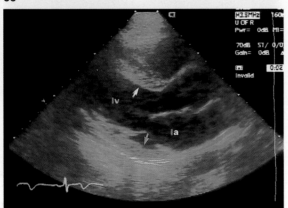

56

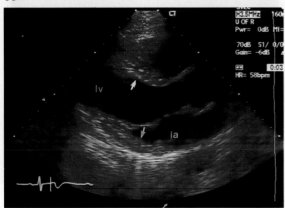

57

Color Plates 55, 56, and 57. Colorization of the two-dimensional image of the left ventricle may help identify endocardial borders (arrow). La, left atrium; lv, left ventricle. (See also Fig. 17-5.)

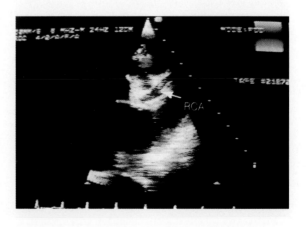

Color Plate 60. Short-axis transesophageal image of the right coronary artery (arrow). RCA, right coronary artery. (From DeBruijn NP, Clements FM. Transesophageal color flow imaging. *In* Doppler Color Flow Imaging. Kisslo J, Adams DB, Belkin RN, eds. NY, Churchill Livingstone; 1988, Fig. 12-5, pg. 170.) (See also Fig. 19-5.)

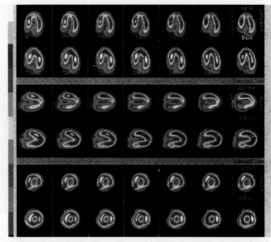

Color Plate 58. Myocardial perfusion SPECT study of left ventricle, indicating a slightly dilated LV with severe and extensive ischemic defect of the interior wall extending to the apex and antero-apical region. (Courtesy Ronald Schwartz, University of Rochester Nuclear Cardiology Department.) (See also Fig. 17-10.)

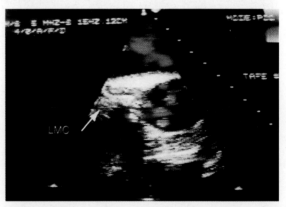

Color Plate 59. Short-axis transesophageal image of the left main coronary artery (arrow). LMC, left main coronary. (From DeBruijn NP, Clements FM. Transesophageal color flow imaging. *In* Doppler Color Flow Imaging. Kisslo J, Adams DB, Belkin RN, eds. NY, Churchill Livingstone; 1988, Fig. 12-5, pg. 170.) (See also Fig. 19-4.)

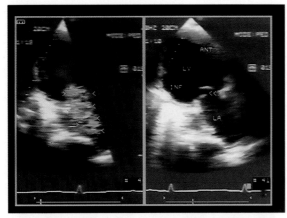

Color Plate 61. Apical two-chamber view (right panel) in a patient with an extensive inferior MI and flail mitral leaflets (arrows) resulting in severe mitral regurgitation (left panel) detected by color flow imaging. LV, left ventricle; LA, left atrium; INF, inferior; ANT, anterior. (See also Fig. 20-8.)

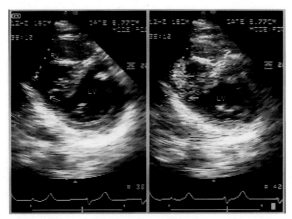

Color Plate 62. Parasternal short axis view of the LV demonstrating thinning of the inferior septum (left panel) and a systolic flow disturbance evident by color flow imaging in a patient with ventricular septal rupture due to an acute inferior MI. (See also Fig. 20-12A.)

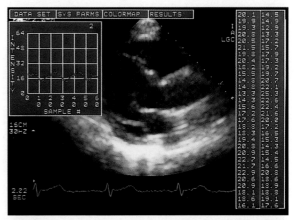

63

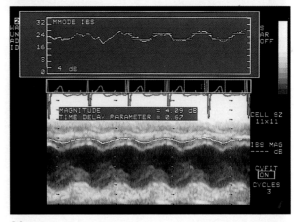

64

Color Plates 63 and 64. (**63**) Parasternal long axis view of the LV employing integrated backscatter imaging. A circular region of interest is positioned in the posterior wall. The graph on the left is the intensity (in decibels) display of the cyclic variation of backscatter, and the graph on the right shows the individual values of backscatter in decibels for 60 samples (See also Fig. 20-13A.) (**64**) M-mode echocardiogram of the septum and left ventricular posterior wall employing integrated backscatter imaging. A region of interest has been traced through the midseptal myocardium with the graphic display of backscatter over time. The average magnitude of cyclic variation was normal (4:1 dB), as was the delay of 0.67 (normal, <1.0). (See also Fig. 20-13B.)

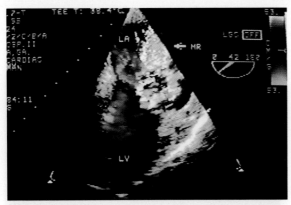

Color Plate 65. This TEE examination reveals the presence of severe mitral valve regurgitation in a patient with ruptured mitral valve leaflet. MV, mitral valve; LV, left ventricle; LA, left atrium. (See also Fig. 23-13*B*.)

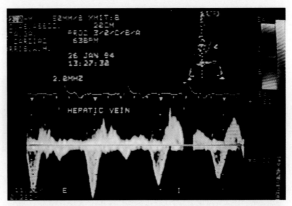

Color Plate 68. Pulsed wave Doppler tracing in the hepatic vein illustrating a restrictive myopathic pattern of flow. Note the increase in diastolic filling and reversed flow during atrial systole. (See also Fig. 24-11.)

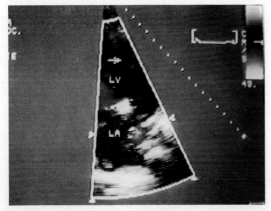

Color Plate 66. Color flow Doppler tracing of a patient with congestive cardiomyopathy. Note the low-velocity flow in the middle to distal left ventricle (LV). See arrow. LA, left atrium. Black-and-white image with spontaneous contrast noted in a patient with DCMP and a low flow state. (See also Fig. 24-3.)

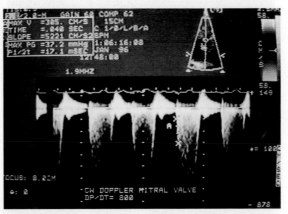

Color Plate 69. This continuous wave Doppler tracing of mitral regurgitation is used to calculate the DP/DT, which is reduced at 800 mm Hg/sec, indicating failing left ventricular systolic function. The DP/DT represents the isovolumic phase index of LV pressure rise (DP/DT) can be estimated. Left atrial pressure does not change significantly during the isovolumic contraction period. Therefore, the MR velocity changes during this period reflect DP/DT. The time interval between 1 and 3 m/sec on the MR velocity integral is measured. The DP/DT is calculated by 32 mm Hg/time (sec). Normal is greater than 1200 mm Hg/sec. The right ventricular DP/DT is derived from the TR jet velocity integral. The time interval between 1 and 2 m/sec is used for the right side. The DP/DT is calculated by 12 mm Hg/time (sec). (See also Fig. 24-13.).

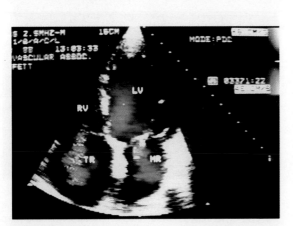

Color Plate 67. Apical four-chamber two-dimensional echocardiogram with color flow Doppler mapping. The patient has mitral (MR) and tricuspid (TR) valve regurgitation. RV, right ventricle; LV, left ventricle. (See also Fig. 24-4.)

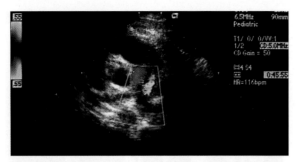

Color Plate 70. Patent ductus arteriosus. Color Doppler demonstrates retrograde diastolic flow in the pulmonary artery originating from the left pulmonary artery. This represents the source of increased pulmonary blood flow seen in these children. (See also Fig. 29-18.)

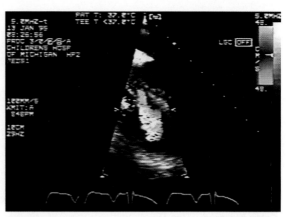

Color Plate 73. Color flow through the ruptured sinus into the right ventricle. The sinus had perforated into both the right ventricle and the right atrium. (See also Fig. 30-7 D.)

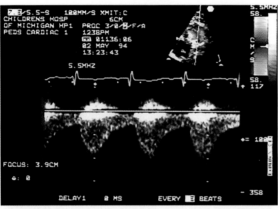

Color Plate 71. Continuous wave Doppler across the co-arctation demonstrating the typical "sawtooth" appearance. (See also Fig. 30-6 B.)

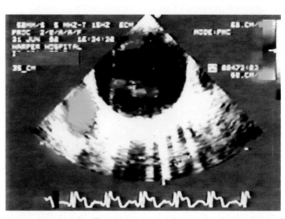

Color Plate 74. Transesophageal longitudinal view of aortic dissection. Color Doppler demonstrating flow from the true to the false lumen in this short axis view. (See also Fig. 30-12 C.)

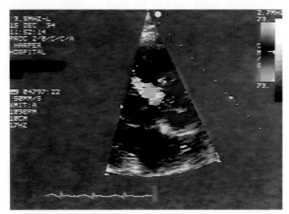

Color Plate 72. Color flow through ruptured right sinus of Valsalva aneurysm. (See also Fig. 30-7 B.)

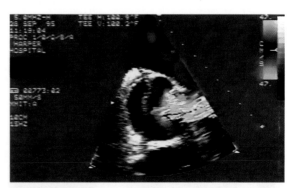

Color Plate 75. A proximal dissection with a highly mobile flap; color Doppler shows aortic regurgitation in the patient. There was intermittent prolapse of the flap through the aortic valve. (See also Fig. 30-13 B.)

PART IV

Acquired Valvular Disease

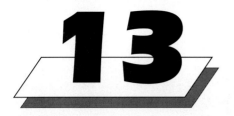

13

The Mitral Valve

DARREL LEWIS and MARK N. ALLEN

Introduction

Echocardiography is the method of choice in evaluating mitral valve disease. Its noninvasive nature, user-friendly interface, and cost effectiveness are useful in the evaluation of cardiac valves. The combination of imaging techniques and Doppler-derived information provides a tremendous amount of information on valvular structure and hemodynamics. Over the last few years, newer techniques and procedures have provided more reliable quantitative information about mitral valve pathology.

Mitral Annular Calcification

Mitral annular calcification is a degenerative process seen frequently in older patients.[15,67,84,135,219] The degree of calcification can vary from very mild to very severe. The precise cause of mitral annular calcification is not fully known. One theory is that it is a natural step in the degeneration of the cardiovascular fibrous tissue that occurs in the older population. Predisposing factors include advanced age, female gender, and diseases that increase the stress on the mitral valve apparatus.[67]

A number of diseases are frequently associated with mitral annular calcification, including aortic stenosis,[11,67] hypertrophic cardiomyopathy,[84] arterial hypertension,[11] mitral valve disease,[6,84,114] conduction disturbances,[9,135,180] and stroke.[4,5,7,15,84,186] Infective endocarditis has also been reported in association with mitral annular calcification.[24,50,67] Some of these disease states suggest a direct cause-and-effect relationship, whereas others may occur as a direct result of mitral annular calcification. Hypertension, aortic stenosis, and hypertrophic cardiomyopathy elevate left ventricular systolic pressure, which in turn increases stress on the mitral apparatus. Diseases such as mitral valve prolapse, mitral valve replacement, and regurgitation exert stress on the mitral valve because of abnormal mitral motion.

Conditions such as conduction disturbances, stroke, and infective endocarditis may be caused by mitral annular calcification. Calcific deposits may extend into the membranous portion of the interventricular septum, involving the atrioventricular node and bundle of His and causing conduction disturbances. In one study, 51% of patients with mitral annular calcification had evidence of atrioventricular or intraventricular block.[67] Atrial fibrillation is another conduction abnormality encountered in patients with mitral annular calcification.[9]

Some studies have shown that patients with mitral annular calcification are twice as likely to have a thromboembolic event as patients without this condition, in the absence of other potential sources.[7,5,15] Embolic events can be due either to the effects of mitral annular calcification on other structures such as left atrial enlargement, resulting in atrial fibrillation,[5] or to calcific emboli,[15] or both.

239

Endocarditis involving a heavily calcified mitral annulus is a rare finding. Most reported cases demonstrate the vegetation attached to the base of the posterior leaflet, with burrowing abscesses around the calcified annulus.[24,50]

Echocardiography is ideal for identifying mitral annular calcification and some of the complications associated with it. A calcified mitral annulus appears as a bright band of echoes (Fig. 13-1). With heavy calcification, mitral leaflet motion can be obscured or hampered (Fig. 13-2), particularly in the posterior leaflet. The presence or severity of mitral regurgitation can also be obscured by shadowing associated with the calcific region. Interrogation of the left atrium from all possible views should be performed in order to evaluate mitral regurgitation.

Recognizing mitral annular calcification by echocardiography is important since its presence can lead to confusion. Mitral annular calcification can mimic mitral stenosis,[46,49,69] pericardial effusion,[46] or masses. Calcification can also extend throughout the base of the heart, and can involve the aortic[8] and mitral valve leaflets as well. Echocardiography also identifies complications associated with mitral annular calcification, such as left atrial enlargement,[9,5,67,135,180] left ventricular enlargement,[135,180] mitral regurgitation,[4] and mitral stenosis.[84,219] In cases where calcium deposits have infiltrated the mitral valve leaflets, causing stenosis, Doppler echocardi-

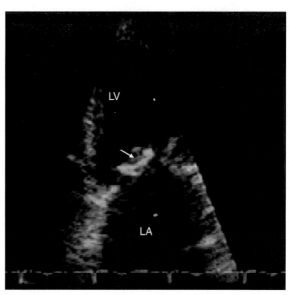

Figure 13-2. Heavy mitral annular calcification (arrow). In this patient the annular calcification is so severe that there is valvular involvement. Leaflet separation is not appreciated.

ography is ideally suited to help make this distinction and grade the severity of the condition.[114]

Mitral Stenosis

CLINICAL CONSIDERATIONS

Mitral valve stenosis occurs when scarring or some other process obstructs blood flow through the mitral valve. The most common cause of mitral stenosis is rheumatic endocarditis. Other rare causes include congenital mitral stenosis, calcification of the mitral annulus that involves the mitral leaflets, thrombus, vegetations, atrial myxomas, and parachute mitral valve deformity.[23,47,84,138,145,187,229]

In rheumatic mitral stenosis the leaflets and chordae tendineae become scarred and contracted. Adhesions cause fusion of the commissures of the valve, restricting motion of both leaflets. As a result of this process, the leaflets become tethered in a downward position, creating a funnel-shaped structure. The orifice becomes narrowed, inhibiting normal flow from the left atrium to the ventricle. The stenotic valve therefore becomes a barrier to normal flow of blood. The result is an increase in left atrial pressure. As the left atrial pressure rises, a number of secondary changes can be observed.

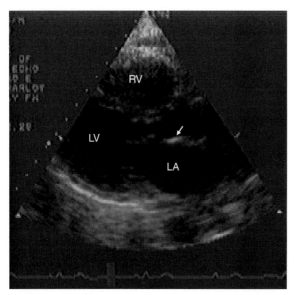

Figure 13-1. Parasternal long axis view demonstrating mitral annular calcification. In this case the amount of calcification is mild.

Normally, the area of the mitral orifice is 4 to 6 cm². A decrease in mitral orifice area causes a diastolic pressure gradient between the left atrium and left ventricle, leading to left atrial hypertension. When the valve area is 2 cm² or more, the transvalvular pressure gradient is only minimally elevated and the patient is usually asymptomatic. When the mitral valve area becomes less than 2 cm², a significant pressure gradient usually develops (Fig. 13-3). A significant pressure gradient across the mitral valve leads to pressure overload of the left atrium, pulmonary vasculature, and right ventricle.[107]

The increase in the pressure of the left atrium may lead to atrial enlargement. Atrial fibrillation is usually associated with mitral stenosis because of the increase in atrial pressure. As the heart rate increases the diastolic filling period decreases, causing the transvalvular pressure gradient to increase further. With chronic elevation of left atrial pressure, structural and functional changes occur in the pulmonary vasculature. The elevated left atrial pressure causes an increase in pulmonary resistance, leading to reduced lung compliance and difficulty in breathing. The right heart, in turn, has to work harder to pump blood to the lungs. Over time the right heart may go into failure. Once the right heart is affected by mitral stenosis, tricuspid regurgitation usually develops.[68]

Other serious complications of mitral stenosis include thrombus formation within the left atrium, mitral regurgitation, pulmonary hypertension, and decreased cardiac output. The combination of a dilated left atrium and the resulting loss of function and stasis of blood creates an ideal situation for the formation of a thrombus (Fig. 13-4). The left atrial appendage is a common site for thrombus formation. With left atrial enlargement the annulus becomes stretched, leading to mitral regurgitation. Pulmonary hypertension develops because of the increased resistance to pulmonary venous flow.

Clinical symptoms of mitral stenosis include dyspnea at rest,[175,181,228] pulmonary edema,[181] palpitations, fatigue, chest pain, hemoptysis,[181] hoarseness,[68] and stroke.[13] Dyspnea and pulmonary edema occur because of the changes in the pulmonary vasculature, which reduce lung compliance. Atrial fibrillation contributes to the loss of atrial function, which eventually leads to palpitations and fatigue. The increased pulmonary pressure results in the rupture of pulmonary capillaries, leading to bleeding or hemotysis. Pulmonary hypertension can contribute to chest pain. As the left atrium enlarges, it may impinge upon the laryngeal nerve, causing hoarseness.

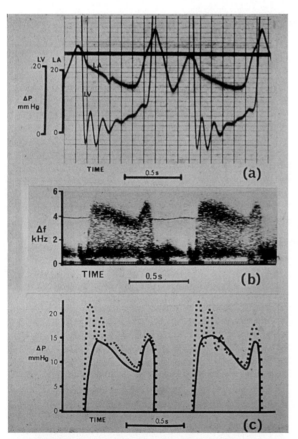

Figure 13-3. Simultaneous pressure recordings across and transmitral velocity profiles in a patient with mitral stenosis. (**A**) The left atrial (LA) pressure remains elevated relative to the left ventricular pressure (LV). (**B,C**) Note the similarities in the timing and magnitude of the transmitral pressure gradient. Left atrial pressure (solid line) remains high throughout diastole.

ECHOCARDIOGRAPHIC FEATURES

M-Mode

Before the advent of two-dimensional imaging and Doppler, M-mode was used in evaluating the presence of stenosis. From the parasternal window the cursor is placed through the anterior and posterior mitral valve leaflets. Normally, the anterior mitral valve tracing resembles the letter M in diastole, while the tracing of the posterior leaflet resembles a W (Fig. 13-5*A*). To best understand the anatomic

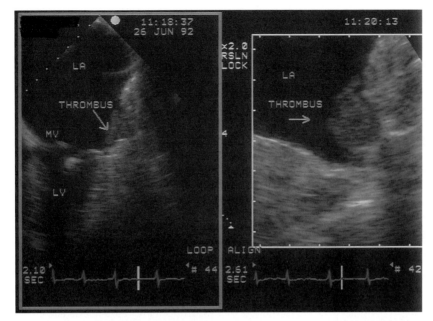

Figure 13-4. A complication of mitral stenosis. Low-flow state in the left atrium sets the stage for thrombus formation. Transesophageal view of a patient with mitral stenosis and a clot in the left atrial appendage. TEE is the method of choice in evaluating the left atrium and its appendage in this clinical setting. LA, left atrium; MV, mitral valve; LV, left ventricle.

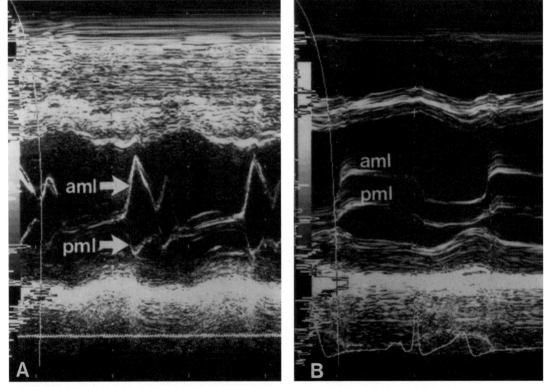

Figure 13-5. (**A**) M-mode scan across a normal mitral valve. Notice the typical M shape of the anterior leaflet (aml) and the typical W shape of the posterior leaflet (pml). (**B**) M-mode scan across a stenotic mitral valve. The posterior leaflet is drawn anteriorly and there is a characteristic flattening of both leaflets, with a loss of the normal configuration. The leaflets appear thickened as well.

and physiologic event that occurs at each point, each event is identified by a letter. The point at which the mitral valve begins to open is the D point. The E point is identified as the moment when the valve reaches its maximum excursion. Following the E point is the F point, which is the lowest point reached after initial closure. The E-F slope is determined by drawing a line from the E to the F point, which is steep in the normal valve. During atrial systole the point at which the valve opens again and reaches a peak is labeled A. Point C is located where the valve closes.

Classic M-mode tracings of mitral stenosis include (1) flattening of the E-F slope, (2) anterior motion of the posterior leaflet, (3) decreased A wave of the mitral leaflet (Fig. 13-5*B*), (4) left atrial enlargement, (5) paradoxical septal wall motion (due to right ventricular volume overload), and (6) thickening of the leaflets. There are circumstances that will affect each of these findings. The length of the E-F slope is determined by how long it takes the left atrium to empty. Therefore, the longer it takes the left atrium to empty, the longer the E-F slope. The presence of a flatted E-F slope does not always indicate mitral stenosis. Aortic regurgitation, espe-cially if the jet is directed toward the anterior mi-tral valve leaflet, will result in E-F flattening (Fig. 13-6), as will an elevated end-diastolic pressure within the left ventricle. Therefore, it is important to have a thorough understanding of the patient's clinical history.

Two-Dimensional Echocardiography

Two-dimensional echocardiography is useful in assessing mitral stenosis because it may provide information on the cause. In rheumatic mitral stenosis, the process begins at the tips of the mitral leaflets and spread toward the annulus along the chordae throughout the submitral apparatus. The leaflets may be thin but dome-shaped throughout diastole. Other causes of mitral stenosis, although rare, can be identified by two-dimensional imaging. Calcific mitral stenosis can be identified by the thickened mitral annular region; it lacks the characteristic doming appearance of rheumatic mitral stenosis.

Two-dimensional imaging allows assessment of left atrial size; enlargement is caused by elevated pressures due to the narrow opening. Another important observation is leaflet doming (hockey stick appearance); this is a result of high pressure overload

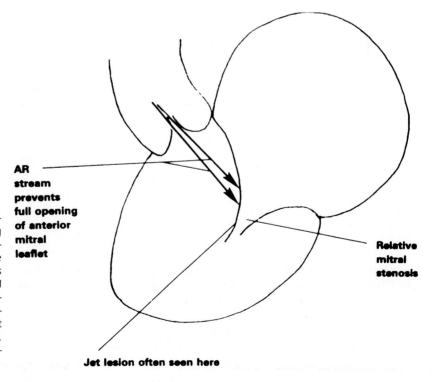

AR stream prevents full opening of anterior mitral leaflet

Relative mitral stenosis

Jet lesion often seen here

Figure 13-6. Aortic insufficiency (AR) may cause flattening of the mitral valve leaflets, particularly if the jet directly strikes the anterior mitral valve leaflet. This clinical scenario can mimic mitral valve stenosis, so careful attention to the patient's clinical condition is important. (From Constant J. Bedside Cardiology, 4th ed. Boston, Little, Brown; 1993:Reprinted with permission.)

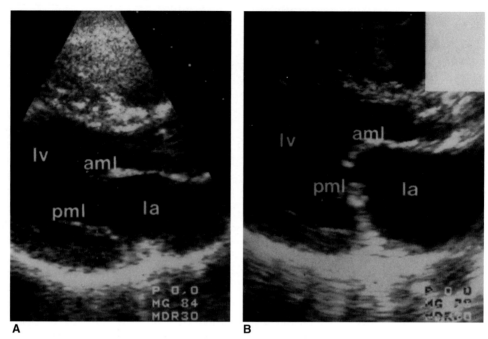

A   B

Figure 13-7. Two-dimensional echocardiogram of normal (**A**) and abnormal (**B**) mitral valve leaflets. In a normal mitral valve the leaflets are thin and separate widely in diastole. In mitral stenosis (**B**) the leaflets dome because they fuse with one another. The classic hockey stick appearance can be appreciated in the stenotic valve. Notice the difference in left atrial size between the patient with (**B**) and without mitral stenosis (**A**). La, left atrium; lv, left ventricle; aml, anterior mitral valve leaflet; pml, posterior mitral valve leaflet.

in the left atrium and also of fusion between the tissues of the leaflets. These signs are seen in at least moderate stenosis (Fig. 13-7*A,B*).

CALCULATING MITRAL VALVE AREAS

Two-Dimensional Planimetry

Mitral valve areas can be measured directly from two-dimensional images. The mitral valve orifice is best visualized from a parasternal short-axis view, with the mitral opening centered in the imaging sector. The transducer is angled superior and inferior between the cardiac base and apex until the very tips of the mitral valve leaflets are appreciated. The measurement is performed at the beginning of diastole when the mitral valve is at its widest excursion[198] (Fig. 13-8). The valve area is traced using the ultrasound system's calipers. The tracing is made along the inside border of the mitral orifice. This method has correlated well with surgical findings,[90] hemodynamic data,[127,140,221,225] and autopsy findings.[221,225]

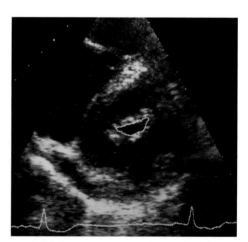

Figure 13-8. Parasternal short-axis view of the mitral valve in mitral stenosis. Beginning in a parasternal short-axis view at the base of the heart, the transducer is angled toward the apex of the left ventricle and then back toward the base. Once the tips of the mitral valve come into the field of view, the area is traced using on-line calipers. Careful attention to gain settings is very important in this measurement.

PITFALLS. Although two-dimensional planimetry is considered the echocardiographic procedure of choice by many in determining mitral valve area, there are problems with this method, including (1) improper imaging plane, (2) inappropriate system gain settings, (3) poor lateral resolution, (4) shadowing from associated calcification, and (5) mitral commissurotomy. Improper imaging planes usually reveal an orifice area that seems to be larger than it actually is.[90] Improper rotation, angulation, or transducer placement can contribute to this error. Great care must be taken to ensure that these errors do not occur. Gain settings that are too high will result in underestimation of the valve area because the extra echoes will fill in the opening, effectively reducing the orifice area[127,140] (Fig. 13-9 *A,B*). Conversely, gain settings that are too low will result in the dropout of echoes, and the sonographer will need to guess where the borders are located. This will result in the overestimation of valve areas. The lateral resolution of ultrasound systems may have some limitations and consequently result in echo dropout, which in turn leaves the sonographer guessing where the borders are located. Heavy calcification of the valve leaflets or annulus may result in extensive shadowing of the orifice. In these situations, accurate area tracings are not possible and should not be attempted if the orifice area cannot be clearly seen.[90] Following a mitral valve commissurotomy or balloon valvuloplasty, the mitral valve area is no longer elliptical and the incised or fractured commissure may not be clearly seen. Due to the distortion of the valve leaflets following these procedures, planimeterization can underestimate the area of the orifice.

Despite these limitations two-dimensional assessment continues to be a reliable method of mitral valve area determination because this method comes closest to measuring true anatomic dimensions and is not influenced by changes in hemodynamic conditions brought about by regurgitation or other changes in loading conditions. Great care should be taken in planimeterizing the mitral valve orifice. At least three measurements should be taken and averaged in patients in normal sinus rhythm, and an average of five tracings should be calculated in patients in atrial fibrillation.[198] Most systems have a playback mode that allows for the proper timing of the maximal orifice excursion.

Doppler Techniques

Doppler measurements allow the calculation of peak and mean gradients, as well as valve area calculations. Several Doppler-derived techniques can be used to calculate the valve area, including the pressure half-time method,[192,197] deceleration time index,[83] continuity equation method,[121,137] proxi-

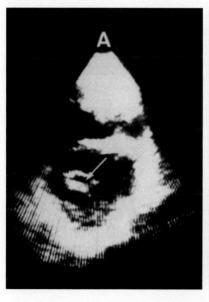 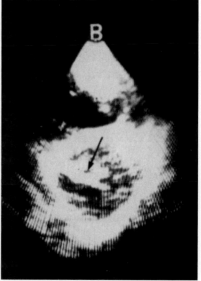

Figure 13-9. Parasternal short-axis view of the mitral valve in mitral stenosis. In this particular case the gain settings are too high (**B**), resulting in an underestimation of valve area. The proper gain settings allow all borders to just be seen (**A**). Gain settings that are too low will lead to dropout of echoes, resulting in overestimation of valve area. (From Feigenbaum H. Echocardiography, 5th ed. Baltimore: Williams & Wilkins, 1994; 243.)

mal isovelocity surface area,[166] and proximal flow convergence.[172] Each of these methods has advantages and disadvantages, and all yield rather good correlations. Apical views are typically used to assess mitral stenosis by Doppler due to blood flow that is nearly parallel to the sound wave.

PRESSURE HALF-TIME. The pressure half-time method has gained widespread acceptance in calculating valve areas of native as well as prosthetic valves. The basic concept was first described in 1976 by Holen et al.[92] and was later modified by Hatle et al.[86] This method measures the time required for the peak gradient to fall by one-half. When the mitral valve area is 1.0 cm^2, it takes roughly 220 msec for the pressure gradient to drop to half of its initial valve (pressure half-time). This calculation is relatively simple and is performed with calipers on most current ultrasound systems. Pressure or pressure difference within the heart is the force driving blood flow. Therefore, the maximum velocity of blood is directly related to the maximum pressure. This relationship is best demonstrated by the Bernoulli equation, which states that pressure is equal to four times velocity squared ($\Delta P = 4V^2$). This is a measure of the rate at which the pressure difference between the left atrium and left ventricle decreases or decays. This decrease or decay will obviously take less time if the valve is wide open and blood flows between the two chambers unimpeded, but if the opening is small, blood flow will be prolonged, thereby maintaining a higher pressure difference between the two chambers over a longer period of time.

In order to obtain an adequate Doppler signal, the cursor is positioned as parallel as possible across the mitral valve. Color Doppler echocardiography can be used to help identify the jet (Fig. 13-10). In mitral stenosis, the jet across the valve may be eccentric. The Doppler signal should be well demarcated, with a clear, crisp audio sound. Once acceptable signals are obtained, the peak velocity is identified and the velocity representing one-half of the original pressure gradient is determined by dividing the peak velocity by the square root of 2 or 1.4 (or multiplying it by 0.71). A line is drawn along the slope, beginning at the peak and intercepting the half-value. Vertical lines are then drawn from the peak to the baseline hash markers, and another vertical line is drawn from the half-value to the baseline.

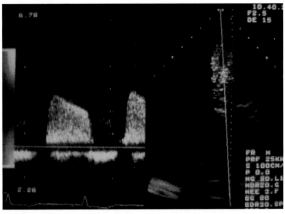

Figure 13-10. In mitral stenosis, pathology of the valve may result in an eccentric jet. The use of color flow Doppler echocardiography may help align the continuous wave (CW) Doppler cursor with the jet, allowing an adequate spectral display. (See also Color Plate 38.)

The distance between these two lines represents time on a Doppler spectral display and is equal to the pressure half-time for the valve (Fig. 13-11). This number is then divided into 220, and the valve area is calculated. This technique has correlated very well with the Gorlin equation used in catheterization laboratories.[26,85,194]

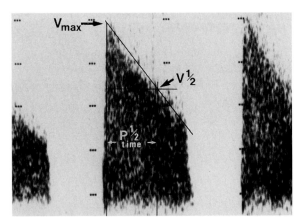

Figure 13-11. Continuous wave Doppler recording across the mitral valve in a patient with mitral stenosis. The mitral valve area is calculated using the pressure half-time method. The maximum early diastolic velocity is identified (V_{max}) and is divided by the square root of 2. This will give the velocity at which the pressure value falls to half of its original value ($V_{1/2}$). A line is drawn intersecting these two points, and the distance between the two points represents the pressure half-time/($P_{1/2}$). The mitral valve area is calculated by dividing 220 by the obtained half-time value.

PITFALLS. Although this method has proven to be useful in the evaluation of mitral stenosis, conditions that alter either pressure or compliance may result in an inaccurate measurement or area calculation. Since this measurement is dependent on pressure differences, distortion of left atrial or ventricular pressure may result in over- or underestimation of mitral valve area. Aortic insufficiency essentially increases pressure within the left ventricle due to the increased volume within the chamber. This tends to shorten the pressure half-time, which in turn leads to overestimation of the mitral valve area.[74,137] An increased left ventricular end-diastolic pressure may also adversely affect the pressure half-time measurement. A stiff or noncompliant left ventricle will also shorten the pressure half-time and overestimate the mitral valve area.[105] Immediately following balloon mitral valvotomy, dramatic differences in left atrial pressure and volume occur, invalidating the pressure half-time calculation.[136] The presence of significant mitral regurgitation increases the initial peak gradient, and the correlation of the Gorlin and pressure half-time methods is poor.[192] The frequent atrial contractions present in atrial fibrillation or flutter may make pressure half-time measurements difficult. In spite of these limitations, the pressure half-time method is widely accepted and is used to measure mitral valve areas. It is an easily performed,

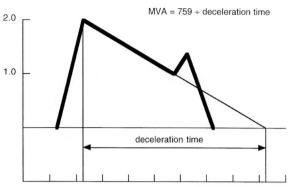

Figure 13-13. A simpler version of the pressure half-time measurement is the deceleration time method. In this measurement, the time taken for the pressure to fall to zero is calculated. A line is drawn from the peak diastolic velocity to the baseline. The time difference is then divided into 750 in order to calculate the mitral valve area.

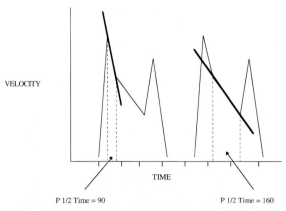

Figure 13-12. Illustration of two different measurements of a stenotic mitral valve spectral display. In the left panel the pressure half-time measurement is taken at the early diastolic peak, resulting in a low-pressure half-time and underestimation of mitral valve area. The right panel demonstrates the correct method of measuring the pressure half-time.

noninvasive test that has good correlation in the absence of atrial fibrillation or flutter. Another potential for error occurs in patients with Lutenbachers syndrome, which is a rare condition in which there is an atrial septal defect associated with mitral valve stenosis. In this clinical setting, the pressure within the left atrium may not increase since blood crosses the interatrial septum. Doppler-derived gradients may not, therefore, be accurate.

The Doppler signal across a stenotic mitral valve is usually linear, but it may demonstrate an early diastolic peak followed by a more linear decay.[86] In this situation, the measurement is obtained from the more dominant slope and the early diastolic peak is ignored (Fig. 13-12). Transesophageal echocardiography (TEE) may have a role in evaluating the mitral valve anatomy more closely. Doppler measurements across the valve from a TEE approach may also be performed; however, a significant angle of incidence may result in an underestimation of valve area in 21 to 32% of patients.[197]

MITRAL DECELERATION TIME. This method is a simpler version of the pressure half-time measurement. It determines the amount of time required for the pressure to fall to zero and is calculated by measuring the time from the peak diastolic velocity to the baseline[234] (Fig. 13-13). The mitral valve area is calculated from the following equation:

$$MVA = \frac{750}{DC}$$

DOPPLER ECHOCARDIOGRAPHY
CONTINUITY EQUATION

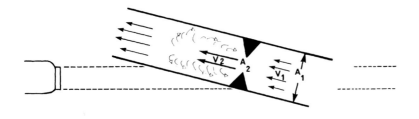

$$A_1 \times V_1 = A_2 \times V_2$$

$$A_2 = \frac{A_1 \times V_1}{V_2}$$

Figure 13-14. Method for calculating mitral valve areas from the continuity equation. (From Feigenbaum H. Echocardiography, 5th ed. Baltimore: Williams & Wilkins; 1994:247. Reprinted with permission.)

where DC is the deceleration time. This measurement follows the same logic as the mitral valve pressure half-time and is therefore susceptible to the same hemodynamic variables.

CONTINUITY EQUATION. The continuity equation is also used to calculate mitral valve area. This equation is based on the principle of conservation of mass and energy where flow in a tube is equal to the product of the mean velocity and the cross-sectional area (Fig. 13-14). Theoretically, this method is independent of transvalvular gradients and atrioventricular compliance and is therefore less likely to be influenced by changing hemodynamic states.[57,105,230] It is reliable and accurate in calculating mitral valve area.[57,105] Three measurements are required to calculate mitral valve area using the continuity equation (see Chapter 14):

1. Velocity time integral (VTI) trace of the spectral Doppler display from the mitral inflow site using continuous wave Doppler.
2. VTI trace of the spectral Doppler display from the mitral outflow site (usually the left ventricular outflow tract [LVOT]) using pulsed wave Doppler. (Taken at the same level as the LVOT diameter measurement.)
3. Diameter of the mitral outflow tract used in the above measurement in systole (widest diameter). Once these measurements are obtained they are substituted in the equation

$$MVA = \frac{LVOT_{VTI} \times LVOT_{diameter}}{MV_{VTI}}$$

PITFALLS. The continuity equation reflects the hemodynamic area of the mitral valve, not the anatomic area. Therefore, for the continuity equation to be accurate, the flow volume across the stenotic valve and the reference valve or LVOT must be equal.[105,137] In the presence of moderate to severe mitral regurgitation, the stroke volume will be inaccurate and will result in underestimation of the mitral valve area. In the presence of severe aortic insufficiency, the stroke volume will be increased, leading ultimately to overestimation of the mitral valve area.[21,105] Other problems with mitral valve area calculated from the continuity equation are associated with the number of calculations required, especially the inherent problems associated with measuring outflow tract diameters (areas). Slight errors in measuring outflow tract diameters lead to large errors in calculating areas.

Proximal Flow Convergence—Proximal Isovelocity Surface Area (Acceleration)

This method is based on the principle of conservation of mass. Color flow Doppler is used to observe flow convergence toward the mitral valve orifice. As flow travels from a large area to a progressively smaller one, flow converges toward the opening, forming concentric isovelocity layers (*iso* = same). Following the principle of conservation of mass, the flow at all of the concentric layers must be equal to the flow in the orifice. Flow at each layer can be calculated by multiplying its velocity by its area[172] (Fig. 13-15). Color flow Doppler recordings are obtained from an apical four-chamber view. The ra-

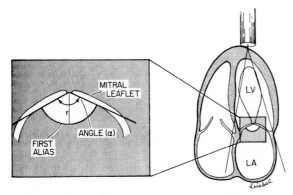

Figure 13-15. Because of the funnel shape of the stenotic mitral orifice, flow cannot converge along hemispheric surfaces, and hence some correction must be introduced to allow for the constriction of the flow field by the mitral leaflets. This diagram illustrates the method for calculating the angle subtended by the stenotic valve, which is then used to correct for the actual deviation from the ideal hemispheric surface. LV, left ventricle; LA, left atrium. (From Weyman AE. Principles and Practice of Echocardiography, 2nd ed. Philadelphia, Lea & Febiger; 1994: 415. Reprinted with permission.)

dius of the flow convergence (Fig. 13-16) is measured at its peak diastolic value from the narrowest portion of the flow convergence, or what is called the *vena contracta*, to the first color alias.[172] The measurement is taken at the vena contracta because this is the narrowest region, where velocities are highest. The anatomic area tends to be larger; there-

fore, if the measurement is taken at the orifice rather than at the vena contracta, the valve area may be inaccurate.[235] Flow rate is calculated by assuming uniform radial flow, but since a stenotic mitral valve is funnel-shaped, the angle must be corrected. The following equation provides the mitral valve area:

$$MVA = 2\pi r^2 \times (\text{angle} \div 180 \text{ degrees})$$
$$\times (V \text{ aliased} \div V \text{ peak})$$

The aliased velocity is obtained from the system's color bar, which indicates the velocity at which aliasing occurs. The color hemisphere can be optimized by shifting the baseline.[14,161,166,170]

PITFALLS. Correlation with planimeterized mitral valve area is excellent.[172] The major limitation of this technique is the relative complexity of the measurements without appropriate software (available currently on some ultrasound systems). Many aspects of this technique require meticulous measuring[166] and may not be appropriate in all clinical settings. The small size of the proximal flow convergence can lead to inaccurate measurements. Baseline shifting can lead to selective suppression of low velocities by the color wall filter. Finally, variations in leaflet geometry may not be accounted for in the simple angle correction measurement made.[172]

Despite these limitations, the proximal flow convergence method allows accurate assessment of

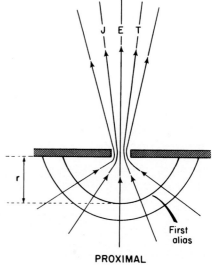

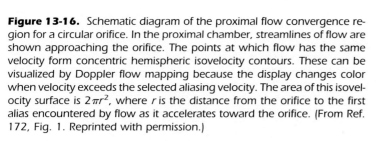

Figure 13-16. Schematic diagram of the proximal flow convergence region for a circular orifice. In the proximal chamber, streamlines of flow are shown approaching the orifice. The points at which flow has the same velocity form concentric hemispheric isovelocity contours. These can be visualized by Doppler flow mapping because the display changes color when velocity exceeds the selected aliasing velocity. The area of this isovelocity surface is $2\pi r^2$, where r is the distance from the orifice to the first alias encountered by flow as it accelerates toward the orifice. (From Ref. 172, Fig. 1. Reprinted with permission.)

mitral stenosis and is not influenced by mitral regurgitation or irregular rhythms.[166] This method offers yet another way to calculate mitral valve area in the setting of stenosis.[172] Table 13-1 summarizes some of the methods and the pitfalls for calculating mitral valve areas.

Percutaneous Balloon Mitral Valvotomy

Once the diagnosis of mitral stenosis is made, the decision to replace or repair the valve by mitral commissurotomy is based upon the severity of the stenosis and the patient's symptoms. Mitral commissurotomy is a process whereby the mitral valve area is enlarged. This method is preferred over valve replacement because of its lower incidence of mortality, morbidity, and postoperative complications.[87] Recently, a new nonsurgical technique has been used to treat patients with mitral stenosis. Valve area is increased by inflating a balloon catheter that has been passed across the interatrial septum and positioned in the mitral valve orifice. The balloon is then inflated, splitting the valve along the commissures without causing traumatic damage to the valve leaflets. This procedure is called *percutaneous mitral balloon valvotomy*. Echocardiography is useful in this procedure by guiding the transseptal catheter and helping to visualize the placement of the balloon in the mitral orifice,[146,149,160,196,202,212] as well as assessing the outcome, identifying complications, and assessing valve area after the procedure.[55,56,80,120,136,144,158,169,171,176,203,213,227] In addition, the extent of the resulting interatrial defect[12,94,168,204] and screening for atrial thrombus before the procedure[38,44,124,167,201] can all be performed by a TEE exam.

TEE is a safe, effective, and valuable tool to monitor each step of the balloon valvotomy. It shortens the time required for the procedure and improves the results.[160] Because the catheter is passed across the atrial septum, an atrial septal defect is created. Examination of the atrial septal defect by TEE can help follow its course and determine the degree of shunting.[12,168] Studies have demonstrated that these defects are minimal and usually disappear in the majority of cases by 3 months.[12,168] Under constant TEE monitoring of the transseptal puncture, balloon placement and follow-up of the valve area can be achieved (Fig. 13-17*A–C*).

Echocardiography is used not only during percutaneous mitral balloon valvotomy and postopera-

◢◢◢ TABLE 13-1. METHODS OF MITRAL VALVE AREA CALCULATIONS

Method	Modality	Pitfalls	Problem
Planimetry	Two-dimensional	High gains	Underestimates
		Low gains	Overestimates
		Commissurotomy	Distorts area
		Improper planes	Under- or overestimates
			Poor visualization
		Shadowing	Overestimates
		Poor lateral resolution	
Pressure half-time (deceleration time method)	Doppler (CW)	Severe AI	Overestimates
		Inc. LVEDP	Overestimates
		Mitral regurgitation	
		A-fib	Too much signal variation
Continuity equation	Doppler (CW, PW)	Severe MR	Underestimates
	Two-dimensional	Severe AI	Overestimates
		Measurement	Erroneous areas
		Cal. errors	
Proximal flow convergence	Color flow Doppler	Complex measurement	Errors if not careful
		Baseline shifting	May overestimate
	Two-dimensional measurement	Variations in leaflet geometry	Errors in angle corrections
		Radius drawn from orifice instead of from vena contracta	Inaccurate area

AI, aortic insufficiency; LVEDP, left ventricular end-diastolic pressure; A-fib, atrial fibrillation; CW, continuous wave Doppler; PW, pulsed wave Doppler.

tive follow-up, but also prior to the procedure to determine appropriate candidates. Contraindications to balloon valvotomy include the presence of severe mitral regurgitation, significant mitral apparatus calcification, severe disease of other valves, and the presence of left atrial thrombus.[160] The presence of an atrial thrombus does not completely rule out the procedure and is usually vigorously treated with anticoagulant therapy, and subsequent resolution of the thrombus is documented by TEE.[142] Wilkins et al.[226] established criteria to help determine which patients can benefit from this procedure.

Morphologic features of the valve, such as leaflet mobility, thickening, degree of calcification, and subvalvular involvement, have been shown to aid in the identification of suitable patients. Echocardiography also identifies associated findings such as mitral and aortic regurgitation, aortic stenosis, tricuspid stenosis and regurgitation, pulmonary hypertension, left atrial thrombus, left and right ventricular function, and the presence of pericardial effusions. Morphologic features of the leaflet, such as thickening, mobility, and calcification, are appreciated from parasternal long and short axis views, as well as apical views. The degree of involvement of the subvalvular structures is investigated from apical views, with attention to the papillary muscles and chordal structures.[226] The valve is scored using the criteria in Table 13-2. Using a scale from 0 to 16, the valve is scored, with the higher scores indicating more severe disease. These criteria have proven to be better predictors of the outcome of percutaneous mitral balloon valvotomy than other clinical or hemodynamic variables. Patients whose valvular score is 8 or less have a favorable outcome, while those with a score of 9 or higher usually do not. However, a high score does not necessarily preclude a good outcome. Statistically, these criteria have proved to be better predictors of the outcome than any other evaluation tool, but they do not reliably predict postdilatation mitral regurgitation.[1,226] Of all these criteria, the presence of diffuse calcification involving most of the mitral apparatus predicts a suboptimal outcome.

Echocardiographically Derived Values for Mitral Stenosis

Values for mitral stenosis derived from echocardiographic examinations are as follows:

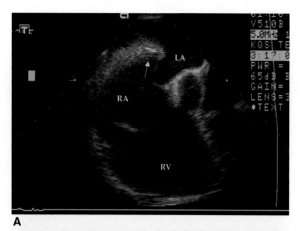

A

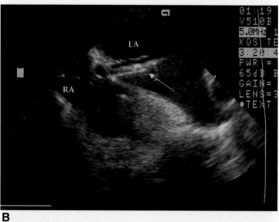

B

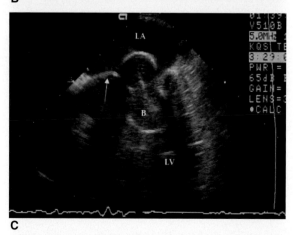

C

Figure 13-17. TEE scan of a patient with mitral stenosis undergoing a percutaneous mitral valve balloon valvotomy. (**A**) The catheter is guided across the interatrial septum (arrow). (**B**) The catheter has crossed the interatrial septum and is noted in the left atrium. (**C**) The catheter is guided across the mitral valve and the balloon is inflated (B), creating a larger mitral valve area (arrow). TEE or TTE can then be used to calculate the valve area. LA, left atrium; LV, left ventricle; RA, right atrium; RV, right ventricle.

TABLE 13-2. GRADING OF MITRAL VALVE CHARACTERISTICS FROM THE ECHOCARDIOGRAPHIC EXAMINATION

Grade	Mobility	Subvalvular Thickening	Thickening	Calcification
1	Highly mobile valve with only leaflet tips restricted	Minimal thickening just below the mitral leaflets	Leaflets near normal in thickness (4–5 mm)	A single area of increased echo brightness
2	Leaflet mild and base portions have normal mobility	Thickening of chordal structures extending up to one-third of the chordal length	Midleaflets normal, considerable thickening of margins (5–8 mm)	Scattered areas of brightness confined to leaflet margins
3	Valve continues to move forward in diastole, mainly from the base	Thickening extending to the distal third of the chords	Thickening extending through the entire leaflet (5–8 mm)	Brightness extending into the midportion of the leaflets
4	No or minimal forward movement of the leaflets in diastole	Extensive thickening and shortening of all chordal structures extending down to the papillary muscles	Considerable thickening of all leaflet tissue (>8–10 mm)	Extensive brightness throughout much of the leaflet tissue

Note: The total echocardiographic score was derived from an analysis of mitral leaflet mobility, valvular and subvalvular thickening, and calcification, which were graded from 0 to 4 according to the above criteria. This gave a total score of 0 to 16.

Source: Ref. 26.

MITRAL VALVE AREA

Normal	>2.5 cm^2
Mild	1.5 to 2.5 cm^2
Moderate	1.0 to 1.5 cm^2
Severe	<1.0 cm^2

PRESSURE HALF-TIME

Normal	30 to 60 msec
Mild	90 to 150 msec
Moderate	150 to 219 msec
Severe	≥220 msec

MEAN PRESSURE GRADIENT

Mild	≤5 mm Hg
Moderate	6 to 12 mm Hg
Severe	>12 mm Hg

Mitral Regurgitation

Echocardiography is ideal for evaluating the presence of mitral regurgitation, as well as for grading its severity. In addition, echocardiography can be used to help identify the etiology of the regurgitant lesion. Mitral regurgitation can be caused by a number of pathologic conditions such as rheumatic mitral valve disease, mitral valve prolapse,[65,218] myocardial infarction (papillary muscle dysfunction),[17,75,103] rup-tured chordae tendineae, flail mitral valve leaflets, mitral valve vegetations, heart transplant,[163] dilated cardiomyopathies,[101] and left ventricular outflow tract obstructions.[222] Mitral valve regurgitation can also be found in patients with normal "echocardiographic" hearts.[117,207]

ECHOCARDIOGRAPHIC VIEWS

The mitral valve can be viewed from a number of acoustic windows that allow a thorough assessment of its structure and hemodynamic characteristics. Two-dimensional echocardiography may allow suspicion of mitral regurgitation, but for quantification, Doppler echocardiography is ideal. A number of techniques and measurements can be used to assess the severity of regurgitation. The effects of mitral regurgitation on other cardiac chambers and vessels may also provide some idea of the severity of the lesion. Factors such as jet size (length and width), area, and volume can be assessed using echocardiography. A great deal of research has been done in an effort to find quantitative methods to help assess the severity of mitral regurgitation.

SECONDARY FINDINGS

Left Atrium and Ventricle

Mitral regurgitation may be chronic or acute. In acute mitral regurgitation, there is usually no significant change in the size or function of either the left atrium or left ventricle.[216] In chronic mitral regurgitation, left atrial and ventricular volume increases.[25,238] As a result, left ventricular end-diastolic and end-systolic dimensions increase, ultimately increasing left ventricular mass calculations. If this condition is left untreated, left ventricular function may become impaired due to the volume overload. The treatment of clinically significant mitral regurgitation includes mitral valve replacement or repair.[216] Following valve repair or replacement, left ventricular function, as measured by the ejection fraction, improves and left ventricular dimensions decrease.[238] Dilated left atrial dimensions, as measured anteroposteriorly and superoinferiorly, correlate very well with severe mitral regurgitation.[25] Left ventricular systolic function and left atrial dimension are widely used as prognostic indicators in patients with significant mitral regurgitation.[162]

ASSESSING MITRAL REGURGITATION

Assessment of the severity of mitral regurgitation is clinically important. A number of techniques have been developed to help find a reproducible and reliable, noninvasive method of doing so. Echocardiographic techniques range from visual estimations of color flow Doppler jet size, shape, and area to more involved quantitative measures and calculations. Correlation of these various procedures with gold standard techniques is good, but regardless of the reported literature, internal validation should always be obtained prior to routine reporting. In addition, the pitfalls of each technique should be well appreciated in order to avoid making erroneous diagnoses.

Pulsed Wave Doppler

From apical views, pulsed wave Doppler echocardiography can be used to map the left atrium for the presence of mitral regurgitation. This procedure requires point-by-point assessment of the entire left atrium with the range gate using the pulsed wave technique. The interrogation begins by positioning the sample volume immediately above the mitral valve in the left atrium and systematically swinging the sample volume to the left or toward the interatrial septum and back to the right. This is done at each level of the atrium until the top of the chamber is reached[2,152,159] (Fig. 13-18). Scoring of the degree of mitral valve regurgitation is based on the level at which a regurgitant signal is detected. Mitral regurgitation localized near the mitral leaflets is considered mild, while regurgitation detected near the top of the chamber is considered severe.

PITFALLS. There are several limitations to this technique. First, this process is laborious since the entire left atrium must be mapped. Second, atrial dilatation may lead to overestimation of the severity of mitral regurgitation. Third, eccentric jets may be missed, leading to underestimation of the severity of regurgitation. Finally, effects of attenuation, especially from the far field, may result in weak or missed signals, leading to underestimation of severity. With the advent of color Doppler echocardiography, this technique is seldom used except when color is not available.

Continuous Wave Doppler

Continuous wave Doppler echocardiography has been used to grade the severity of mitral valve regurgitation by studying the intensity of the Doppler signals[209] or the backscatter power.[122] Theoretically, the signal intensity contains information regarding the number of moving particles or scatters encountered within the sound beam.[22] The degree of regurgitation is estimated by visual estimation of the Doppler signal. Low-intensity continuous wave Doppler signals result from jet flow with a small number of scatters, while high-intensity continuous wave Doppler signals contain a large number of scatters[209] (Fig. 13-19). The continuous wave Doppler signal correlates well with the severity of mitral regurgitation.[122,209]

PITFALLS. Using this method to assess the severity of mitral regurgitation does not account for the various anatomic, attenuation, or hemodynamic factors. Additionally, system settings must be constant in order to establish a standard, which is nearly impossible because of patient variability. Still, the results of this method have correlated well with those of other studies, but further work is needed.

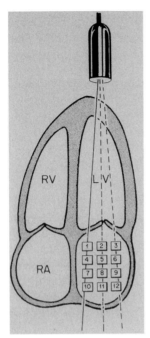

Figure 13-18. Pulsed wave Doppler method of determining the degree of mitral regurgitation. The pulsed wave range gate is positioned at different spots in the left atrium, using an apical view, and systematically swept from one side to the other at different levels until the entire left atrium has been interrogated. RA, right atrium; RV, right ventricle, LA, left atrium; LV, left ventricle. (From Weyman AE. Principles and Practice of Echocardiography, 2nd ed. Philadelphia, Lea & Febiger; 1994. Reprinted with permission.)

Color Flow Doppler

Color flow Doppler provides a quick and relatively accurate assessment of the severity of mitral valve regurgitation.[115,132,170] Color Doppler evaluation of mitral regurgitation can and should be performed from a number of echocardiographic planes (Fig. 13-20*A,B*). The parasternal short-axis, apical four-chamber, apical two-chamber, and apical long axis views and the subcostal four-chamber view allow a better appreciation of the regurgitant jet than imaging in any single plane. The color patterns of mitral regurgitation depend upon the degree of turbulence and the direction of the jet relative to the transducer. From an apical view, jets directed away from the transducer will be blue, but there may also be a mosaic pattern if turbulence exists. From a parasternal long-axis view, the jet may be red or blue,

depending on its angle of flow relative to the position of the transducer.

Jet length, width, and area should be considered together if one is estimating the severity of mitral regurgitation visually. These dimensions are influenced by ultrasound system gain settings such as those involving wall filters, gain, pulse repetition, color maps, and transducer frequency. In addition, constraints of the left atrium and eccentric jets may lead to inaccurate assessment of severity.[170] Still, this method is used in most clinical settings because it allows the echocardiographer to integrate information on jet dynamics and chamber geometry in determining severity.[170] The grade of mitral regurgitation is based on similar characteristics of pulsed wave Doppler. A small color jet noted just above the valve is generally considered mild; a jet that is seen one-third to midway into the left atrium, but that is "full," may be considered mild to moderate; a full jet seen halfway into the left atrium is generally considered moderate; a color jet observed halfway to two-thirds of the way into the left atrium is considered moderate to severe; and a mitral valve regurgitant jet seen filling the entire left atrium and extending to the far wall is generally considered

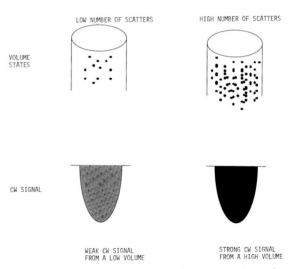

Figure 13-19. Continuous wave Doppler displays of a weak mitral regurgitant signal (left panel) and a strong regurgitant signal (right panel). The signal strength can be used to help grade the severity of the regurgitation because the signal strength is based in part on the number of scatterers (volume) within the sound beam. (Modified from Ref. 208. Reprinted with permission.)

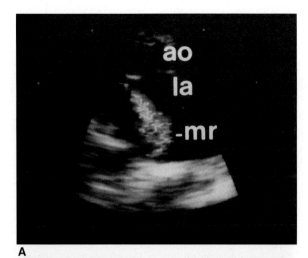

A

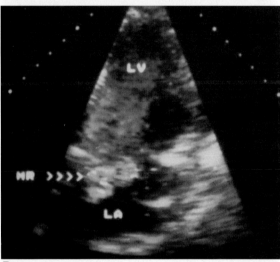

B

Figure 13-20. In assessing the degree of mitral regurgitation by color flow Doppler, a number of imaging planes should be used in order to get a better appreciation of the degree of regurgitation and the secondary findings associated with it. (**A**) Parasternal long-axis view of a patient with mild mitral regurgitation. (**B**) Apical four-chamber view of a patient who also has mild mitral regurgitation. (See also Color Plates 39 and 40.)

severe[185] (Fig. 13-21). In each of these cases, the jet's length, width, and area relative to the left atrium are considered in making the diagnosis. Mitral regurgitant jet areas are measured using the area calipers available on most ultrasound systems.

Jet area is also used as a reference for mitral regurgitation severity. The actual jet is planimeterized and can be reported as an absolute number or as a ratio of the left atrial area as determined from the same plane, but it does not provide a volume calculation. The mitral regurgitation jet area is divided by the left atrial area. A ratio of 0.2 or less is consistent with mild mitral regurgitation, 0.2 to 0.4 is moderate, and 0.4 or greater is severe.[89] This procedure can easily be performed using transthoracic echocardiography (TTE) as well as TEE, with similar results.[30] Inherent in this method is temporal variation in mitral regurgitant jets.[191] The maximal jet can appear during early, middle, or late systole. In addition, jet persistence varies markedly. The relevance of this variation in determining severity is unknown, but it has profound effects on area measurements, so several beats of mitral regurgitant jets should be averaged.

PITFALLS. Major pitfalls associated with this method include the presence of an eccentric jet (Fig. 13-22), in which jet size cannot be fully appreciated.[33,58] System settings will also vary from operator to oper-

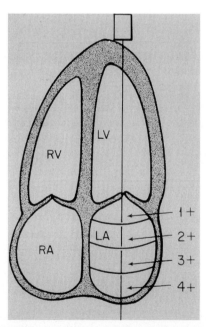

Figure 13-21. Grading used in evaluating the degree of mitral regurgitation by color Doppler echocardiography. 1+, mild; 2+, mild to moderate; 3+, moderate to severe; 4+, severe. LA, left atrium; LV, left ventricle; RA, right atrium; RV, right ventricle. (From Weyman AE. Principles and Practice of Echocardiography, 2nd ed. Philadelphia, Lea & Febiger; 1994:434. Reprinted with permission.)

ator and from patient to patient. Improper gain settings can underestimate the severity if too low or overestimate it if too high. In addition, left atrial compliance will affect the jet geometry.

Jet Width

Jet width alone has also been reported to be an accurate method for the assessment of mitral regurgitation,[63,205] provided that the width of the jet is measured at its origin or at the vena contracta. The best views used to make this measurement are the apical views.[63] The procedure involves a simple diameter measurement of the mitral regurgitation. Cutoff for differentiating mild and moderate from severe degrees of regurgitation range from 3 mm[104] to 6.5 mm.[63,205] The advantages of this method, unlike area determination, is that jet width is independent of flow volume and is not influenced by eccentric jets, and the system's color flow settings can be standardized for this measurement.[63]

Flow Convergence

Accelerating flow proximal to regurgitant orifices such as stenotic and regurgitant lesions has been observed with color flow Doppler echocardiography.[14,34,128,237] The presence of this flow can be used to determine the severity of regurgitation. Using the basis behind the continuity equation, the flow going into the regurgitant orifice must be equal to the flow going out. With this in mind, if flow proximal to the valve can be determined, then flow distal to the leak can be calculated, thereby providing a quantitative measure of severity.[14] In patients with mild regurgitation, flow convergence is typically not observed.[34] It has been suggested that the size of the flow convergence indicates the severity of the regurgitation[34,128,231,237] (Fig. 13-23). Apical views are best suited to identify proximal flow convergence. Proper velocity scales and gain settings are also important in visualizing the color area. The effects of mitral valve prolapse and eccentric jets on the accuracy of this method are still not completely clear, but they may influence the proximal jet size.[34] This method may provide a quick assessment of the severity of mitral regurgitation and may be of particular importance in the assessment of mitral prosthetic regurgitation.[237] The

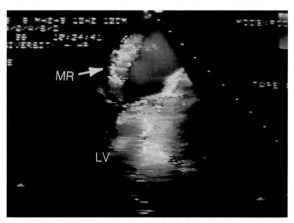

Figure 13-22. TEE scan with color flow Doppler demonstrating an eccentric mitral regurgitant jet in the left atrium (top). MR, mitral regurgitation; LV, left ventricle. (See also Color Plate 41.)

materials that make up prosthetic mitral valves typically shadow the left atrium, making detection and assessment of regurgitation by TTE difficult, if not impossible. Because this technique evaluates flow in the visual field above the mitral valve, flow can be well delineated. Convergence as noted by color Doppler echocardiography is used to evaluate further the severity of mitral regurgitation. This topic is covered in more detail in the next section.

Proximal Isovelocity Surface Area

Limitations of simple color Doppler interrogation of mitral valve regurgitation have led to more quantitative assessments of regurgitation. Most Doppler methods are influenced by hemodynamic changes and so may not provide an accurate assessment of severity. The effective regurgitant orifice area, on the other hand, is less likely to be influenced by these changes and therefore provides a more realistic assessment of the severity of regurgitation.[235,236] The effective regurgitant orifice area is a measure of the severity of mitral regurgitation and is also a major determinant of left atrial and ventricular enlargement in the setting of mitral regurgitation.[61,209] The proximal isovelocity surface area (PISA) appears to hold the promise of becoming a reliable and reproducible method in assessing the degree of mitral regurgitation and can be used to

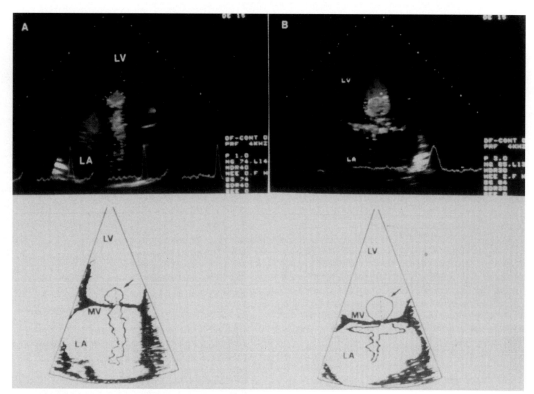

Figure 13-23. Color Doppler echocardiograms obtained from the apical approach. Flow convergence region (FCR) is represented as a homogeneous blue flow pattern located on ventricular side of mitral valve (MV), with a central aliased zone, immediately proximal to orifice, that is yellow-red (arrow). First aliasing limit is shifted to 38 cm/sec. Panel **A**: Moderate to severe mitral regurgitation in a patient with central jet. Measured FCR radius is 11 mm. Panel **B**: Severe mitral regurgitation in a patient with eccentric jet. Measured radius is 18 mm. LA, left atrium; LV, left ventricle. (From Ref. 14, Fig. 3. Reprinted with permission.)

calculate effective regurgitant orifice area.[61,72,81,161,189,209,233,237] This technique, unlike others, evaluates flow proximal to the regurgitant orifice, where it remains laminar and therefore more predictable. Measurements for this technique are relatively simple but do require careful attention to detail. The ideal echocardiographic views for obtaining the necessary measurements are the apical views, particularly the apical four-chamber view.

As blood approaches a regurgitant orifice such as a mitral valve, its velocity increases, forming concentric hemispheres. The velocity of blood at any spot in a given hemisphere is the same (Fig. 13-24). The hemispheres closest to the orifice have the highest velocity, while their surface area decreases. Using color Doppler, these hemispheres can be differentiated from one another due to

aliasing at particular velocities. To identify these hemispheres traveling at different velocities, the baseline is shifted downward to display a red-blue transition. The velocity at which this transition occurs is the aliased velocity at the hemisphere, or V_n (Fig. 13-25). The instantaneous flow across the orifice can be calculated by multiplying V_n by the area of the hemisphere. The area of the hemisphere is calculated as $2\pi r^2$. To determine the area of the hemisphere, the radius is measured from the first aliased transition to the vena contracta or *pinch point*. The radius is then multiplied by 6.283 (2 × π or 2 × 3.14) and then squared. The effective regurgitant orifice area is calculated by dividing the peak regurgitant velocity obtained by continuous wave Doppler scanning across the mitral valve into the product of the aliased velocity and the hemi-

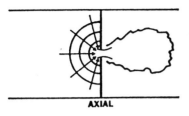

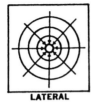

Figure 13-24. Diagrammatic representation of velocity relations for flow through circular orifice visualized in axial direction (top) and in lateral direction (bottom). Velocity along streamlines is constant at any point along any concentric hemispheric surface. According to the continuity principle, flow volume is the same at any hemispheric surface proximal to and at the orifice. (From Ref. 161, Fig. 1. Reprinted with permission.)

spheric area.[189,233] The necessary measurements for this calculation are illustrated in Figure 13-26.

In order to optimize these measurements, do the following important steps. First, optimize the appearance of the proximal flow convergence zone by "zooming" the image. Second, lower the velocity scale and baseline shift in order to enhance the red-blue alias from a distance far enough away from the orifice to allow two-dimensional measurements. Third, use an apical four-chamber view and adjust the gray scale gain controls to optimize the color display. Finally, as with all two-dimensional or Doppler calculations, it is important to use several beats and take the average in making calculations; this increases accuracy.

PITFALLS. The results of PISA appear to correlate with those obtained by other techniques. However, this technique has limitations. The major problems are related to the geometric assumption made about flow convergence. Flow convergence is assumed to be hemispheric. This may not always be the case since the hemispheres tend to flatten out the closer they come to the orifice. This leads to an underesti-

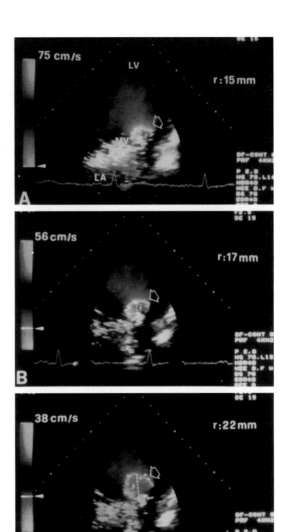

Figure 13-25. Systolic images in a patient with severe mitral regurgitation. Flow convergence region (open arrow) is clearly visible proximal to regurgitant orifice. Zero-line (arrowhead) is progressively shifted to decrease first aliasing limit. Panel **A**: Aliasing limit, 75 cm/sec; *r*, 15; calculated regurgitant flow rate, 1,059 ml/sec. LV, left ventricle; LA, left atrium. Panel **B**: Aliasing limit, 56 cm/sec; *r*, 17 mm; calculated regurgitant flow rate, 1,034 ml/sec. Panel **C**: Aliasing limit, 38 cm/sec; *r*, 22 mm; calculated regurgitant flow rate, 1,155 ml/sec. (From Ref. 14, Fig. 2. Reprinted with permission.)

Mitral Regurgitation Worksheet
PISA Method

Step 1. Color Doppler PISA Measurement

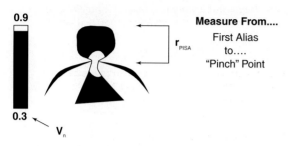

Measure From....
First Alias
to....
"Pinch" Point

Tips

- A4C View
- Adjust color Doppler velocity baseline so V_n is about 0.3 m/s.
- Measure r_{PISA} from first alias to pinch point.

1. The **instantaneous regurgitant flow rate** by PISA is equal to the area of the isovelocity surface area multiplied by the instantaneous flow velocity value (Nyquist velocity).

$$Q_{PISA} = A_{PISA\ SURFACE} * V_n$$
$$Q_{PISA} = 2\pi (r_{PISA})^2 * V_n$$

2. The **instantaneous regurgitant flow rate** can also be calculated from the product of the effective regurgitant orifice area and the instantaneous CW velocity.

$$Q_{MR\ CW} = A_{MR\ EOA} * V\ MR_{max} = Q_{PISA}$$

3. The **regurgitant effective orifice area** is calculated by the quotient of the PISA instantaneous regurgitant flow rate and the instantaneous velocity.

$$A_{MR\ EOA} = Q_{PISA} / V\ MR_{max}$$
$$A_{MR\ EOA} = 2\pi (r_{PISA})^2 * V_n / V\ MR_{max}$$

Step 2. CW Doppler Velocity Measurement

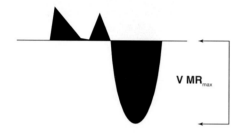

$V\ MR_{max}$

Measurements:

r_{PISA}	_____	cm
$V\ MR_{max}$	_____	cm/sec
V_n	_____	cm/sec

Calculations:

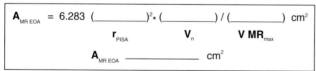

$$A_{MR\ EOA} = 6.283\ (\underline{\hspace{1.5cm}})^2 * (\underline{\hspace{1.5cm}}) / (\underline{\hspace{1.5cm}})\ cm^2$$

r_{PISA} V_n $V\ MR_{max}$

$$A_{MR\ EOA}\ \underline{\hspace{2cm}}\ cm^2$$

Figure 13-26. Worksheet demonstrating the proper calculations for determining the effective regurgitant orifice area ($A_{MR\ EOA}$) using the PISA method. Step 1: Adjust the color baseline to find the first alias. The radius of the PISA (r_{PISA}) is then measured from the vena contracta pinch point to the first aliased velocity. The instantaneous regurgitant flow rate Q_{PISA} is equal to the product of the PISA area and the Nyquist velocity (V_n). Step 2: The maximum velocity across the mitral regurgitation (V MR_{max}) is measured using continuous wave (CW) Doppler. Step 3: Once the three measurements are made, the numbers are substituted into the above equation and the effective regurgitant orifice area is calculated. (Created by Dr. Karl Schwarz, University of Rochester.)

Mitral Regurgitation Worksheet
PWD Doppler Method

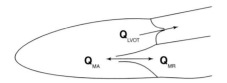

Tips

- Use the lowest possible velocity scale when measuring the VTI at the mitral annulus.
- Measure the mitral annulus in more than one apical view if there is significant calcification.

Grade	RV	$A_{MR\ EOA}$
I	< 30 ml	< 0.2 cm^2
II	30 – 44	0.2 – 0.3
III	45 – 59	0.3 – 0.4
IV	≥ 60 ml	> 0.4 cm^2

1. Mitral **Regurgitant volume** is equal to the difference between total diastolic mitral annular flow and systolic LVOT Flow.
$$RV = Q_{MA} - Q_{LVOT}$$

2. **Regurgitant volume** is also equal to the product of regurgitant effective orifice area and the regurgitant flow velocity integral.
$$RV = A_{MR\ EOA} \times VTI_{MR\ CW}$$

3. **Regurgitant effective orifice area** can be calculated from the quotient of the regurgitant volume and the regurgitant flow velocity integral.
$$A_{MR\ EOA} = RV / VTI_{MR\ CW}$$

4. **Regurgitant fraction** is the regurgitant volume divided by the total diastolic annular flow.
$$RF = RV / Q_{MA}$$

Measurements:

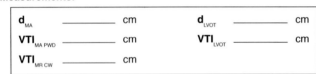

$Q_{MA} = 1/4\ \pi\ (d_{MA})^2 * VTI_{MA\ PWD} = 0.785\ (\underline{\hspace{2cm}})^2 * (\underline{\hspace{2cm}}) = \underline{\hspace{2cm}}$ ml
$\qquad\qquad\qquad\qquad\qquad\qquad\qquad\quad d_{MA} \qquad\quad VTI_{MA\ PWD} \qquad Q_{MA}$

$Q_{LVOT} = 1/4\ \pi\ (d_{LVOT})^2 * VTI_{LVOT} = 0.785\ (\underline{\hspace{2cm}})^2 * (\underline{\hspace{2cm}}) = \underline{\hspace{2cm}}$ ml
$\qquad\qquad\qquad\qquad\qquad\qquad\qquad\quad d_{LVOT} \qquad\quad VTI_{LVOT} \qquad Q_{LVOT}$

$RV = Q_{MA} - Q_{LVOT} = (\underline{\hspace{2cm}}) - (\underline{\hspace{2cm}}) = \underline{\hspace{2cm}}$ ml
$\qquad\qquad\qquad\qquad\qquad Q_{MA} \qquad\quad Q_{LVOT} \qquad RV$

$A_{MR\ EOA} = RV / VTI_{MR\ CW} = (\underline{\hspace{2cm}}) / (\underline{\hspace{2cm}}) = \underline{\hspace{2cm}}$ cm^2
$\qquad\qquad\qquad\qquad\qquad\quad RV \qquad\quad VTI_{MR\ CW} \qquad A_{MR\ EOA}$

$RF = (Q_{MA} - RV) / Q_{MA} = (\underline{\hspace{2cm}}) / (\underline{\hspace{2cm}}) = \underline{\hspace{2cm}}$
$\qquad\qquad\qquad\qquad\qquad\quad RV \qquad\qquad Q_{MA} \qquad RF$

Figure 13-27. Worksheet demonstrating the steps involved in calculating the effective regurgitant orifice area ($A_{MR\ EOA}$) and the regurgitant volume (RV). There are essentially five measurements for this method: the mitral valve annulus (d_{MA}) measured at the annulus level from a four chamber view, the velocity time integral (VTI $_{MA\ PWD}$) using pulsed wave Doppler and positioned at the mitral annulus level, the velocity time integral of the mitral regurgitant signal measured with continuous wave Doppler (VTI $_{MR\ VTI}$), the diameter of the left ventricular outflow tract (d_{LVOT}), and the velocity time integral of the left ventricular outflow tract (VTI $_{LVOT}$). Once these numbers are obtained, they can substituted into the equation, and regurgitant volume and regurgitant area can be calculated. Valves and their corresponding severity are illustrated. (Created by Dr. Karl Schwarz, University of Rochester.)

mation of flow rate. Additionally, the spherical shape of the flow convergence zone may be distorted by geometric constraints such as left ventricular walls or severe mitral regurgitation, causing an overestimation of flow rate.[209] These problems can be overcome by adjusting the aliasing velocity.

Regurgitant Volume

The regurgitant volume provides a quantitative assessment of the degree of mitral regurgitation. It is equal to the difference between systolic flow across the left ventricular outflow tract and diastolic flow across the left ventricular inflow tract. Figure 13-27 illustrates the steps needed to make this calculation.

PULMONARY VENOUS VELOCITIES

Normal Doppler signals across the pulmonary veins demonstrate a biphasic pattern with forward-flow signals observed during both ventricular systole and ventricular diastole[29] (Fig. 13-28). This normal pattern can become altered with atrial fibrillation,[108] left ventricular systolic and diastolic dysfunction,[109,110] constrictive pericarditis,[182] pulmonary venous obstruction,[42] and severe mitral regurgitation.[152] The flow patterns observed in patients with increasingly severe mitral regurgitation included an increase in peak diastolic velocity and diastolic velocity integral and a decrease in peak systolic velocity and systolic velocity integral. In severe mitral regurgitation, the systolic signal may become reversed[29] (Fig. 13-29). In one study the sensitivity of reversed systolic flow in severe mitral regurgitation was 90%.[29]

The pulmonary arteries can be seen by TTE and are normally seen from an apical four-chamber view. Poor acoustic windows and attenuation make clear delineation of flow signals difficult in some patients. TEE tends to provide a much clearer view of the vessels.

TABLE 13-3. METHODS FOR DETERMINING SEVERITY OF MITRAL REGURGITATION

Method	Modalities	Pitfalls	Problem
Pulsed mapping	Pulsed wave Doppler	Tedious	Underestimates
		Attenuation	Underestimates
		Dilated LA	Underestimates
		Eccentric jets	Underestimates
Continuous wave Doppler	Continuous wave spectral display	Needs constant gain settings	Inaccurate if gain settings are changed
		No account for hemodynamic changes	
Color flow Doppler		Eccentric jets	Underestimates
		High color gain	Overestimates
		Low color gain	Underestimates
		High system gain	Masks— underestimates
Flow convergence	Color flow Doppler	Not seen in mild MR or all cases	
PISA	Color Doppler Pulsed wave	Improper radius measurement	Under- or overestimates
		Geometric errors	Overestimates
		Flattened hemisphere	Underestimates
Pulmonary venous flow	Pulsed wave Doppler	Attenuation	No or weak signal
		Improper range gate size	No or weak signal
		Limited grading	Poor signal
			Changes in flow signal seen only in severe MR

LA, left atrium; MR, mitral regurgitation; PISA, proximal isovelocity surface area.

Table 13-3 summarizes some of the methods and the pitfalls for evaluating mitral regurgitation.

TEE AND CONTRAST ECHOCARDIOGRAPHY

Assessment of mitral regurgitation by TEE color Doppler[143,177,185,238] and transpulmonary contrast echocardiography[214,215] can be performed accurately and may be valuable in patients with poor transthoracic windows. TEE allows a more thorough evaluation of the left atrium in the presence of a prosthetic mitral valve. Criteria for grading mitral regurgitation by TEE have been proposed (Table 13-4). The area ratio method described above can

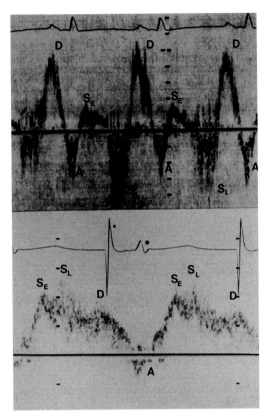

Figure 13-29. Upper panel: Pulmonary venous flow pattern in a patient with severe mitral regurgitation. Note the positive (forward) early systolic wave (S_E) and the negative (regurgitant) flow during ventricular systole (S_L). Lower panel: Pulmonary venous flow in the same patient after mitral valve replacement. Systolic regurgitant flow is absent and the peak diastolic velocity (D) is lower. Postoperatively the patient was on a dual chamber pacemaker. A, atrial contraction wave; *, atrial pacing spike; •, QRS complex. (From Ref. 29, Fig. 3. Reprinted with permission.)

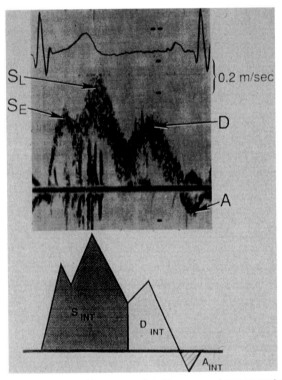

Figure 13-28. Upper panel: Left upper pulmonary vein flow in a normal subject. Note the quadraphasic flow pattern. Lower panel: Schematic diagram indicating how the Doppler velocity signals were analyzed. A, peak velocity corresponding to atrial contraction; A_{INT}, time-velocity integral of reversed flow corresponding to atrial contraction; D, peak diastolic velocity; D_{INT}, time-velocity integral of the forward flow during ventricular diastole; S_E, early systolic velocity; S_L, late systolic velocity; S_{INT}, time-velocity integral of the forward flow during ventricular systole. (From Ref. 29, Fig. 1. Reprinted with permission.)

also be applied. TEE interrogation of mitral regurgitation may not provide a view of the entire left atrium in one plane, but with careful probe manipulation this limitation can be overcome. In severe mitral regurgitation, reversed flow can be noted in the pulmonary veins. TEE allows better interrogation of these vessels than does TTE.

Transpulmonary contrast echocardiography improves the signal-to-noise ratio and significantly enhances both spectral and color Doppler signals.[214,215] This technique has proven to be safe and well tolerated by patients. It is particularly useful in patients with poor acoustic windows where clear mitral regurgitant signals are weak. Contrast agents

TABLE 13-4. Criteria for Assessing Severity of Mitral Regurgitation (MR) Evaluated by TEE

Degree of MR	TEE-MR Area	TF	SBF
Mild	1–3 cm²	–	–
Mild to moderate	3 cm²	–	–
Moderate to severe	3 cm²	+	–
Severe	3 cm²	+	+

TF, turning flow in the left atrium; SBF, systolic backward flow in the pulmonary veins.
Source: Modified from Ref. 177.

capable of passing through the pulmonary vasculature and surviving long enough to opacify the left heart are becoming available. This technique shows great promise in the future.

DIASTOLIC MITRAL REGURGITATION

Mitral regurgitation is typically a systolic event. However, under various conditions, mitral regurgitation can be noted during diastole (Fig. 13-30). Diastolic regurgitation usually occurs during atrioventricular block,[148] but it has also been observed in atrial fibrillation or flutter, severe aortic insufficiency, and diastolic left ventricular abnormalities.[173] This

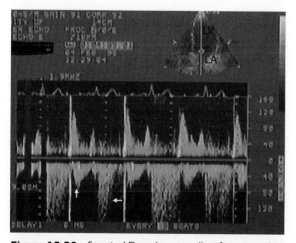

Figure 13-30. Spectral Doppler recording from a patient with both systolic (horizontal arrow) and diastolic (vertical arrow) mitral regurgitation. The systolic mitral regurgitation begins immediately following the QRS. The diastolic regurgitation begins after the P wave.

condition occurs because left atrial pressure is allowed to fall below left ventricular pressure.

Mitral Valve Prolapse

Mitral valve prolapse (MVP) is characterized by protruding or buckling of one or both mitral leaflets into the left atrium in systole in varying degrees.[184] The leaflets extend above the plane of the mitral valve annulus. However, mild posterior displacement of the leaflets may be considered normal, requiring rather strict criteria for the diagnosis of this disease. Since a diagnosis of mitral valve prolapse carries with it a need for antibacterial prophylaxis (antibiotics), as well as the emotional burden of having "heart disease," it is important not to overdiagnose.[184] The need for strict criteria comes from the fact that the mitral valve leaflets may appear large and "redundant" in normal individuals. This is a function of the relatively large size of the leaflets compared to the small left ventricles.[45,134] MVP has also been noted in ballet dancers,[40] as well as in patients with anorexia nervosa.[129] It may be frequently diagnosed to explain such symptoms as arrhythmias, chest pain, "panic attacks," and systemic emboli because MVP is frequently associated with such findings.[184]

MVP is relatively common in thin, young women[220] and in patients with Marfan's syndrome.[199] The major complication of MVP is varying degrees of mitral regurgitation.[78,155] However, there are patients with MVP who do not have significant mitral regurgitation. Bacterial endocarditis is another complication associated with MVP, presumably due to leaflet thickening.[126] Other complications include flail mitral valve[184] and sudden death from ventricular tachycardia or fibrillation.[27,239]

Clinically, the diagnosis of MVP is based on the auscultative findings of a systolic click and an apical systolic murmur. Echocardiographic definition of MVP is fairly pronounced. First, there is late systolic bulging or buckling of one or both leaflets posterosuperior to the plane of the mitral annulus. Generally, if the leaflets prolapse ≥3 mm beyond the mitral annulus late in systole, the diagnosis of MVP is made[64,153,184] (Fig. 13-31). This condition is seen using either M-mode or two-dimensional echocardiography from a left parasternal long-axis view. Holosystolic displacement of the mitral valve may also be seen, but it does not necessarily indicate pro-

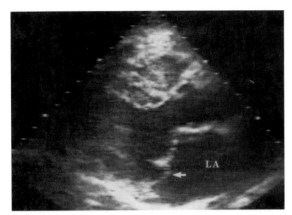

Figure 13-31. Two-dimensional echocardiogram of classic mitral valve prolapse, the mitral valve leaflets are seen buckling above the plane of the mitral annulus. (From Jawad IA. Practical Guide to Echo & Cardiac Doppler, 2nd ed. Reprinted with permission.)

lapse.[82] Second, the leaflets are typically thickened in MVP. This finding can be difficult to make by echocardiography, since structural thickness can be influenced by gain settings. It is therefore important that the sonographer use appropriate gain settings and compare the thickness of other structures at the same depth, such as the aortic valve cusps, to that of the mitral leaflets.[184]

The two-dimensional parasternal long-axis view is ideally suited to make this diagnosis because the mitral valve is perpendicular to the sound beam. The apical views have been proposed as appropriate views as well. However, recent work has shown the mitral annulus to be saddle-shaped rather than flat or circular, and its connection to the skeletal structure of the heart tends to be high in the anterior and posterior segments and lower in the medial and lateral segments.[118,119] Therefore, the leaflets can appear to be above the annular plane if imaged through the medial and lateral low points, indicating prolapse, or can appear to be below the mitral annulus if imaged through the high points[118,119] (Fig. 13-32). Therefore, apical views may lead to the overdiagnosis of MVP.[179]

M-mode has long been used to diagnose MVP. With the M-mode cursor positioned at the tips of the mitral valve leaflets, the prolapsing commissures are seen to be displaced posteriorly in midsystole (Fig. 13-33). However, one must exercise caution

when using M-mode to evaluate for MVP. If the transducer is positioned too low on the chest, prolapse may be missed. If the transducer is placed too high on the chest and angled downward, false MVP can be created. To avoid these potential errors, the sonographer should pay close attention to the ap-

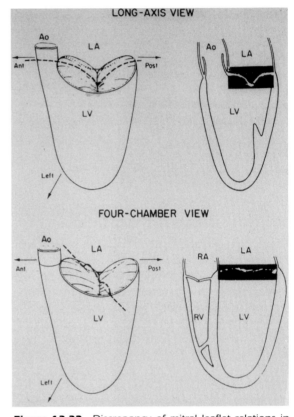

Figure 13-32. Discrepancy of mitral leaflet relations in two-dimensional echocardiographic views (long axis and four chamber) of an in vitro model (left) with a saddle-shaped annulus and leaflets that are concave toward the left ventricle (LV), reflecting its distending pressure. The highest points of the saddle (farthest from the apex) are considered to be located anteriorly (Ant.) and posteriorly (Post.), with medial and lateral low points consistent with in vivo observations. The heavy interrupted lines on the left indicate the plane of view. On the right, echocardiographic images of the model are shown, along with diagrams of surrounding structures. The dotted lines in the echocardiographic images demarcate an apparent annular plane in each view; they are manually placed with the aid of the echocardiographic instrument. Of note, the leaflets lie below the annular plane in the long axis view and above the plane in the four-chamber view. Ao, aorta; LA, left atrium; RA, right atrium; RV, right ventricle. (Ref. 118, Fig. 17-18. Reprinted by permission of the American Heart Association, Inc.)

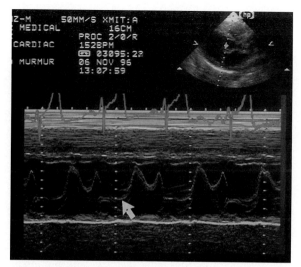

Figure 13-33. M-mode echocardiogram of MVP. The diagnosis is based on the scooped effect of the leaflets at their closure line (arrow) in systole.

pearance of surrounding structures to ensure the use of correct echocardiographic planes.[125,224]

Echocardiography, especially two-dimensional echocardiography, is a valuable tool in the evaluation of the mitral valve for prolapse. Color flow Doppler is useful in assessing the severity of associated mitral regurgitation. It is important, however, to establish strict echocardiographic criteria for its diagnosis and to be aware of the potential for error using this method.

Flail Leaflets and Aneurysms of the Mitral Valve

Flail mitral valve leaflets demonstrate a whipping motion and are seen prolapsing well into the left atrium.[131] In diastole the flail leaflet is seen in the left ventricle, and in systole it is seen in the atrium. Because there is a loss of coaptation between the two leaflets, there is usually significant mitral regurgitation. The parasternal and apical views should be used to evaluate flail leaflets since its whipping motion may cause it to move into and out of the plane.

Aneurysms of the mitral valve are uncommon and usually occur in association with infective endocarditis.[157] Aneurysm can affect either leaflet but is more common on the anterior leaflet. This is

thought to occur because the primary site of infection is the aortic valve, which results in aortic insufficiency. The aortic insufficiency jet strikes the anterior leaflet, producing jet lesions and consequent leaflet infection. Mitral valve aneurysms appear as localized bulges arising from the mitral leaflet and extending for a variable distance (Fig. 13-34A,B). There may also be perforations that allow blood to flow across the valve. These can be visualized on color flow Doppler (Fig. 13-34C). These

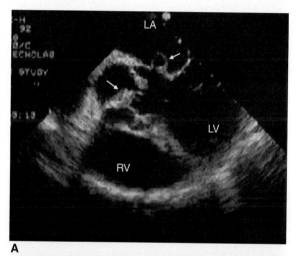

A

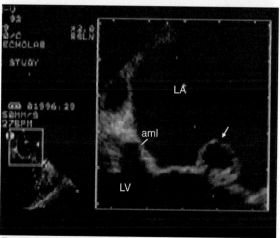

B

Figure 13-34. TEE scans of a patient with infective bacterial endocarditis that originated on the aortic valve. An aortic insufficiency jet lesion is believed to be responsible for the anterior mitral valve leaflet aneurysm (arrow). (**A**) The aneurysm demonstrates the classic bulge. (**B**) Magnified image of the aneurysm. (continues)

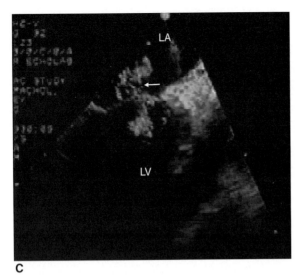

C

Figure 13-34. (Continued) **(C)** Color Doppler can be seen across the aneurysm. (See also Color Plate 42.) This patient also had an aortic root abscess.

patients are usually in very critical condition because the aneurysms may rupture, causing catastrophic mitral regurgitation. Aneurysms can be detected using TTE, but TEE exams usually allow a more detailed look at the lesion.

REFERENCES

1. Abascal VM, Wilkins GT, Choong CY, et al. Mitral regurgitation after percutaneous mitral valvuloplasty in adults: Evaluation by pulsed Doppler echocardiography. J Am Coll Cardiol. 1988;11: 257–263.

2. Abbasi AS, Allen MW, DeCristofara D, et al. Detection and estimation of the degree of mitral regurgitation by range-gated pulsed Doppler echocardiography. Circulation. 1980;61:143.

3. Alam M, Sun I. Superiority of transesophageal echocardiography in detecting ruptured mitral chordae tendineae. Am Heart J. 1991;121(6): 1819–1821.

4. Aronow WS. Usefulness of M-mode, 2-dimensional, and Doppler echocardiography in the diagnosis, prognosis, and management of valvular aortic stenosis, aortic regurgitation, and mitral annular calcium in older patients. J Am Geriatr Soc. 1995; 43:295–300.

5. Aronow WS, Koenigsberg M, Kronzon I, et al. Association of mitral annular calcium with new thromboembolic stroke and cardiac events at 39-month follow-up in elderly patients. Am J Cardiol. 1990; 65:1511–1512.

6. Aronow WS, Kronzon I. Correlation of prevalence and severity of mitral regurgitation and mitral stenosis determined by Doppler echocardiography with physical signs of mitral regurgitation and mitral stenosis in 100 patients aged 62 to 100 years with mitral annular calcium. Am J Cardiol. 1987; 60:1189–1190.

7. Aronow WS, Schoenfeld MR, Gutstein H. Frequency of thromboembolic stroke in persons ≥60 years of age with extracranial carotid arterial disease and/or mitral annular calcium. Am J Cardiol. 1992; 70:123–124.

8. Aronow WS, Schwartz KS, Koenigsberg M. Correlation of aortic cuspal and aortic root disease with aortic systolic ejection murmurs and mitral annular calcium in persons older than 62 years in a long-term health care facility. Am J Cardiol. 1986;58: 651–652.

9. Aronow WS, Schwartz KS, Koenigsberg M. Correlation of atrial fibrillation with presence or absence of mitral annular calcium in 604 persons older than 60 years. Am J Cardiol. 1987;59:1213–1214.

10. Aronow WS, Schwartz KS, Koenigsberg M. Correlation of murmurs of mitral stenosis and mitral regurgitation with presence of mitral annular calcium in persons older than 62 years in a long-term health care facility. Am J Cardiol. 1987;59:181–182.

11. Aronow WS, Schwartz KS, Koenigsberg M. Correlation of serum lipids, calcium and phosphorus, diabetes mellitus, aortic valve stenosis and history of systemic hypertension with presence or absence of mitral annular calcium in persons older than 62 years in a long-term health care facility. Am J Cardiol. 1987;59:381–382.

12. Arora R, Jolly N, Kalra GS, et al. Atrial septal defect after balloon mitral valvuloplasty: A transesophageal echocardiographic study. Angiology. 1993; 44(3):217–221.

13. Baker CG, Finnegan TRL. Epilepsy and mitral stenosis. Br Heart J. 1957;19:159–163.

14. Bargiggia GS, Tronconi L, Sahn DJ, et al. A new method for quantitation of mitral regurgitation based on color flow Doppler imaging of flow convergence proximal to regurgitant orifice. Circulation. 1991;84(4):1481–1489.

15. Benjamin EJ, Plehn JF, D'Agostino RB, et al. Mitral annular calcification and the risk of stroke in an elderly cohort. N Engl J Med. 1992;6:371–379.

16. Bernstein NE, Tunick PA, Freedberg RS, et al. Presumed single-leaflet mitral valve: Recognition by transthoracic and transesophageal echocardiography. Am Heart J. 1994;127:216–219.

17. Bhatnagar SK, Al Yusuf AR. Significance of a mitral regurgitation systolic murmur complicating a first acute myocardial infarction in the coronary care unit—assessment by colour Doppler flow imaging. Eur Heart J. 1991;12:1311–1315.

18. Biasucci LM, Lombardo A, Rossi E, et al. Color Doppler study of mitral regurgitation during percutaneous transluminal coronary angioplasty. Am Heart J. 1993;127(6):1491–1496.

19. Black IW, Hopkins AP, Lee L, et al. Left atrial spontaneous echo contrast: A clinical and echocardiographic analysis. J Am Coll Cardiol. 1991;18(2):398–404.

20. Bonow RO, et al. Reversal of left ventricular dysfunction after aortic valve replacement for chronic aortic regurgitation: Influence of duration of preoperative left ventricular dysfunction. Circulation. 1984;70:570–579.

21. Braverman AC, Thomas JD, Lee RT. Doppler echocardiographic estimation of mitral valve area during changing hemodynamic conditions. Am J Cardiol. 1991;68:1485–1490.

22. Brody WR, Meindl JD. Theoretical analysis of the CW Doppler ultrasonic flowmeter. IEEE Trans Biomed Engl. 1974;21:183–192.

23. Buchbinder NA, Roberts WC. Left-sided valvular active infective endocarditis: A study of forty-five necropsy patients. Am J Med. 1972;53:20–35.

24. Burnside JW, Desanctis RW. Bacterial endocarditis on calcification of the mitral annulus fibrosus. Ann Intern Med. 1972;76:615–618.

25. Burwash IG, Blackmore GL, Koilpillai CJ. Usefulness of left atrial and left ventricular chamber sizes as predictors of the severity of mitral regurgitation. Am J Cardiol. 1992;70:774–779.

26. Byrg RJ, Williams GA, Labovitz AJ, et al. Effects of atrial fibrillation and mitral regurgitation on calculated mitral valve area in mitral stenosis. Am J Cardiol. 1986;57:634.

27. Campbell RWF, Goodman MG, Fiddler GI, et al. Ventricular arrhythmias in syndrome of balloon deformity of mitral valve. Definition of possible high-risk group. Br Heart J. 1976;38:1053.

28. Carabello BA. What exactly is 2+ to 3+ mitral regurgitation? J Am Coll Cardiol. 1992;19(2):339–440.

29. Castello R, Pearson AC, Lenzen P, et al. Effect of mitral regurgitation on pulmonary venous velocities derived from transesophageal echocardiography color-guided pulsed Doppler imaging. J Am Coll Cardiol. 1991;17(7):1499–1506.

30. Castello R, Lenzen P, Aguirre F, et al. Variability in the quantitation of mitral regurgitation by Doppler color flow mapping: Comparison of transthoracic and transesophageal studies. J Am Coll Cardiol. 1992;20(2):433–438.

31. Chen C, Schneider B, Koschyk D, et al. Biplane transesophageal color Doppler echocardiography for assessment of mitral valve area with mitral inflow jet widths. J Am Soc Echocardiogr. 1995;8(2):121–131.

32. Chen CJ, Rodriguez L, Letho JP, et al. Continuous wave Doppler echocardiography for noninvasive assessment of left ventricular dP/dt and relaxation time constant from mitral regurgitant spectra in patients. J Am Coll Cardiol. 1994;23(4):970–976.

33. Chen C, Thomas JD, Anconina J, et al. Impact of impinging wall jet on color Doppler quantification of mitral regurgitation. Circulation. 1991;84:712–720.

34. Chen C, Koschyk D, Brockhoff C, et al. Noninvasive estimation of regurgitant flow rate and volume in patients with mitral regurgitation by Doppler color mapping of accelerating flow field. J Am Coll Cardiol. 1993;21(2):374–383.

35. Cheriex EC, Pieters FA, Janssen JH, et al. Value of exercise Doppler-echocardiography in patients with mitral stenosis. Int J Cardiol. 1994;45:219–226.

36. Chiang CW, Kuo CT, Chen WJ, et al. Comparisons between female and male patients with mitral stenosis. Br Heart J. 1994;72:567–570.

37. Chiang CW, Lo SK, Kuo CT, et al. Noninvasive predictors of systemic embolism in mitral stenosis: An echocardiographic and clinical study of 500 patients. Chest. 1994;106(2):396–399.

38. Chirillo F, Ramondo A, Dan M, et al. Successful emergency percutaneous balloon mitral valvotomy in a patient with massive left atrial thrombosis: Utility of transesophageal echocardiographic monitoring. Cardiology. 1991;79:161–164.

39. Chow WH, Chow L, Ng W. Free-floating but immobile ball thrombus in left atrium: Diagnosis aided by transesophageal echocardiography. Int J Cardiol. 1993;39:213–215.

40. Cohen JL, Austin SM, Segal KR, et al. Echocardiographic mitral valve prolapse in ballet dancers: A function of leanness. Am Heart J. 1987;113:341.

41. Cohen ID, Sand ME, Sandelski J, et al. Doppler echocardiographic evaluation of severe rheumatic submitral valve stenosis. J Am Soc Echocardiogr. 1994;7(5):542–546.

42. Cooper SG, Sullivan ID, Bull C, et al. Balloon dilatation of pulmonary venous pathway obstruction after Mustard repair for transposition of the great arteries. J Am Coll Cardiol. 1989;14:194–198.

43. Dahan M, Paillole C, Martin D, et al. Determinants of stroke volume response to exercise in patients

with mitral stenosis: A Doppler echocardiographic study. J Am Coll Cardiol. 1993;21(2):384–389.

44. Cormier B, Vahanian A, Lung B, et al. Influence of percutaneous mitral commissurotomy on left atrial spontaneous contrast of mitral stenosis. Am J Cardiol. 1993;71:842–847.

45. Darsee JR, Mikolich R, Nicoloff NB, et al. Prevalence of mitral valve prolapse in presumably healthy young men. Circulation. 1979;59:619.

46. Dashkoff N, Karacuschansky M, Come PC, et al. Echocardiographic features of mitral annulus calcification. Am Heart J. 1977;94:585.

47. da Silva CL, Edwards JE. Parachute mitral valve in the adult. Arq Bras Cardiol. 1973;26:149.

48. David D, Lang RM, Marcus RH, et al. Doppler echocardiographic estimation of transmitral pressure gradients and correlations with micromanometer gradients in mitral stenosis. Cardiology. 1991; 67:1161–1164.

49. D'Cruz IA, Cohen HC, Prabhu R, et al. Clinical manifestations of mitral annulus calcification, with emphasis on its echocardiographic features. Am Heart J. 1977;94:367.

50. D'Cruz IA, Collison HK, Gerrardo L, et al. Two-dimensional echocardiographic detection of staphylococcal vegetation attached to calcified mitral anulus. Am Heart J. 1982;103:295–298.

51. DeDomenico R, Gheno G, Cucchini F. Double orifice in prolapsing mitral valve. Int J Cardiol. 1993; 41:171–172.

52. Enomoto K, Kaji Y, Mayumi T, et al. Frequency of valvular regurgitation by color Doppler echocardiography in systemic lupus erythematosus. Am J Cardiol. 1991;67:209–211.

53. Enriquez-Sarano M, Kaneshige AM, Tajik AJ, et al. Amplitude-weighted mean velocity: Clinical utilization for quantitation of mitral regurgitation. J Am Coll Cardiol. 1993;22(6):1684–1690.

54. DeMaria AN, Smith MD. Quantitation of Doppler color flow recordings: An oxymoron? J Am Coll Cardiol. 1992;20(2):439–440.

55. Derumeaux G, Bonnemains T, Remadi F, et al. Non-invasive assessment of mitral stenosis before and after percutaneous balloon mitral valvotomy by Doppler continuity equation. Eur Heart J. 1992; 13:1034–1039.

56. Desideri A, Vanderperren O, Serra A, et al. Long-term (9 to 33 months) echocardiographic follow-up after successful percutaneous mitral commissurotomy. Am J Cardiol. 1992;69:1602–1606.

57. Dumesnil JG, Honos GN, Lemieux M, et al. Validation and applications of mitral prosthetic valvular areas calculated by Doppler echocardiography. Am J Cardiol. 1990;65:1443–1448.

58. Enriquez-Sarano M, Tajik AJ, Bailey KR, et al. Color flow imaging compared with quantitative Doppler assessment of severity of mitral regurgitation: Influence of eccentricity of jet and mechanism of regurgitation. J Am Coll Cardiol. 1993;21(5): 1211–1219.

59. Enriquez-Sarano M, Tajik AJ, Schaff HV, et al. Echocardiographic prediction of left ventricular function after correction of mitral regurgitation: Results and clinical implications. J Am Coll Cardiol. 1994;24(6):1536–1543.

60. Enriquez-Sarano M, Tajik AJ, Schaff HV, et al. Echocardiographic prediction of survival after surgical correction of organic mitral regurgitation. Circulation. 1994;90(2):830–837.

61. Enriquez-Sarano M, Seward JB, Bailey KR, et al. Effective regurgitant orifice area: A noninvasive Doppler development of an old hemodynamic concept. J Am Coll Cardiol. 1994;23(2):443–451.

62. Eusebio J, Louie EK, Edwards LC, et al. Alterations in transmitral flow dynamics in patients with early mitral valve closure and aortic regurgitation. Am Heart J. 1994;128(5):941–947.

63. Fehske W, Omran H, Manz M, et al. Color-coded Doppler imaging of the vena contracta as a basis for quantification of pure mitral regurgitation. Am J Cardiol. 1994;73:268–274.

64. Feigenbaum H. Echocardiography in management of mitral valve prolapse. Aust NZ J Med. 1992;22: 550–555.

65. Folger GM, Hajar R, Robida A, et al. Occurrence of valvular heart disease in acute rheumatic fever without evident carditis: Colour flow Doppler identification. Br Heart J. 1992;67:434–438.

66. Freeman WK, Schaff HV, Khandheria BK, et al. Intraoperative evaluation of mitral valve regurgitation and repair by transesophageal echocardiography: Incidence and significance of systolic anterior motion. J Am Coll Cardiol. 1992;20(3):599–609.

67. Fulkerson PK, Beaver BM, Auseon JC, et al. Calcification of the mitral annulus: Etiology, clinical associations, complications and therapy. Am J Med. 1979;66:967–977.

68. Gaasch WH, O'Rourke RA, Cohn LH, et al. Mitral valve disease. *In* Schlant R, Alexander RW, O'Rourke RA, et al. (eds): Hurst's The Heart, 8th ed. New York, McGraw-Hill; 1994:1483–1518.

69. Gabor GE, Mohr BD, Goel PC, et al. Echocardiographic and clinical spectrum of mitral annular calcification. Am J Cardiol. 1979;44:31.

70. Ge Z, Zhang Y, Fan D, et al. Simultaneous measurement of left atrial pressure by Doppler echocardiography and catheterization. Int J Cardiol. 1992; 37:243–251.

71. Geibel A, Gornandt L, Kasper W, et al. Reproducibility of Doppler echocardiographic quantification of aortic and mitral valve stenoses: Comparison between two echocardiography centers. Am J Cardiol. 1991;67:1013–1021.

72. Giesler M, Crossman G, Schmidt A, et al. Color Doppler echocardiographic determination of mitral regurgitant flow from the proximal velocity profile of the flow convergence region. Am J Cardiol. 1993;71:217–224.

73. Giesler M, Hombach V. Determination of mitral regurgitant flow rate from color flow maps of the regurgitant flow convergence region. J Am Coll Cardiol. 1993;22(5):1554–1555.

74. Gillam LD, Choong CY, Wilkins GT, et al. The effect of aortic insufficiency on Doppler pressure half-time calculations of mitral valve area in mitral stenosis. Circulation. 1986;74(suppl 2):2–217.

75. Goldman AP, Glover MU, Mick W, et al. Rose of echocardiography/Doppler in cardiogenic shock: Silent mitral regurgitation. Ann Thorac Surg. 1991; 52:296–299.

76. Gorcsan J, Blanc MS, Reddy S, et al. Hemodynamic diagnosis of mitral valve obstruction by left atrial myxoma with transesophageal continuous wave Doppler. Am Heart J. 1993;124(4):1109–1112.

77. Gorcsan J, Snow FR, Paulsen W, et al. Noninvasive estimation of left atrial pressure in patients with congestive heart failure and mitral regurgitation by Doppler echocardiography. Am Heart J. 1991; 121(3):858–863.

78. Grayburn PA, Berke MR, Spain MG, et al. Relation of echocardiographic morphology of the mitral apparatus to mitral regurgitation in mitral valve prolapse: Assessment by Doppler color flow imaging. Am Heart J. 1990;119:1095.

79. Grayburn PA, Fehske W, Omran H, et al. Multiplane transesophageal echocardiographic assessment of mitral regurgitation by Doppler color flow mapping of the vena contracta. Am J Cardiol. 1994; 74:912–917.

80. Grayburn PA. Southwestern internal medicine conference: Clinical applications of transesophageal echocardiography. Am J Med Sci. 1994;307(2): 151–161.

81. Grossman G, Giesler M, Schmidt A, et al. Quantification of mitral regurgitation by colour flow Doppler imaging—value of the "proximal isovelocity surface area" method. Int J Cardiol. 1993;42: 165–173.

82. Haikal M, Alpert MA, Whiting RB, et al. Sensitivity and specificity of M-mode echocardiographic signs of mitral valve prolapse. Am J Cardiol. 1982;50: 185.

83. Halbe D, Bryg RJ, Labovitz AJ. A simplified method for calculating mitral valve area using Doppler echocardiography. Am Heart J. 1988;116: 877.

84. Hammer WJ, Roberts WC, deLeon AC. "Mitral stenosis" secondary to combined "massive" mitral annular calcific deposits and small, hypertrophied left ventricles: Hemodynamic documentation in four patients. Am J Med. 1978;64:371–376.

85. Hatle L, Angelsen B. Doppler Ultrasound in Cardiology: Physical Principles and Clinical Applications, 2nd ed. Philadelphia, Lea & Febiger; 1985.

86. Hatle L, Brubakk A, Tromsdal A, et al. Noninvasive assessment of pressure drop in mitral stenosis by Doppler ultrasound. Br Heart J. 1978;40:131.

87. Heger JJ, Wann LS, Weyman AE, et al. Long-term changes in mitral valve area after successful mitral commissurotomy. Circulation. 1979;59:443.

88. Heinle SK, Tice FD, Kisslo J. Effect of dobutamine stress echocardiography on mitral regurgitation. J Am Coll Cardiol. 1995;25(1):122–127.

89. Helmcke F, Nanda NC, Hsiung MC, et al. Color Doppler assessment of mitral regurgitation with orthogonal planes. Circulation. 1987;75:175–183.

90. Henry WL, Griffith MS, Michaelis MD, et al. Measurements of mitral orifice area in patients with mitral valve disease by real-time two-dimensional echocardiography. Circulation. 1975;51:827.

91. Himelman RB, Kusumoto F, Oken K, et al. The flail mitral valve: Echocardiographic findings by precordial and transesophageal imaging and Doppler color flow mapping. J Am Coll Cardiol. 1991; 17(1):272–279.

92. Holen J, Aaslid R, Landmark K, et al. Determination of pressure gradient in mitral stenosis with a non-invasive ultrasound Doppler technique. Acta Med Scand. 1976;199:455–460.

93. Holen J, Simonsen S. Determination of pressure gradient in mitral stenosis with Doppler echocardiography. Br Heart J. 1979;41:529.

94. Hung JS, Fu M, Yeh KH, et al. Usefulness of intracardiac echocardiography in transseptal puncture during percutaneous transvenous mitral commissurotomy. Am J Cardiol. 1993;72(11):853–854.

95. Hwang JJ, Chen JJ, Lin SC, et al. Diagnostic accuracy of transesophageal echocardiography for detecting left atrial thrombi in patients with rheumatic heart disease having undergone mitral valve operations. Am J Cardiol. 1993;72:677–681.

96. Hwang JJ, Kuan P, Lin SC, et al. Reappraisal by transesophageal echocardiography of the significance of left atrial thrombi in the prediction of systemic arterial embolization in rheumatic mitral valve disease. Am J Cardiol. 1992;70:769–773.

97. Hwang JJ, Kuan P, Chen JJ, et al. Significance of left atrial spontaneous echo contrast in rheumatic mitral valve disease as a predictor of systemic arterial embolization: A transesophageal echocardiographic study. Am Heart J. 1994;127(4):880–885.

98. Hwang JJ, Shyu KG, Hsu KL, et al. Significant mitral regurgitation is protective against left atrial spontaneous echo contrast formation, but not against systemic embolism. Chest. 1994;106(1): 8–12.

99. Jolly N, Mohan JC, Arora R. Transesophageal Doppler pulmonary venous flow pattern and left atrial spontaneous contrast in mitral stenosis. Int J Cardiol. 1992;36:357–360.

100. Jordon RA, Scheifley CH, Edwards JE. Mural thrombosis and arterial embolism in mitral stenosis. A clinicopathologic study of fifty-one cases. Circulation. 1951;33:363–367.

101. Junker A, Thayssen P, Nielsen B, et al. The hemodynamic and prognostic significance of echo-Doppler-proven mitral regurgitation in patients with dilated cardiomyopathy. Cardiology. 1993;83: 14–20.

102. Kalman JM, Jones EF, Lubicz S, et al. Evaluation of mitral valve repair by intraoperative transesophageal echocardiography. Aust NZ J Med. 1993;23: 463–469.

103. Kamp O, DeCock CC, Van Eenige MJ, et al. Influence of pacing-induced myocardial ischemia on left atrial regurgitant jet: A transesophageal echocardiographic study. J Am Coll Cardiol. 1994;23(7): 1584–1589.

104. Kamp O, Dijkstra JW, Huitink H, et al. Transesophageal color flow Doppler mapping in the assessment of native mitral valvular regurgitation: Comparison with left ventricular angiography. J Am Soc Echocardiogr. 1991;4:598–606.

105. Karp K, Teien D, Bjerle P, et al. Reassessment of valve area determinations in mitral stenosis by the pressure half-time method: Impact of left ventricular stiffness and peak diastolic pressure difference. J Am Coll Cardiol. 1989;13:594.

106. Kawahara T, Yamagishi M, Seo H, et al. Application of Doppler color flow imaging to determine valve area in mitral stenosis. J Am Coll Cardiol. 1991; 18(1):185–192.

107. Kennedy JW, Yarnall SR, Murray JA, et al. Quantitative angiocardiography: IV. Relationships of left atrial and ventricular pressure and volume in mitral valve disease. Circulation. 1970;41:817–824.

108. Keren G, Bier A, Sherez J, et al. Atrial contraction is an important determinant of pulmonary venous flow. J Am Coll Cardiol. 1986;7:693–695.

109. Keren G, Sonnenblick EH, Le Jemtel TH, et al. Mitral annulus motion: Relation to pulmonary venous and transmitral flows in normal subjects and in patients with dilated cardiomyopathy. Circulation. 1988;78:621–629.

110. Klein AL, Hatle LK, Burstow DJ, et al. Doppler characterization of left ventricular diastolic function in cardiac amyloidosis. J Am Coll Cardiol. 1989; 13:1017–1026.

111. Klein AL, Stewart WJ, Bartlett J, et al. Effects of mitral regurgitation on pulmonary venous flow and left atrial pressure: An intraoperative transesophageal echocardiographic study. J Am Coll Cardiol. 1992;20(6):1345–1352.

112. Klein AL, Obarski TP, Stewart WJ, et al. Transesophageal Doppler echocardiography of pulmonary venous flow: A new marker of mitral regurgitation severity. J Am Coll Cardiol. 1991;18(2): 518–526.

113. Labovitz AJ. Mitral stenosis and left atrial thrombus: Rose of transesophageal echocardiography. Chest. 1993;103(2):331–332.

114. Labovitz AJ, Nelson JG, Windhorst DM, et al. Frequency of mitral valve dysfunction from mitral annular calcium as detected by Doppler echocardiography. Am J Cardiol. 1985;55:133–137.

115. Lesbre JP, Tribouilloy C. Echo-Doppler quantitative assessment of non-ischemic mitral regurgitation. Eur Heart J. 1991;12(suppl B):10–14.

116. Lai LP, Shyu KG, Chen JJ, et al. Usefulness of pulmonary venous flow pattern and maximal mosaic jet area detected by transesophageal echocardiography in assessing the severity of mitral regurgitation. Am J Cardiol. 1993;72:1310–1313.

117. Lavie CJ, Hebert K, Cassidy M. Prevalence and severity of Doppler-detected valvular regurgitation and estimation of right-sided cardiac pressures in patients with normal two-dimensional echocardiograms. Chest. 1993;103(1):226–231.

118. Levine RA, Triulzi MO, Harrigan P, et al. The relationship of mitral annular shape to the diagnosis of mitral valve prolapse. Circulation. 1987;75:756.

119. Levine RA, Sanfilipo AJ, Marshall JE, et al. Three-dimensional echocardiographic reconstruction of the mitral valve, with implications for the diagnosis of mitral valve prolapse. Circulation. 1989;80:589.

120. Levin TN, Feldman T, Bednarz J, et al. Transesophageal echocardiographic evaluation of mitral valve morphology to predict outcome after balloon mitral valvotomy. Am J Cardiol. 1994;73:707–710.

121. Loperfido F, Laurenzi F, Gimigliano F, et al. A comparison of the assessment of mitral valve area by continuous wave Doppler and cross-sectional echocardiography. Br Heart J. 1987;57:348.

122. MacIsaac AI, McDonald IG, Kirsner RL, et al. Quantification of mitral regurgitation by integrated

Doppler backscatter power. J Am Coll Cardiol. 1994;24(3):690–695.

123. McCully RB, Enriquez-Sarano M, Tajik AJ, et al. Overestimation of severity of ischemic/functional mitral regurgitation by color Doppler jet area. Am J Cardiol. 1994;74:790–793.

124. Manning WJ, Reis GJ, Douglas PS. Use of transesophageal echocardiography to detect left atrial thrombi before percutaneous balloon dilatation of the mitral valve: A prospective study. Br Heart J. 1992;67:170–173.

125. Markiewicz W, London E, Popp RL. Effect of transducer placement on echocardiographic mitral valve motion. Am Heart J. 1978;96:555.

126. Marks AR, Choong CY, Chir MB, et al. Identification of high-risk and low-risk subgroups of patients with mitral valve prolapse. N Engl J Med. 1989; 320:1031.

127. Martin RP, Rakowski H, Kleiman JA, et al. Reliability and reproducibility of two-dimensional echocardiographic measurement of the stenotic mitral valve orifice area. Am J Cardiol. 1979;43:560.

128. Mele D, Vandervoort P, Palacios I, et al. Proximal jet size by Doppler color flow mapping predicts severity of mitral regurgitation. Circulation. 1995; 91(4):746–754.

129. Meyers DG, Starke H, Pearson PH, et al. Mitral valve prolapse in anorexia nervosa. Ann Intern Med. 1986;105:384.

130. Minagoe S, Yoshikawa J, Yoshida K, et al. Obstruction of inferior vena caval orifice by giant left atrium in patients with mitral stenosis: A Doppler echocardiographic study from the right parasternal approach. Circulation. 1992;86(1):214–225.

131. Mintz GS, Kotler MN, Segal BL, et al. Two-dimensional echocardiographic recognition of ruptured chordae tendineae. Circulation. 1978;57:244.

132. Miyatake K, Izumi S, Okamato M, et al. Semiquantitative grading of severity of mitral regurgitation by real-time two-dimensional Doppler flow imaging. J Am Coll Cardiol. 1986;7:82.

133. Mizushige K, Shiota T, Paik J, et al. Effects of pulmonary venous flow direction on mitral regurgitation jet area as imaged by color Doppler flow mapping: An in vitro study. Circulation. 1995;91(6): 1834–1839.

134. Morise AP, Gibson TC, Davis SM, et al. The effect of amyl nitrate on the mitral valve echocardiogram in presumably healthy young adults. Chest. 1982; 81:483.

135. Nair CK, Thomson W, Pyschon K, et al. Long-term follow-up of patients with echocardiographically detected mitral annular calcium and comparison with age- and sex-matched control subjects. Am J Cardiol. 1989;63:465–470.

136. Nakatani S, Nagata S, Beppu S, et al. Acute reduction of mitral valve area after percutaneous balloon mitral valvuloplasty: Assessment with Doppler continuity equation method. Am Heart J. 1991;121: 770–775.

137. Nakatani S, Masuyama T, Kodama K, et al. Value and limitation of Doppler echocardiography in the quantification of stenotic mitral valve area: Comparison of the pressure half-time and continuity equation methods. Circulation. 1988;77:78.

138. Nasser WK, Davis RH, Dillon JC, et al. Atrial myxomas: Clinical and pathological features in nine cases. Am Heart J. 1972;83:694–704.

139. Nishimura RA, Rihal CS, Tajik AJ, et al. Accurate measurement of the transmitral gradient in patients with mitral stenosis: A simultaneous catheterization and Doppler echocardiographic study. J Am Coll Cardiol. 1994;24(1):152–158.

140. Nichol PM, Gilbert BW, Kisslo JA. Two-dimensional echocardiographic assessment of mitral stenosis. Circulation. 1977;55:120.

141. Nishimura RA, Schwartz RS, Tajik AJ, et al. Noninvasive measurement of rate of left ventricular relaxation by Doppler echocardiography: Validation with simultaneous cardiac catheterization. Circulation. 1993;88(1):146–155.

142. Olson LJ, Freeman WK, Enriquez-Sarano M, et al. Transesophageal echocardiographic evaluation of native valvular heart disease. *In* Freeman WK, Seward JB, Khandheria BJ, et al (eds): Transesophageal Echocardiography. Boston, Little, Brown; 1994:187–242.

143. Omoto R, Shunei K, Matsumura M, et al. Evaluation of biplane color Doppler transesophageal echocardiography in 200 consecutive patients. Circulation. 1992;85:1237–1247.

144. O'Shea JP, Abascal VM, Wilkins GT, et al. Unusual sequelae after percutaneous mitral valvuloplasty: A Doppler echocardiographic study. J Am Coll Cardiol. 1992;19(1):186–191.

145. Osterberger LE, Goldstein S, Khaja F, et al. Functional mitral stenosis in patients with massive mitral annular calcification. Circulation. 1981;64:472–476.

146. Otto CM, Davis KB, Holmes DR, et al. Methodologic issues in clinical evaluation of stenosis severity in adults undergoing aortic or mitral balloon valvuloplasty. Am J Cardiol. 1992;69:1607–1616.

147. Pai RG, Pai SM, Bodenheimer MM, et al. Estimation of rate of left ventricular pressure rise by Doppler echocardiography: Its hemodynamic validation. Am Heart J. 1993;126(1):240–242.

148. Panidis JP, Munley B, Facc JR, et al. Diastolic mitral

regurgitation in patients with atrioventricular conduction abnormalities: A common finding by Doppler echocardiography. J Am Coll Cardiol. 1986;7:768.

149. Parro A, Helmcke F, Mahan EF, et al. Value and limitations of color Doppler echocardiography in the evaluation of percutaneous balloon mitral valvuloplasty for isolated mitral stenosis. Am J Cardiol. 1991;67:1261–1267.

150. Pearlman AS. Role of echocardiography in the diagnosis and evaluation of severity of mitral and tricuspid stenosis. Circulation. 1991;84(3):I-193–I-197.

151. Pearlman AS, et al. Echocardiographic detection of mitral regurgitation in mitral valve prolapse. *In* CT Lancee (ed): Echocardiography. The Hague, Martinus Nijhoff; 1979.

152. Pearson AC, Castello R, Wallace PM, et al. Effect of mitral regurgitation on pulmonary venous velocities derived by transesophageal echocardiography (abstract). Circulation. 1989;80(suppl II):II-571.

153. Petrone RK, Klues HG, Panza JA, et al. Coexistence of mitral valve prolapse in a consecutive group of 528 patients with hypertrophic cardiomyopathy assessed with echocardiography. J Am Coll Cardiol. 1992;20(1):55–61.

154. Pieper E, Hellemans IM, Hamer H, et al. Additional value of biplane transesophageal echocardiography in assessing the genesis of mitral regurgitation and the feasibility of valve repair. Am J Cardiol. 1995;75:489–493.

155. Pini R, Devereux RB, Greppi B, et al. Comparison of mitral valve dimensions and motion in mitral valve prolapse with severe mitral regurgitation to uncomplicated mitral valve prolapse and to mitral regurgitation without mitral valve prolapse. Am J Cardiol. 1988;62:257.

156. Pini R, Greppi B, Roman MJ, et al. Time-motion reconstruction of mitral leaflet motion from two-dimensional echocardiography in mitral valve prolapse. Am J Cardiol. 1991;68:215–220.

157. Pocock WA, Lakier JB, Hitchcock JF, et al. Mitral valve aneurysm after infective endocarditis in the billowing mitral leaflet syndrome. Am J Cardiol. 1977;40:130.

158. Prasad K, Radhakrishnan S. Echocardiographic variables affecting surgical outcome in patients undergoing closed mitral commissurotomy. Int J Cardiol. 1992;87:237–242.

159. Quinones MA, Young JB, Waggoner AD, et al. Assessment of pulsed Doppler echocardiography in the detection and quantification of aortic and mitral regurgitation. Br Heart J. 1980;44:612.

160. Ramondo A, Chirillo FA, Dan M, et al. Value and limitations of transesophageal echocardiographic monitoring during percutaneous balloon mitral valvotomy. Int J Cardiol. 1991;31:223–234.

161. Recusani F, Bargiggia GS, Yoganathan AP, et al. A new method for quantification of regurgitant flow rate using color Doppler flow imaging of the flow convergence region proximal to a discrete orifice: An in vitro study. Circulation. 1991;83(2):594–604.

162. Reed D, Abbott RD, Smucker ML, et al. Prediction of outcome after mitral valve replacement in patients with symptomatic chronic mitral regurgitation. The importance of left atrial size. Circulation. 1991;84:23.

163. Rees AP, Milani RV, Lavie CJ, et al. Valvular regurgitation and right-sided cardiac pressures in heart transplant recipients by complete Doppler and color flow evaluation. Chest. 1993;104(1):82–87.

164. Reid CL, Rahimtoola SH. The role of echocardiography/Doppler in catheter balloon treatment of adults with aortic and mitral stenosis. Circulation. 1991;84(3)I-240–I-249.

165. Rey S, Tunon J, Vinolas X, et al. Free-floating left atrial thrombus and its mechanical interaction with mitral regurgitant jet assessed by color Doppler echocardiography. Am Heart J. 1992;123(4):1067–1069.

166. Rifkin RD, Harper K, Tighe D. Comparison of proximal isovelocity surface area method with pressure half-time and planimetry in evaluation of mitral stenosis. J Am Coll Cardiol. 1995;26(2):458–465.

167. Rittoo D, Sutherland GR, Currie P, et al. A prospective study of left atrial spontaneous echo contrast and thrombus in 100 consecutive patients referred for balloon dilation of the mitral valve. J Am Soc Echocardiogr. 1994;7(5):516–527.

168. Rittoo D, Sutherland GR, Shaw T. Quantification of left-to-right atrial shunting and defect size after balloon mitral commissurotomy using biplane transesophageal echocardiography, color flow Doppler mapping, and the principle of proximal flow convergence. Circulation. 1993;87(5):1591–1603.

169. Rittoo D, Sutherland GR, Currie P, et al. The comparative value of transesophageal and transthoracic echocardiography before and after percutaneous mitral balloon valvotomy: A prospective study. Am Heart J. 1993;125(4):1094–1105.

170. Rivera JM, Vandervoort PM, Morris E, et al. Visual assessment of valvular regurgitation: Comparison with quantitative Doppler measurements. J Am Soc Echocardiogr. 1994;7(5):480–487.

171. Rodriguez L, Monterroso VH, Abascal VM, et al. Does asymmetric mitral valve disease predict an adverse outcome after percutaneous balloon mitral

valvotomy? An echocardiographic study. Am Heart J. 1992;123(6):1678–1682.

172. Rodriguez L, Thomas JD, Monterroso V, et al. Validation of the proximal flow convergence method: Calculation of orifice area in patients with mitral stenosis. Circulation. 1993;88(3):1157–1165.

173. Rokey R, Murphy DJ, Nielsen AP, et al. Detection of diastolic atrioventricular valvular regurgitation by pulsed Doppler echocardiography and its association with complete heart block. Am J Cardiol. 1986;57:692.

174. Ross RS. Right ventricular hypertension as a cause for precordial pain. Am Heart J. 1961;61:134–137.

175. Rowe JC, Bland EF, Sprague HB, et al. The course of mitral stenosis without surgery: Ten and twenty year perspectives. Ann Intern Med. 1960;52:741–749.

176. Ruiz CE, Zhang HP, Gamra H, et al. Late clinical and echocardiographic follow up after percutaneous balloon dilatation of the mitral valve. Br Heart J. 1994;71:454–458.

177. Sadoshima J, Koyanagi S, Sugimachi M, et al. Evaluation of the severity of mitral regurgitation by transesophageal Doppler flow echocardiography. Am Heart J. 1992;123(5):1245–1251.

178. Samstad SO, Rossvoll O, Torp HG, et al. Cross-sectional early mitral flow-velocity profiles from color Doppler in patients with mitral valve disease. Circulation. 1992;86(3):748–755.

179. Sasaki H, Ogawa S, Handa S, et al. Two-dimensional echocardiographic diagnosis of mitral valve prolapse syndrome in presumably healthy young students. J Cardiogr. 1982;12:23–31.

180. Savage DD, Garrison RJ, Castelli WP, et al. Prevalence of submitral (annular) calcium and its correlates in a general population-based sample (The Framingham Study). Am J Cardiol. 1983;51:1375–1378.

181. Selzer A, Cohn KE. Natural history of mitral stenosis: A review. Circulation. 1972;45:878–890.

182. Schiavone WA, Calafiore PA, Currie PJ, et al. Doppler echocardiographic demonstration of pulmonary venous flow velocity in three patients with constrictive pericarditis before and after pericardiectomy. Am J Cardiol. 1989;63:145–147.

183. Schwartz R, Meyerson RM, Lawrence LT, et al. Mitral stenosis, massive pulmonary hemorrhage and emergency valve replacement. N Engl J Med. 1966;272:755–758.

184. Shah PM. Echocardiographic diagnosis of mitral valve prolapse. J Am Soc Echocardiogr. 1994;7(3):286–293.

185. Sheikh KH, Bengtson JR, Rankin JS, et al. Intraoperative transesophageal Doppler color flow imaging used to guide patient selection and operative treatment of ischemic mitral regurgitation. Circulation. 1991;84(2):594–604.

186. Sherman DG, Dyken ML, Fisher M, et al. Cerebral embolism. Chest. 1986;89:82S–98S.

187. Shone JD, Sellers RD, Anderson RC, et al. The developmental complex of "parachute mitral valve," supravalvular ring of left atrium, subaortic stenosis and coarctation of aorta. Am J Cardiol. 1963;11:714–725.

188. Shyu KG, Lei MH, Hwang JJ, et al. Morphologic characterization and quantitative assessment of mitral regurgitation with ruptured chordae tendineae by transesophageal echocardiography. Am J Cardiol. 1992;70:1152–1156.

189. Simpson IA, Sahn DJ. Quantification of valvular regurgitation by Doppler echocardiography. Circulation. 1991;84(3):I-188–I-192.

190. Smith MD, Cassidy JM, Gurley JC, et al. Echo Doppler evaluation of patients with acute mitral regurgitation: Superiority of transesophageal echocardiography with color flow imaging. Am Heart J. 1995;129(5):967–974.

191. Smith MK, Kwan OL, Spain MG, et al. Temporal variability of color Doppler jet areas in patients with mitral and aortic regurgitation. Am Heart J. 1992;123(4):953–960.

192. Smith MD, Wisenbaugh T, Grayburn PA, et al. Value and limitations of Doppler pressure half-time in quantifying mitral stenosis: A comparison with micromanometer catheter recordings. Am Heart J. 1991;121(2):480–488.

193. Sochowski RA, Chan KL, Ascah KJ, et al. Comparison of accuracy of transesophageal versus transthoracic echocardiography for the detection of mitral valve prolapse with ruptured chordae tendineae (flail mitral leaflet). Am J Cardiol. 1991;67:1251–1255.

194. Stamm RB, Martin RP. Quantification of pressure gradients across stenotic valves by Doppler ultrasound. J Am Coll Cardiol. 1983;2:707.

195. Stewart WJ, Currie PJ, Salcedo EE, et al. Evaluation of mitral leaflet motion by echocardiography and jet direction by Doppler color flow mapping to determine the mechanism of mitral regurgitation. J Am Coll Cardiol. 1992;20(6):1353–1361.

196. Stewart WJ, Salcedo EE, Cosgrove DM. The value of echocardiography in mitral valve repair. Cleve Clin J Med. 1991;58:177–183.

197. Stoddard MF, Prince CR, Tuman WL, et al. Angle of incidence does not affect accuracy of mitral stenosis area calculation by pressure half-time: Application to Doppler transesophageal echocardiography. Am Heart J. 1994;127(6):1562–1572.

198. Stoddard MF, Prince CR, Ammash NM, et al. Two-

dimensional transesophageal echocardiographic determination of mitral valve area in adults with mitral stenosis. Am Heart J. 1994;127(5):1348–1353.

199. Tahernia AC. Cardiovascular anomalies in Marfan's syndrome: The role of echocardiography and B-blockers. South Med J. 1993;86(3):305–310.

200. Taylor J, Rodger JC. Floppy mitral valves in elderly patients: Clinical features and associated echocardiographic findings. Age Ageing. 1991;20:80–84.

201. Tessier P, Mercier LA, Burelle D, et al. Results of percutaneous mitral commissurotomy in patients with a left atrial appendage thrombus detected by transesophageal echocardiography. J Am Soc Echocardiogr. 1994;7(4):394–399.

202. Thomas MR, Monaghan MJ, Smyth DW, et al. Comparative value of transthoracic and transesophageal echocardiography before balloon dilatation of the mitral valve. Br Heart J. 1992;68:493–497.

203. Thomas MR, Monaghan MJ, Michalis LK, et al. Echocardiographic restenosis after successful balloon dilatation of the mitral valve with the Inoue balloon: Experience of United Kingdom centre. Br Heart J. 1993;69:418–423.

204. Thomas MR, Monaghan MJ, Metcalfe JM, et al. Residual atrial septal defects following balloon mitral valvuloplasty using different techniques. Eur Heart J. 1992;13:496–502.

205. Tribouilloy C, Shen WF, Quere JP, et al. Assessment of severity of mitral regurgitation by measuring regurgitant jet width at its origin with transesophageal Doppler color flow imaging. Circulation. 1992;85(4):1248–1253.

206. Tribouilloy C, Shen WF, Rey JL, et al. Mitral to aortic velocity-time integral ratio: A non-geometric pulsed-Doppler regurgitant index in isolated pure mitral regurgitation. Eur Heart J. 1994;15:1335–1339.

207. Tribouilloy C, Shen WF, Slama MA, et al. Non-invasive measurement of the regurgitant fraction by pulsed Doppler echocardiography in isolated pure mitral regurgitation. Br Heart J. 1991;66:290–294.

208. Utsunomiya T, Patel D, Doshi R, et al. Can signal intensity of the continuous wave Doppler regurgitant jet estimate severity of mitral regurgitation? Am Heart J. 1992;123(1):166–171.

209. Vandervoort PM, Rivera JM, Mele D, et al. Application of color Doppler flow mapping to calculate effective regurgitant orifice area: An in vitro study and initial clinical observations. Circulation. 1993;88(3):1150–1156.

210. Reference deleted.

211. Vigna C, deRito V, Criconia GM, et al. Left atrial thrombus and spontaneous echo-contrast in non-anticoagulated mitral stenosis: A transesophageal echocardiographic study. Chest. 1993;103(2):348–352.

212. Vilacosta I, Iturralde E, San Roman JA, et al. Transesophageal echocardiographic monitoring of percutaneous mitral balloon valvulotomy. Am J Cardiol. 1992;70:1040–1044.

213. Villanova C, Melacini P, Scognamiglio R, et al. Long-term echocardiographic evaluation of closed and open mitral valvulotomy. Int J Cardiol. 1993;38:315–321.

214. von Bibra H, Sutherland G, Becher H, et al. Clinical evaluation of left heart Doppler contrast enhancement by a saccharide-based transpulmonary contrast agent. J Am Coll Cardiol. 1995;25(2):500–508.

215. von Bibra H, Becher H, Firschke C, et al. Enhancement of mitral regurgitation and normal left atrial color Doppler flow signals with peripheral venous injection of a saccharide-based contrast agent. J Am Coll Cardiol. 1993;22(2):521–528.

216. Vuille C, Weyman A. Left ventricle I: General considerations, assessment of chamber size and function. *In* Weyman A (ed): Principles and Practice of Echocardiography, 2nd ed. Philadelphia, Lea & Febiger; 1994:616–617.

217. Waggoner AD, Barzilai B, Miller JG, et al. On-line assessment of left atrial area and function by echocardiographic automatic boundary detection. Circulation. 1993;88(3):1142–1149.

218. Waller BF, Morrow AG, Maron BJ, et al. Etiology of clinically isolated, severe, chronic, pure mitral regurgitation: Analysis of 97 patients over 30 years of age having mitral valve replacement. Am Heart J. 1982;104:276–288.

219. Waller BF, Roberts WC. Cardiovascular disease in the very elderly: Analysis of 40 necropsy patients aged 90 years or over. Am J Cardiol. 1983;51:403–421.

220. Wann LS, Grove JR, Hess TR, et al. Prevalence of mitral valve prolapse by two-dimensional echocardiography in healthy young women. Br Heart J. 1983;49:334.

221. Wann LS, Weyman AE, Dillon JC, et al. Determination of mitral valve area by cross-sectional echocardiography. Ann Intern Med. 1978;88:337.

222. Webster PJ, Raper RF, Ross DE, et al. Pharmacologic abolition of severe mitral regurgitation associated with dynamic left ventricular outflow tract obstruction after mitral valve repair: Confirmation by transesophageal echocardiography. Am Heart J. 1993;126(2):480–483.

223. Weis AJ, Salcedo EE, Stewart WJ, et al. Anatomic explanation of mobile systolic clicks: Implications for the clinical and echocardiographic diagnosis of mitral valve prolapse. Am Heart J. 1995;129(2): 314–320.

224. Weiss AN, Mimbs JW, Ludbrook PA, et al. Echocardiographic detection of mitral valve prolapse: Exclusion of false positive diagnosis and determination of inheritance. Circulation. 1975;52:1091.

225. Weyman AE, Wann LS, Rogers EW, et al. Five-year experience in corresponding cross-sectional echocardiographic assessment of the mitral valve area with hemodynamic valve area determinations (abstract). Am J Cardiol. 1979;43:386.

226. Wilkins GT, et al. Percutaneous balloon dilatation of the mitral valve: An analysis of echocardiographic variables related to outcome and the mechanism of dilatation. Br Heart J. 1988;60:299.

227. Wisenbaugh T, Berk M, Essop R, et al. Effect of mitral regurgitation and volume loading on pressure half-time before and after balloon valvotomy in mitral stenosis. Am J Cardiol. 1991;67:162–168.

228. Wood P. An appreciation of mitral stenosis. Br Med J. 1954;1:1051–1063.

229. Wooley CF, Baba N, Kilman JW, et al. Thrombotic calcific mitral stenosis: Morphology of the calcific mitral valve. Circulation. 1974;49:1167–1174.

230. Wranne B, Ask P, Loyd D. Analysis of different methods of assessing the stenotic mitral valve area with emphasis on the pressure gradient half-time concept. Am J Cardiol. 1990;66:614–620.

231. Wu YT, Chang AC, Chin AJ. Semiquantitative assessment of mitral regurgitation by Doppler color flow imaging in patients aged <20 years. Am J Cardiol. 1993;71:727–732.

232. Xiao HB, Jin XY, Gibson DG. Doppler reconstruction of left ventricular pressure from functional mitral regurgitation: Potential importance of varying orifice geometry. Br Heart J. 1995;73:53–60.

233. Xie GY, Berk MR, Hixson CS, et al. Quantification of mitral regurgitant volume by the color Doppler proximal isovelocity surface area method: A clinical study. J Am Soc Echocardiogr. 1995;8:48–54.

234. Yang SS, Gholdberg H. Simplified Doppler estimation of mitral valve area. Am J Cardiol. 1985;56: 488.

235. Yoran C, Yellin EL, Becker RM, et al. Dynamic aspects of acute mitral regurgitation: Effects of ventricular volume, pressure and contractility on the effective regurgitant orifice area. Circulation. 1979; 60:170–176.

236. Yoran C, Yellin EL, Becker RM, et al. Mechanism of reduction of mitral regurgitation with vasodilator therapy. Am J Cardiol. 1979;43:773–777.

237. Yoshida K, Yoshikawa J, Akasaka T, et al. Value of acceleration flow signals proximal to the leaking orifice in assessing the severity of prosthetic mitral valve regurgitation. J Am Coll Cardiol. 1992;19(2): 333–338.

238. Zile MR, Gaasch WH, Carroll JD, et al. Chronic mitral regurgitation: Predictive value of preoperative echocardiographic indexes of left ventricular function and wall stress. J Am Coll Cardiol. 1984; 3:235.

239. Zuppiroli A, Mori F, Favilli S, et al. Arrhythmias in mitral valve prolapse: Relation to anterior mitral leaflet thickening, clinical variables, and color Doppler echocardiographic parameters. Am Heart J. 1994;128(5):919–927.

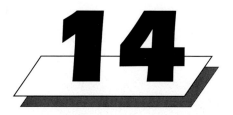

14

Aortic Valve Disease

MARK HARRY

Historically, the quantitative assessment of aortic valve disease has usually been based on data obtained during a cardiac catheterization procedure. However, cardiac catheterization is an expensive, invasive procedure that does not lend itself to serial follow-up studies. Over the past decade, echocardiography has gained popularity as a noninvasive method for the evaluation of aortic valve disease. Integrated, comprehensive exams utilizing two-dimensional echocardiography, color flow Doppler and spectral Doppler can often provide the morphologic and hemodynamic information necessary to determine the etiology and severity of aortic stenosis and/or regurgitation. Several studies have validated the use of echocardiography for the diagnosis and serial assessment of patients with aortic valve disease.[2,3,14] This chapter will explore the uses and limitations of the various echocardiographic methods that are part of a comprehensive assessment of aortic stenosis and aortic regurgitation. The technical considerations applicable to these methods will also be discussed.

Aortic Stenosis

The clinical symptoms of aortic stenosis often include chest pain, shortness of breath, and sometimes syncope. Most patients do not develop these classic symptoms until the degree of aortic stenosis is at least moderate to severe. In infants, children, and young adults, symptoms are often absent even when the aortic stenosis is severe.[1,7,23] Common causes of aortic stenosis include degenerative changes in the valve, congenital abnormalities, or rheumatic etiologies. Degenerative calcification of the aortic valve leaflets is the most common cause of aortic stenosis in elderly patients. Patients with a bicuspid aortic valve tend to develop calcific aortic stenosis at an earlier age than patients with normal aortic valve anatomy.[18] The most common indication for echocardiography is the presence of a harsh systolic ejection murmur heard at the right sternal border that may radiate up the carotids.

ECHOCARDIOGRAPHIC FEATURES

The normal aortic valve has three leaflets that are thin, pliable, and can be seen opening widely in the parasternal long and short axis views. When a patient has calcific aortic stenosis, the aortic valve leaflets are thickened and dense, with evidence of decreased motion in the two-dimensional parasternal long and short axis views (Fig. 14-1). In patients with congenital or rheumatic aortic stenosis, the body of the aortic valve leaflets can be thin and pliable and appears to move normally on M-mode images, while two-dimensional images reveal that the tips of the leaflets are tethered, resulting in restricted opening of the aortic valve at the leaflet tips. The tethered aortic valve can best be seen as early systolic doming of the leaflets in the parasternal and apical long axis views.

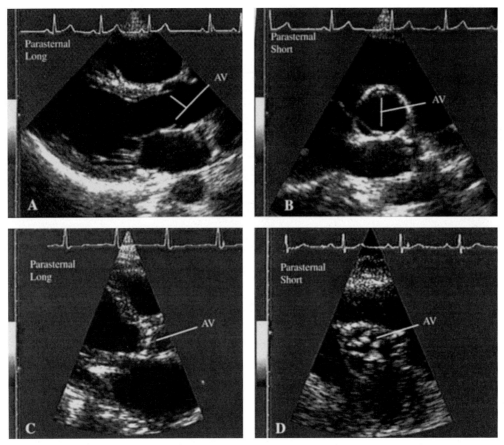

Figure 14-1. Two-dimensional images of a normal thin, pliable aortic valve (**A**, **B**) and a densely calcified aortic valve (**C**, **D**). In the upper parasternal views the normal aortic valve leaflets can be seen opening widely in these early systolic frames. In the lower parasternal views the heavily calcified aortic valve leaflets demonstrate significantly reduced opening in these early systolic frames. AV, aortic valve.

Most patients with aortic stenosis will develop left ventricular hypertrophy. This is secondary to pressure overload on the left ventricle. As the severity of aortic stenosis increases, so does the degree of left ventricular hypertrophy. When left ventricular systolic performance is normal, the pressure gradient across the aortic valve will increase in proportion to the degree of reduction in the aortic valve area. The response of the left ventricle to this increase in resistance is an increase in muscle mass, much as a body builder increases muscle mass by increasing the amount of weight he or she can lift. When left ventricular function is normal, a peak instantaneous gradient (80 mm Hg) or a mean gradient (50 mm Hg) is consistent with severe aortic

stenosis.[11] However, if the patient is in a low cardiac output state, the peak gradient, mean gradient, and aortic valve area may not be reliable indicators of the severity of aortic stenosis.

In echocardiography the area of the aortic valve is calculated using the continuity equation, which is based on the principle of the conservation of mass. All blood flowing through the left ventricular outflow tract must also cross the aortic valve. The stroke volume across the left ventricular outflow tract will equal the stroke volume across the aortic valve, provided that there is no membranous ventricular septal defect. The continuity equation calculates the effective valve area. When a patient is in a low cardiac output state (low driving pressure), the aortic valve may open only partially, resulting in an underestimation of the aortic valve area (effective valve area) using the continuity equation. A dobutamine stress test can be performed to increase the patient's cardiac output and the driving pressure across the aortic valve. During dobutamine infusion the patient's peak and mean gradient will increase significantly and the aortic valve area will remain small if the patient does indeed have significant aortic stenosis.[10] There will be a relatively small increase in the peak and mean gradient and a significant increase in the valve area if the effective aortic valve area was reduced due to depressed left ventricular function.

The severity of aortic stenosis cannot be determined reliably by transthoracic two-dimensional echocardiographic assessment of the aortic valve leaflet opening. Recently, transesophageal echocardiographic images of the aortic valve have been used to assess the aortic valve area in some patients.[20] However, in most patients, transesophageal echocardiography is not necessary. A systematic comprehensive color and spectral Doppler evaluation of the aortic valve and the left ventricular outflow tract using standard transthoracic echocardiographic methods provides an accurate determination of aortic valve area and aortic stenosis severity.

THE ECHOCARDIOGRAPHIC EXAM

The echocardiographic examination should be a comprehensive assessment of multiple parasternal, apical, subcostal, and suprasternal views. The patient's height, weight, age, heart rate, and blood pressure should be recorded at the time of the exam. These data are useful for serial echocardiographic follow-up and comparison with cardiac catheterization data. There will be a significant difference between the echocardiographic and catheterization data if there was a significant difference in the heart rate and/or blood pressure (loading conditions) during the two studies. Various medications and contrast agents administered during the cardiac catheterization procedure can have a profound effect on afterload and preload, resulting in data that do not correlate with the findings on the echocardiogram.

Parasternal Views

Two-dimension and/or M-mode linear measurements of the left ventricle, chamber size, and wall thickness should be obtained. Figure 14-2 illustrates the short axis view, which can be used for measuring left ventricular global function, chamber size, and wall thickness. Figure 14-1*A* and 14-1*B* shows the parasternal views that are generally used to measure aortic root diameter, aortic valve cusp separation, and left atrial diameter. Technically, the parasternal short axis view should be used to make M-mode measurements of the aortic valve, aortic root, and left atrium because the M-mode cursor can be more accurately aligned through the center of these structures.

It is important to note that M-mode dimensions can be unreliable and are subject to significant error if a patient has asymmetric hypertrophy and/or regional wall motion abnormalities. Despite these limitations, M-mode measurements generally provide reliable data for serial follow-up of chamber size and wall thickness.[5] A single M-mode trace is generally not useful for determining aortic valve leaflet excursion since reduction in stroke volume may reduce the leaflet excursion and only two of the three aortic valve leaflets can be seen on a single M-mode trace.

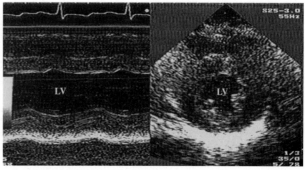

Figure 14-2. Two-dimensional and M-mode images in a patient with calcific aortic stenosis. Images from the parasternal short axis view at papillary level demonstrate significant left ventricular hypertrophy. LV, left ventricle.

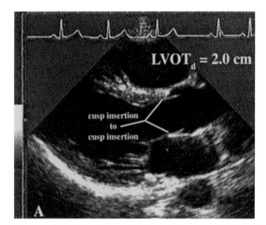 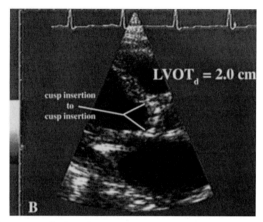

Figure 14-3.   Left ventricular outflow tract (LVOT) diameter technique in a patient with a normal aortic valve (**A**) and in a 75-year-old female with calcific aortic stenosis (**B**).

The parasternal long axis view is ideal for measuring left ventricular outflow tract diameter, which is one component of the continuity equation. This is measured from the insertion of the anterior coronary cusp (generally the right coronary cusp) to the insertion of the posterior coronary cusp (generally the noncoronary cusp) (Fig. 14-3). The cross-sectional area of the left ventricular outflow tract = 3.141 × the left ventricular outflow tract radius squared (r^2) or 0.785 × the left ventricular outflow tract diameter squared. We assume that the left ventricular outflow tract has a circular shape. It is important to remember that any error made in measuring the left ventricular outflow tract diameter will be squared, causing a significant error in the calculation of the aortic valve area. The left ventricular outflow tract diameter should not be measured if the parasternal window is poor and/or there is heavy calcification of the aortic valve extending into the outflow tract. A simple outflow tract/aortic valve ratio may be sufficient for assessment of the severity of aortic stenosis. This ratio will be discussed later.

Apical Views

Flow velocity patterns associated with aortic stenosis and aortic regurgitation are generally most parallel with the ultrasound transducer in the apical views. Pulsed wave Doppler, continuous wave Doppler, and color flow Doppler cursors can easily be aligned with the blood flow being measured using a duplex transducer. In patients with aortic stenosis, the peak left ventricular outflow tract gradient, velocity time integral, peak instantaneous aortic valve gradient, and mean aortic valve gradient are commonly obtained using a left ventricular outflow view (Fig. 14-4). It is important to remember that if the ultrasound beam is not sampling the flow velocities within 20 degrees of parallel, the gradient and velocity time integral will be significantly underestimated (Fig. 14-5). In many patients, the ultrasound trans-

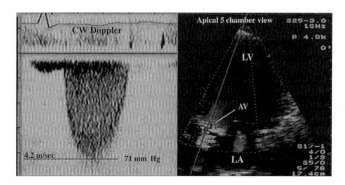

Figure 14-4.   Continuous wave (CW) Doppler in a patient with calcific aortic stenosis. A peak gradient of 71 mm Hg and a mean gradient of 40 mm Hg indicate significant obstruction of the aortic valve (AV). LV, left ventricle; LA, left atrium.

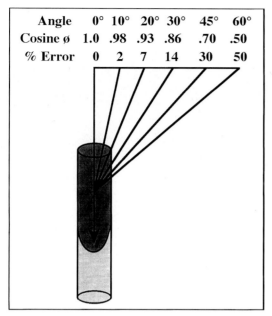

Figure 14-5. The Doppler equation that ultrasound systems use to calculate velocities assumes that the cosine of the angle is zero unless the sonographer uses the angle correction function. Angle correction is not generally used in echocardiography. This illustration clearly shows that there is very little error (underestimation) of velocities when blood flow is sampled between 0 degrees and 20 degrees.

ducer usually has to be positioned laterally and toward the axilla to obtain a position parallel to flow. Patients with congenital aortic stenosis will frequently have eccentric stenotic jets, which may require the use of a nonstandard view to obtain the position most parallel to that of the flow. Apical, right parasternal, suprasternal, and subcostal views of the aortic valve should be interrogated with continuous wave Doppler to ensure that the highest velocity across the aortic valve has been obtained (Fig. 14-6).[24]

The duplex transducer is more convenient to use than the nonimaging continuous wave Doppler transducer but can lack the sensitivity and access that a nonimaging continuous wave Doppler transducer provides. The nonimaging continuous wave Doppler transducer requires considerable skill and practice to use effectively, but its benefits outweigh its inconvenience.[21] When imaging a patient with multiple valvular abnormalities, care must be taken to identify the Doppler flow patterns accurately. Aortic stenosis, mitral regurgitation, and tricuspid regurgitation all occur in systole; thus timing and waveform characteristics are key in the identification process (Fig. 14-7).

Figure 14-6. Multiple windows should be interrogated with continuous wave Doppler to ensure that the highest velocities across the aortic valve have been recorded.

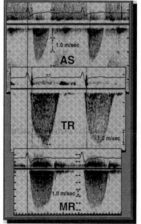

R to onset = 70 msec
Ejection time = 200 msec
Peak velocity = 2.7 m/sec

R to onset = 40 msec
Regurge time = 360 msec
Peak velocity = 4.0 m/sec

R to onset = 40 msec
Regurge time = 320 msec
Peak velocity = 5.6 m/sec

Figure 14-7. Continuous wave Doppler tracings in a patient with mitral regurgitation, aortic stenosis, and tricuspid regurgitation. The aortic stenosis continuous wave Doppler trace can easily be differentiated from the tricuspid regurgitation and mitral regurgitation traces if all three traces are recorded and compared. Notice that the aortic stenosis trace does not start until the end of the isovolumic contraction period, and the aortic ejection time is significantly shorter than the tricuspid regurgitation or mitral regurgitation time.

Most cardiac catheterization laboratories still report a peak-to-peak aortic valve gradient instead of a peak instantaneous gradient. The peak-to-peak gradient is the difference between the peak left ventricular pressure and the peak aortic pressure. It is usually lower than the peak instantaneous gradient (Fig. 14-8).

Generally, the greater the severity of aortic stenosis, the greater the delay between the peak left ventricular and peak aortic valve pressures; thus there can be as much as 30 mm Hg difference between the peak-to-peak gradient and the peak instantaneous gradient. If a patient's heart rate, blood pressure, and cardiac output are the same during cardiac catheterization and echocardiography, then the patient's mean aortic valve gradient and aortic valve area should be very similar. Figure 14-9 is an example of the cardiac catheterization and echocardiographic data in an elderly patient with calcific aortic stenosis.

If the peak velocity across the left ventricular outflow tract (V_1) is less than 1.0 m/sec, the simplified form of the Bernoulli equation ($4 \times V^2_2$) can be used to calculate the peak instantaneous aortic valve gradient. If V_1 is greater than or equal to 1.0 m/sec, the modified form of the Bernoulli equation ($4 \times (V^2_2 - V^2_1)$) should be used to calculate the peak instantaneous aortic valve outflow (Fig. 14-10). The peak instantaneous aortic valve gra-

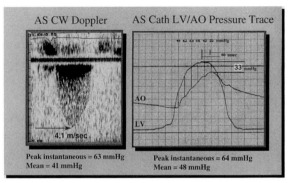

Peak instantaneous = 63 mmHg
Mean = 41 mmHg

Peak instantaneous = 64 mmHg
Mean = 48 mmHg

Figure 14-9. The continuous wave (CW) Doppler trace across this patient's aortic valve and the cardiac catheter pressure tracings were taken 7 days apart. The patient's heart rate and blood pressure were similar during both studies. Notice the 60-msec delay between the peak left ventricular (LV) pressure and the aortic (AO) peak pressure and the 31-mm Hg difference between the peak-to-peak and peak instantaneous aortic valve gradient.

dient for the patient data shown in Figure 14-10 would be as follows:

$$4(3.2^2 - 1.0^2) = (10.24 - 1.0) = 4 \times 9.24$$
$$= 37 \text{ mm Hg}$$

Normally, the stroke volume is the same across all four heart valves. This continuity of flow is the basis for calculation of the aortic valve area. Using the area × length formula, we can calculate the stroke volume across the left ventricular outflow tract and the aortic valve. The cross-sectional area of a cylinder times the length of that cylinder equals the volume of the cylinder. The cross-sectional area of the left ventricular outflow tract or aortic valve times the distance the column of blood travels past the left ventricular outflow tract or the aortic valve during one cardiac cycle (stroke distance) equals the stroke volume across the left ventricular outflow tract or aortic valve. The velocity time integral is a measure of stroke distance. The left ventricular outflow tract stroke volume divided by the aortic valve velocity time integral equals the aortic valve area in square centimeters[10,13,19,22] (Fig. 14-11).

If the velocities in the left ventricular outflow tract are over- or underestimated, the aortic valve area will be under- or overestimated, respectively. There are a number of technical factors that may cause the pulsed wave Doppler data from the left ventricular outflow tract to be inaccurate. The

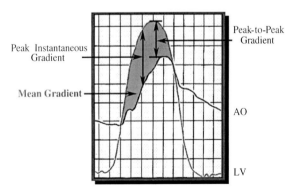

Figure 14-8. This stylized cardiac catheterization trace illustrates the difference between the peak-to-peak and peak instantaneous left ventricular (LV), aortic (AO) gradient.

Figure 14-10. Pulsed wave and continuous wave Doppler data from a 75-year-old female patient with calcific aortic stenosis. The peak left ventricular outflow tract (LVOT) velocity (1.0 m/sec) was obtained by positioning a pulsed wave Doppler sample gate about 1.0 cm below the aortic valve in the LVOT (**A**). The peak instantaneous aortic valve velocity was obtained from the same apical position with the continuous wave Doppler directed across the aortic valve (**B**).

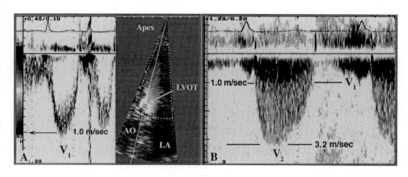

velocities will be too high if the pulsed wave Doppler sample volume is positioned in the region of prestenotic flow acceleration in front of the aortic valve. The velocities will be too low if the pulsed wave Doppler sample volume is positioned too low in the left ventricular outflow tract (Fig. 14-12). Respiration and translation of the aortic valve annulus during the cardiac cycle can make it difficult to select the appropriate pulsed wave Doppler trace to measure because the pulsed wave Doppler sample volume is constantly moving up and down and/or from side to side in the left ventricular outflow tract. These problems can be overcome by asking the patient to hold his or her breath briefly while the pulsed wave Doppler data are being obtained and by measuring an average of three to five quality tracings.

When a patient is in atrial fibrillation, it will be difficult to measure an appropriate left ventricular outflow tract peak velocity since the left ventricular outflow tract and aortic valve peak velocities are commonly measured at different times. The stroke volume can vary significantly from beat to beat because the R-R intervals can vary significantly. A number of methods can be employed to increase the accuracy of the left ventricular outflow tract velocity data when a patient is in atrial fibrillation.

Ten consecutive beats can be averaged. R-R matched left ventricular outflow tract and aortic valve tracings can be used or the left ventricular outflow tract and aortic valve velocities can be measured simultaneously using continuous wave Doppler scanning.

The left ventricular outflow tract and aortic valve components, V_1 and V_2, are commonly seen in continuous wave Doppler tracings across the aortic valve.[6] Figure 14-10 is an example of simultaneous left ventricular outflow tract (V_1) velocities and aortic valve (V_2) velocities. Notice that the peak velocity of the left ventricular outflow tract component in the continuous wave Doppler trace is the same as the pulsed wave Doppler peak left ventricular outflow tract velocity. Figure 14-13 illustrates why the left ventricular outflow tract velocities can be seen in continuous wave Doppler tracings of the aortic valve from the apical window.

It is important to remember that the continuous wave Doppler gain must not be set too high; if this happens, the volume–intensity relationships will not be appreciated in the continuous wave Doppler tracings. If significant color flow Doppler flow acceleration is seen in the left ventricular outflow tract because of asymmetric septal hypertrophy, the simultaneous method should not be used.

$$(\text{LVOT}_{CSA} \times \text{LVOT}_{VTI}) \div \text{AV}_{VTI} = \text{AV}_{CSA} \ (\textbf{Aortic Valve Area cm}^2)$$

$$(0.785 \times \text{LVOT}_d^2 \times \text{LVOT}_{VTI}) \div \text{AV}_{VTI} = \textbf{Aortic Valve Area cm}^2$$

Figure 14-11. Continuity equation for calculation of the aortic valve area (AVA). In most cases, the peak left ventricular outflow tract (LVOT) velocity V_1 and peak aortic valve (AV) velocity V_2 can be substituted in the continuity equation for the velocity time integral. The continuity equation would then be (0.785 × LVOT_d^2 × LVOT V_1) ÷ AV V_2 = AVA cm^2).

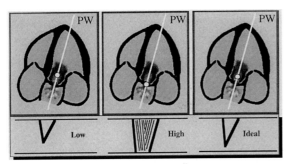

Figure 14-12. *The correct method for positioning the pulsed wave (PW) Doppler sample volume in the left ventricular outflow tract in a patient with aortic stenosis.*

Also, if the line separating the left ventricular outflow tract component and the aortic valve (AV) component is not clearly seen, then the simultaneous method should not be used. Spectral Doppler gain should be set only as high as is necessary to clearly measure the spectral Doppler trace. If the gain is set too high, the velocity time integral and gradients may be overestimated. The spectral Doppler filters should be increased when interrogating the high-velocity, low-volume flow across the AV component with continuous wave Doppler. The spectral Doppler filters should be set low when interrogating the low-velocity, high-volume flow in the left ventricular outflow tract.

When it is technically difficult to measure the left ventricular outflow tract diameter, a simple left ventricular outflow tract/aortic valve velocity ratio can be helpful in determining if a patient has an aortic valve area less than 0.75 cm^2.[10] A left ventricular outflow tract/aortic velocity or velocity time integral ratio of 0.20 is consistent with an aortic valve area less than 0.75 cm^2 when the patient has an average left ventricular outflow tract diameter of 2.0 to 2.2 cm (Fig. 14-14). The left ventricular outflow tract/aortic valve ratio can be useful for determining the systolic performance of a prosthetic aortic valve. Numerous published studies have attempted to document the normal peak and mean gradients across the various types and sizes of prosthetic aortic valves. Unfortunately, changes in stroke volume due to changing loading conditions may make the peak and mean gradients less useful for serial follow-up studies. The left ventricular outflow tract/aortic valve ratio will not change unless there is a change in the size of the left ventricular outflow tract (which is rare) or obstruction of the prosthetic aortic valve (Fig. 14-15).

Most of the anatomic and hemodynamic information for assessing the severity of aortic stenosis is obtained from the parasternal and apical views, with the exception of aortic valve velocities. It is not uncommon to obtain the highest aortic valve velocity from either the subcostal, right paraster-

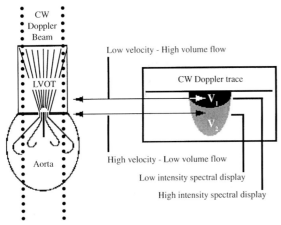

Figure 14-13. *Apical window continuous wave (CW) Doppler tracings across a calcified, stenotic aortic valve or a prosthetic aortic valve can show two distinct envelopes. The darker inner envelope represents the low-velocity, high-volume flow in the left ventricular outflow tract (V_1). The lighter outer envelope represents the high-velocity, low-volume flow crossing the stenotic aortic valve (V_2).*

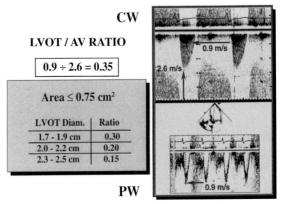

Figure 14-14. *This patient has a left ventricular outflow tract (LVOT) diameter of 2.0 cm and a calculated aortic valve (AV) area of 1.09 cm². The LVOT/AV velocity ratio in this patient is consistent with mild to moderate aortic stenosis. The LVOT/AV ratio is not a true dimensionless ratio. When a patient's LV function is normal and the LVOT is large, the velocities in the LVOT will be significantly lower than those of a patient with the same LV function, a smaller LVOT diameter, and the same body surface area.*

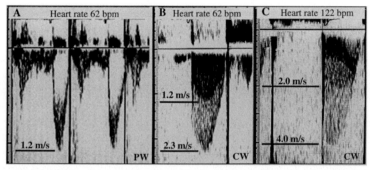

Figure 14-15. These Doppler data are from a dobutamine study on a patient with a Medtronic Hall aortic valve (AV) replacement. The first panel (**A**) shows the resting pulsed wave Doppler trace from the left ventricular outflow tract (LVOT) at a level just below the aortic valve (AV). The second panel (**B**) is the resting continuous wave (CW) Doppler trace across the LVOT and AV. V_1 and V_2 can be clearly seen. The resting LVOT/AV ratio is 0.52. The third panel (**C**) shows the CW Doppler trace across the LVOT and AV during infusion of dobutamine at 30 μg/min. Again, V_1 and V_2 can be clearly seen. Also, notice the darker late-peaking mid-LV obstruction component associated with increased LV contraction. The LVOT/AV ratio is 0.50 at 30 μg/min. Even though the heart rate and gradients nearly doubled, the LVOT/AV ratio stayed essentially the same.

nal, or suprasternal view, particularly in patients with noncalcific aortic stenosis. The range of normal and abnormal echocardiographic values for the assessment of aortic stenosis are shown in Table 14-1.

All aortic valve areas should be indexed using body surface area. A patient with a large body surface area (greater than 2.0 m2) may be symptomatic with a valve area greater than 0.75 cm2 while a patient with a small body surface area (less than 2.0 m2) may be asymptotic with a valve area less than 0.75 cm2. If the calculated aortic valve area divided by the body surface area is less than or equal to 0.45 cm2 the aortic stenosis can be considered severe.

Aortic Regurgitation

The most common indication for echocardiographic assessment of aortic regurgitation is the presence of a high-pitched, diastolic decrescendo blowing murmur heard at the left sternal border during auscultation. Symptoms of aortic regurgitation include dyspnea, orthopnea, paroxysmal nocturnal dyspnea, and signs of congestive heart failure. Patients with chronic aortic regurgitation may be relatively asymptomatic for a long period of time, but when symptoms of heart failure develop, mortality increases if there is no surgical intervention.[9] If the patient with chronic aortic regurgitation has

TABLE 14-1. RANGE OF VALUES BASED ON A REVIEW OF PAST AND CURRENT LITERATURE

	NORMAL VALUES	
Valve area 2.5–4.5 cm²	LVOT diameter 1.8–2.4 cm	LVOT VTI 18–22 cm
	VALVE AREA	
Mild AS 1.1–1.9 cm²	Mod AS 0.75–1.0 cm²	Severe AS <0.75 cm²
	PEAK GRADIENT	
Mild AS 16–36 mm Hg	Mod AS 36–79 mm Hg	Severe AS ≥80 mm Hg
	MEAN GRADIENT	
Mild AS <20 mm Hg	Mod AS 20–49 mm Hg	Severe AS ≥50 mm Hg

Abbreviations: LVOT, left ventricular outflow tract; AS, aortic stenosis.

significant coronary artery disease or atrial fibrillation, the presence of symptoms of heart failure may complicate the clinical outcome. When left ventricular enlargement and reduced systolic function are present, surgery will involve higher risk to the patient and the postoperative benefits may be reduced due to permanent left ventricular dysfunction.[17] Cardiac catheterization has been the method of choice for determining the severity of aortic regurgitation. Cardiac catheterization measurements of the aortic pulse pressure and left ventricular end diastolic pressure, as well as subjective assessment of the degree of contrast in the left ventricle during aortic root contrast injection, are used to determine the severity of aortic regurgitation (Fig. 14-16).

ECHOCARDIOGRAPHIC FEATURES

The etiology of aortic regurgitation can be subdivided into two groups involving the aortic valve and the aorta. Aortic valve abnormalities include rheumatic involvement, endocarditis, degenerative changes, and calcific and congenital malformation. Etiologies involving the aorta include idiopathic dilatation and Marfan's syndrome. Transthoracic and transesophageal images are useful for detecting the above-mentioned structural abnormalities and complement Doppler techniques for assessing the severity of aortic regurgitation. Two-dimensional echocardiographic and/or M-mode measures of left ventricular size and wall stress may be helpful in determining which patients need surgical intervention.

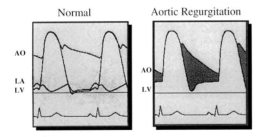

Figure 14-16. The stylized cardiac catheterization tracings on the left represent the normal aortic root (AO), left atrial (LA) pressure, and left ventricular (LV) pressure. The stylized tracings on the right represent the AO and LV pressures in a patient with significant aortic regurgitation. The pressure gradient between the LV and the AO drop off rapidly during diastole when there is significant aortic regurgitation.

If the end-diastolic left ventricular diameter exceeds 70 mm or the end-systolic left ventricular diameter exceeds 50 mm or the fractional shortening drops below 30% or the wall stress (systolic blood pressure × [end-diastolic radius ÷ wall thickness]) is above 600 mm Hg, surgical correction should be considered.[19] Until the advent of color flow imaging, echocardiographic assessment of aortic regurgitation severity was difficult at best. Several studies comparing aortic angiography with the dimensions of the color flow Doppler aortic regurgitant jet in the left ventricular outflow tract have shown favorable results.[4,15] The height and area of the color Doppler aortic regurgitant jet just below the aortic valve in the left ventricular outflow tract appear to be directly proportional to the size of the regurgitant orifice.

PARASTERNAL VIEWS

Two-dimensional and/or M-mode measurements of left ventricular systolic function, left heart chamber sizes, and left ventricular wall thickness are commonly obtained from the parasternal views. The left ventricular outflow tract systolic diameter measured from the parasternal long axis view is used in combination with pulsed wave Doppler to calculate the aortic valve stroke volume, regurgitant volume, and regurgitant fraction. The parasternal long axis view is ideal for measuring the anteroposterior diameter of the color Doppler aortic regurgitant jet at a level just below the aortic valve. The aortic regurgitant jet diameter divided by the diastolic left ventricular outflow tract diameter provides a regurgitant jet/left ventricular outflow tract diameter ratio. If this diameter ratio was greater than 40%, Dolan et al. reported 94% sensitivity and 97% specificity for 3 to 4 + aortic regurgitation compared to angiography.[4] Generally, a regurgitant jet/left ventricular outflow tract diameter ratio less than 30% is consistent with mild aortic regurgitation; between 30–50%, moderate regurgitation; and greater than 50%, severe regurgitation (Fig. 14-17). The regurgitant jet/left ventricular outflow tract diameter ratio method may not be reliable if the aortic regurgitant jet is eccentric or does not have a circular cross-sectional shape.

The aortic regurgitant jet area measured from the parasternal short axis view can also be used to assess the severity of aortic regurgitation. The regurgitant jet area measured just below the aortic valve

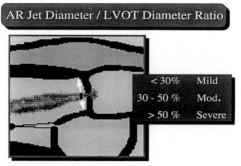

Figure 14-17. *The aortic regurgitation/left ventricular outflow tract (AR/LVOT) diameter ratio is measured from the parasternal long axis view. The LVOT diameter is measured from the cusp insertion to the cusp insertion of the aortic valve leaflets in diastole. The AR jet diameter is measured just below the aortic valve. This method is ideal for central AR jets that have a circular cross-sectional shape.*

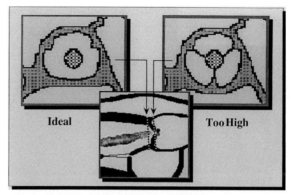

Figure 14-18. *The left ventricular outflow tract/aortic regurgitation (LVOT/AR) area ratio is measured from the parasternal short axis view. The LVOT and AR area should be traced at a level just below the aortic valve in diastole. The short axis view shown here on the right is at a more proximal aortic root level. An LVOT area traced at this level will result in a significant overestimation of the LVOT area. The short axis view shown here on the left is the proper level for tracing the LVOT and AR areas.*

divided by the left ventricular outflow tract area provides a regurgitant jet/left ventricular outflow tract area ratio. A ratio greater than 25% has been shown to be 92% sensitive and 97% specific for 3 to 4+ aortic regurgitation compared to angiography.[4]

The difference between the cutoff points for 3 and 4+ aortic regurgitation using the diameter ratio method and the area ratio method is most likely due to the fact that the left ventricular outflow tract area can be technically difficult to trace even under ideal circumstances. If the left ventricular outflow tract area is measured at a level where the aortic valve cusps can be clearly seen, the outflow tract area will be overestimated since this is actually at the level of the aortic root. The left ventricular outflow tract area should be measured just below the aortic valve where the basal portion of the anterior mitral valve leaflet can be visualized along the posterior portion of the image (Fig. 14-18). Calcification of the subaortic region or lateral and medial dropout of the two-dimensional image may make it impossible to trace accurately the left ventricular outflow tract area. To overcome the above-mentioned problems, we have employed a simplified method involving calculation of the diastolic left ventricular outflow tract area. The square of the diastolic left ventricular outflow tract diameter (measured from cusp insertion to cusp insertion) multiplied by 0.785 equals the left ventricular outflow tract diastolic area. We have found that the calculated area ratio method is more similar to the

diameter ratio in central circular aortic regurgitant jets than is the traced area ratio method (Fig. 14-19).

Before the advent of color Doppler, pulsed and continuous wave Doppler were used to quantitate the severity of aortic regurgitation. Pulsed wave Doppler mapping was tedious, and in most cases the extent to which the aortic regurgitant jet extended into the left ventricle was not a sensitive indicator of aortic regurgitation severity. The slope of

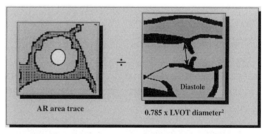

Ratio < 30% Mild   Ratio > 50 % Severe

(Not Validated)

Figure 14-19. *In this simplified aortic regurgitation/left ventricular outflow tract (AR/LVOT) area ratio method the LVOT area is calculated instead of traced. The AR jet area trace on the left is divided by the calculated LVOT area on the right.*

the continuous wave Doppler velocity trace has been shown to be a reasonable indicator of aortic regurgitation severity.[4,8] As the severity of aortic regurgitation increases, so does the diastolic pressure in the left ventricle. This increase in left ventricular diastolic pressure results in a progressive drop in the continuous wave aortic regurgitant velocities. The deceleration rate and pressure half-time have been used as an indicator of aortic regurgitation severity (Figs. 14-20 and 14-21).

Several technical factors should be taken into consideration when using the half-time or deceleration rate. The velocity scale should be set to at least 5.0 m/sec when attempting to record the diastolic jet of aortic regurgitation. The diastolic pressure in the aorta is generally about 80 mm Hg, and the diastolic pressure in the left ventricle is generally about 10 mm Hg (80 − 10 = 70 mm Hg); therefore the early diastolic velocity will be at least 4 m/sec. Doppler filters should be set high (at least 800 Hz), and the Doppler gain should be optimized. The high-velocity portion of the aortic regurgitant trace can be a useful indicator of aortic regurgitation severity. If the intensity of the high-velocity portion of the aortic regurgitant envelope is similar to that of the aortic outflow envelope, then the aortic regurgitation may be severe. Occasionally the aortic regurgitant jet will be very eccentric, particularly in patients with a bicuspid aortic valve. When the regurgitant jet is eccentric, the continuous wave Doppler may be more parallel to the aortic regurgitant jet in the parasternal, subcostal, or suprasternal view instead of the more commonly seen apical view (Fig. 14-22).

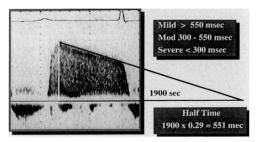

Figure 14-21. *This is an example of a continuous wave Doppler trace taken from the apical window in a patient with moderate aortic regurgitation. The pressure half-time is calculated by multiplying the deceleration time in milliseconds by 0.29.*

APICAL VIEWS

Color flow Doppler recordings of mild to moderate aortic regurgitant jets are often very impressive in the apical views because the Doppler beam is parallel to the high-velocity regurgitant jet (high aortic diastolic driving pressure is 60–70 mm Hg). The aortic regurgitant jet may extend to the left ventricular apex but may still be only mild to moderate in severity.[12] The deceleration time and pressure half-time can be poor discriminators of the degree of aortic regurgitation.[4] Left ventricular diastolic compliance, left atrial pressure, and heart rate can significantly alter the left ventricular diastolic filling pressure, causing the deceleration rate and half-time method to be an unreliable discriminator of aortic regurgitation severity. If the continuous wave Doppler beam does not remain within the regurgitant jet throughout the diastolic period the slope will be significantly increased, causing overestimation of aortic regurgitation severity (Fig. 14-23).

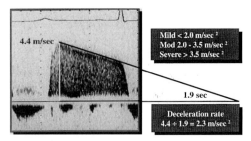

Figure 14-20. *This is an example of a continuous wave Doppler trace taken from the apical window in a patient with moderate aortic regurgitation. The deceleration rate is calculated by dividing the peak aortic regurgitation velocity by the deceleration time measured from the point of the peak aortic regurgitation velocity along the aortic regurgitation slope all the way to the baseline.*

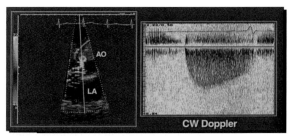

Figure 14-22. *This is a two-dimensional Doppler frame (left panel) and a continuous wave (CW) Doppler trace (right panel) from the left parasternal window in a patient with a bicuspid aortic valve and severe aortic regurgitation. LA, left atrium; AO, aorta.*

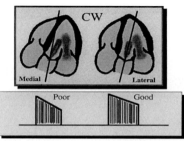

Figure 14-23. The continuous wave (CW) Doppler alignment shown on the left is from a more medial chest position. Patient respiration and cardiac motion cause translation of the aortic valve, which prevents the CW Doppler beam from staying aligned with the regurgitant jet throughout diastole. The CW Doppler alignment shown on the right is from a more lateral chest position where the CW Doppler is aligned with the regurgitant jet throughout the diastolic period.

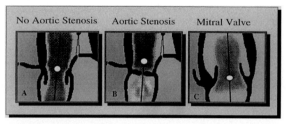

Figure 14-25. When measuring the stroke volume (SV) across the aortic valve (AV) in a patient without aortic stenosis (AS), the pulsed wave (PW) Doppler sample volume is positioned at the AV level (**A**). If the patient has AS the PW Doppler sample volume is positioned about 1 cm below the AV (**B**). When measuring the SV across the mitral valve (MV) the PW Doppler sample volume is positioned at the level of the mitral valve annulus (**C**).

Doppler-derived regurgitant volumes can be useful for quantification of aortic regurgitation if there is minimal or absent mitral regurgitation and no subaortic obstruction.[16] The stroke volume across the aortic valve minus the stroke volume across the mitral valve equals the regurgitant volume. A regurgitant volume greater than 60 to 65 ml is consistent with severe aortic regurgitation.[10] The regurgitant volume divided by the aortic valve stroke volume equals the regurgitant fraction (Fig. 14-24).

Calculation of stroke volumes can be technically demanding. A small error in the measurement of the systolic left ventricular outflow tract diameter and/or diastolic mitral valve diameter can result in a significant error in the regurgitant volume or fraction because the diameter of the left ventricular outflow tract and the mitral valve annulus are squared. If the pulsed wave Doppler sample volume is not positioned properly, the aortic valve and/or mitral

valve velocity time integral will be inaccurate (Fig. 14-25). A regurgitant fraction between 0% and 20% is consistent with little or no regurgitation. A regurgitant fraction between 20% and 30% is consistent with mild regurgitation; between 30% and 50%, moderate regurgitation; and greater than 50%, severe regurgitation.

There is a learning curve for calculating regurgitant volumes and fractions. The method should be evaluated in at least 20 patients with no aortic or mitral regurgitation, and one should be able to obtain stroke volumes across both valves that are within 15% of each other. Figures 14-26, 14-27, and 14-28 show data on a patient with severe aortic regurgitation.

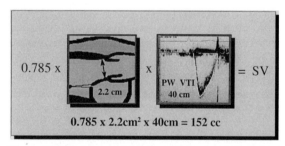

Figure 14-26. The stroke volume (SV) across this patient's aortic valve (AV) is 152 cc. The left ventricular outflow tract diameter is measured from the parasternal long axis view. The AV velocity time integral (VTI) is measured with pulsed wave Doppler from an apical outflow view, with the sample volume placed at the level of the AV. The AV VTI trace should be made along the outer edge of the Doppler spectrum or the VTI will be underestimated. Normally the AV VTI is 18 to 22 cm.

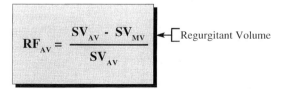

$$RF_{AV} = \frac{SV_{AV} - SV_{MV}}{SV_{AV}} \quad \leftarrow \boxed{\text{Regurgitant Volume}}$$

Figure 14-24. The aortic valve regurgitant volume and fraction can be calculated using this formula. A regurgitant volume greater than or equal to 65 cc is consistent with severe aortic regurgitation. A regurgitant fraction greater than 50% is consistent with severe aortic regurgitation. RF, regurgitant volume; SV, stroke volume.

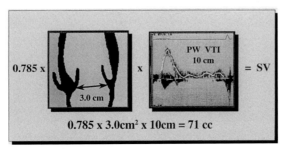

Figure 14-27. The stroke volume (SV) across this patient's mitral valve (MV) is 71 cc. The MV diameter is measured from the apical four-chamber view. The MV velocity time interval (VTI) is measured with pulsed-wave Doppler from the apical four-chamber view with the sample volume placed at the level of the MV annulus. The MV VTI trace should be made along the modal (most intense) portion of the Doppler spectrum or the VTI will be overestimated. Normally, the MV VTI is 10 to 12 cm.

SUPRASTERNAL WINDOW

The descending aorta can be visualized from the suprasternal window in most patients. Normally there is a brief period during early diastole when blood flow reverses in the descending aorta followed by continued forward flow down the descending aorta. This normal brief reversal of flow is due to the elastic recoil of the aorta and the movement of blood from the smaller-diameter descending aorta toward the larger-diameter ascending aorta after aortic valve closure. When a patient has moderate to severe aortic regurgitation, there will be holodiastolic flow reversal in the descending aorta (Fig. 14-29).

As the severity of aortic regurgitation increases, so does the holodiastolic velocity in the descending aorta. Although not validated, we have found that if the velocity time integral of the holodiastolic reversal velocities exceeds 15 cm, the degree of aortic

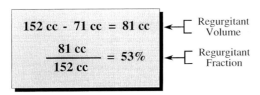

Figure 14-28. Both the regurgitant volume and regurgitant fraction in this patient are consistent with severe aortic regurgitation.

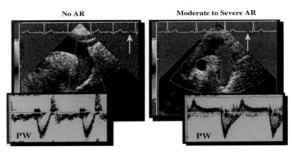

Figure 14-29. The panel on the left shows the typical two-dimensional and pulsed wave (PW) Doppler findings from the descending aorta in a patient with no aortic regurgitation (AR). The panel on the right shows the typical two-dimensional and PW Doppler findings from the descending aorta in a patient with moderate to severe AR.

regurgitation is generally severe compared to other validated echocardiographic measures of aortic regurgitation such as regurgitant jet/left ventricular outflow tract diameter ratios and regurgitant fractions (Fig. 14-30).

SUBCOSTAL WINDOW

The abdominal aorta can be visualized in most adult patients from the subcostal window or left lateral flank approach. The abdominal aorta is best imaged at a level that is slightly lower than the standard position used to obtain cardiac images. Generally, it is not possible to obtain spectral Doppler recordings

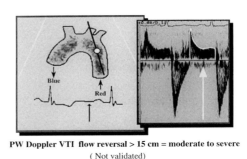

Figure 14-30. The panel on the left illustrates the correct position for sampling the descending aorta with pulsed wave (PW) Doppler. The medium-sized PW sample gate is positioned just below the origin of the left subclavian artery. The panel on the right shows how to trace the holodiastolic reversal velocities to obtain the velocity time interval (VTI).

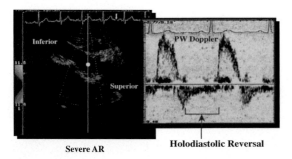

Figure 14-31. Two-dimensional Doppler (left) and pulsed wave Doppler (right) from the subcostal window, abdominal aorta, in a patient with severe aortic regurgitation.

that are parallel to the abdominal aorta; thus the color flow and spectral Doppler velocities will be significantly lower than the descending aortic velocities. We have found that the presence of holodiastolic reversal of the color Doppler signal in the abdominal aorta is sensitive in discriminating between mild to moderate and moderate to severe regurgitation. The accuracy of this method may be limited if the patient has a thoracic or abdominal aortic aneurysm or a severely calcified, narrow aorta. (Figs. 14-31 and 14-32).

Over the past decade, advances in technology have made echocardiography the most commonly used noninvasive method for the evaluation of aortic valve disease. As technology has advanced, so has the sophistication of the instrumentation on most of today's ultrasound systems. To obtain the best possible echocardiographic assessment, the sonographer must possess considerable technical skill and have the ability to adapt the various echocardiographic techniques and methods to each individual patient.

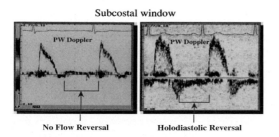

Figure 14-32. The panel on the left is an abdominal pulsed wave Doppler trace from a patient with no aortic regurgitation. The panel on the right is from a patient with severe aortic regurgitation.

REFERENCES

1. Bengur AR, Snider R, Meliones JN, et al. Doppler evaluation of aortic valve area in children with aortic stenosis. J Am Coll Cardiol. 1991;18:1499–1505.
2. Callahan MJ, Tajik AJ, Su-Fan Q, et al. Validation of instantaneous pressure gradients measured by continuous wave Doppler in experimentally induced aortic stenosis. Am J Cardiol. 1985;56:989–993.
3. Currie PJ, Seward JB, Reeder GS, et al. Continuous wave Doppler echocardiographic assessment of severity of calcific aortic stenosis: Simultaneous Doppler-catheter correlative study in 100 adult patients. Circulation. 1985;71:1162–1169.
4. Dolan MS, Castello R, St Vrain JE, et al. Quantitation of aortic regurgitation by Doppler echocardiography: A practical approach. Am Heart J. 1995;129:1014–1020.
5. Feigenbaum H. Echocardiography, 5th ed. Philadelphia, Lea & Febiger; 1994.
6. Harry MJ, et al. Beat to beat Doppler method for evaluating the systolic performance of native and prosthetic aortic valves. J Am Soc Echocardiogr. 1993;6:S26.
7. Kennedy KD, Nishimura RA, Holmes DR, et al. Natural history of moderate aortic stenosis. J Am Coll Cardiol. 1991;17:313–319.
8. Labovitz AJ, Ferrara RP, Kern MJ, et al. Quantitative evaluation of aortic insufficiency by continuous wave Doppler echocardiography. J Am Coll Cardiol. 1986;8:1341–1347.
9. Oakley CM, et al. Optimal timing of surgery for chronic mitral or aortic regurgitation. J Heart Valve Dis. 1993;2:223–229.
10. Oh JK, et al. The Echo Manual. Boston, Little, Brown; 1994.
11. Oh JK, Taliercio CP, Homes DR, et al. Prediction of the severity of aortic stenosis by Doppler aortic valve area determination: Prospective Doppler-catheterization correlation in 100 patients. J Am Coll Cardiol. 1988;11:1227–1234.
12. Omoto R, et al. The development of real time two dimensional Doppler echocardiography and its clinical significance in acquired valvular diseases. Jpn Heart J. 1984;25:325–340.
13. Otto CM, Pearlman AS, Comess XA, et al. Determination of the stenotic aortic valve area in adults using Doppler echocardiography. J Am Coll Cardiol. 1986;7:509–517.
14. Otto CM, Nishimura RA, Davis KB, et al. Doppler echocardiographic findings in adults with severe symptomatic valvular aortic stenosis. Am J Cardiol. 1991;68:1477–1484.
15. Perry GJ, Helmcke F, Nanda NC, et al. Evaluation of aortic insufficiency by Doppler color flow mapping. J Am Coll Cardiol. 1987;9:952–959.

16. Rokey R, et al. Determination of regurgitant fraction in isolated mitral or aortic regurgitation by pulsed Doppler two-dimensional echocardiography. J Am Coll Cardiol. 1986;7:1273–1278.

17. Samuels DA, Curfman GD, Friedlich AL, et al. Valve replacement for aortic regurgitation: Long term follow up with factors influencing the results. Circulation. 1979;60:647–654.

18. Shintaro B, Suzuki S, Matsada H, et al. Rapidity of progression of aortic stenosis in patients with congenital bicuspid aortic valves. Am J Cardiol. 1993; 71:322–327.

19. Skjaerpe T, Hegrenaes L, Hathe L, et al. Noninvasive estimation of valve area in patients with aortic stenosis by Doppler ultrasound and two-dimensional echocardiography. Circulation. 1985;72:810–818.

20. Stoddard MF, Arce J, Liddell NE, et al. Two-dimensional transesophageal echocardiographic determination of aortic valve area in adults with aortic stenosis. Am Heart J. 1991;122:1415–1422.

21. Tavli T, et al. Doppler-derived aortic valve gradients: Imaging versus non-imaging techniques. J Heart Valve Dis. 1993;2:253–256.

22. Teirstein P, Yeager M, Yock PG, et al. Doppler echocardiographic measurement of aortic valve area in aortic stenosis: A noninvasive application of the Gorlin formaula. J Am Coll Cardiol. 1986;8: 1059–1065.

23. Vaslef SN, Roberts WC. Early descriptions of aortic valve stenosis. Am Heart J. 1993;125:1465–1474.

24. Williams GA, Labovitz AJ, Nelson JG, et al. Value of multiple echocardiographic views in the evaluation of aortic stenosis in adults by continuous-wave Doppler. Am J Cardiol. 1985;55:445–449.

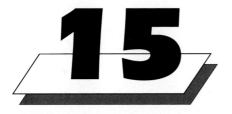

15

Right Heart Valve Disease

MARK N. ALLEN

Introduction

The anatomy of the right-sided valves was described in Chapter 1. This chapter discusses the pathologic processes that affect the tricuspid and pulmonic valves. Most discussion on the pathology of the heart valves focuses on the left heart valves. However, there are conditions that predispose to the right-sided valves that can be detected echocardiographically. Diseases that primarily affect the left-sided valves may also affect the right-sided valves, but much less frequently.

Tricuspid Valve

ECHOCARDIOGRAPHIC VIEWS

There are several optimal views or acoustic windows that can be used to evaluate the tricuspid valve by two-dimensional echocardiography. A modification of the standard left parasternal long-axis view allows visualization of the tricuspid valve and the right ventricular inflow tract (Fig. 15-1). This view is obtained by placing the transducer at the level of the third or fourth intercostal space, with the reference mark pointed toward the patient's right shoulder (long axis orientation). The transducer is rotated slightly counterclockwise and angled posteriorly. Figure 15-1 illustrates this modified view, demonstrating the right atrium, tricuspid valve, and right ventricle.

A parasternal short axis view will also demonstrate the tricuspid valve (Fig. 15-2). From this view, the valve is best seen with the transducer positioned at the base of the heart and angled posteriorly and medially toward the right side of the patient's body, as described in Chapter 10. From this view, the doming characteristics of a stenotic valve can be appreciated. In addition, the direction of blood flow is toward and parallel to the transducer, accommodating Doppler interrogation.

The apical four-chamber view allows visualization of the mitral and tricuspid valves in the same plane (Fig. 15-3). The sonographer should attempt to locate the point of maximum impulse (PMI) using two fingers. Once the PMI is located, the transducer is placed on this point and minor rotations or angulations, as described in Chapter 10, may be necessary to optimize the image. However, while this view will aid in the visualization of the tricuspid valve, the direction of blood flow will not be parallel to the sound beam in most patients. This problem can be corrected by using a modification of the view just described. Using this orientation as a starting point, the transducer is slid up one interspace toward the patient's midline. This will align the Doppler cursor parallel to flow across the tricuspid valve.

The subcostal long axis view will allow visualization of the right ventricle, right atrium, and tricuspid valve (Fig. 15-4). Although the flow of blood from this view will typically be at an angle of 20 degrees or more, careful angulation of the transducer may allow

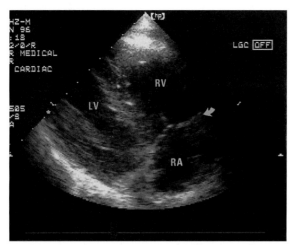

Figure 15-1. Modified left parasternal long axis view demonstrating the right ventricular inflow tract and tricuspid valve. RA, right atrium; RV, right ventricle; LV, left ventricle; arrow, tricuspid valve.

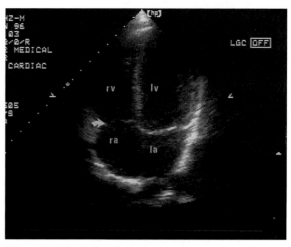

Figure 15-3. Apical four-chamber view demonstrating the tricuspid valve (arrow). ra, right atrium; rv, right ventricle; la, left atrium; lv, left ventricle.

Doppler interrogation of the valve with near-parallel orientation. In patients with chronic obstructive pulmonary disease (COPD), other acoustic windows will typically be very poor and a subcostal approach may be the only available window.

The stand-alone Doppler probe can also be used to evaluate the tricuspid valve. A poor-quality image will not necessarily provide a poor Doppler signal. Becoming proficient with a pencil or pedoff probe is important because it can be a powerful tool in the echocardiography lab. Starting in an apical

position, the sonographer uses the pencil probe to locate the mitral flow signal. With a slight posterior angulation the tricuspid valve signal can be identified. The tricuspid regurgitant signal can be differentiated from the aortic signal in that the former will last throughout most of systole and will peak more slowly. Differentiating the tricuspid regurgitant signal from mitral regurgitation can be more difficult. When using this technique, it is important to identify the mitral valve inflow, which usually has a higher velocity than the tricuspid valve inflow.

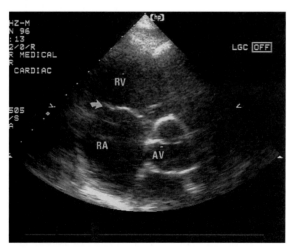

Figure 15-2. Left parasternal short axis view demonstrating tricuspid valve (arrow). RA, right atrium; RV, right ventricle; AV, aortic valve.

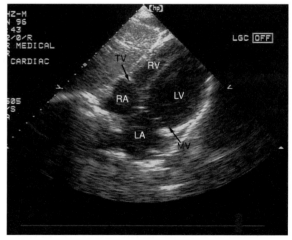

Figure 15-4. Subcostal four-chamber view demonstrating the tricuspid valve (arrows). RA, right atrium; RV, right ventricle; LA, left atrium; LV, left ventricle; MV, mitral valve.

This technique is particularly important in patients who have poor imaging windows and where the presence and severity of tricuspid regurgitation, as well as the determination of systolic pulmonary artery pressures, are important diagnostic questions.

Tricuspid Stenosis

Tricuspid stenosis is most often caused by rheumatic heart disease.[31] It can also be caused by other conditions, such as systemic lupus erythematosus, carcinoid heart disease, Loeffler's endocarditis, metastatic melanoma, and congenital heart disease.[26,31,42,68,76,84] The diagnosis of tricuspid stenosis may be overlooked clinically because the characteristic physical signs can be masked by concurrent mitral valve disease[21,31,38,71]; consequently, it is important for the echocardiographer to have a thorough understanding of the patient's history.

RHEUMATIC TRICUSPID STENOSIS

The reported incidence of tricuspid valve involvement in patients with rheumatic mitral valve disease varies from 3% to 67%.[1,12,19,21,24,31,36,71] Isolated rheumatic tricuspid stenosis almost never occurs.[1,12,21,31,36,71] Significant tricuspid stenosis occurs in roughly 3–5% of patients with rheumatic

disease.[58] The diagnosis of tricuspid stenosis is important because undetected and uncorrected tricuspid stenosis can lead to an increase in operative morbidity and mortality in patients who undergo surgery for left-sided valve disease.[4,47,86] Uncorrected rheumatic tricuspid stenosis can lead to chronic elevation in right atrial pressure and low cardiac output despite successful surgical correction of the left-sided valves.[47]

Echocardiography is useful in the detection of tricuspid stenosis.[24,38,58] Although the M-mode findings in rheumatic tricuspid stenosis are similar to those in rheumatic mitral stenosis, the accuracy of the former is far lower. The M-mode criteria for rheumatic tricuspid stenosis include (1) diminished EF slope, (2) anterior displacement of the posterior leaflet, and (3) thickening of valve leaflets and apparatus.[58] However, in rheumatic heart disease, there is frequently concurrent pulmonary hypertension and right ventricular hypertrophy, which also lead to a diminished EF slope.[33] Anterior displacement of the posterior leaflet cannot always be well visualized and is therefore not a reliable finding.[58]

Two-dimensional echocardiography is a more reliable technique in the diagnosis of rheumatic tricuspid stenosis.[4,47,86] Two-dimensional criteria for rheumatic tricuspid stenosis include (1) doming of the tricuspid valve leaflets in diastole, typically more

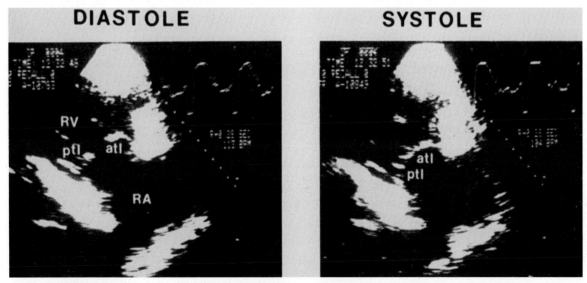

Figure 15-5. Two-dimensional echocardiographic study of a patient with rheumatic tricuspid stenosis. Diastolic (left) and systolic (right) frames of a thickened tricuspid valve. RA, right atrium; RV, right ventricle; atl, anterior leaflet; ptl, posterior leaflet. (Reprinted by permission of the publisher from Daniels SJ, Mintz GS, Kotler M. Rheumatic Tricuspid Valve Disease: 2D Echocardiographic hemodynamic and angiographic correlations. The American Journal of Cardiology, Vol: 54, p 493. Copyright 1983 by Excerpta Medica Inc.)

toward the tips of the leaflets, (2) thickening and reduced excursion of the posterior or septal leaflets, or both, and (3) reduced tricuspid orifice diameter relative to the diameter of the tricuspid annulus in the same scan plane[38] (Fig. 15-5).

Doppler echocardiography can be used to qualify and quantitate the severity of tricuspid stenosis. The Doppler signals in tricuspid stenosis are similar in appearance to those in mitral stenosis.[62] With the Doppler sample placed across the tricuspid valve, the Doppler signal will have a higher diastolic velocity than normal and will demonstrate turbulent flow. There will also be prolonged reduction in velocity throughout diastole.[63] Velocities across the tricuspid valve can be higher than normal in the presence of tricuspid regurgitation but do not usually exceed 0.7 m/sec. Velocities across a stenotic tricuspid valve will be close to or higher than 1 m/sec[62] (Fig. 15-6). Calculating the area of a valve is more difficult due to the anatomic structure of the valve and the lack of reliable data. Planimeterization by two-dimensional echocardiography is difficult, due in part to the inability to view the tricuspid valve in a cross-sectional plane. A Doppler-derived valve area can be calculated using the pressure half-time method, but insufficient data exist on the validity of these numbers. At present, the quantifiable data are limited to the peak velocities and the peak and mean gradients across the tricuspid valve.

Color Doppler flow can be helpful in guiding the continuous or pulsed wave Doppler cursors by locating the turbulent diastolic jet. This can be done from a number of imaging planes, such as in the left parasternal short axis and apical four-chamber views.

CARCINOID HEART DISEASE

Carcinoid heart disease results from the presence of carcinoid tumors, which are found predominantly in the gastrointestinal tract. These tumors produce vasoactive substances that ultimately cause endothelial damage to the right side of the heart.[72] The primary tumors can be small, with hepatic metastases noted in most patients who demonstrate cardiac involvement. Involvement of the heart occurs late in the progression of the disease in nearly half of those with carcinoid syndrome.[68,72] Clinical symptoms include episodes of facial flushing with stimuli, abdominal pain, diarrhea, and renal and hepatic failure. Hepatomegaly is usually associated with later stages of the disease. Cardiac signs include elevated venous pressure and systolic and diastolic murmurs.[41,72]

The two-dimensional echocardiographic signs of carcinoid heart disease are distinctive and are usually restricted to the right heart. These findings include (1) dilation of the right ventricle with abnormal septal motion, indicative of right ventricular volume overload, (2) thickened tricuspid valve leaflets that are retracted, with foreshortened chordae, and (3) thickened, retracted pulmonic valve cusps. The tricuspid valve leaflets usually do not coapt completely and remain open throughout the cardiac cycle (Fig. 15-7).[5,13,30] The Doppler signs of carcinoid heart disease include (1) tricuspid regurgitation, which is the most prevalent finding, (2) increased diastolic velocities across the tricuspid valve, (3) increased diastolic velocities across the pulmonic valve, and (4) pulmonic insufficiency. Although these findings are similar to those of rheumatic tricuspid steno-

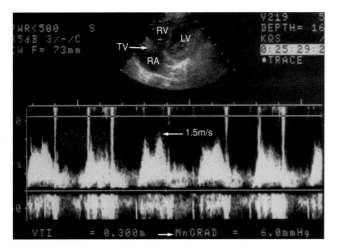

Figure 15-6. Doppler and two-dimensional images of a patient with rheumatic tricuspid stenosis (arrows). Continuous Doppler signal from a modified apical view across the tricuspid valve. Note the mean gradient of 6 mm Hg and the peak velocity of >1.5 m/sec (bottom arrow). *RA,* right atrium; *RV,* right ventricle; *LV,* left ventricle; *TV,* tricuspid valve.

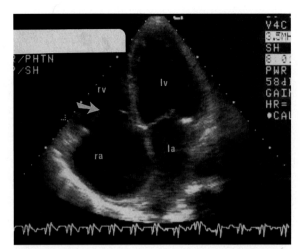

Figure 15-7. Patient with carcinoid heart disease. The tricuspid valve is retracted and foreshortened and remains open in systole (arrow). ra, right atrium; rv, right ventricle; la, left atrium; lv, left ventricle.

sis, carcinoid heart disease is differentiated by the lack of left-sided valvular involvement.[13,25,30,66,78]

TRICUSPID REGURGITATION

A common abnormality associated with the tricuspid valve in the adult population is the presence of tricuspid regurgitation. This is caused by two general mechanisms. First, it can be caused secondary to right heart chamber abnormalities such as right atrial and ventricular enlargement or right ventricular infarction.[32] Right atrial enlargement causes dilatation of the tricuspid annulus, preventing the leaflets from closing completely.[16] Enlargement of the right ventricle is associated with conditions that cause a volume or pressure overload of the right ventricle. These conditions include aortic and mitral valve disease, especially mitral stenosis, in which the left-sided pressure elevates to a level that causes pulmonary hypertension. Pulmonic and tricuspid valve insufficiency, the latter being caused by a number of factors, including the presence of a pacer wire, cardiac transplant,[56] or tricuspid valve disease, also cause RV dilation. Other causes of RV dilation include congenital heart disease such as partial anomalous venous return. Dilatation of the right ventricle as a consequence of volume overload is thought to alter the tricuspid apparatus, distorting its relation with the valve leaflets.[32] Right ventricular infarction has been associated with tricuspid regurgitation.[59] The posterior papillary muscle of the right ventricle

is frequently involved in right ventricular infarction, and it is this muscle that attaches to the posterior and septal leaflets of the tricuspid valve.[27]

The second, and less common, mechanism of regurgitation across the tricuspid valve occurs as a consequence of actual tricuspid valve disease, including rheumatic tricuspid disease, tricuspid valve prolapse, endocarditis, ruptured papillary muscles or chordae, carcinoid heart disease, congenital defects of the tricuspid valve such as tricuspid valve dysphasia, and Ebstein's anomaly and trauma.[80,81]

Assessing the cause of tricuspid regurgitation will aid in patient management. However, tricuspid regurgitation is frequently noted in patients with structurally normal hearts.[11,17,43,64,85] Two-dimensional echocardiography allows the visualization of the valve and can help identify valvular abnormalities or secondary causes such as annular dilatation. The severity of tricuspid regurgitation is best detected using Doppler echocardiography techniques. Several methods provide some qualitative measure in assessing the severity of tricuspid regurgitation. Jet size is perhaps the most common method used. Color Doppler echocardiography provides sensitivity and specificity in the detection and assessment of tricuspid regurgitation allowing the jet to be visualized from a variety of tomographic planes[56] (Fig. 15-8A–C). Color Doppler provides a rapid assessment of the severity of tricuspid regurgitation.[18] Jet size, in terms of length and area, correlates reasonably well with angiographic grades.[53] The larger the jet, the more severe the lesion. Typically, the jet is considered mild if it is noted to be within one-third of the right atrium, moderate if it is within the first half and severe if it fills the right atrium (Fig. 15-9). Although this is less than precise, a rough correlation does exist between the size of the color jet and the severity of the regurgitation.[29] The severity can also be determined by calculating the ratios of right atrial area to areas of the color jet.[56] Despite the good correlations, one must keep in mind that the color jet is a velocity jet, not a volume jet; furthermore, the jet is influenced by other factors, including pressures, atrial size, and technical variations among laboratories. Factors such as gain settings and system configurations can also affect the visualization of regurgitant jets. It is important to use a variety of scanning planes and acoustic windows when evaluating tricuspid regurgitation.

Another method used to assess tricuspid severity is to observe the pattern of flow within the he-

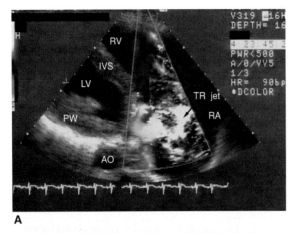

A

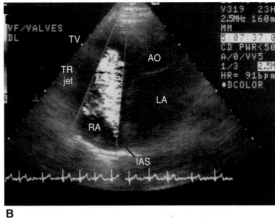

B

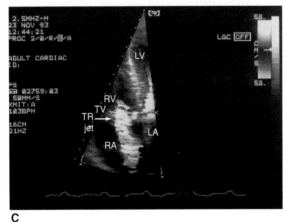

C

Figure 15-8. (**A**) Modified left parasternal long axis or right ventricular inflow view of a patient with significant tricuspid regurgitation (arrow). RA, right atrium; RV, right ventricle; LV, left ventricle; IVS, interventricular septum; PW, posterior wall; Ao, descending thoracic aorta; TR, tricuspid regurgitation. (**B**) Left parasternal short axis view of a patient with significant tricuspid regurgitation (TR) (arrow). Note the enlarged right and left atria. RA, right atrium; RV, right ventricle; LV, left ventricle; LA, left atrium; IAS, interatrial septum; TV, tricuspid valve. (**C**) Apical four-chamber view of a patient with tricuspid regurgitation (arrow). RA, right atrium; RV, right ventricle; LA, left atrium; LV, left ventricle; TV, tricuspid valve.

patic veins and inferior vena cava. From a subcostal transducer position, the hepatic veins and inferior vena cava can be seen emptying into the right atrium. Blood flows from these vessels into the right atrium during systole when right atrial pressure falls as a result of atrial relaxation. In patients with severe tricuspid regurgitation, retrograde flow is noted in

the hepatics and inferior vena cava as systolic flow reversal (Fig. 15-10). This pattern of flow in not noted in patients considered to have mild or moderate tricuspid regurgitation.[82]

The quantitative methods described for mitral regurgitation (see Chapter 13) can also be applied to the evaluation of tricuspid regurgitation. How-

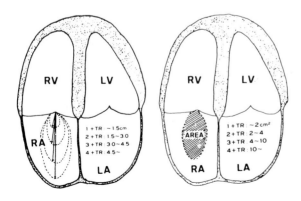

Figure 15-9. Method for quantifying tricuspid regurgitation (TR) jet area and volume. RA, right atrium; RV, right ventricle; LA, left atrium; LV, left ventricle. (From Miyatake K. Evaluation of tricuspid regurgitation by pulsed doppler and 2D echocardiography. Circulation. Vol. 66, p. 777. Copyright 1982 by American Heart Association.)

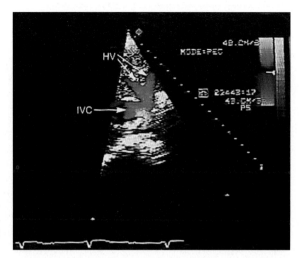

Figure 15-10. Subcostal view of hepatic veins and inferior vena cava (IVC) in a patient with significant tricuspid regurgitation. Note the systolic reflux flow in these vessels (red flow). HV, hepatic vein. (See also Color Plate 46.)

ever, further data are needed to validate these approaches to tricuspid regurgitation.

Figures 15-8A to 15-8C demonstrate some of the views used to assess tricuspid regurgitation. The apical four-chamber view allows visualization of the tricuspid valve. It may not always be possible to see the tricuspid valve clearly in this view, especially in conditions where the left heart is dilated, in patients with COPD, or in those with poor acoustic windows. The parasternal short axis view, with the transducer angled toward the base of the heart and tilted toward the right, will also allow visualization of the tricuspid valve. From a high parasternal long axis view, visualization of the right ventricular inflow and the tricuspid valve is possible. These views, like the apical views, may not always be available. However, the subcostal view can also be used to evaluate the tricuspid regurgitation jets. A subcostal four-chamber view and a subcostal short axis view can be obtained and will allow assessment of the jets, although it may be difficult to determine the severity from these views, especially if the entire right atrium is not well seen. From the subcostal position, the hepatic veins and inferior vena cava can be seen. As stated earlier, when there is severe tricuspid regurgitation, flow in these vessels can be reversed throughout systole.

Determining the severity of tricuspid regurgitation can be helpful in deciding to repair or replace the tricuspid valve in patients having surgery for other cardiac abnormalities.[16] However, the most common reason to identify and define tricuspid regurgitation is the determination of systolic pulmo-

nary pressures. Although color Doppler can help identify and assess the severity, the velocity of the tricuspid regurgitation jet; therefore, the pressures can be assessed only by continuous Doppler echocardiography. Pulsed wave Doppler can also identify the presence of regurgitation, but it cannot determine pressure gradients if the velocities are higher than the Nyquist limit. In the presence of tricuspid regurgitation, the pressure gradients can be calculated using the Bernoulli equation, discussed in Chapter 15. Once the pressure gradient is calculated, the systolic pulmonary artery pressures can be calculated by adding the right atrial pressure to the peak gradient across the tricuspid valve. Normal right atrial pressures range from 10 to 14 mm Hg.[28] Frequently, the pulmonary artery pressure is calculated by adding 10 mm Hg to the peak tricuspid valve pressure gradient. Another method used to calculate systolic pulmonary artery pressure is to multiply the tricuspid valve pressure gradient by 25% and add that number to the tricuspid regurgitation gradient. This method may provide a more accurate right atrial pressure in patients with significantly increased pulmonary artery pressures. Figure 15-11 demonstrates these two formulas.

The detection of tricuspid regurgitation can be difficult in some patients, so calculating pulmonary artery pressures using this technique may not be possible. Flow across the pulmonic valve can be used to assess the presence and, to some degree, the severity of the systolic pulmonary artery pressure. Measuring the acceleration time, the preejection period, and the ejection time of the Doppler signal

Assuming RA pressure is 10 mm Hg
PAP = RVSP = 4 v2 + RA pressure

v = peak velocity of TR jet
RA pressure = jugular venous pressure

Assuming RA pressure is 25% of regurgitant pressure
PAP = RVSP = 4 v2 + RA pressure
PAP = RVSP = 4 v2 + 25%(v)

Figure 15-11. Formula for calculating tricuspid regurgitation gradients and pulmonary artery pressures.

can help detect the presence and, to some degree, the severity of pulmonary hypertension. The combination of the various echocardiographic techniques has proven useful in the detection and assessment of tricuspid regurgitation. Two-dimensional echocardiography helps to determine the cause of the regurgitant lesion. Color Doppler aids in detection and assessment, and continuous wave Doppler helps in the evaluation of pulmonary artery pressure in the presence of regurgitation. The color map is useful in identifying the jets and can be used to guide the continuous wave cursor into the proper position to obtain pressure gradients.

Detection of tricuspid regurgitation is not always easy due to factors such as poor acoustic windows, technical difficulties, and trivial regurgitant jets. Contrast echocardiography has been useful in enhancing tricuspid regurgitation.[3,8,15,23,40,46,51,77,79]

When agitated saline solution is injected into a peripheral vein, microbubbles are noted in the right atrium and ventricle. In the presence of tricuspid regurgitation, the Doppler signal from the regurgitant jet is enhanced (Fig. 15-12*A,B*).

TRICUSPID VALVE PROLAPSE

Tricuspid valve prolapse is a condition in which the tricuspid valve buckles into the right atrium during systole. This occurs in conjunction with mitral valve prolapse, and some studies have shown that tricuspid valve prolapse occurs in as many as 54% of patients with mitral valve prolapse.[2,14,35,48,69] The diagnosis of tricuspid valve prolapse is difficult due to the lack of echocardiographic criteria and problems inherent in visualizing all the leaflets of the tricuspid valve from standard views. The diagnosis can be made by observing the tricuspid valve leaflets prolapsing past the tricuspid valve annulus during systole.[60] The ideal approach to analyzing tricuspid valve motion with reference to its attachment to the valve ring is the parasternal long axis view of right ventricular inflow, which allows visualization of the anterior and posterior leaflets. The apical four-chamber view may also be used, allowing evaluation of the anterior and septal leaflets.[74] Transesophageal echocardiography may have an increasingly important role in identifying and determining the severity of tricuspid valve prolapse[45] (Fig. 15-13).

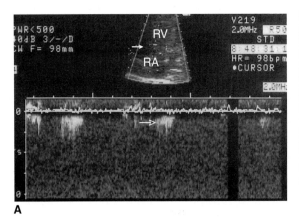
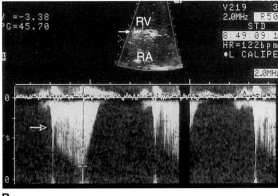

A   **B**

Figure 15-12. Frame **A** in a patient with trivial tricuspid regurgitation and a weak tricuspid regurgitation Doppler signal. With contrast enhancement (frame **B**) the tricuspid regurgitation is well demonstrated by color Doppler (open arrow) and the continuous wave Doppler signal is well demarcated (closed arrow). RA, right atrium; RV, right ventricle. (See also Color Plates 47 and 48.)

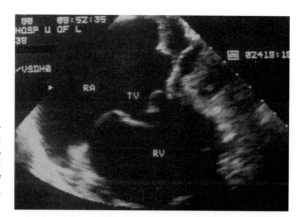

Figure 15-13. Transesophageal echocardiogram of a patient with tricuspid valve (TV) prolapse. Note the systolic collapse of the valve leaflets behind the plane of the valve annulus. RA, right atrium; RV, right ventricle. (From Liddell N et al. Transesophageal Echocardiographic Diagnosis of Isolated Tricuspid Valve Prolapse with Severe Tricuspid Regurgitation. American Heart Journal 1992:231.)

TRICUSPID ENDOCARDITIS

Endocarditis of the tricuspid valve is rare. It occurs primarily in the setting of intravenous drug abuse but may also occur with alcoholism and congenital defects such as ventral septal defect.[6,9] Typical clinical findings in patients with infective endocarditis involving the right-sided valves include (1) temperature above 100° F, (2) positive blood cultures—usually *Staphylococcus aureus*, and (3) murmurs of tricuspid or pulmonic insufficiency.[6,9] Pulmonary infiltrates can also be seen on chest roentgenograms or computed tomography scans (Fig. 15-14A,B).

The diagnosis of tricuspid endocarditis by two-dimensional echocardiography can be made by the appearance of a dense mass or masses that are highly mobile. The mass may appear shaggy, involving the entire valve (Fig. 15-15A,B), or as a

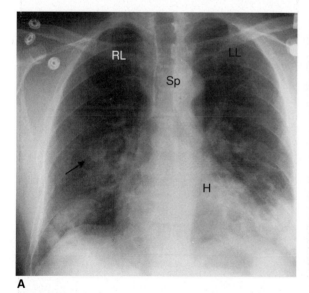

A

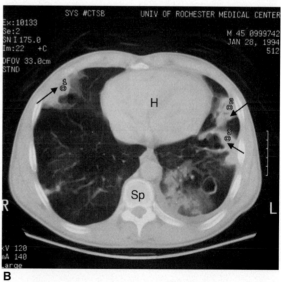

B

Figure 15-14. Chest film (**A**) and computed tomography scan (**B**) of a patient with bacterial endocarditis demonstrating lung infiltrates (arrows). RL, right lung; LL, left lung; H, heart; Sp, spine.

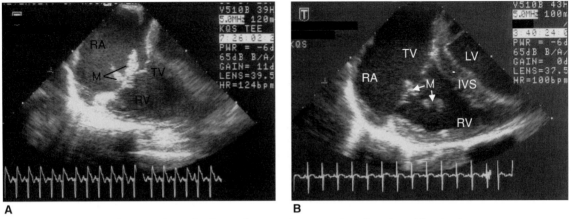

Figure 15-15. (**A,B**) Transesophageal echocardiogram demonstrating the tricuspid valve in patients with a history of intravenous drug use and tricuspid endocarditis. Note the shaggy appearance of these vegetations (M). RA, right atrium; RV, right ventricle; LV, left ventricle; TV, tricuspid valve; IVS, interventricular septum.

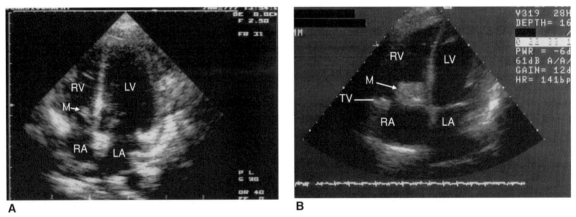

Figure 15-16. (**A,B**) Apical four-chamber views demonstrating the right atrium (RA) and right ventricle (RV) in a patient with tricuspid endocarditis. Note the polyploid appearance of these vegetations (M). LA, left atrium; LV, left ventricle; TV, tricuspid valve.

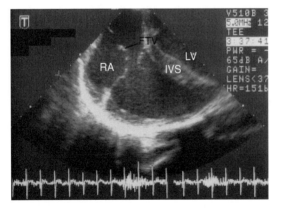

Figure 15-17. Transesophageal echocardiogram demonstrating the right atrium (RA) and right ventricle (RV) in a patient with a history of intravenous drug use and tricuspid endocarditis. Note the flail tricuspid valve (FTV), a complication of tricuspid endocarditis. IVS, interventricular septum.

polypoid structure attached to a single leaflet[9,52] (Fig. 15-16*A,B*). Tricuspid valve vegetations may be differentiated on two-dimensional echocardiography by either transthoracic or transesophageal echocardiography from masses such as myxomas by observing their anatomic location.[20] Myxomas typically have a stalk attached to the interatrial septum, while vegetations move in concert with the valve throughout the cardiac cycle. The most common anatomic complications of tricuspid endocarditis are tricuspid regurgitation and, more rarely, flail tricuspid valve[6,61] (Fig. 15-17). The diagnosis of flail tricuspid valve leaflet may be an important indication for early valvulectomy in the setting of endocarditis.[7]

Pulmonic Valve Disease

The pulmonic valve can be seen from different transthoracic positions; the left parasternal short-axis view is perhaps the best. From this position the transducer is angled slightly to the left, toward the left shoulder. A subcostal short axis window also provides a view of the pulmonic valve (Fig. 15-18). This view is best obtained by placing the transducer in a standard subcostal four-chamber view and rotating it toward the patient's left shoulder, revealing a short axis orientation.

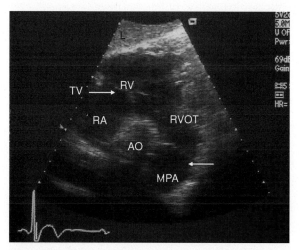

Figure 15-18. *Short axis subcostal view of the pulmonic valve (arrows). RA, right atrium; RV, right ventricle; TV, tricuspid valve; RVOT, right ventricular outflow tract; Ao, aorta; MPA, main pulmonary artery; L, liver.*

PULMONIC STENOSIS

In the adult, acquired pulmonic valve stenosis is rare. Pulmonary stenosis is a congenital disease and is discussed in detail in Chapter 29.

PULMONIC REGURGITATION

Pulmonic valve regurgitation is commonly noted in adults,[11] although its clinical significance is not well defined. It is recognized originating from the pulmonic valve as turbulent flow traveling into the right ventricular outflow tract during diastole. Color Doppler echocardiography is the ideal method for detecting the regurgitant jet. From a parasternal short axis view, the regurgitant flow is seen as a red mosaic jet traveling into the right ventricular outflow tract in diastole (Fig. 15-19). From this same position, pulsed and continuous wave Doppler demonstrate a wideband turbulent signal above the Doppler baseline in diastole.

In normal subjects, the diastolic signals of pulmonic regurgitation have the following characteristics: (1) long duration in diastole; (2) centrally located jet, originating from the valve coaptation point and directed toward the right ventricular outflow tract; and (3) flow velocities that are nearly the same as the transpulmonary pressure difference.[75] The causes of pulmonic valve insufficiency in the otherwise normal patient are still unclear. However, it is believed that it may be caused by the anatomic characteristics of the valve, which are different from those of the aortic valve in that the cusps of the pulmonic valve are thinner, have a less tight fibrous ring, and have shallower sinuses. Additionally, the retrograde pressure gradient from the pulmonary artery in diastole may not be sufficient to close the valve tightly enough to prevent regurgitation.[37,70]

Pulmonic valve regurgitation can be caused by numerous cardiac pathologies, including (1) pulmonary hypertension, (2) bacterial endocarditis, (3) pulmonary valvotomy, (4) congenital defects, (5) carcinoid heart disease, and (6) trauma.[83] Some early studies suggested that by examining the velocity profile of the regurgitant jet[54,75] and the distance traveled by the jet,[75] it is possible to differentiate between physiologic or normal pulmonic regurgitation and that caused by cardiac pathology. The velocity of the pulmonic regurgitant jet reflects the transpulmonary pressure difference during diastole. In a normal person with pulmonic regurgitation, the transpulmonary gradient is small, in the range

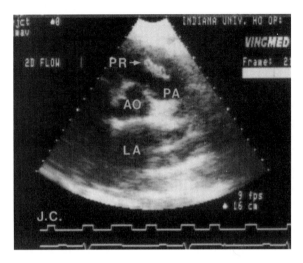

Figure 15-19. Left parasternal short axis view of the pulmonic valve with regurgitation (PR). LA, left atrium; AO, aorta; PA, pulmonary artery. (From Feigenbaum H. Echocardiography, 5th ed. Baltimore: Williams & Wilkins, 1994: 300.)

of 9 mm Hg (velocity of 1.5 m/sec). In patients with pulmonary hypertension this gradient is significantly greater.[75] Further, pulsed wave Doppler signals of the pulmonic regurgitant jet in patients with normal pulmonary artery pressures (<18 mm Hg) tend to peak early in diastole and then gradually slows in later diastole. In patients with higher pulmonary artery pressures (>25 mm Hg) the velocity profile exhibits a wideband spectrum that is sustained throughout diastole.[54]

The maximum distance traveled by the regurgitant jet may help differentiate clinically significant pulmonary regurgitation. In patients with no significant cardiac abnormalities (i.e., significant pulmonary hypertension), the distance traveled by the regurgitant jet is less than 10 mm. In patients with underlying cardiac pathology such as pulmonary hypertension, the regurgitant jet travels more than 20 mm.[75]

The regurgitant index and regurgitant fraction have also been used to assess the severity of pulmonic insufficiency[34,49] (Table 15-1). One must remember, however, that in the presence of pulmonic stenosis or aortic insufficiency, these values are less useful. Although these measurements may help to distinguish between physiologic and pathologic pulmonic insufficiency, further validation is needed.

PULMONIC ENDOCARDITIS

Endocarditis of the pulmonic valve is rare.[10,22,67] M-mode and two-dimensional echocardiography are useful in evaluating for endocarditis. Two-dimensional echocardiography provides spatial information on the valvular structures, allowing a more complete assessment of valve structures, and is therefore superior to M-mode in evaluating right-

TABLE 15-1. Measures of Severity of Pulmonic Valve Insufficiency

Degree of Pulmonary Insufficiency	Jet Distance (mm)	Regurgitant Index (cm^{2-}/m^2)	Regurgitant Fraction (%)
Mild	<10	0.64 +/− 0.60	<40%
Moderate	10–20	1.07 +/− 0.63	40–60%
Severe (clinically significant)	>20	2.2 +/− 1.67	>60%

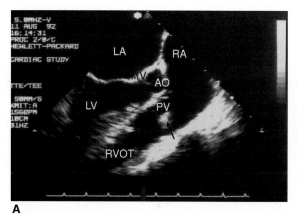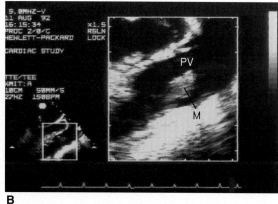

A **B**

Figure 15-20. (**A**) Transesophageal view of the pulmonic valve (PV) in a patient with pulmonic endocarditis. (**B**) The "res" function is used to enhance the image and to better demonstrate the point of attachment of the mass (arrow). LA, left atrium; LV, left ventricle; RVOT, right ventricular outflow tract; MV, mitral valve; RA, right atrium; M, mass.

sided valvular lesions.[10] Transesophageal echocardiography is even more sensitive in detecting vegetations of the valves, particularly in prosthetic valves.[55] The ability to visualize vegetations by transthoracic and transesophageal echocardiography is directly related to the size of the vegetations. The presence of vegetations on the pulmonic valve can be detected as shaggy echoes or localized echoes that are attached to or appear to replace normal valve tissue[39,50,57,65,73] (Fig. 15-20*A*,*B*).

The principal causes of pulmonic endocarditis include (1) congenital heart disease and (2) opiate addiction (intravenous drug abuse).[10] Congenital defects most often associated with pulmonic valve endocarditis include those in which a left-to-right shunt is a predisposing factor: (1) subpulmonary or subcristal ventral septal defect, (2) patient ductus arteriosus, (3) tetralogy of Fallot, (4) atrial septal defect, and (5) pulmonic stenosis.[10,39,57,73] In opiate addicts, infective endocarditis of the tricuspid valve is 10 times more common than that of the pulmonic valve.[57] In the case of intracardiac shunting, vegetations usually develop on the low-pressure side of the defect with endocardial trauma and downstream from the site of the lesions.[57] Regardless of the cause, these patients usually present with high fever.[10,50,55,57,73] A careful clinical history and physical examination are essential in these patients. Complications of pulmonic valve endocarditis include pulmonic valve insufficiency, rupture of the pulmonic valve, and premature opening of the valve.[10,22,44]

REFERENCES

1. Aceves S, Carral R. The diagnosis of tricuspid valve disease. Am Heart J. 1947;34:114–130.
2. Ainsworth RP, Hartamann AF, Aker U, et al. Tricuspid valve prolapse with late systolic tricuspid insufficiency. Radiology. 1973;107:309.
3. Amano K, Sakamoto T, Hada Y, et al. Detection of tricuspid regurgitation by contrast echocardiography. Japanese Circulation J. 1982;46:395–401.
4. Austen WG, De Sanctis RW, Sanders GA, et al. The surgical treatment of acquired trivavular disease. J Thorac Cardiovasc Surg. 1965;49:640.
5. Baker CJ, McNee VD, Scovil JA, et al. Tricuspid insufficiency in carcinoid heart disease: An echocardiographic description. Am Heart J. 1981;101:107–108.
6. Banks T, Fletcher R, Ali N. Infective endocarditis in heroin addicts. Am J Med. 1973;55:444–451.
7. Bates ER, Sorkin RP. Echocardiographic diagnosis of flail anterior leaflet in tricuspid endocarditis. Am Heart J. 1983;106:161–163.
8. Beard JT, Beard BF. Saline contrast enhancement of trivial tricuspid regurgitant signals for estimating pulmonary pressures. Am J Cardiol. 1988;62:486–488.
9. Berger M. Two-dimensional echocardiographic findings in right-sided infective endocarditis. Circulation. 1980;61:855–861.
10. Berger M, Wilkes HS, Gallerstein PE, et al. M-mode and two-dimensional echocardiographic findings in pulmonic valve endocarditis. Am Heart J. 1984;107:391–393.
11. Berger M, Hecht SR, Van-Tosh A, et al. Pulsed and continuous wave Doppler echocardiographic assess-

ment of valvular regurgitation in normal subjects. J Am Coll Cardiol. 1989;13:1540.

12. Braunwald E. Valvular heart disease. *In* Braunwald E (ed): Heart Disease. A Textbook of Cardiovascular Medicine. Philadelphia, WB Saunders; 1980: 1147–1149.

13. Callahan JA, Wroblewski EM, Reeder GS, et al. Echocardiographic features of carcinoid heart disease. Am J Cardiol. 1982;50:762–768.

14. Chandraratna PAN, Lopez JM, Fernandez JI, et al. Echocardiographic detection of tricuspid valve prolapse. Circulation. 1975;51:823.

15. Chen CC. Tricuspid regurgitation in tricuspid valve prolapse demonstrated with contrast cross-sectional echocardiography. Am J Cardiol. 1980;46: 983–987.

16. Child JS. Improved guides to tricuspid valve repair: Two-dimensional echocardiographic analysis of tricuspid annulus function and color flow imaging of severity of tricuspid regurgitation. JACC. 1989;14: 1275–1277.

17. Choong CY, Abasacal VM, Weyman J, et al. Prevalence of valvular regurgitation by Doppler echocardiography in patients with structurally normal hearts by two-dimensional echocardiography. Am Heart J. 1989;117:636.

18. Chopra HK, Nanda NC, Fan P, et al. Can two-dimensional echocardiography and Doppler color flow mapping identify the need for tricuspid valve repair? JACC. 1989;14:1266–1274.

19. Clausen BJ. Rheumatic heart disease: An analysis of 796 cases. Am Heart J. 1940;20:454–474.

20. Come PC, Kurland GS, Vine HS. Two-dimensional echocardiography in differentiating right atrial and tricuspid valve mass lesions. Am J Cardiol. 1979;44: 1207–1212.

21. Cooke W, White PD. Tricuspid stenosis with particular reference to diagnosis and prognosis. Br Heart J. 1941;3:147.

22. Cremieux AC, et al. Clinical and echocardiographic observations in pulmonary valve endocarditis. Am Heart J. 1985;56:610–613.

23. Curtis JM, Thyssen M, Berner HM, et al. Doppler versus contrast echocardiography for the diagnosis of tricuspid regurgitation. Am J Cardiol. 1985;56: 333–336.

24. Daniels SJ, Mintz GS, Kotler MN. Rheumatic tricuspid valve disease: Two-dimensional echocardiographic, hemodynamic, and angiographic correlations. Am J Cardiol. 1983;51:492–496.

25. Davies MK. Cross sectional echocardiographic feature in carcinoid heart disease. A mechanism for tricuspid regurgitation in this syndrome. Br Heart J. 1984;51:355–357.

26. Deconomos NS, Camilaris DH, Petritis J, et al. Congenital tricuspid valvular stenosis. J Thorac Cardiovasc Surg. 1975;16:100.

27. Erhardt LR. Clinical and pathological observations on different types of acute myocardial infarction: A study of 84 patients after treatment in a coronary care unit. Acta Med Scand. 1974;560(suppl):1–78.

28. Feigenbaum H. Echocardiography, 5th ed. Philadelphia, Lea & Febiger; 1994:294.

29. Feigenbaum H. Echocardiography, 5th ed. Philadelphia, Lea & Febiger; 1994:196.

30. Forman MB. Two-dimensional echocardiography in the diagnosis of carcinoid heart disease. Am Heart J. 1984;107:492–496.

31. Gibson R, Wood P. The diagnosis of tricuspid stenosis. Br Heart J. 1955;17:552.

32. Gibson TC, Foale RA, Guyer DE, et al. Clinical significance of incomplete tricuspid valve closure seen on two-dimensional echocardiography. JACC. 1984;4:1052–1057.

33. Goldberg E, Chaithiraehan S. Severe pulmonary hypertension echocardiographic pseudostenosis of mitral and tricuspid valve. NY State J Med. 1975:1772.

34. Goldberg SJ, Allen HD. Quantitative assessment of Doppler echocardiography of pulmonary or aortic regurgitation. Am J Cardiol. 1985;56:131.

35. Gooch AS, Maranhao V, Scampardonis G, et al. Prolapse of both mitral and tricuspid leaflets in systolic murmur-click syndrome. N Engl J Med. 1972;287: 1218.

36. Goodwin JF, Rab SM, Sinha AK, et al. Rheumatic tricuspid stenosis. Br Med J. 1957;2:1383–1389.

37. Gross L, Kugel MA. Topographic anatomy and histology of the valves in the human heart. Am J Pathol. 1931;7:445–473.

38. Guyer DE, et al. Comparison of the echocardiographic and hemodynamic diagnosis of rheumatic tricuspid stenosis. JACC. 1984;3:1135–1144.

39. Harasawa Y, et al. Two-dimensional echocardiographic demonstration of flail pulmonic valve due to infective endocarditis. Am Heart J. 1984;108: 1552–1554.

40. Himelman RB, Stulbarg M, Kircher B, et al. Noninvasive evaluation of pulmonary artery pressure during exercise by saline enhanced Doppler echocardiography in chronic pulmonary disease. Circulation. 1989; 79:863–871.

41. Kaplan EL. The carcinoid syndromes. *In* Friesen SR (ed): Surgical Endocrinology: Clinical Syndromes. Philadelphia: JB Lippincott, 1978:120–144.

42. Kitchin A, Turner R. Diagnosis and treatment of tricuspid stenosis. Br Heart J. 1964;26:354–379.

43. Kostucke W, Vandenbossche JL, Friart A, et al. Pulsed Doppler regurgitant flow patterns of normal valves. Am J Cardiol. 1986;58:309.

44. Kramer NE, Gill SS, Patel R, et al. Pulmonary valve vegetations detected with echocardiography. Am J Cardiol. 1977;39:1064.

45. Liddell NE. Transesophageal echocardiographic diagnosis of isolated tricuspid valve prolapse with severe tricuspid regurgitation. Am Heart J. 1992;123:230–232.

46. Lieppe W, Behar VS, Scallion R, et al. Detection of tricuspid regurgitation with two-dimensional echocardiography and peripheral veins injections. Circulation. 1978;57:128–132.

47. Lillehei CW, Gannon PG, Levy MJ, et al. Valve replacement for tricuspid stenosis or insufficiency associated with mitral valvular disease. Circulation. 1966;33:34.

48. Maranhao V, Gooch AS, Yang SS. Prolapse of the tricuspid leaflets in the systolic murmur-click syndrome. Cathet Cardiovasc Diagn. 1975;1:81.

49. Marx GR, Hicks RW, Allen HD, et al. Noninvasive assessment of hemodynamic response to exercise in pulmonary regurgitation after operations to correct pulmonary outflow obstruction. Am J Cardiol. 1988;61:595.

50. Mehlman DJ, Furey W, Phair J, et al. Two-dimensional echocardiographic features diagnostic of isolated pulmonic valve endocarditis. Am Heart J. 1982;103:137–139.

51. Meltzer RS, Vered Z, Benjamin P, et al. Diagnosing tricuspid regurgitation by direct imaging of the regurgitant flow in the right atrium using contrast echocardiography. Am J Cardiol. 1983;52:1050–1053.

52. Mintz GS, et al. Comparison of two-dimensional and M-mode echocardiography in the evaluation of patients with infective endocarditis. Am J Cardiol. 1979;43:738.

53. Miyatake K, et al. Evaluation of tricuspid regurgitation by pulsed Doppler and two-dimensional echocardiography. Circulation. 1982;66:777.

54. Miyatake K, Okamoto M, Kinoshita N, et al. Pulmonary regurgitation studied with the ultrasonic pulsed Doppler technique. Circulation. 1982;65:969–976.

55. Mügge A, Daniel WG, Frank G, et al. Echocardiography in infective endocarditis: Reassessment of prognostic complications of vegetation size determined by transthoracic and transesophageal approach. J Am Coll Cardiol. 1989;14:631.

56. Mügge A, Werner DG, Herrmann G, et al. Quantification of tricuspid regurgitation by color Doppler mapping after cardiac transplantation. Am J Cardiol. 1990;66:884–886.

57. Nakamura K, et al. Clinical and echocardiographic features of pulmonary valve endocarditis. Circulation. 1983;67:198–204.

58. Nanna M. Value of two-dimensional echocardiography in detecting tricuspid stenosis. Circulation. 1983;67:221–224.

59. Nixon JV. Right ventricular myocardial infarction. Arch Intern Med. 1982;141:945–947.

60. Ogawa S. Evaluation of combined valvular prolapse syndrome by two-dimensional echocardiography. Circulation. 1982;65:174–180.

61. Oliver J. Echocardiographic findings in ruptured chordae tendineae of the tricuspid valve. Am Heart J. 1983;105:1033–1035.

62. Parris TM. Doppler echocardiographic findings in rheumatic tricuspid stenosis. Am J Cardiol. 1987;60:1414–1416.

63. Perez JE, Ludbrook PA, Ahumada GG. Usefulness of Doppler echocardiography in detecting tricuspid valve stenosis. Am J Cardiol. 1985;55:601.

64. Pollack SJ, et al. Cardiac evaluation of women distance runners by echocardiographic color Doppler flow mapping. J Am Coll Cardiol. 1988;11:89.

65. Puleo JA, Shammas NW, Kelly P, et al. Lactobacillus isolated pulmonic valve endocarditis with ventricular septal defect by transesophageal echocardiography. Am Heart J. 1994;128:1248–1250.

66. Reid CL, et al. Echocardiographic features of carcinoid heart disease. Am Heart J. 1984;107:801–803.

67. Roberts WC, Buchbinder NA. Right-sided valvular infective endocarditis—A clinicopathologic study of twelve necropsy patients. Am J Med. 1972;53:7–19.

68. Roberts WC, Sjoerdsma A. The cardiac disease associated with carcinoid syndrome. Am J Med. 1964;36:5–34.

69. Scampardonis G, Yang SS, Maranhao V, et al. Left ventricular abnormalities in prolapsed mitral leaflet syndrome. Circulation. 1973;48:287.

70. Silver MM. Gross examination and structure of the heart. In Silver MD (ed): Cardiovascular Pathology, New York, Edinburgh, London, Melbourne: Churchill Livingstone; 1983:13.

71. Smith JA, Levine SA. The clinical features of tricuspid stenosis. Am Heart J. 1942;23:739–760.

72. Sokolow M, McIlroy MB (eds). Clinical Cardiology. Los Altos, CA, Lange; 1979:450.

73. Suwa M, et al. Two-dimensional echocardiography of ruptured pulmonic valve with infective endocarditis. Am Heart J. 1984;107:1027–1029.

74. Tajik AJ, et al. Two-dimensional real-time ultrasonic imaging of the heart and great vessels. Mayo Clin Proc. 1978;53:271.

75. Takao S, Miyatake K, Izumi S, et al. Clinical implications of pulmonary regurgitation in healthy individuals: Detection by cross-sectional pulsed Doppler echocardiography. Br Heart J. 1988;59:542–550.

76. Thomas JH, Pandussopoulos DG, Jewell WR, et al. Tricuspid stenosis secondary to metastatic melanoma. Cancer. 1977;39:1732.

77. Torres F, Tye T, Gibbons R, et al. Echo contrast increases the yield of signals for right ventricular pres-

sure measurement by Doppler ultrasound (abstract). Circulation. 1988;78(suppl II):II–548.

78. Trell E, Rausing A, Ripa J, et al. Carcinoid heart disease. Clinicopathologic findings and follow-up in 11 cases. Am J Med. 1973;54:433.

79. Waggoner AD, Barzilai B, Perez JE. Saline contrast enhancement of tricuspid regurgitant jets detected by Doppler color flow imaging. Am J Cardiol. 1990; 65:1368–1371.

80. Wantanabe T. Ruptured chordae tendineae of the tricuspid valve due to nonpenetrating trauma. Chest. 1981;80:751–753.

81. Weyman A. Principles and Practice of Echocardiography, 2nd ed. Philadelphia, Lea & Febiger; 1994: 840.

82. Weyman A. Principles and Practice of Echocardiography, 2nd ed. Philadelphia, Lea & Febiger; 1994: 836.

83. Weyman A. Principles and Practice of Echocardiography, 2nd ed. Philadelphia, Lea & Febiger; 1994: 873.

84. Weyman AE, Rankin R, King H. Loeffler's endocarditis presenting as mitral and tricuspid stenosis. Am J Cardiol. 1977;40:438.

85. Yock PG, Naasz C, Schnittger I, et al. Doppler tricuspid and pulmonic regurgitation in normals: Is it real? Circulation. 1984;70(suppl 2):II–40.

86. Yu PN, Harken DE, Lovejoy FW, et al. Clinical and hemodynamic studies on tricuspid stenosis. Circulation. 1956;13:680.

16

Prosthetic Heart Valves

CRISTY DAVIS

Introduction

Valvular heart disease has plagued humankind for centuries. Using surgery to correct mitral disease was predicted in 1889 by D.W. Samways, M.D., who wrote, "some of the severest cases of mitral stenosis will be relieved by slightly notching the mitral valve."[1] It wasn't until some 60 years later, in the 1950s, when cardiopulmonary bypass was introduced, that the era of open heart surgery began.

In the early days of valvular surgery, stenosis was corrected by attempting to remove the calcium deposits on the native valve.[2] It became apparent rather quickly, however, that a prosthesis for total valve replacement was necessary.

Several investigators are credited with developing various types of prosthetic heart valves. J.M. Campbell, M.D., and Charles Hufnagel, M.D., pioneered the idea of using a caged ball valve mechanism in the descending aorta to treat aortic insufficiency in the early 1950s.[3,4] In 1960, Harkin et al.[5] reported the survival of two patients in whom ball-type valves had been implanted. Albert Starr, M.D., and M.L. Edwards, M.D.,[6] first described their ball-and-cage prosthesis the following year. They were the first to implant a caged ball successfully in the mitral position using a design that didn't mimic native valve anatomy. It was the Starr-Edwards prosthetic valve that brought prosthetic heart valves into widespread clinical use. Carpentier et al.[7] introduced a glutaraldehyde-treated porcine (pig) heterograft (nonhuman tissue) in 1969. Others investigated the use of other types of tissue including autologous (a person's own tissue) fascia lata and homografts (tissue from another human being). Inoescu et al. reported their results using frame-supported fascia lata and bovine (cow) pericardial grafts in 1972.[8] They found that by using bovine pericardial tissue, they could fashion valves of any size necessary, thereby avoiding the problem of small aortic valve heterografts. Other investigators of the era include such notables as Beall, Barnard, Bjork, Braunwald, Cooley, Kay, Lillehei, Magovern, Smeloff, and Wada.

Assessing prosthetic heart valves is undoubtedly one of the greatest challenges that cardiac sonographers face. Echocardiography and phonocardiography have been used to evaluate prosthetic valves since the early 1970s.[9–19] Although phonocardiography is no longer available in most laboratories, transthoracic and transesophageal two-dimensional echocardiography, M-mode echocardiography, and Doppler echocardiography are now routinely used to evaluate prosthetic valve function.

When assessing the heart with a prosthetic valve, an integrated, comprehensive echocardiographic exam should always be performed. While each echo modality by itself provides valuable information on the heart and the prosthetic valve, an integrated examination, including transthoracic and transesophageal echocardiography, provides information that was previously elicited by cardiac catheterization alone. This includes ventricular size and function, prosthetic valve structural information, and hemodynamics.

Types of Prosthetic Valves

MECHANICAL VALVES

A variety of valves constructed of artificial materials, including pyrolitic carbon, silastic, and titanium have been implanted. The four basic types of mechanical valvular prostheses are the caged ball high-profile valve, the caged disc low-profile valve, the tilting disc low-profile valve, and the bileaflet low-profile valve (Table 16-1).

Caged ball valves consist of a ball enclosed in a high-profile (tall) cage with a fabric-covered sewing ring. In the mitral position, the ball is pushed to the apex of the cage (toward the apex of the heart) during diastole. This allows blood to flow through the base of the cage, which is in the mitral annulus position, and around the sides of the ball. During ventricular systole, left ventricular pressure forces the ball back toward the base of the cage to occlude the orifice (Fig. 16-1).

Problems with early caged ball valves included elevated pressure gradients, ball variance, and relatively high rates of thromboembolic complications. The early metal ball/metal cages were criticized for being noisy. The early silastic balls were criticized for cracking and sticking due to lipid absorption. Finally, the early cloth-covered cages had problems with wear and fraying, which resulted in embolism.

Only the Starr-Edwards caged ball valve (models 1200 and 1260 for aortic valves and model 6120 for mitral valves) remains available for implantation.[20] These models have closed, bare metal cages and properly fabricated salistic balls that reduce wear and ball variance (Fig. 16-2).

Caged disc valves, used extensively in the 1970s, are similar to caged ball valves; however, instead of a ball, they have a disc enclosed in a low-profile (short) cage that is attached to a fabric-covered sewing ring. These valves were introduced mainly to reduce the valve profile, or height, thereby helping to decrease ball variance.

As with the caged ball prosthesis, when in the mitral position, the disc is pushed to the apex of the cage during diastole. This allows blood to flow through the base of the cage and around the sides of the disc. During ventricular systole, left ventricular

TABLE 16-1. TYPES OF MECHANICAL PROSTHETIC VALVES

CAGED BALL (HIGH PROFILE)
Starr-Edwards
Smeloff-Cutter
Brunwald-Cutter
Harkin*
Magovern-Cromie
Edwards*
Stuckey*
Ellis*
Hufnagel*
DeBakey-Surgitool*
Cooley-Liotta-Cromie*
Serville-Arbonville*

TILTING DISC (LOW PROFILE)
Bjork-Shiley
Medtronic-Hall
Lillehei-Kaster
Omniscience
Wada-Cutter*
Pierce*
Alvarez*
Cruz-Kaster*
Pierce*
OmniCarbon*
Sorin Biomedica*
Bicer-Valve*

CAGED DISC OR FLOATING DISC (LOW PROFILE)
Beall-Surgitool (no longer used)
Kay-Suzuki
Cooley-Cutter*
Kay-Shiley*
Cross-Jones*
Starr-Edwards*
Barnard-Goosen*
Harken-Cromie*
Hufnagel-Conrad*
Cooley-Bloodwell-Cutter*
Lillehei-Nakib*
Hammersmith*
Woodward*
Davila*
UCT-Barnard*
Serville-Arbonville*
Teardrop Discoid*
Pin Teardrop*

BILEAFLET
St. Jude Medical
Gott-Daggett*
Kalke-Lillehei*
Duromedics*
CarboMedics*

* Valves marked with an asterisk are not presented in this chapter since they are rarely seen.

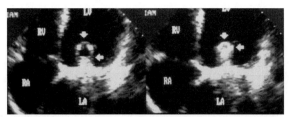

Figure 16-1. Two (left and right panels) two-dimensional echocardiographic four-chamber view images showing a caged ball prosthesis seated in the mitral position. The left panel shows the prosthesis during systole when the ball is seated in the base of the cage. The right panel shows the ball placement during diastole. The ball is seated in the apex of the cage. Horizontal arrow, leading echo from the ball; vertical arrow, leading echo from the cage; LV, left ventricle; LA, left atrium; RV, right ventricle; RA, right atrium.

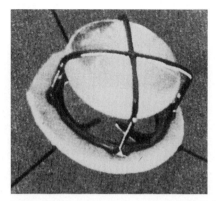

Figure 16-3. Kay-Suzuki (mitral position) low-profile disc prosthesis. (From Hagan A, DeMaria A. *Clinical Applications of Two-Dimensional Echocardiography and Cardiac Doppler*, 2nd ed. Boston, Little Brown; 1989:427, panel H. Reprinted with permission.)

pressure forces the disc back toward the base of the cage to occlude the orifice.

Disc thickness and cage design vary from one valve type to another. For example, the Beall-Surgitool caged disc has a pyrolite carbon disc that is thinner than a Kay-Suzuki disc. Note that the Kay-Suzuki low-profile cage (Fig. 16-3) looks very similar to the Starr-Edwards (caged ball) high-profile cage. The Cross-Jones valve has an open-ended titanium cage with a silastic disc. The cage looks very similar to the Braunwald-Cutter and Smeloff-Cutter (caged ball) cages (Fig. 16-4), except that it is low in profile.

The Beall-Surgitool (model 103) cage design consists of two struts that are bent toward the center of the apex but do not touch each other (Fig. 16-5). Another model of the Beall-Surgitool valve is similar, but the struts are not bent toward the center of the apex (Fig. 16-6). With both Beall valves, the struts and discs are made of carbon-coated pyrolite.

Problems with caged disc valves occurred because blood flow has to change direction around the occluder. This noncentral flow is the cause of high-pressure gradients, blood turbulence, and cell

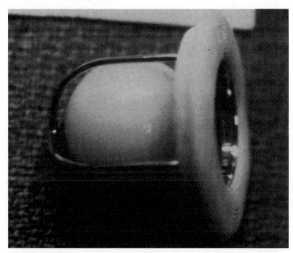

Figure 16-2. Starr-Edwards (model 6120) high-profile caged ball prosthesis.

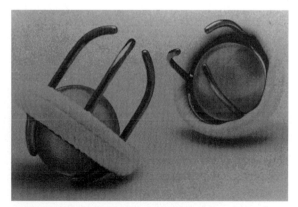

Figure 16-4. Smeloff-Cutter caged ball prosthesis.

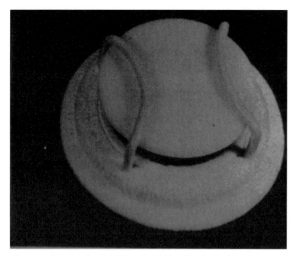

Figure 16-5. Beall (Model 103, mitral position) caged disk prosthesis.

damage. Additionally, some of the caged disc valves had structural failure and high wear.

The problems associated with lateral flow (caged disc) valves led to the development during the late 1960s and early 1970s of tilting disc or pivoting disc valves. *Tilting disc* valves are similar to caged disc valves in that they too utilize a disc rather than a ball; however, the supporting structure for tilting disc valves is very different from the previously described cage. The Bjork-Shiley (Fig. 16-7) and Lillehei-Kaster (Figs. 16-9 and 16-10) valves

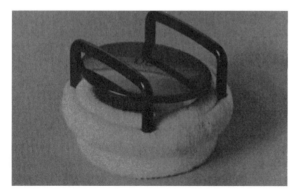

Figure 16-6. Beall-Surgitool caged disk prosthesis.

were the most commonly used tilting disc valves in the 1970s and 1980s.

Both the Lillehei-Kaster and Bjork-Shiley tilting disc valves employ a pivoting disc design with no fixed hinges. The disc rotates freely within the housing and pivots on two side struts or two U-shaped struts extending into the orifice. The disc is retained within the housing by two prongs or by the outflow strut that extends into a circular depression on the disc's outflow surface.[20]

The Bjork-Shiley valve is a low-profile tilting disc valve in which the pyrolytic carbon disc is suspended in a cage made of steilite. This prosthetic valve has been described as looking like a toilet seat in that one edge of the disc moves about 60 degrees up to the open position while the other edge stays fixed. The amount of excursion varies with the size of the prosthesis.

The Lillehei-Kaster and Medtronic-Hall tilting disc valves both utilize a pivoting disc technology. Due to its design with a central perforation, the Medtronic-Hall (Fig. 16-8) disc pivots more toward the center of the valve than does the Lillehei-Kaster disc (Fig. 16-9). Although echocardiographically similar to the Bjork-Shiley valve, the Lillehei-Kaster valve has two spine-like projections as part of the cage (Fig. 16-10). The disc is suspended in a titanium housing encircled by a knitted Teflon sewing ring.

Second-generation tilting disc valves were designed to overcome the problems of high-pressure gradients (particularly in small valves) and high thromboembolic complication rates. Second-generation valves include the Bjork-Shiley with a convex/concave disc, the Bjork-Shiley Monostrut, the Medtronic-Hall, the Omniscience, and the Omnicarbon. The Omniscience and Omnicarbon valves both also utilize a convex/concave disc with two rounded elevations replacing the struts. Of these second-generation valves, only the Medtronic-Hall and Omniscience II are currently marketed in the United States.[20]

Bileaflet tilting disc valves were also developed in the early 1960s. Early valves had two leaflets attached to a center bar by two stainless steel pins that were held by a molded superstrut. Unfortunately, blood flow characteristics around the central strut caused stasis and turbulent flow downstream, which in turn caused embolic problems.

Current bileaflet tilting disc valves consist of two equal-sized semicircular discs attached to a frame in-

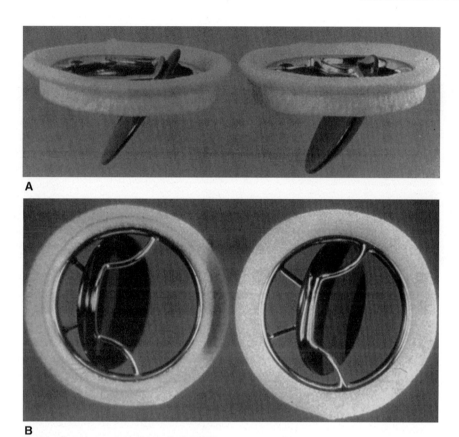

Figure 16-7. Bjork-Shiley low-profile tilting disc prosthesis.

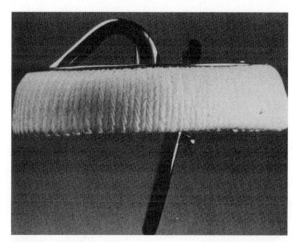

Figure 16-8. Medtronic-Hall disc prosthesis. (From Hagan A, DeMaria A. *Clinical Applications of Two-Dimensional Echocardiography and Cardiac Doppler*, 2nd ed. Boston, Little, Brown; 1989:426, Fig. 13-16, panel L. Reprinted with permission.)

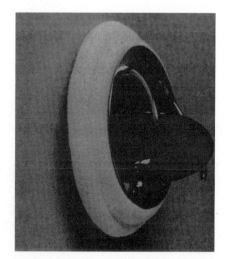

Figure 16-9. Lillehei-Kaster tilting disc prosthesis.

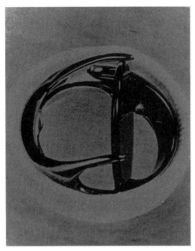

Figure 16-10. Lillehei-Kaster tilting disc prosthesis (side view).

side the sewing ring. The discs are constructed of py-rolite carbon. The St. Jude bileaflet valve (Fig. 16-11) operates similarly to a native valve in that the leaflets (or discs) are horizontal to the annulus plane during systole and parallel to the annulus plane during diastole. When the leaflets are open, blood flows through the three-channeled orifice, with very little obstruction to flow by the discs themselves. The St.

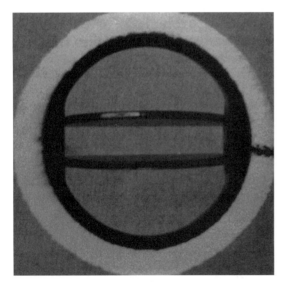

Figure 16-11. St. Jude bileaflet prosthesis.

Jude valve is currently the only bileaflet disc valve available in the United States.[20]

BIOPROSTHETIC VALVES

Compared to the variety of mechanical prosthetic valves that have been implanted, relatively few tissue-type prosthetic valves are currently available (Table 16-2). All bioprosthetic valves, whether heterografts, homografts, or allografts, are made from biologic tissue. Heterografts are made of porcine tissue or bovine pericardial tissue. Most homografts are aortic valves harvested at autopsy that have been cryopreserved. Allografts are made from the patient's own tissue.

All bioprosthetic valves are made to resemble the native aortic valve and are composed of three leaflets mounted on a cloth-covered metal ring that functions as the annulus. Raised stents that resemble a crown are found at each of the three commissures (Fig. 16-12). When the valve is open (during diastole when in the mitral position and during systole when in the aortic position), the orifice is round and blood flow is laminar. It should also be noted that bioprosthetic valves are associated with a lower incidence of thromboembolism than mechanical valves.[21]

The *heterograft* or *xenograft* valves that are most commonly used are the Hancock and Carpentier-Edwards valves. Both types use porcine tissue (aortic valve) covered with woven Dacron, which is pre-

◢◢◢ TABLE 16-2. TYPES OF BIOPROSTHETIC VALVES

HETEROGRAFTS (NONHUMAN TISSUE)
Hancock (porcine)
Carpentier-Edwards (porcine)
Carpentier-Edwards (pericardial)
Ionescu-Shiley (bovine pericardial)
AUTOGRAFTS (THE PATIENT'S OWN TISSUE)
Fascia lata*
HOMOGRAFTS OR XENOGRAFTS (TISSUE FROM ANOTHER HUMAN)
Stented (aortic)*
Unstented (aortic)*
Dura Mater*

* Valves marked with an asterisk are not presented in this chapter since they are rarely seen.

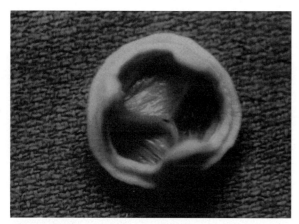

Figure 16-12. Hancock heterograft (mitral position) bioprosthetic valve.

served with glutaraldehyde solution until implantation. The Hancock valve (Fig. 16-12) has three flexible polypropylene stents supported on a stellite ring, while the Carpentier-Edwards valve is mounted on a Elgiloy frame. The Ionescu-Shiley valve (Fig. 16-13) uses bovine pericardium rather than porcine tissue and is also mounted on an Elgiloy frame.

Homograft valves are usually harvested aortic valves that may be stented or unstented. Aortic ho-mografts are used to replace the aortic or pulmonic valve but are rarely used to replace an atrioventricular valve. The aortic valve, ascending aorta, and anterior mitral leaflet are harvested at the time of autopsy and preserved as a block so that they may be trimmed to fit at the time of implantation. Homografts may also be made of dura mater, the outer membrane that covers the spinal cord and brain.

Autograft valves are made from the patient's own tissue and have been used in the mitral valve position. Autografts are usually made of fascia lata, the fibrous membrane that covers and supports the thigh muscles.

Other Prosthetic Devices

Valved conduits are used to repair some types of congenital heart disease. The conduit may be a homograft or an artificial material such as Gore-Tex or Dacron. The conduit may have a mechanical valve or a biologic valve. Blood flow through a valved conduit is similar to blood flow through a valve implanted in the annulus position.

Whenever possible, native valve repair is preferred to valve replacement. In certain situations, a *Carpentier ring* is used to repair native atrioventricular valves. This is a flexible ring that is sewn into the annulus position to help support the native annulus and attached valve leaflets. Echocardiographically, the Carpentier ring resembles a calcified annulus.

Echocardiographic Evaluation of Prosthetic Valves

Transthoracic and transesophageal two-dimensional and Doppler echocardiography are the current methods of choice for evaluating prosthetic valves. Whether using transthoracic or transesophageal echocardiography, the combined use of all echo modalities (i.e., two-dimensional, M-mode, and Doppler echocardiography) is necessary so that spatial, structural, and quantitative information regarding flow characteristics can be gathered.

Two-dimensional echocardiography is used to evaluate the valve structure and its relationship to the rest of the heart. Although technically challenging due to the reverberations and acoustic shadow-

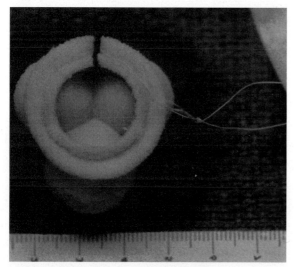

Figure 16-13. Ionescu-Shiley xenograft (using bovine pericardial tissue) bioprosthetic valve.

ing caused by the metal in the prosthesis, transthoracic two-dimensional imaging of mechanical prosthetic valves is still very useful. Not only does two-dimensional echocardiography provide real-time visualization of leaflet motion and qualitative data for evaluating left ventricular performance, it also shows characteristic patterns of leaflet motion. Both of these features help identify the presence of thrombus, vegetations, pannus ingrowth of tissue, and calcific changes in the leaflet tissue or native annulus.

It is important to remember that occluder motion and the presence of vegetations or thrombi are not the only aspects of prosthetic valve assessment for which two-dimensional echocardiography is used. This method allows direct visualization of any abnormal rocking of the prosthesis within the annulus and also helps the clinician assess hemodynamic parameters in order to evaluate the patient's overall condition.

While large, pedunculated vegetations are easily seen with transthoracic echocardiography due to the shadowing and reverberations, many abnormalities, including thrombus, vegetations, flail leaflets, and abscesses may be impossible to detect with transthoracic two-dimensional echocardiography. For example, using the standard apical four-chamber view and the two-chamber view for assessing the atrial side of a mitral prosthetic valve for vegetations or thrombus is futile because of the shadowing and reverberations. In these cases, one should attempt to use nonstandard echo views in order to visualize the left atrium.

M-mode echocardiography is useful when assessing either mechanical or bioprosthetic valves. It is of great benefit when trying to differentiate among thrombus, focal calcification, and endocarditis on bioprosthetic leaflets. M-mode imaging of mechanical valves is used to assess occluder motion. When assessing prosthetic valves with M-mode echocardiography, atypical M-mode windows are frequently used.

Perivalvular leaks, valve regurgitation, and valve stenosis can be assessed with transthoracic Doppler echocardiography. In fact, Doppler has proven invaluable for assessing valve dehiscence. Because regurgitation may be either valvular or perivalvular, the use of color flow Doppler is essential when identifying the location of any regurgitant jet.

In addition to the basic cardiac hemodynamic information that Doppler provides, pulsed wave (PW) Doppler combined with 2-D echocardiography should always be used when evaluating prosthetic valves in order to determine the area of the valve.

The locations of the transducer used to record flow across prosthetic valves are similar to those used for native valves. However, it is important to remember that the direction of flow across a prosthetic valve may not be central to the valve ring. With a caged ball prosthesis, flow must go around the ball. Tilting disc valves, except for the St. Jude valve with double discs, may produce two jets (on either side of the disc).

Therefore, as with M-mode, nontraditional Doppler windows are frequently used to ensure that the Doppler signal is parallel to blood flow. For example, under normal circumstances the parasternal long-axis view would not be used to assess mitral flow since the Doppler signal is perpendicular to mitral flow using this window. When assessing prosthetic mitral flow, however, the parasternal window may actually be the best window to use, depending on the type of prosthesis and the position of the prosthetic valve within the heart.

The transthoracic approach is also useful when evaluating mechanical valves in the aortic position. The apical four-chamber, apical two-chamber, and parasternal long-axis views are used to evaluate the subaortic region in these cases. Additional views used to assess this region include the parasternal short-axis, subcostal four-chamber, and subcostal short-axis views at the base.

While it is possible to determine the type of valve (caged ball, caged disc, tilting disc, or bileaflet) with transthoracic echocardiography, the same information may be gleaned by reading the patient's chart or by talking with the patient.

Transesophageal two-dimensional and Doppler echocardiography are the newest echocardiographic techniques utilized to evaluate prosthetic valve function. Because transesophageal echocardiography views cardiac structures from the back of the heart, the technical problems, including reverberations and shadowing in the left atrium, are avoided. Therefore, transesophageal echocardiography is the modality of choice in those cases where prosthetic valves are being assessed for thrombus, vegetations, abscess, or flail leaflets.

Perivalvular leaks are seen better with transesophageal echo, and since transthoracic echocardiography tends to underestimate the degree of mitral regurgitation, transesophageal echo is the modality of choice for evaluating mitral regurgitation.

Transesophageal echo is of little benefit, however, when evaluating a mechanical aortic prosthesis due to shadowing of the left ventricular outflow tract when using this approach.

Echocardiography Calculations

Various echocardiography calculations are routinely used when assessing prosthetic valves. The modified Bernoulli equation (pressure gradient = 4 × velocity^2) is used to estimate pressure gradients in native valves as well as prosthetic valves. It is important to remember that normal Doppler velocities are higher in prosthetic valves than in native valves (Tables 16-3 to 16-6). When calculating effective valve orifice areas, it has been reported that the standard pressure half-time calculation is not accurate with prosthetic valves. This is thought to be due to the fact that the constant 220 used in calculating pressure half-time was derived for stenotic native valves rather than prosthetic valves. Therefore, using pressure half-time to estimate valve areas in prosthetic valves may grossly overestimate the area of a mitral prosthesis.

Pressure half-time estimates of bioprosthetic valve orifice areas should be accurate since they depend on the time course of the velocity decline relative to the maximum velocity rather than on the velocity itself. The formula for calculating pressure half-time in prosthetic mitral valves is the same formula used in calculating pressure half-time in native valves.

The continuity equation is the calculation of choice for determining the area of mitral and aortic prostheses when there is no significant mitral or aortic regurgitation. Using the continuity equation for bioprosthetic valve replacements is fairly accurate since the flow profile through a bioprosthetic valve is similar to the flow profile through a native valve.

Using the continuity equation for a mechanical valve, however, may be problematic since the equation assumes a flat flow velocity profile through the valve orifice as well as proximal to the valve. Obviously, a flat flow velocity profile is not seen in bileaflet valves. Due to the high velocities through the central orifice of a bileaflet valve, a significant error in measurement of volume flow rate will occur, resulting in underestimation of the valve area. Fortunately, tilting disc valves and caged ball valves don't have the same flow problems as bileaflet valves. The formula for prosthetic mitral valve area is:

$$
\begin{aligned}
\text{MVR area} &= \text{LVOT area} \\
&\quad \times (\text{LVOT TVI/MP TVI}) \\
&= \text{LVOT diameter}^2 \times 0.785 \\
&\quad \times (\text{LVOT TVI/MP TVI})
\end{aligned}
$$

TABLE 16-3. NORMAL DOPPLER VALUES FOR MITRAL VALVE PROSTHESES

Valve Type	No. of Pts	V Max (m/s)	Peak Grad (mm Hg)	Mean Vel (m/s)	Mean Grad (mm Hg)	MVA (cm^2)
CAGED BALL						
Starr-Edwards	43	1.9 ± 0.4	14.6 ± 5.5	1.1 ± 0.3	4.6 ± 2.4	2.0 ± 0.5
CAGED DISC						
Beall	13	1.8 ± 0.2	13.4 ± 4.0	1.2 ± 0.2	6.0 ± 2.0	1.70 ± 0.2
TILTING DISC						
Bjork-Shiley	128	1.6 ± 0.3	10.7 ± 2.7	0.8 ± 0.3	2.9 ± 1.6	2.4 ± 0.6
Lillehei-Kaster	10	1.8	13.5	0.9	2.9 ± 1.6	1.9 ± 0.2
BILEAFLET TILTING DISC						
St. Jude	156	1.6 ± 0.3	10.0 ± 3.6	0.9 ± 0.2	3.5 ± 1.3	2.9 ± 0.6
BIOPROSTHETIC						
Hancock	114	1.5 ± 0.3	9.7 ± 3.2	1.1 ± 0.3	4.3 ± 2.1	1.7 ± 0.4
Carpentier-Edwards	75	1.8 ± 0.2	12.5 ± 3.6	1.3 ± 0.2	6.5 ± 2.1	2.5 ± 0.7
Ionescu-Shiley	29	1.5 ± 0.3	8.5 ± 2.9	0.9 ± 0.2	3.3 ± 1.2	2.4 ± 0.8

Note: Values shown are mean ± 1 SD.
Source: Modified from Refs. 34 and 35.

TABLE 16-4. Normal Doppler Values for Aortic Valve Prostheses

Valve Type	No. of Pts	V Max (m/s)	Peak Grad (mm Hg)	Mean Vel (m/s)	Mean Grad (mm Hg)
Caged Ball					
Starr-Edwards	56	3.1 ± 0.5	38.6 ± 11.7	2.5 ± 0.2	24.0 ± 4.0
Tilting Disc					
Bjork-Shiley	102	2.6 ± 0.4	23.8 ± 8.8	1.8 ± 0.3	14.3 ± 5.5
Bileaflet Tilting Disc					
St. Jude	70	2.4 ± 0.3	25.5 ± 5.1	1.7 ± 0.5	12.5 ± 6.4
Bioprosthetic					
Carpentier-Edwards (porcine)	143	2.4 ± 0.5	23.2 ± 8.7	1.9 ± 0.4	14.4 ± 5.7
Hancock (porcine)	91	2.4 ± 0.4	23.0 ± 6.7	1.7 ± 0.2	11.0 ± 2.3
Ionescu-Shiley (bovine pericardial)	32	2.5 ± 1.7	24.7 ± 7.7	1.9 ± 0.3	14.0 ± 4.3
Homograft		1.8 ± 0.4			7.0 ± 3.0

Note: Values shown are mean ± 1 SD.
Source: Modified from Refs. 34–39.

TABLE 16-5. Normal Doppler Values for Aortic Prostheses According to Size

Valve Type	Size (mm)	Ref	No. of Pts	V Max (m/s)	Peak Grad (mm Hg)	Size (mm)	Ref	No. of Pts	Mean Vel (m/s)	Mean Grad (mm Hg)
Mechanical										
St. Jude	19	26, 27	6	3.0 ± 0.8	31.2 ± 17.3	19	27, 28	5	2.4 ± 0.6	22.2 ± 11.0
	21	26, 28, 29	14	2.7 ± 0.3	30.0 ± 5.7	21	27, 29	11	1.9 ± 0.3	14.4 ± 5.0
	23	26, 27	17	2.3 ± 0.6	23.2 ± 11.5	23	27, 28	19	1.6 ± 0.5	10.8 ± 6.3
	25	26, 27	12	2.2 ± 0.5	19.8 ± 8.2	25	27	9	1.2 ± 0.5	11.0 ± 6.0
Bjork-Shiley						19	28	3	2.3 ± 0.4	21.0 ± 7.0
	21	30	4	2.8 ± 0.9	30.5 ± 19.9	21	28	1	2.0	16.0
	23	20, 30	11	2.6 ± 0.4	27.3 ± 8.7	23	20, 28	20	1.9 ± 0.3	14.0 ± 5.0
	25	20, 30	13	2.1 ± 0.3	18.4 ± 5.3	25	20, 28	13	1.8 ± 0.2	13.3 ± 2.5
	27	20, 30	10	1.9 ± 0.2	14.6 ± 3.1	27	20, 28	7	1.6 ± 0.2	9.7 ± 2.5
	29	30	2	1.9 ± 0.2	14.0 ± 2.5	29	30	2	1.3 ± 0.6	7.0 ± 6.0
Bioprosthetic										
Hancock	21	30	1	3.5	49.0					
	23	20, 30	10	2.4 ± 0.2	23.0 ± 4.6	23	20	7	1.7 ± 0.1	12.0 ± 2.0
	25	20, 30	22	2.3 ± 0.3	20.7 ± 4.6	25	20	10	1.7 ± 0.2	11.0 ± 2.0
	27	20, 30	18	2.1 ± 0.4	20.5 ± 5.7	27	20	5	1.6 ± 0.2	10.0 ± 3.0
	29	30	2	2.2 ± 0.4	19.9 ± 7.1					
Carpentier-Edwards	19	26, 31	11	2.8 ± 0.7	31.6 ± 14.9	19	31	3	2.0 ± 0.1	16.5 ± 1.4
	21	31	7	2.7 ± 0.4	27.3 ± 9.9	21	31	7	1.9 ± 0.4	14.5 ± 6.0
	23	26, 30, 31	28	2.6 ± 0.4	26.6 ± 8.9	23	31, 32	13	1.8 ± 0.4	12.7 ± 5.7
	25	26, 30, 31	27	2.5 ± 0.4	34.4 ± 7.9	25	28, 31	6	1.6 ± 0.2	10.4 ± 2.3
	27	26, 30, 31	28	2.4 ± 0.4	23.6 ± 7.2	27	28, 31	3	1.6 ± 0.1	9.9 ± 1.0
	29	30, 31	12	2.4 ± 0.4	22.8 ± 8.4	29	31	1	1.7	11.6
	31	30	5	2.4 ± 0.4	22.3 ± 8.1					

Source: Modified from Ref. 34.

TABLE 16-6. NORMAL DOPPLER VALUES FOR TRICUSPID VALVE PROSTHESES

Valve Type	V Max (m/s)	Mean Grad (mm Hg)	Pressure Half-Time (m/sec)
CAGED BALL Starr-Edwards	1.3 ± 0.2	3.2 ± 0.8	140 ± 48
TILTING DISC Bjork-Shiley	1.3	2.2	144
BILEAFLET TILTING DISC St. Jude	1.2 ± 0.3	2.7 ± 1.1	108 ± 32
BIOPROSTHETIC Heterograft	1.3 ± 0.2	3.2 ± 1.1	145 ± 37

Source: Modified from Connolly HM. Doppler hemodynamic profiles of eighty-six normal tricuspid valve prostheses. *J Am Coll Cardiol* 1991;17:69A. (Abstract)

where MVR = mitral valve replacement, LVOT TVI = left ventricular outflow tract time velocity integral, and MP TVI = time velocity integral of the mitral prosthesis velocity obtained by continuous wave (CW) Doppler.

The formula for calculating aortic prosthetic valve area using the continuity equation is:

$$AVR = LVOT \text{ area} \times (LVOT\ TVI/AP\ TVI)$$
$$= SRID^2 \times 0.785$$
$$\times (LVOT\ TVI/AP\ TVI)$$

where AVR = aortic valve replacement and SRID = sewing ring inner diameter. TVI is obtained from CW Doppler velocity of the aortic valve.

Another method of evaluating prosthetic valves for stenosis is to measure the "step-up" in velocity across the valve. In the aortic position, the ratio of outflow tract velocity to aortic jet velocity reflects the degree of stenosis. The ratio will be close to 1 if no obstruction to flow exists; however, the ratio becomes less than 1 when narrowing increases. The normal velocity ratio across an aortic prosthesis ranges from 0.35 to 0.50 compared with 0.75 to 0.90 for native aortic valves.

The velocity ratio method is useful because it takes volume flow rate into account and does not require a diameter measurement. Ideally, a baseline normal Doppler exam will be performed and subsequent velocity ratios can be compared to the baseline ratio.

Just as all prosthetic valves exhibit higher flow velocities than native valves, normal prosthetic valves exhibit some regurgitation. The same criteria for determining the amount of regurgitation in native valves is used for prosthetic valves.

1. Normal prosthetic valve regurgitation has the following characteristics:
   - Mitral regurgitant jet area of <2 cm² and a jet length of less than 2.5 cm
   - Aortic regurgitant jet area of less than 1 cm² and a jet length of less than 1.5 cm
2. Severe aortic prosthetic regurgitation has the following characteristics:
   - A pressure half-time of the regurgitant jet of 250 m/sec or lower
   - Restrictive mitral inflow pattern (acute aortic insufficiency)
   - Holodiastolic reversals in the descending thoracic aorta
   - Regurgitant fraction of 55% or higher
3. Severe mitral prosthetic regurgitation has the following characteristics:
   - Increased mitral inflow peak velocity and normal mitral inflow pressure half-time
   - Dense mitral regurgitant CW Doppler signal
   - Regurgitant fraction of 55% or higher

Normal Two-Dimensional and M-mode Echo Findings in Mechanical Valves

Transthoracic two-dimensional and M-mode echocardiography can be used to evaluate all mechanical and bioprosthetic valves that are used to replace any native valve within the heart. Although mitral and aortic valve replacement is more common than right heart valve replacement, occasionally prosthetic tricuspid valves are implanted; however, pulmonic valve replacement is much less common.

Because echocardiographic images of mechanical valves in the mitral position are generally technically superior to images from valves in the aortic or tricuspid position, most of the following illustrations involve mitral prosthetic valves.

Figures 16-14 and 16-15 show typical normal transthoracic two-dimensional echocardiograms from a patient with a caged ball prosthesis in the mitral position. In this example, the cage itself can be seen on the ventricular side of the mitral annulus

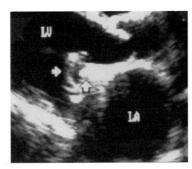

Figure 16-14. Two-dimensional echocardiogram of a caged ball prosthetic valve in the mitral position utilizing the parasternal long-axis window. Horizontal arrow, cage; vertical arrow, ball and artifact; LV, left ventricle; LA, left atrium.

in the parasternal long-axis view (see Fig. 16-14) and in the apical four-chamber view (see Fig. 16-15). Other two-dimensional views to utilize when assessing a caged ball prosthesis include the apical two-chamber view, the apical long-axis view, and the subcostal four-chamber view. Due to different positioning of the valve during implantation, it may be necessary to angulate the transducer slightly in order to record an optimum image of the prosthesis.

In this example, an echo from the leading edge of the ball can be easily seen moving within the cage in real time and is seen as a bright echo within the cage in this still frame image (arrows). Notice the reverberations and acoustic shadowing within the left atrium.

In order to assess ball excursion within the cage of a caged ball valve in the mitral position, M-mode

echocardiography utilizing the apical window should be used. Figure 16-16 shows a typical M-mode image obtained from the apical window. Although this recording resembles an M-mode tracing of the aortic valve, the most anterior bright echo represents the cage of the prosthetic valve, while the most posterior bright echo represents the valve sewing ring. The motion of these parallel echoes mimics the motion of the native valve annulus to which the valve is sutured. The bright echo moving away from the transducer just before the electrocardiographic (ECG) T wave is the leading edge of the ball as it moves toward the mitral annulus (systole.) The M-mode recording of a normal caged ball prosthesis will show rapid, brisk movements of the ball within the cage with sharp rather than rounded edges. No echo is recorded from the posterior surface of the ball; however, dense linear echoes are recorded posterior to the prosthesis and represent reverberations from the valve material.

Occasionally, a caged ball will be seen in the aortic position. The echocardiographic views to use in assessing aortic prostheses are the parasternal long-axis view, the apical long-axis or five-chamber view, and the subcostal long-axis or five-chamber view. It is often difficult to obtain adequate images using these views since these valves are smaller and therefore more difficult to see; in addition, as with

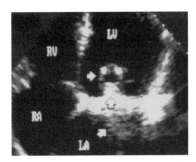

Figure 16-15. Two-dimensional echocardiogram of a caged ball prosthetic valve in the mitral position utilizing the apical four-chamber view. Horizontal arrow, cage; vertical arrow, ball; angled arrow, reverberation artifact; LV, left ventricle; LA, left atrium; RV, right ventricle; RA, right atrium.

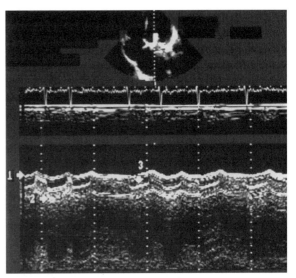

Figure 16-16. M-mode echocardiogram of a caged ball prosthetic valve in the mitral position utilizing the apical four-chamber window. 1, cage; 2, valve sewing ring; 3, leading edge of ball during diastole.

any mechanical valve, reverberations and acoustic shadowing can be problematic.

M-mode echocardiography of the caged ball placed in the aortic position should be accomplished using the apical long-axis view in which the ultrasonic beam is parallel to the movement of the ball within the cage. The M-mode appearance of the aortic caged ball valve will be identical to that of a caged ball valve in the mitral position.

When a caged ball prosthesis is implanted in the tricuspid position, the views that produce the best images of the valve include the parasternal long-axis view of the tricuspid valve (medially angulated from the parasternal long-axis view), the apical four-chamber view, and the subcostal four-chamber view. For M-mode assessment, the apical four-chamber view is the best since the ultrasonic beam is parallel to the ball excursion.

Low-profile caged disc prostheses are echocardiographically very similar to caged ball prostheses. The cage and disc may be seen with two-dimensional echocardiography from the parasternal window and from the apical window when the prosthesis is located either in the mitral, tricuspid, or aortic position. Again, the parasternal long-axis medially angulated view of the tricuspid valve is excellent for evaluating a prosthetic tricuspid valve. Because the cage is shorter, it may be more difficult to distinguish between the cage, the disc, and the sewing ring.

Again, to assess the excursion of the disc within the cage in either mitral, tricuspid, or aortic valve replacements, M-mode echocardiography utilizing the apical window should be performed. The short-axis view at the base of the heart may also prove useful when interrogating the prosthetic tricuspid valve. The appearance of the disc within the cage will be identical to the M-mode recording of the caged ball, except that the bright echoes from the cage will be closer together.

The Bjork-Shiley tilting disc prosthesis is probably the most frequent tilting disc valve prosthesis seen with echocardiography. Usually the best echocardiographic windows to use when evaluating a tilting disc prosthesis in either the mitral, tricuspid, or aortic position with two-dimensional echocardiography are the parasternal window (long-axis view) and the apical window (four-chamber, five-chamber, apical long-axis, or two-chamber view). Slight angulation of the transducer may be necessary to

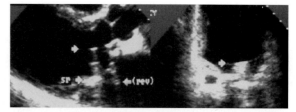

Figure 16-17. Parasternal long-axis view and apical four-chamber view from a patient with a tilting disc prosthesis in the mitral position. Horizontal arrows show the leading edge of the disc. Sr, sewing ring; rev, reverberations.

record the full excursion of the disc since valve placement and orientation will vary from patient to patient.

Figure 16-17 shows a typical transthoracic two-dimensional echocardiogram from a patient with a tilting disc prosthesis in the mitral position. In this example, the prosthesis is easily recorded from the parasternal and apical windows. Although the disc housing is not easily identifiable, dense linear echoes from the sewing ring are seen, and the leading edge of the disc can be seen as bright linear echoes when the valve is open during diastole (arrows). Reverberations from the valve material are seen within the left atrium.

To assess the disc excursion from a tilting disc valve in the mitral or aortic position, M-mode echocardiography is performed utilizing the parasternal window.

As mentioned previously, slight angulation of the transducer may be necessary to optimize the recording of the disc excursion.

When using M-mode to evaluate a Bjork-Shiley valve located in the tricuspid position, full disc excursion may be difficult to obtain. As with native tricuspid valves, angulating the transducer to position the ultrasonic beam perpendicular to the leaflets as they open and close can be very difficult. Using an apical four-chamber view or a basal short-axis view to interrogate the disc excursion of a tilting disc tricuspid valve with M-mode echocardiography generally proves to be as futile as interrogating a native tricuspid valve from these views. Although leaflet motion is recorded, full excursion of the leaflet cannot be appreciated.

Using the parasternal window from a low intercostal space can sometimes be helpful. Also, depending on how the patient's heart lies within the thorax, a medially angulated right-sided long-axis view may prove beneficial. Frequently, M-mode scanning from the subcostal four-chamber view provides the best results since the ultrasonic beam can usually be directed perpendicular to the disc from this window.

Figure 16-18 shows a typical M-mode tracing obtained from the parasternal window in a patient with a tilting disc prosthesis in the mitral position. M-mode scanning from this window will show multiple dense linear echoes originating from the sewing ring and reverberations from the sewing ring during systole. When the disc tilts to open, there is rapid anterior motion into the left ventricular cavity followed by gradual posterior motion that parallels the posterior motion of the sewing ring and mitral annulus in diastole. The M-mode recording of a normal tilting disc prosthesis will show rapid, brisk opening and closing movements.

The transthoracic two-dimensional echocardiographic recordings of a normal St. Jude bileaflet tilting disc valve is seen in Figure 16-19. The image was recorded from the parasternal long-axis view. Other views to use when evaluating a St. Jude valve in the mitral or aortic position are the parasternal short-axis view and the standard apical and subcostal views.

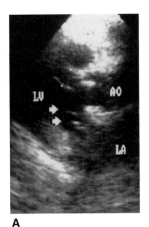
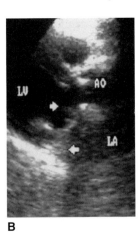

Figure 16-19. (**A**) Parasternal long-axis image (diastole) from a patient with a normal St. Jude valve in the mitral position. Both discs are seen as parallel lines during diastole. LV, left ventricle; LA, left atrium; AO, aortic root. (**B**) Parasternal long-axis image (systole) from the same patient. Top arrow shows side lobe artifact; bottom arrow shows reverberations; LV, left ventricle; LA, left atrium; AO, aortic root.

In this example (Fig. 16-19*A*), notice that when the valve is open, both discs tilt and become parallel to each other. The two leaflets (discs) can be seen as parallel linear echoes during diastole (bottom arrow). Notice the side-lobe artifact generated from the bright echo of the anterior leaflet (top arrow), which should not be mistaken for a pedunculated vegetation. When the valve is closed, the discs rest within the sewing ring and are no longer seen in the echo image. Reverberations from the sewing ring are noted within the left atrium (arrow). As with the mono-leaflet tilting disc valve (Bjork-Shiley), the orientation of the prosthetic valve will vary from patient to patient. Therefore, it is important to angulate the transducer to visualize the leaflets adequately with transthoracic two-dimensional echocardiography.

Figure 16-20 is an example of a St. Jude valve in the aortic position being assessed with the parasternal short-axis view and the parasternal long-axis view. In both views, the bileaflet valve is easily identified as two parallel lines seen during systole.

The transesophageal image of the St. Jude mitral valve in Figure 16-21 shows why transesophageal echocardiography is so useful when evaluating prosthetic valves. The open leaflets, seen as two parallel lines during diastole, are readily identifiable (arrows). Notice that reverberations within the left

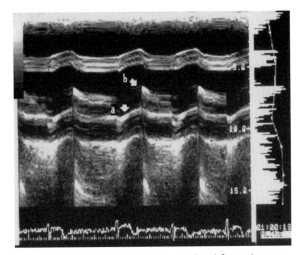

Figure 16-18. M-mode image obtained from the parasternal window in a patient with a tilting disc prosthesis in the mitral position. During systole (**A**), the sewing ring is seen as a dense linear echo. The disc tilts open during early diastole (**B**) and is seen as rapid anterior motion with a gradual posterior motion as the disc "drifts" closed throughout diastole.

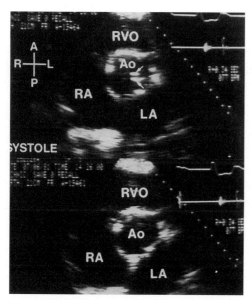

Figure 16-20. Parasternal short-axis view at the base in a patient with a St. Jude medical prosthesis in the aortic position during systole (upper panel) showing parallel reflectance (arrows) from the bileaflet valve. During diastole (lower panel) there is no reflectance from the closed valve. RVO, right ventricular outlet; LA, left atrium; RA, right atrium; Ao, aorta. (From Hagan A, DeMaria A. *Clinical Applications of Two-Dimensional Echocardiography and Cardiac Doppler.* Boston, Little, Brown; 1989:427, Fig. 13-13. Reprinted with permission.)

atrium are not a factor when utilizing transesophageal echocardiography since the heart is imaged from the left atrial side.

Figure 16-22 is a normal M-mode tracing from a patient with a St. Jude prosthesis in the mitral

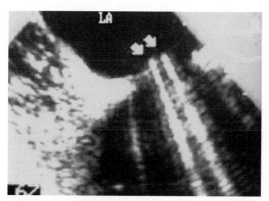

Figure 16-21. Transesophageal image of a St. Jude prosthesis in the mitral position. Arrows show the open leaflets as two parallel lines. LA, left atrium.

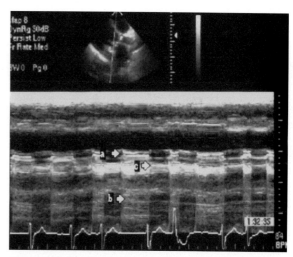

Figure 16-22. M-mode tracing from the parasternal window in a patient with a St. Jude valve in the mitral position. a, open discs during diastole; b, reverberation from sewing ring; c, sewing ring during systole.

position. The recording was obtained from the parasternal long-axis position. Two parallel bright echoes from both discs are seen in diastole (a) when the valve is open. Reverberations from the sewing ring are also prominent during diastole (b) and are generated from the sewing ring. During systole, echoes from the discs are not seen; however, the thick, bright linear echo that represents the sewing ring should be noted.

Normal Two-Dimensional and M-mode Echo Findings in Bioprosthetic Valves

Bioprosthetic valves are trileaflet valves attached to a sewing ring with three stents. A bioprosthetic valve implanted in the aortic position appears similar to a native aortic valve; however, increased thickness in the left ventricular outflow tract and the ascending aorta at the suture sites is usually seen. Figure 16-23 illustrates a porcine valve in the aortic position (a) during systole and (b) during diastole. The valve leaflets are not seen in frame a; however, the increased thickness of the sewing ring is easily visualized. Frame b represents early diastole just prior to mitral valve opening. The aortic valve appears much thicker with the valve closed, although the leaflets are difficult to identify due to the reflectivity of the sewing ring. Reverberation from the valve prosthesis is seen in the left atrium.

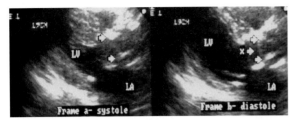

Figure 16-23. Long-axis images from a patient with a porcine aortic valve. Arrows a and b point to prominent sewing ring echoes. X, closed aortic valve leaflets; LV, left ventricle; LA, left atrium.

When implanted in the mitral position, bioprosthetic valves may initially be mistaken for caged ball valves due to the appearance of the stents; however, the similarities end there.

Figure 16-24 illustrates a porcine valve in the mitral position. In this case, the leaflets can be easily visualized within the stents in the apical four-chamber (left panel) view during diastole (arrow). The leaflets are more difficult to see in the still frame of the parasternal long-axis view (right panel). Frequently, visualization of the leaflets may be limited due to the presence of the sewing ring and stents. When seen, normal bioprosthetic leaflets appear very similar to native valve leaflets.

Evaluation with two-dimensional or M-mode echocardiography of a bioprosthetic valve is identical to evaluation of a native valve. Standard parasternal long-axis and short-axis views and apical five-chamber or long-axis views are used to see the valve leaflets and the motion of the aortic valve. M-mode scanning through the aortic valve utilizing the parasternal window will produce the typical box-like opening in systole that is seen in native valves (Fig. 16-25).

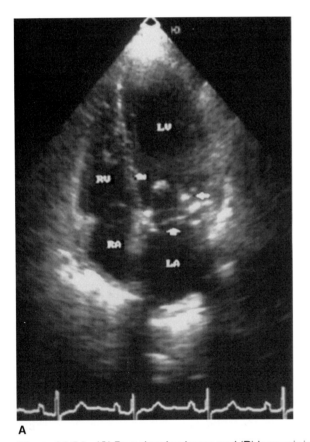

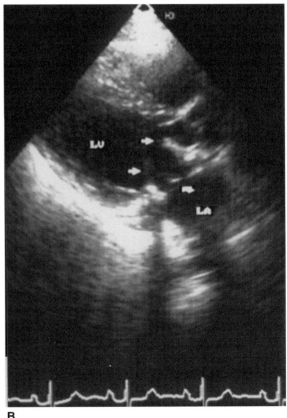

A B

Figure 16-24. **(A)** Four-chamber image and **(B)** long-axis image from a patient with a porcine mitral valve. Horizontal arrows point to stents. Vertical arrow points to valve leaflet. LV, left ventricle; LA, left atrium; RV, right ventricle; RA, right atrium.

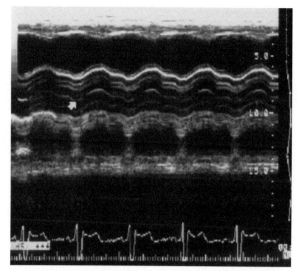

Figure 16-25. *M-mode echocardiogram from a patient with a porcine aortic valve. Arrow points to the typical aortic valve opening "box" seen during systole.*

Standard two-dimensional echocardiographic views are also used to evaluate a bioprosthetic valve in the mitral position. Again, as with native valves, M-mode echocardiography is performed using the parasternal long-axis view, in which the valve leaflets

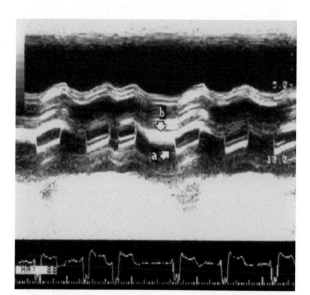

Figure 16-26. *M-mode tracing of a porcine mitral valve. a, valve leaflet in systole; b, stent of prosthesis and valve leaflet during diastole. Note that the structure of the stent cannot be distinguished from the leaflet due to artifact from the stent itself.*

appear box-like during systole. Echoes returning from the sewing ring and stents are very prominent and appear similar to the echoes from a calcified mitral annulus (Fig. 16-26).

Normal Two-Dimensional Findings in Carpentier Rings and Valved Conduits

As noted previously, Carpentier rings in the mitral position echocardiographically appear similar to a calcified mitral annulus. The best views to utilize in documenting the presence of a Carpentier ring are those that show the mitral annulus, such as the parasternal long-axis view and the apical four-chamber view. The ring may also be visualized with the parasternal short-axis view with the sound beam cutting across at the annulus level.

Figure 16-27 shows two parasternal long axis views in a patient with mitral valve prolapse. Panel a is the long-axis image acquired prior to the placement of a Carpentier ring in the annulus. Notice the prolapsing posterior mitral leaflet and the left atrial and left ventricular enlargement.

Panel B is the long-axis image acquired after the placement of the Carpentier ring (arrows). Notice that after surgery, the ventricle and atrium have decreased in size and the cross-sectional diameter of the mitral annulus is appreciably reduced.

Two-dimensional imaging of valved conduits is generally even more challenging technically than imaging of prosthetic valves. This is due in part to the differing locations of the conduits and the technical limitations imposed by the conduit material.

In general, all echocardiographic windows should be used when evaluating any conduit with two-dimensional echocardiography. Transducer an-

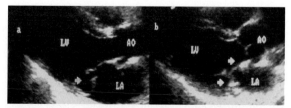

Figure 16-27. *Two parasternal long-axis images from a patient with a repaired mitral valve. (**A**) An arrow points to the native prolapsing mitral valve leaflet. (**B**) The repaired mitral valve with the arrows pointing to the Carpentier ring. LV, left ventricle; LA, left atrium; AO, aorta.*

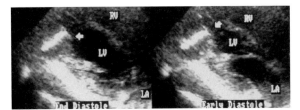

Figure 16-28. Two modified parasternal long-axis images from a patient with aortic atresia. The arrow points to the conduit attached at the apex. The conduit itself is seen as a bright linear echo outside of the left ventricle. LV, left ventricle; LA, left atrium; RV, right ventricle.

gulation may be necessary to record nonstandard views that show the conduit attachments. Remember that conduit placement will vary from patient to patient.

Figure 16-28 shows a modified parasternal long-axis view from a patient with aortic valve atresia. One end of the conduit is attached near the apex of the left ventricle, while the opposite end is attached to the ascending aorta in order for blood to flow from the left heart through the systemic system. A valve (not seen due to reflectance of the conduit material) is located at the apical end of the conduit to prevent backflow of blood into the left ventricle.

The conduit (arrow) is noted as a bright linear echo outside of the ventricle. Due to the position of the conduit, Doppler interrogation of the conduit valve was technically inadequate. Likewise, the conduit attachment into the ascending aorta was never adequately visualized with two-dimensional echocardiography.

Normal Doppler Findings in All Types of Prosthetic Valves

Because the effective orifice area of any prosthetic valve is smaller than the orifice area of a normal native valve, some obstruction to flow is always present with prosthetic valves. As a result, slightly higher forward flow velocities are recorded when prosthetic valves are interrogated with Doppler echocardiography. The Doppler velocities, calculated pressure gradients, and valve areas obviously depend not only on the type of prosthesis, but also on the size and position of the valve. Normal Doppler flow velocities through various types of prosthetic valves are summarized in Table 16-3 to 16-6.

As one might expect, flow profiles across bioprosthetic valves appear similar to flow profiles across native valves. Because all tissue valves are trileaflet and have a central orifice, blood flow is laminar, with a blunt profile in a normal bioprosthetic valve. Like native valves, a high percentage of normally functioning bioprosthetic valves also have a small amount of regurgitation.

Flow profiles across mechanical valves, however, vary with the type of valve and never resemble the flow across a native valve. Like bioprosthetic valves, normally functioning mechanical valves also exhibit a small amount of regurgitation.

Color Doppler not only allows one to detect regurgitant flow, it also enables one to appreciate the normal direction of blood flow through different types of mechanical prostheses. Although the ultrasound windows used to record flow across prosthetic valves are similar to those used for native valves, the operator must be aware that the direction of flow across a prosthetic valve may not be central to the valve ring (Fig. 16-29). Also, the blood flow stream into the ventricle through any mitral prosthesis, regardless of type, is directed toward the septum rather than toward the apex. This is due to the

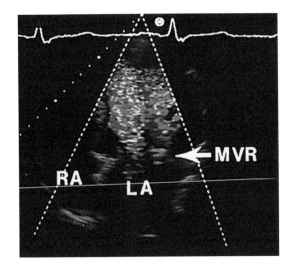

Figure 16-29. Apical four-chamber view from a patient with a porcine mitral valve replacement (MVR) showing color flow toward the apex along the septal wall and flow toward the base along the lateral wall. This pattern is the opposite of the color flow pattern through a normal native valve. RA, right atrium; LA, left atrium. (From Otto CM, Pearlman AS. *Textbook of Clinical Echocardiography.* Philadelphia, WB Saunders; 1995: Fig. 11-13. Reprinted with permission.) (See also Color Plate 49.)

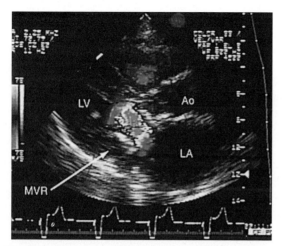

Figure 16-30. Parasternal long-axis image from a patient with a porcine mitral valve replacement (MVR) showing a normal left ventricular color flow pattern through the valve. LV, left ventricle; LA, left atrium; Ao, aorta. The jet (shown in blue due to aliasing) is directed toward the septum. (From Otto CM, Pearlman AS. *Textbook of Clinical Echocardiography.* Philadelphia, WB Saunders; 1995: Fig. 11-12. Reprinted with permission.) (See also Color Plate 50.)

orientation of the implanted prosthesis (Fig. 16-30).

With a caged ball valve, blood flows across the sewing ring and around all sides of the ball when the valve is in the open position. When in the closed position, the ball is seated in the sewing ring and a small amount of regurgitation may be seen around the ball.

An open tilting disk valve has two orifices. Because one is larger than the other, the flow profile appears to be asymmetrical as blood accelerates along the surface of the tilted disk. Regurgitation occurs at the closure line when the disk closes and is directed away from the sewing ring at the edge of the larger of the two orifices (Fig. 16-31A).

The Doppler flow profile across bileaflet mechanical valves has three peaks that correspond to the two large lateral orifices and the small central slit-like orifice present when the valve is in the open position (Fig. 16-31B). Higher flow velocities occur in the center of each orifice. It should be noted that localized high-pressure gradients are seen within the small central orifice and are fre-

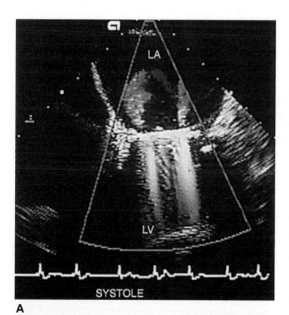

A SYSTOLE

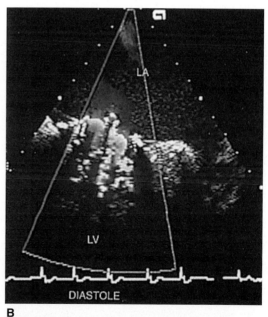

B DIASTOLE

Figure 16-31. (**A**) Systolic color flow image of a bileaflet mitral valve prosthesis showing two normal jets of regurgitation. LA, left atrium; LV, left ventricle. (**B**) Diastolic color flow image of a bileaflet mitral valve prosthesis showing the three peaks that correspond to the two large lateral orifices and the smaller central slit-like orifice. LA, left atrium; LV, left ventricle. (From Otto CM, Pearlman AS. *Textbook of Clinical Echocardiography.* Philadelphia, WB Saunders; 1995: Fig. 11-5, top and bottom panels. Reprinted with permission.) (See also Color Plates 51 and 52.)

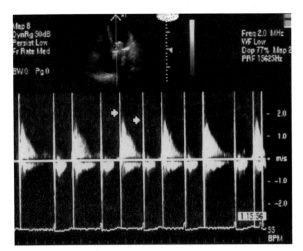

Figure 16-32. Spectral Doppler tracing from a patient with a caged ball mitral valve prosthesis. The arrows point to the high-intensity clicks produced by the opening and closing of the valve.

quently substantially higher than the overall pressure gradient across the valve. Two crisscross jets of regurgitation are seen when the bileaflet valve closes. These regurgitant jets are seen in the plane parallel to the leaflet opening plane. Additionally, two smaller regurgitant jets are seen in the plane perpendicular to the leaflet opening plane.

The opening and closing sounds of prosthetic valves create brief, intense signals that are easily recorded with Doppler imaging. These "clicks" appear as a dark, narrow band of short duration on the spectral display. Usually both opening and closing valve clicks are seen and are similar to those seen with native valves but are of greater intensity (Fig. 16-32). As one would expect, metallic valves produce much higher signals than tissue valves. Additionally, the motion of the ball or disc may result in color flow artifact, in which inconsistent color signals cover large areas of the two-dimensional sector.

Other Echocardiographic Findings Associated with Prosthetic Valves

Most changes that the heart has undergone in order to compensate for the hemodynamic overload caused by diseased native valves will regress following valve replacement. The amount of improvement depends on how well the heart functioned before the valve was replaced.

In cases of severe aortic stenosis where left ventricular hypertrophy has occurred as a result of longstanding increased afterload, the change observed in patients following surgery can be quite dramatic. Serial echocardiograms performed over several months will show regression of left ventricular hypertrophy and improvement in contractility.

A gradual decrease in left atrial size may be noted following replacement of a stenotic mitral valve since left atrial pressure that was previously elevated will decrease following valve replacement. However, the left atrium will always remain larger than normal.

When regurgitant aortic or mitral valves are replaced, the volume overload on the left ventricle is alleviated. While the ventricular size may decrease, it will always be larger than normal and contractility may not improve. Occasionally, left ventricular function may worsen immediately after valve replacement.

Another echocardiographic finding associated with prosthetic valves is the atypical or paradoxical motion of the interventricular septum. Although not related specifically to valve replacement, this paradoxical motion is frequently noted following open heart surgery and is thought to be related to postoperative adhesions along the anterior border of the chest wall.

Prosthetic Valve Dysfunction

Prosthetic valve diseases are quite different from native valvular diseases and may be classified into two categories of prosthetic valve dysfunction: mechanical failure and tissue degeneration. *Mechanical failure* refers to any problem with the prosthetic valve structure itself (either mechanical valves or bioprosthetic valves) and may be due to ball or disc variance, thrombus formation, pannus ingrowth around the valve, or endocarditis. *Tissue degeneration* refers to any problem with the tissue of the bioprosthetic valve or the surrounding tissue of either the mechanical or bioprosthetic valve. Tissue degeneration may be caused by infective endocarditis or abscess, loose or torn sutures, or calcific changes within the native annulus. All prosthetic valve dysfunction is readily detectable by comprehensive transthoracic and transesophageal echocardiographic exams.

Disc or ball variance refers to changes in the silastic disc or ball, probably due to abrasion and deposits of blood lipids. As a result, the disc or ball increases in size, or its normal contour is distorted. Any such alteration results in uneven stress, cracking, tearing, or grooving of the prosthesis (Fig. 16-33). A decrease in the size of the disc or ball could cause it to break loose from the struts or the cage, resulting in acute severe regurgitation. An increase in the size of the ball or disc, or a distortion in contour, could cause it to stick to the struts or cage in the open position, also causing regurgitation. These complications are less frequently encountered with newer models of mechanical prostheses.

Thromboembolic complications in patients with prosthetic valves are probably related to the blood flow characteristics through the valve. Areas of blood stagnation, eddies, or high shear stress con-

tribute to blood clotting, which may result in embolic events in various organs. A thrombus on the valve is more commonly seen on the valve housing rather than on the disc, ball, or leaflet due to the intricate design of the housing.[24]

A thrombus on the valve housing may also continue to adhere to the valve surface and continue to attract more fibrin and blood cells until it becomes big enough to cause valve thrombosis (Fig. 16-34). When this occurs, the normal function of the disc or ball is altered. It may fail to open completely or it may stick in one position, obstructing blood flow. Unlike native valve stenosis, this functional obstruction occurs relatively rapidly, and there is not enough time for the normal cardiac adaptive mechanisms to respond to the new overload. If the disc

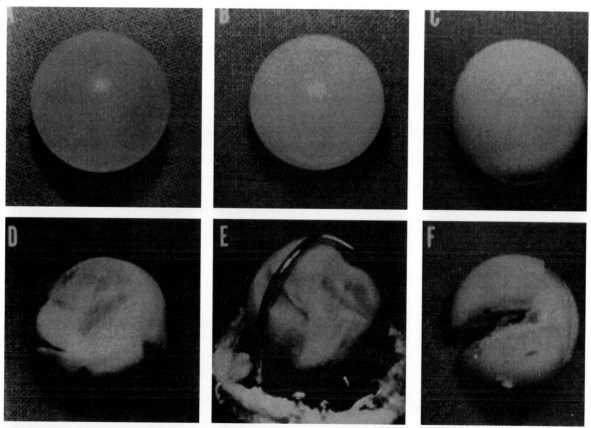

Figure 16-33. Examples of ball variance. **(A)** Normal silastic poppet 1.5 years after implantation. **(B)** Opaque ball after 3 years in situ. **(C)** Slightly eccentric and grooved ball, removed after 3 years. **(D)** Grooved poppet. **(E)** Grooved poppet stuck in the open position. **(F)** Cracked ball removed 4 years after insertion.

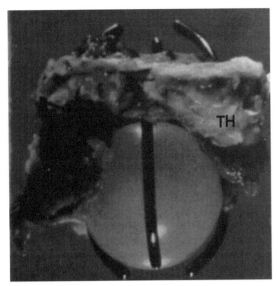

Figure 16-34. Excised caged ball prosthesis with a large thrombus attached to the valve housing. (From Salcedo E. Atlas of Echocardiography, 2nd ed. Philadelphia, WB Saunders, 1987:185.)

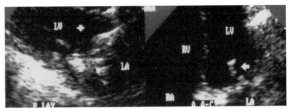

Figure 16-35. Parasternal long-axis image and apical four-chamber image from a patient with a large, pedunculated vegetation (arrow) attached to the mitral prosthesis within the left ventricle. LV, left ventricle; LA, left atrium; RV, right ventricle; RA, right atrium.

or ball fails to close properly, significant regurgitation may occur.

Thrombi adhering to prosthetic valve structures are often difficult to identify with transthoracic echocardiography.

Pannus ingrowth around the valve refers to newly formed vascular tissue around the prosthetic valve. Pannus ingrowth causes problems similar to those associated with thrombi. The newly formed tissue may impair the disc or ball excursion and closure, thereby causing regurgitation, stenosis, or both.

Infective endocarditis occurs in approximately 2% of patients with prosthetic valves because prosthetic valves are foreign bodies and, as such, are targets for infection. Endocarditis in patients with prosthetic valves is a very serious complication. Patients with endocarditis occurring relatively soon after implantation have a reportedly high mortality rate.

Endocarditis in patients with either mechanical or bioprosthetic valvular prostheses may result in vegetations similar to those seen on a native valve; however, with a mechanical valve, the infection is often paravalvular, and no vegetation may be present. Additionally, there is a higher incidence of abscess formation, which may cause dehiscence of the prosthesis from bacterial endocarditis in patients with prosthetic valves rather than in patients with vegetations on native valves. Paravalvular regurgitation may develop following paravalvular infection, abscess formation, or suture rupture caused by tissue degeneration.

Relatively large vegetations may restrict normal valve closure (similar to thrombus formation on a prosthetic valve), causing regurgitation. As the vegetation continues to increase in size, progressive regurgitation is quite common.

Like thrombus formations on mechanical valves, vegetations are also frequently difficult to identify with transthoracic echocardiography; however, large, mobile vegetations may be seen prolapsing back and forth across the sewing ring or even moving within the left ventricle or left atrium. Figure 16-35 shows a large, pedunculated vegetation attached to the mitral prosthesis within the left ventricle. A smaller vegetation attached to an aortic valve prosthesis is seen within the left ventricle in Figure 16-36.

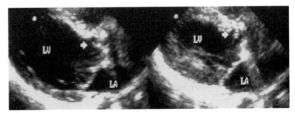

Figure 16-36. Parasternal long-axis images from a patient with a prosthetic aortic valve showing a vegetation attached to the valve leaflet (arrows). The vegetation can be seen in diastole (left panel) and systole (right panel). LV, left ventricle; LA, left atrium.

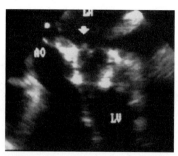

Figure 16-37. Transesophageal echocardiogram from a patient with a prosthetic mitral valve. The arrows point to a small, mobile mass attached to the atrial side of the prosthesis. LA, left atrium; LV, left ventricle; AO, aorta.

Like vegetations on mechanical valves, small vegetations on the stents of a bioprosthetic valve are difficult to identify. Vegetations on the tissue leaflets themselves, however, appear echocardiographically similar to vegetations on native cardiac valves.

Due to the acoustic shadowing and reverberations seen within the left atrium with transthoracic echocardiography, transesophageal echocardiography is frequently performed in order to better assess the prosthesis that is suspected of being infected. In Figure 16-37, a small, mobile mass is seen attached to the atrial side of a mitral valve prosthesis.

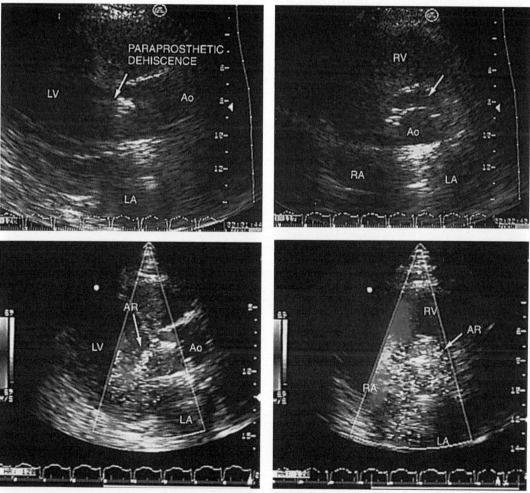

Figure 16-38. Two-dimensional (above) and color flow Doppler (below) images in parasternal long-axis (left) and short-axis (right) views in a patient with aortic valve dehiscence due to endocarditis and paraprosthetic aortic regurgitation. Two-dimensional imaging shows an echolucent space anterior to the sewing ring. Color flow imaging shows flow anterior to the prosthesis in a long-axis view with a circumferential pattern of regurgitation seen in the short-axis view. LV, left ventricle; LA, left atrium; RV, right ventricle; RA, right atrium, Ao, aorta; AR, aortic regurgitation. (From Otto CM, Pearlman AS. *Textbook of Clinical Echocardiography.* Philadelphia, WB Saunders; 1995: Fig. 11-18. Reprinted with permission.) (See also Color Plates 53 and 54.)

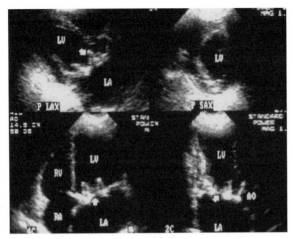

Figure 16-39. Two-dimensional echocardiogram from a patient with a bioprosthetic mitral valve. Calcific changes in the mitral valve leaflet (arrows) result in thickened, less mobile leaflets. PLAX, parasternal long axis; PSAX, parasternal short axis; 4C, four chamber; 2C, two chamber; LV, left ventricle; LA, left atrium; RV, right ventricle; RA, right atrium; AO, aorta.

In addition to providing a better acoustic window, transesophageal echocardiography utilizes a higher-frequency transducer, which is helpful when attempting to identify small structures.

Abscess formation along the sewing ring may be identified as a localized area of ultrasound density different from the surrounding tissue. Dehiscence of the prosthetic implant is not uncommon in such conditions.

Antibiotics alone may not be adequate to control the infection. In cases of progressive regurgitation, fungal endocarditis, persistent infection, ring abscess, repeated major embolization, and relapse due to endocarditis, surgical removal and replacement of the infected prosthesis is necessary.

Dehiscence refers to the rupture of one or more sutures that anchor the sewing ring of the prosthesis to the native annulus. Dehiscence of the prosthesis is frequently a complication that occurs early after surgery, or it may result from abscess formation at the valve annulus in patients with bacterial endocarditis. Regardless of the cause of dehiscence, paravalvular regurgitation is very common, and surgery must be performed to correct the problem (Fig. 16-38).

With dehiscence, exaggerated motion of the prosthetic valve relative to the valve annulus is seen on two-dimensional echocardiography. A rocking motion of the prosthesis, in which the sewing ring prolapses outside the plane of the valve annulus throughout the cardiac cycle, may be seen in extreme cases. This rocking motion frequently suggests significant dehiscence.

In addition to the tissue degeneration caused by infection, tissue degeneration includes calcific changes and weakening of the bioprosthetic tissue of the leaflets themselves or the native annulus tissue.

The calcific changes that occur in bioprosthetic valve leaflets lead to progressive thickening and reduced mobility of the leaflets (Fig. 16-39). As in native valves, the reduced mobility ultimately leads to stenosis of the valve, with relative obstruction to flow. Calcific changes in the annulus may result in regurgitation.

The chemical treatment of bioprosthetic valve tissue eventually causes the tissue to degenerate. Fenestration (small holes) and occasional rupture of a bioprosthetic valve leaflet (flail leaflet) due to degeneration of the tissue 5 to 10 years after implantation is not unusual (Fig. 16-40).

Normal bioprosthetic leaflets are usually faintly visualized on routine echocardiography and appear very similar to native valve leaflets. Fenestration of a bioprosthetic leaflet is very difficult to visualize

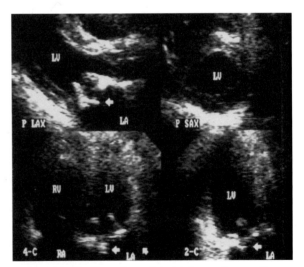

Figure 16-40. Two-dimensional echocardiogram from a patient with a degenerative bioprosthetic mitral valve leaflet. Arrows point to the flail posterior leaflet. PLAX, parasternal long axis; PSAX, parasternal short axis; 4C, four chamber; 2C, two chamber; LV, left ventricle; LA, left atrium; RV, right ventricle; RA, right atrium.

with two-dimensional echocardiography; however, the resultant regurgitation is fairly easily detectable with Doppler echocardiography. As with native valves, progressive deposition of calcium makes the leaflets of bioprosthetic valves more echogenic.

Other Echocardiographic Findings in Prosthetic Valve Dysfunction

In addition to assessing the actual prosthetic valve with two-dimensional and Doppler echocardiography, several other findings associated with cardiac dysfunction should be integrated into the final analysis.

As previously noted, the normal cardiac response to valve replacement is an improvement in chamber size and systolic function. For this reason, a baseline echocardiogram should be obtained relatively soon after surgery to document any changes that occur. Subsequent echocardiograms should include information regarding the response of the cardiac chambers, such as size, hypertrophy, and systolic function. While it may be difficult to decide whether changes are due to persistent postoperative abnormalities or new pathology, any differences noted in subsequent echo examinations should be of concern.

Signs of prosthetic valve dysfunction include:

- Reduced or compromised cardiac output
- An increase in antegrade velocity across the valve
- A decrease in valve area
- Increased regurgitation (by color flow)
- An increase in intensity of the CW Doppler regurgitant signal
- Progressive increase in chamber size
- Persistent left ventricular hypertrophy
- Recurrent pulmonary hypertension following an initial decline in pulmonary pressures

For example, if left ventricular hypertrophy is a persistent two-dimensional echocardiographic finding following aortic valve replacement, one should consider the possible development of prosthetic aortic stenosis. If the ventricle dilates, the possibility of volume overload (aortic regurgitation or mitral regurgitation) should be considered. If the ventricle was previously normal and exhibits a new hyperdynamic status, mitral regurgitation may be present. A decrease in cardiac output may also signal prosthetic valve dysfunction; however, temporary worsening of left ventricular function may be noted immediately after valve replacement.

Additional information can be gleaned from the Doppler exam when assessing the antegrade velocity across the prosthetic valve. For example, an increase in antegrade velocity may be due to increased volume (prosthetic regurgitation) rather than stenosis. In this scenario, even though the calculated gradient will be increased, the calculated valve area should remain the same. Keep in mind that an increase in velocity may also be due to an increase in cardiac output. If this is the case, velocities across other valves will also be increased.

Estimated pulmonary artery pressures should be compared to pressures documented in previous studies as well. Recurrent pulmonary hypertension that occurs after an initial decline in pulmonary pressures could signal mitral prosthetic valve dysfunction.

Pseudo-Prosthetic Valve Dysfunction

Occasionally, cardiac dysfunction after valve replacement may be due to the valve replacement, even though the prosthetic valve functions normally. This may occur if the implanted valve is not the correct size for the patient's heart. For example, if an aortic valve replacement is too small for the amount of blood flowing through it, hemodynamic compromise will occur similar to that seen in aortic stenosis. Or if a relatively large ball-and-cage prosthesis is implanted in a small ventricle, the left ventricular outflow tract may be obstructed by the mitral prosthesis.

Prosthetic valve dysfunction may also be suspected from the echocardiographic appearance of the diminished opening of the valve in patients with low cardiac output. In some cases, cardiac output that was impaired due to left ventricular dysfunction before the implant was placed will not return to normal following valve replacement. In these cases, serial echocardiography is useful to help differentiate between existing decreased cardiac output and actual valve dysfunction since left ventricular function will always be impaired.

Blood flow across prosthetic valves in patients with ECG abnormalities such as atrial fibrillation may also mimic valvular dysfunction. For example, in patients with a mitral disc prosthesis and a prolonged PR interval, left ventricular and left atrial pressures equilibrate after atrial contraction. During this time, flow essentially stops and the disc drifts closed. The echocardiographic image of this phenomenon simulates the rounded, closed appearance of the valve that is seen with thrombus formation.

Incidental Echocardiographic Findings in Patients with Prosthetic Devices

Occasionally, incidental findings are noted on echocardiograms performed on patients with prosthetic valves or other prosthetic devices. While not particularly life-threatening, or even considered valvular dysfunction, these findings should be documented with echocardiography when present.

Spontaneous contrast can be seen in patients with prosthetic valves and is similar to the spontaneous contrast seen in patients with an enlarged left atrium and decreased flow; however, in patients with prosthetic valves the implications of this phenomenon are not the same. While patients with spontaneous contrast caused by low-flow states have a higher incidence of thrombus formation than does the general population, such is not the case in patients with prosthetic valve spontaneous contrast.

With prosthetic valves, spontaneous contrast is more commonly seen in mechanical valves than bioprosthetic valves. It is caused by microcavitation downstream from the valve due to the impact of the occluder against the sewing ring (Fig. 16-41).

A *prosthetic valve seated in an abnormal position* is another incidental finding that poses no problem

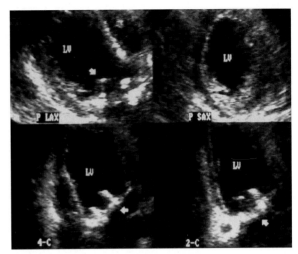

Figure 16-42. Two-dimensional echocardiogram from a patient with a porcine mitral valve replacement. Note the prosthetic valve position (arrows) within the native mitral annulus. PLAX, parasternal long axis; PSAX, parasternal short axis; 4C, four chamber; 2C, two chamber; LV, left ventricle.

for the patient but may pose a problem when interrogating the valve with Doppler. Figure 16-42 shows a porcine mitral valve seated in an abnormal position, and Figure 16-43 shows an abnormally positioned caged ball valve in the mitral position. Notice how the approach to Doppler interrogation of these valves would vary from the usual approach.

A rather uncommon incidental echocardiographic finding in a patient with a prosthetic mitral valve is seen in Figure 16-44. In this patient, the native mitral valve is still in place and causes left ventricular outflow tract obstruction. Because sur-

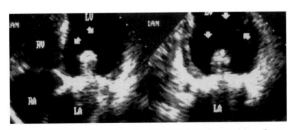

Figure 16-41. Apical images from a patient with a Starr-Edwards mitral valve replacement. Although difficult to appreciate on still frame images, the arrows point to spontaneous contrast in the left ventricle. LV, left ventricle; LA, left atrium; RV, right ventricle; RA, right atrium.

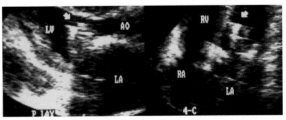

Figure 16-43. Parasternal long-axis image (left) and four-chamber image (right) from a patient with a caged ball valve in the mitral position. Arrows point to the apex of the cage, which is positioned near the interventricular septum in the left ventricular outflow tract. LV, left ventricle; AO, aorta; LA, left atrium; RV, right ventricle; RA, right atrium.

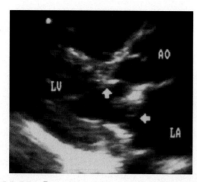

Figure 16-44. Parasternal long-axis images from a patient with a bioprosthetic mitral valve (horizontal posterior arrow) and the native mitral valve (vertical anterior arrow) still in place. LV, left ventricle; LA, left atrium; AO, aorta.

gery on this patient was performed at an outside institution and medical records were not available at the time of this echocardiogram, the reason(s) for leaving the native valve are not clear.

Recommended Transthoracic Echocardiographic Approach to Evaluation of Prosthetic Valves

The key to providing a comprehensive echocardiographic evaluation of prosthetic valves is to remember the concept of the *integrated* examination. Where one modality provides essential image information, another modality provides essential hemodynamic information, and so forth. Therefore, use each echocardiography modality to its fullest potential in order to gather the appropriate data needed for valve assessment.

The echocardiographic windows and technical details of data recording used for both native valve and prosthetic valve evaluation are essentially identical. At times, however, nonstandard imaging planes may be used to better assess the area behind the prosthetic valve since acoustic shadowing and reverberations can be problematic.

The recommended routine for evaluating prosthetic valves is:

1. Perform a standard two-dimensional examination according to the laboratory protocol, paying close attention to:
   - Chamber size, wall thickness, and systolic function
   - Structural integrity of the prosthesis

2. Utilize any and all features available on the ultrasound system to obtain the best image possible of the prosthesis. Pay close attention to gain and power settings to help reduce the amount of acoustic reverberation when possible.
3. If available, utilize the zoom feature on your echocardiographic system to help identify any valvular structural abnormality.
4. Look for evidence of thrombus, vegetation, flail leaflet, calcified leaflets, abnormal rocking of the struts, and so on.
5. Record images of the valve using all possible acoustic windows.
6. Utilize M-mode echocardiography to help identify any abnormal opening or closing patterns and to document valve occluder excursion.
7. Utilize Doppler echocardiography to gather hemodynamic data, including peak flow velocity, maximum and mean gradients, pressure half-time (or deceleration time), effective valve areas, diastolic filling profiles, color-flow jet areas, flow reversals in the pulmonary vein or descending aorta, and regurgitant fraction.
8. Utilize color Doppler and CW Doppler from all acoustic windows to perform a careful search for valvular regurgitation.
9. If regurgitation is found, determine whether it is perivalvular or valvular.
10. If the regurgitation is valvular, document its cause if possible. Look for leaflet tears or ruptures, thrombi, or vegetations.
11. Utilize Doppler echocardiography and perform calculations to determine the presence or absence of valvular stenosis.
12. Compare the current echocardiographic examination to prior exams and document any changes.

REFERENCES

1. Samways DW. Cardiac peristalsis: Its nature and effects. *Lancet.* 1898;1:927.
2. Souttar HS. Surgical treatment of mitral stenosis. *Br Med J.* 1925;2:603.
3. Campbell JM. An artificial aortic valve. *J Thorac Cardiovasc Surg.* 1950;19:312.
4. Hufnagel CA. Aortic plastic valvular prostheses. *Bull Georgetown Univ Med Center.* 1951;4:128.

5. Harken DE, Soroff HS, Taylor WJ, et al. Partial and complete prosthesis in aortic insufficiency. *J Thorac Cardiovasc Surg.* 1960;40:744.

6. Starr A, Edwards ML. Mitral replacement: Clinical experience with a ball-valve prosthesis. *Ann Surg.* 1961;154:726.

7. Carpentier A, Lamaigra G, Robert L, et al. Biological factors affecting long-term results of various heterografts. *J Thorac Cardiovasc Surg.* 1969;58:467.

8. Ionescu MI, Pakrashi BC, Holden MP, et al. Results of aortic valve replacement with frame-supported fascia lata and pericardial grafts. *J Thorac Cardiovasc Surg.* 1972;64:340.

9. Assad-Morell JL, Tajik AJ, Anderson MW, et al. Malfunctioning tricuspid valve prosthesis: Clinical, phonographic, echocardiographic, and surgical findings. *Mayo Clin Proc.* 1973;49:443.

10. Gibson TC, Starek PJ, Moos S, et al. Echocardiographic and phonocardiographic characteristics of the Lillehei-Kaster mitral valve prosthesis. *Circulation.* 1974;49:434.

11. Brodie BR, Grossman W, McLauren L, et al. Diagnosis of prosthetic mitral valve malfunction with combined echophonocardiography. *Circulation.* 1976;53:93.

12. Berndt TB, Goodman DJ, Popp RL. Echocardiographic and phonocardiographic confirmation of suspected cage mitral valve malfunction. *Chest.* 1976; 70:221.

13. Wann LS, Pyhel HJ, Judson WE, et al. Ball variance in a Harken mitral prosthesis: Echocardiographic and phonocardiographic features. *Chest.* 1977;72:785.

14. Estevez R, Mookherjee S, Potts J, et al. Phonocardiographic and echocardiographic features of Lillehei-Kaster mitral prosthesis. *J Clin Ultrasound.* 1977;5: 153.

15. Kotler MN, Segal BL, Parry WR. Echocardiographic and phonocardiographic evaluation of prosthetic heart valves. *Cardiovasc Clin.* 1978;9:187.

16. Waggoner AD, Quinones MA, Young JB, et al. Echo-phonocardiographic evaluation of obstruction of prosthetic mitral valve. *Chest.* 1980;78:60.

17. DePace NL, Kotler MN, Mintz GS, et al. Echocardiographic and phonocardiographic assessment of the St. Jude cardiac valve prosthesis. *Chest.* 1981;80: 272.

18. Mintz GS, Carlson EB, Kotler MN. Comparison of noninvasive techniques in evaluation of the nontissue cardiac valve prosthesis. *Am J Cardiol.* 1982;49:39.

19. Alam M, Garcia R, Goldstein S. Echo-phonocardiographic features of regurgitant porcine mitral and tricuspid valves presenting with musical murmurs. *Am Heart J.* 1983;105:456.

20. Frankl WS, Brest AN (eds). *Valvular Heart Disease: Comprehensive Evaluation and Treatment.* Philadelphia, FA Davis; 1993.

21. Lefrak E, Starr A. *Cardiac Valve Prostheses.* New York, Appleton-Century-Crofts; 1979.

22. Frazier H, Sweeney M, Radovancevic B, et al. Surgical treatment of heart disease. *In* Willerson JT (ed): *Treatment of Heart Diseases.* Gower; 1992:6.1–6.15.

23. Teijeira FJ, Mikhail AA. Cardiac valve replacement with mechanical prostheses: Current states and trends. *In* Hwang NHC, et al. (eds): *Advances in Cardiovascular Engineering.* New York, Plenum Press; 1992:197–226.

24. Teijeira FJ. Mechanical valve prostheses: Mono or bileaflet? Presented at the International Society of Cardio-Thoracic Surgeons Third World Congress, Salzburg, Austria, January 1993.

25. Fiore AC, Naunheim KS, D'Orazio S, et al. Mitral valve replacement: Randomized trial of St. Jude and Medtronic-Hall prostheses. *Ann Thorac Surg.* 1992; 54:68.

26. Antunes MJ. Reoperations on cardiac valves. *J Heart Valve Dis.* 1992;1:15–28.

27. Ryan TJ, Armstron WF, Dillon JC, et al. Doppler echocardiographic evaluation of patients with porcine mitral valves. *Am Heart J.* 1986;111:237.

28. Rashtian MY, Stevenson DM, Allen DT, et al. Flow characteristics of four commonly used mechanical heart valves. *Am J Cardiol.* 1986;58:743.

29. Daniel LB, Grigg LE, Weisel RD, et al. Comparison of transthoracic and transesophageal assessment of prosthetic valve dysfunction. *Echocardiography.* 1990;7:83–95.

30. Otto CM, Pearlman AS. *Textbook of Clinical Echocardiography.* Philadelphia, WB Saunders; 1995.

31. Oh JK, Seward JB, Tajik AJ. *The Echo Manual.* Boston, Little, Brown; 1994.

32. Feigenbaum H. *Echocardiography,* 5th ed. Philadelphia, Lea & Febiger; 1994.

33. Rhodes M. Mitral valve replacement using the Khonsari procedure: Unusual two-dimensional echocardiographic findings. *JDMS* 1995;11:137.

34. Reisner SA, Meltzer RS. Normal values of prosthetic valve Doppler echocardiographic parameters: A review. *J Am Soc Echocardiogr.* 1988;1:201.

35. Zabalgoitia M. Echocardiographic assessment of prosthetic heart valves. *Curr Prob Cardiol.* 1992;17: 269.

36. Sagar KB, Wann S, Paulsen WHJ, et al. Doppler echocardiographic evaluation of Hancock and Bjork-Shiley prosthetic valves. *J Am Coll Cardiol.* 1986;7: 681.

37. Baumgartner H, Khan S, DeRobertis M, et al. Discrepancies between Doppler and catheter gradients

in aortic prosthetic valves in vitro. A manifestation of localized gradients and pressure recovery. *Circulation*. 1990;82:1467.

38. Chafizadeh ER, Zoghbi WA. Doppler echocardiographic assessment of the St. Jude medical prosthetic valve in the aortic position using the continuity equation. *Circulation*. 1991;83:213.

39. Jaffe WM, Coverdale HA, Roche AHG, et al. Doppler echocardiography in the assessment of the homograft aortic valve. *Am J Cardiol*. 1989;63:1466.

40. Miller FA, Callahan JA, Taylor CL, et al. Normal aortic valve prosthesis hemodynamics: 609 prospective Doppler examinations (abstract). *Circulation*. 1989;80(Suppl II):169.

41. Connolly HM, Miller FA Jr, Taylor CL, et al. Doppler hemodynamic profiles of 82 clinically and echocardiographically normal tricuspid valve prostheses. *Circulation*. 1993;88:2722.

42. Cooper DM, Stewart WJ, Schiavone WA, et al. Evaluation of normal prosthetic valve function by Doppler echocardiography. *Am Heart J*. 1987;114:576.

43. Panidis IP, Ross J, Mintz GS. Normal and abnormal prosthetic valve function as assessed by Doppler echocardiography. *J Am Coll Cardiol*. 1986;8:317.

44. Kisanuki A, Tei C, Arikawa K, et al. Continuous wave Doppler echocardiographic assessment of prosthetic aortic valves. *J Cardiogr*. 1986;16:121.

45. Holen J, Simonsen S, Froysaker T. Determination of pressure gradient in the Hancock mitral valve from noninvasive ultrasound Doppler data. *Scand J Clin Lab Invest*. 1981;41:177.

46. Ramirez ML, Wong M, Sadler N, et al. Doppler evaluation of bioprosthetic and mechanical aortic valves: Data from four modes in 107 stable, ambulatory patients. *Am Heart J*. 1988;115:418.

47. Lesbre JP, Chassat C, Lesperance J, et al. Evaluation of new pericardial bioprostheses by pulsed and continuous Doppler ultrasound. *Arch Mal Coeur*. 1986; 79:1439.

48. Kisanuki A, Tei C, Arikawa K, et al. Continuous wave Doppler assessment of prosthetic valves in the mitral position: Comparison of the St. Jude medical mechanical valve and the porcine xenograft valve. *J Cardiogr*. 1985;15:1119.

49. Baumgartner H, Khan S, DeRobertis M, et al. Color Doppler regurgitant characteristics of normal mechanical mitral valve prostheses in vitro. *Circulation*. 1992;85:323.

50. Daniel WG, Mugge A, Grote J, et al. Comparison of transthoracic and transesophageal echocardiography for detection of abnormalities of prosthetic and bioprosthetic valves in the mitral and aortic positions. *Am J Cardiol*. 1993;71:210.

PART V

Echocardiography Evaluation of Cardiac Chambers

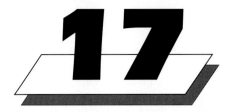

Echocardiographic Assessment of the Left Chambers

CYNTHIA A. HECTOR and MARK N. ALLEN

Introduction

The left ventricle is the largest chamber of the heart and accounts for most of the heart mass. Its role in pumping the blood to all regions of the body accounts for its larger size, relative to other cardiac chambers. The anatomy of the left ventricle is described in detail in Chapter 1. The left atrium receives blood from the lungs. The anatomy of the left atrium is also described in Chapter 1.

Echocardiographic Views

There are several echocardiographic views that allow visualization of the left ventricle. The apical views allow interrogation of the apex, which can be difficult to see in other views. The left ventricle can be seen from the parasternal long- and short-axis orientations, the apical views (including the four-chamber, two-chamber, and apical long-axis views), and the subcostal views. In fact, to examine the left ventricle properly, all these views should be used and recordings made. The specific walls and structures identified by these views are discussed in Chapter 10.

Left Ventricular Measurements

M-MODE MEASUREMENTS

The maximum internal dimensions of the left ventricle can be measured by M-mode or two-dimensional echocardiography. Before two-dimensional

echocardiography, M-mode was used to measure the size of cardiac structures. M-mode measurements are still recorded by many sonographers and are usually done in addition to two-dimensional measurements. For left ventricular dimensions, the M-mode cursor is placed at the base of the left ventricle at the tips of the mitral valve leaflets. Systolic measurements are made at the end of systole and are most accurately recorded at the nadir of the posterior motion of the interventricular septum when septal motion is normal[30] (Fig. 17-1). The wall thickness, as well as the internal diameter of the left ventricle, can be measured. The inward or downward excursion of the interventricular septum does not occur simultaneously with the maximum upward excursion of the posterior wall. The peak upward motion of the posterior wall does not occur until after the second heart sound. Therefore, the peak downward excursion of the interventricular septum corresponds more closely with end systole.[30] However, in patients with abnormal septal motion, the timing is not accurate; therefore, the measurement is best made using the posterior wall as the reference. The diastolic measurements of the left ventricle should be made at end diastole, at the onset of the QRS complex, or at the peak of the R wave (Fig. 17-1).

The major pitfall in using M-mode to make diameter measurements is that the accuracy of measurements depends on the successful alignment of the M-mode cursor so that it is perpendicular to

341

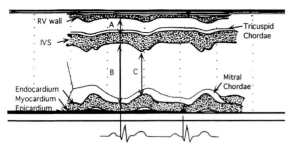

Figure 17-1. M-mode of the left ventricle. (**A**) represents the proper measurement for the right ventricle. (**B**) is the measurements for left ventricular end-diastolic dimensions. (**C**) is left ventricular end-systolic measurements. Left ventricular wall thickness is measured in diastole at the same level for (**B**). RV, right ventricle; IVS, interventricular septum. Note that mitral chordae are seen parallel to the posterior wall. As a general rule, the most rapidly rising structures represent the true posterior left ventricular wall.

two-dimensional measurements is that it can be more difficult to make the measurements at the appropriate times in the cardiac cycle. However, most systems allow the sonographer to loop or scroll the image to the appropriate location in the cardiac cycle. An adequate ECG can help determine the appropriate timing.

The success in obtaining adequate two-dimensional measurements depends on the clarity with which the endocardial borders are defined. In some patients, it can be difficult to define these borders. It is also important to realize that the best measurements will be obtained when the sound waves are aligned perpendicular to the cardiac surfaces. The parasternal long-axis view is the best position to use when measuring left ventricular dimensions (Fig. 17-3). From this position, the sound waves transect

the cardiac structures. In many cases, perpendicular alignment is nearly impossible. Factors such as age, regional or global left ventricular dysfunction, or postoperative status can often affect the size or shape of the heart at the base.[113] Additionally, the intercostal space that is used for transducer placement varies from patient to patient. In patients with technically difficult windows, chronic obstructive pulmonary disease, and pectus excavatum, it is sometimes necessary to use a lower intercostal space, causing the echocardiographic beam to intersect the interventricular septum, posterior walls, and cavity obliquely, resulting in wall measurements that are falsely thick and cavity dimensions that are falsely enlarged.[16] Figure 17-2 clearly demonstrates the problems inherent in M-mode measurements. In experienced hands, M-mode measurements are fairly reproducible in the absence of left ventricular size changes.[28,113] The major advantage of M-mode is its ability to time the cardiac events precisely with the electrocardiogram (ECG).

TWO-DIMENSIONAL MEASUREMENTS

Two-dimensional measurements are very common and in many labs are done exclusively. Unlike M-mode, two-dimensional measurements can be made regardless of the position of the heart. As long as endocardial borders are well defined, measurements can be made, because there is no need to align a cursor with cardiac structures. The major pitfall with

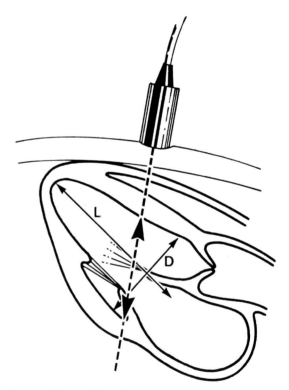

Figure 17-2. Problems inherent in M-mode measurements are usually associated with malalignment of the M-mode cursors so that the structures are not perpendicular to the cursor. These errors result in measurements that are larger than the actual dimensions. L, D, long and minor left ventricular dimensions. (From Feigenbaum H. Echocardiographic Evaluation of Cardiac Chambers. Philadelphia, Lea & Febiger; 1994:137, Fig. 3-7. Reprinted with permission.)

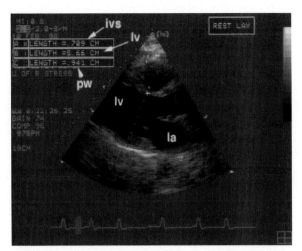

Figure 17-3. Parasternal long-axis view of the left ventricle demonstrating proper techniques in measuring the left ventricular walls and cavity in diastole and in systole.

chamber volume and wall thickness. When pressures within the left ventricle are abnormally elevated for a long period of time, left ventricular walls hypertrophy results in an increase in left ventricular mass. In this case, chamber volume does not change significantly. By contrast, with prolonged volume increases, the increase in mass is due predominantly to the enlargement of the chamber and not necessarily to an increase in wall thickness. Due to this distinction, *mass* is a more precise term in describing the effects of pressure or volume increases in the left ventricle, whereas *left ventricular hypertrophy* is more narrowly defined to include only an increase in wall thickness. Further, elevated left ventricular mass is a stronger predictor, other than age, of

the walls perpendicularly. A parasternal short-axis approach can also be used to obtain two-dimensional measurements. Measurements can also be taken from the apical four-chamber view. However, it must be remembered that from this view the sound waves are parallel to the structures, which may result in artifact. With proper system settings and attention to endocardial borders, errors can be avoided. Figure 17-4 demonstrates the location for making two-dimensional measurements of the left ventricle.[85] The normal values for left ventricular size are listed in Table 17-1.[85,87] Colorization of the two-dimensional image can help define endocardial borders (Fig. 17-5*A–C*).

LEFT VENTRICULAR MASS

Once the left ventricular wall thickness and chamber dimensions are obtained, a left ventricular mass can be calculated. In response to abnormal pressures or volumes, there is an increase in muscular hypertrophy of the left ventricle. The degree of hypertrophy correlates with the severity of the increased load on the ventricle. The echocardiographic finding of left ventricular hypertrophy can be used as a predictor of cardiovascular risk and higher mortality.[105] Anatomically, hypertrophy of the left ventricle is characterized by an increase in muscle weight or mass.[105] Left ventricular mass is defined by two parameters:

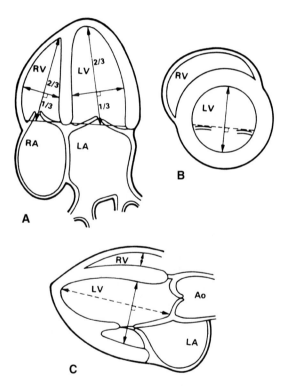

Figure 17-4. Two-dimensional measurements obtained from the apical four-chamber view (**A**), parasternal short-axis view (**B**), and parasternal long-axis view (**C**). In actuality, the superior-inferior dimensions shown here (dashed arrow) in the parasternal long-axis view are difficult to obtain since the apex is seldom seen clearly from this view. On the other hand, the wall thickness and anteroposterior cavity dimensions (solid arrows) are best obtained from this view. Ao, aorta; LA, left atrium; LV, left ventricle; RA, right atrium; RV, right ventricle. (From Ref. 85, p. 360. Reprinted with permission.)

▰▰▰ TABLE 17-1. HEART CHAMBER MEASUREMENTS BY TWO-DIMENSIONAL ECHOCARDIOGRAPHY

View	Normal Range (cm) (Mean ± 2 SD)	Mean (cm)	Index (cm/m²)	Absolute Range (cm)
Apical four-chamber				
LVed major	6.9–10.3	8.6	4.1–5.7	7.2–10.3
LVed minor	3.3–6.1	4.7	2.2–3.1	3.8–6.2
LVes minor	1.9–3.7	2.8	1.3–2.0	2.1–3.9
LV FS	0.27–0.50	38	—	0.26–0.47
RV major	6.5–9.5	8.0	3.8–5.3	6.3–9.3
RV minor	2.2–4.4	3.3	1.0–2.8	2.2–4.5
Parasternal long-axis				
LVed	3.5–6.0	4.8	2.3–3.1	3.8–5.8
LVes	2.1–4.0	3.1	1.4–2.1	2.3–3.9
FS	0.25–0.46	36	—	0.26–0.45
RV	1.9–3.8	2.8	1.2–2.0	1.9–3.9
Parasternal short-axis				
Chordal level				
LVed	3.5–6.2	4.8	2.3–3.2	3.8–6.1
LVes	2.3–4.0	3.2	1.5–2.2	2.6–4.2
LV FS	0.27–0.42	34	—	0.27–0.41
Papillary muscle level				
LVed	3.5–5.8	4.7	2.2–3.1	3.9–5.8
LVes	2.2–4.0	3.1	1.4–2.2	2.5–4.1
LV FS	0.25–0.43	34	—	0.25–0.43

LVed, Left ventricle, end-diastole; *LVes*, left ventricle, end-systole; *LV FS*, left ventricular fractional shortening; *RV*, right ventricle.
   Note: Although it is a common and useful practice in adult cardiology to correct values for body surface area, for pediatric applications, or for smaller or larger than average subjects, charts based on subjects of a wide range of body sizes should be consulted.
   Source: Data from Schnittger I, Gordon EP, Fitzgerald PJ, Popp RI. Standardized intracardiac measurements of two-dimensional echocardiography. J Am Coll Cardiol. 1983;2:934–938. Reprinted with permission.

cardiovascular morbidity and mortality, in men and women.[34,51,54]

A number of methods can be used to calculate left ventricular mass. The simplest and first method is based on wall thickness and is used to estimate left ventricular mass using M-mode or two-dimensional echocardiographic measurements.[23] This method correlates closely with cardiac weights obtained at autopsy. In this method, a simple formula is used to calculate left ventricular mass (LVM) based upon three measurements of the left ventricle[10]:

$$\text{Anatomic LVM} = 1.04[(\text{LVID}_{ED} + \text{PWT}_{ED} + \text{IVS}_{ED})^3 - (\text{LVID}_{ED})^3] - 13.6 \text{ g}$$

These measurements include the interventricular septal thickness (IVS), the internal diameter of the heart (LVID), and the posterior left ventricular wall (PWT), all measured at end diastole. The ideal view for taking these measurements is the left parasternal long-axis view.

Whenever a three-dimensional structure is measured using a one-dimensional technique, certain assumptions are made. With these simple mass calculations, it is assumed that the heart is a prolate ellipsoid with a chamber length equal to twice the diameter, and is measured at the midpapillary level. Wall thicknesses measured at the base are averaged to represent the thickness of all the walls of the left ventricle. In patients with wall motion abnormalities or in those whose hearts deviate from this assumed geometry, the formula is unreliable. In these cases, left ventricular mass should not be reported. Yet, in spite of these inherent difficulties, many labs use this method to record left ventricular mass. Using two-dimensional echocardiography to guide the M-mode cursor can increase the accuracy of these measurements, but even this enhancement has limitations.[92]

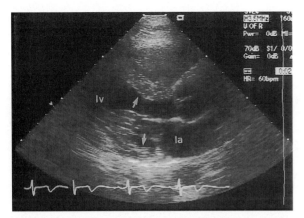

Figure 17-5. Colorization of the two-dimensional image may help identify endocardial borders (arrow). La, left atrium; lv, left ventricle. (See also Color Plates 55, 56, and 57.)

Two-dimensional measurements of left ventricular mass have proven to increase the accuracy of left ventricular mass calculations by echocardiography techniques.[13,17,34,78,86] A number of techniques are used to measure left ventricular mass by two-dimensional echocardiography. Table 17-2 summarizes normal values for left ventricular mass.[40]

Recent advances in three-dimensional echocardiography may prove promising in determining left ventricular mass calculations. The current method of mass calculations requires a standard ultrasound unit, a three-dimensional spatial locator, and a personal computer.[47] One technique used to reconstruct the heart uses a polyhedral surface reconstruction algorithm. Three-dimensional reconstruction of the heart is achieved by using an acoustical spatial locator attached to the imaging

transducer. The spatial locator records the traducer's position and orientation. At the same time, the spatial locator using a set of three sound emitters and a set of four microphone receivers records the image's X, Y, and Z coordinates, ultimately resulting in a three-dimensional reconstruction of the cardiac image.[47]

Early results with this technique compare favorably with the results of other diagnostic tests such as magnetic resonance imaging, as well as measurements of gross anatomic specimen in canine models. Comparisons with one-dimensional and two-dimensional echocardiography indicate that three-dimensional mass determinations have a higher accuracy rate.[34,47] With further refinement of this technique, three-dimensional imaging and calculations may prove very useful in a more practical setting.

VOLUME CALCULATIONS

Volume and global left ventricular systolic function can be calculated most reliably using two-dimensional echocardiography.[65,84,94,98,104] M-mode measurements for these calculations are less reliable, especially in the setting of coronary artery disease.[58,84] Calculation of left ventricular volumes can provide information on left ventricular mass, as well as overall left ventricular systolic function. Numerous methods are used to make these calculations. Some of these are summarized in Figure 17-6.[65] The single-plane or biplane area-length methods and Simpson's method of discs are generally more accurate and widely used for volume and ejection fraction determinations.[85] These calculations are typically performed more easily in a practical setting. All volume calculations make some geometric assumptions, and regional wall motion abnormalities will dramatically affect the results.

Area-Length Method

This method calculates volume from the equation $V = 0.85 \ A^2/L$. The area (A) of the left ventricle is traced from an apical four- or two-chamber view (Fig. 17-7). The system's tracing function is used to trace around the left ventricular cavity, at the border of the cavity-endocardial border. The length measurement is made from the center of the mitral annular plane to the apex.

TABLE 17-2. Left Ventricular Mass (Normal Values): Truncated Ellipsoid Method

Mass	Mean ± SD	
	Males (*n* = 44)	Females (*n* = 40)
Grams	148 ± 26	108 ± 21
Index (gm/m²)	76 ± 13	66 ± 11

Source: Data from Helak JW, Reichek N. Quantitation of human left ventricular mass and volume by two-dimensional echocardiography: In vitro anatomic validation. Circulation. 1981;63:1398–1407. Reprinted with permission.

Algorithm	Formula	Geometric model

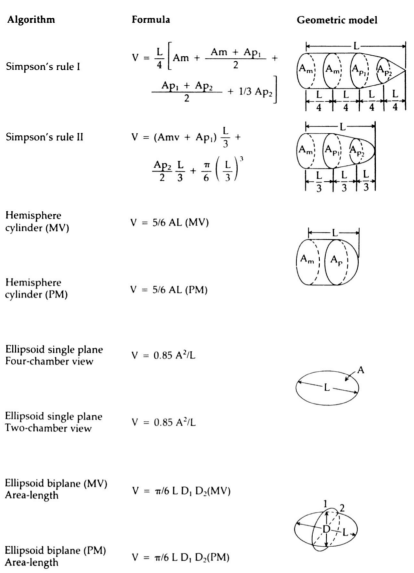

Simpson's rule I

$$V = \frac{L}{4}\left[Am + \frac{Am + Ap_1}{2} + \frac{Ap_1 + Ap_2}{2} + 1/3\ Ap_2\right]$$

Simpson's rule II

$$V = (Amv + Ap_1)\frac{L}{3} + \frac{Ap_2}{2}\frac{L}{3} + \frac{\pi}{6}\left(\frac{L}{3}\right)^3$$

Hemisphere cylinder (MV)

$$V = 5/6\ AL\ (MV)$$

Hemisphere cylinder (PM)

$$V = 5/6\ AL\ (PM)$$

Ellipsoid single plane Four-chamber view

$$V = 0.85\ A^2/L$$

Ellipsoid single plane Two-chamber view

$$V = 0.85\ A^2/L$$

Ellipsoid biplane (MV) Area-length

$$V = \pi/6\ L\ D_1\ D_2(MV)$$

Ellipsoid biplane (PM) Area-length

$$V = \pi/6\ L\ D_1\ D_2(PM)$$

Figure 17-6. Various methods of calculating left ventricular volumes. V, volume; L, longest length from apical four-chamber view; A_m, area of short axis at level of mitral valve; A_p, area of short axis at level of papillary muscle; D_1, diameter of minor axis (right to left); D_2, diameter of minor axis (anteroposterior); PM, papillary muscle; MV, mitral valve. (From Ref. 65, p. 239. Reprinted with permission.)

BY SINGLE PLANE AREA LENGTH

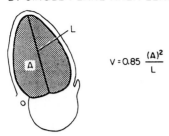

$$V = 0.85 \frac{(A)^2}{L}$$

Figure 17-7. Single-plane area length method for determining left ventricular volume. The cavity area is determined by using the system's on-line calibers to trace the endocardial borders. The length of the left ventricle is measured from the center of the mitral annular plane to the apex of the left ventricle. The same measurements are taken from a four-chamber view as well. The volume is then calculated from the above equation. *A,* area of the left ventricular cavity; *L,* length of the left ventricular cavity. (From Schiller MB et al. Recommendations for quantification of the left ventricle by two-dimensional echocardiography. J Am Soc Echocardiogr 1989;2:362. Reprinted with permission.)

Simpson's Method of Discs

This method divides the left ventricle into a series of cylinders (usually 20) of equal height and sums their areas to calculate left ventricular volume[85] (Fig. 17-8). This method is generally more accurate than other methods because it is not as sensitive to distortions in left ventricular geometry.

Table 17-3 summarizes normal volumes as calculated from these basic methods.[108]

Global Systolic Function

In adult echocardiography, the assessment of the left ventricle systolic function is a common request. Echocardiography is an excellent technique for determining global as well as regional function of the left ventricle. The attributes of high spatial and temporal resolution and the ability to define regional wall thickening, as well as endocardial excursion, make echocardiography extremely useful in defining regional dysfunction due to ischemic disease, cardiomyopathy, contusion, and other disorders. There are a number of measurements that can be used to evaluate the left ventricle using echocardiography. Some measurements are routinely used, whereas others are used more for academic considerations. For the purpose of this text, the more practical and more routinely used measurements will be discussed.

In evaluating the left ventricle, it is important to obtain clear visualization of the endocardial borders. Without a clear delineation of the endocardium, any method used to determine left ventricular systolic function will be fraught with uncertainty and error.

Resolution of the endocardial borders depends to a great degree on the structure's orientation to the sound beam. Targets that are perpendicular to the sound beam are resolved by the system's axial resolution. The sensitivity of axial resolution varies with the machine, but for most systems, structures that are millimeters or fractions of millimeters can be discerned. Structures that are parallel to the sound beam can be distinguished from one another only if they are more than one beam width apart. In addition, when the target moves within the sound beam, the motion may not always be detectable, particularly with structures that are parallel to the sound beam. Unless the targets move to a distance

LV VOLUME

BY METHOD OF DISCS (MODIFIED SIMPSON'S RULE)

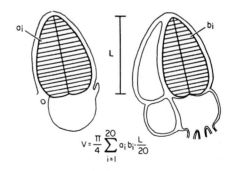

$$V = \frac{\pi}{4} \sum_{i=1}^{20} a_i b_i \cdot \frac{L}{20}$$

BY SINGLE PLANE AREA LENGTH

Figure 17-8. The method of disc or modified Simpson's rule for determining left ventricular volumes. The left ventricle is divided into a series of discs of known diameter and equal height. The number of discs vary from 4 (52) to 256 (R60) and are accounted for in the equation as *n.* The formula is as follows:

$$V = \pi/4 \sum_{i=1}^{n} a_i b_i \, L/n$$

where *n* = the number of discs used, *L* = left ventricular length, and *a* and *b* = diameters of the discs. (From Ref. 85, p. 362. Reprinted with permission.)

TABLE 17-3. LEFT VENTRICULAR END-DIASTOLIC VOLUMES (NORMAL VALUES)

Algorithm	Mean ± SD (Range) ml	Mean ± SD (Range) ml/m²
Four-chamber area length		
Male patients	112 ± 27 (65–193)	57 ± 13 (37–94)
Female patients	89 ± 20 (59–136)	
Two-chamber area length		
Male patients	130 ± 27 (73–201)	63 ± 13 (37–101)
Female patients	92 ± 19 (53–146)	
Biplane disc summation (modified Simpson's rule)		
Male patients	111 ± 22 (62–170)	55 ± 10 (36–82)
Female patients	80 ± 12 (55–101)	

Source: Data from Wahr DW, Wang YS, Schiller NB. Left ventricular volumes determined by two-dimensional echocardiography in a normal adult population. J Am Coll Cardiol. 1983;1:863–868. Reprinted with permission.

greater than the sound beam width, this motion will not be seen. A common problem in assessing the left ventricle for global or regional wall motion is the clear visualization of the lateral wall from the parasternal short-axis and apical four-chamber views. In an apical two-chamber view, the inferior wall can be difficult to see because this structure lies parallel to the path of the sound beam. For this reason, very careful interrogation is required, and only when seen from multiple views should abnormalities be so called.[105]

LEFT VENTRICULAR PERFORMANCE

Left ventricular systolic function can be evaluated by four general methods: stroke volume, ejection fraction, fractional shortening, or velocity of fiber shortening.[105]

Stroke Volume

Stroke volume measures the volume of blood ejected during systole and is the difference between end-diastolic and end-systolic volumes. Two general methods are used for calculating stroke volume (SV) using echocardiography. The first takes advantage of one of the volume calculations described above, but Simpson's method of discs is the usual calculation used. The formula is as follows:

SV = end-diastolic volume − end-systolic volume

Stroke volume can also be calculated using Doppler echocardiography. In this calculation, the flow across the left ventricular outflow tract is equal to the stroke volume. Flow is equal to the velocity time integral obtained by pulsed wave Doppler

times the area of the outflow tract (Fig. 17-9). Cardiac output can then be calculated by multiplying the heart rate by the derived stroke volume. Stroke volume should be calculated at the end of expiration, since it usually decreases during inspiration.

Ejection Fraction

Left ventricular ejection fraction is the single most useful number for describing left ventricular performance. In the normal heart, the ejection fraction is normal between 55% and 78%.[61] It is defined by the following formula:

$$EF = \frac{EDV - ESV}{EDV} \times 100$$

where, EDV is end-diastolic volume and ESV is end-systolic volume.

Several methods are used to calculate ejection fractions using volume determinations and com-

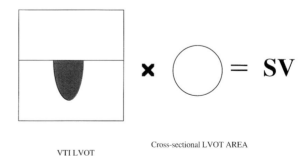

VTI LVOT

Cross-sectional LVOT AREA

Figure 17-9. Stroke volume (SV) calculation using the velocity time integral (VTI) of the left ventricular outflow tract (LVOT) and its cross-sectional area, derived from its diameter measurement.

puter-derived calculations. Most of these methods involve several measurements of the left ventricle from various views and are seldom used. One relatively simple calculation uses the end-diastolic and end-systolic measurements of the left ventricle from a parasternal long-axis view. The formula corrects for the apex by assigning a value of 10% for normal, 5% for hypokinesis, 0% for akinesis, and −5% for dyskinesis.[105] The formula is as follows:

$$EF = \frac{EDD^2 - ESD^2}{EDD^2} \times 100 + K$$

where EDD is end-diastolic dimensions, ESD is end-systolic dimensions, and K is the apex-correction value. This method has proven to be adequate in normal left ventricles, but it cannot be used in patients with wall motion abnormalities.

The most widely used method of reporting the ejection fraction is visual estimation. Visual estimation allows the observer to consider all segments of the left ventricle, not just one plane, as do most measurement techniques. In experienced hands, visual estimation has correlated well with the results of both angiographic[67,97] and radionuclide angiography.[4,67] However, although this method correlates well with other studies, its correlation is not as good between interpreters. Since this method is subjective, it is prone to errors. However, despite these limitations, it is widely used in the clinical setting.

Currently, there are three widely used methods for determining left ventricular ejection fraction. Radionuclide ventriculography is established as a useful and accurate method.[39,89,106] This technique uses a radioactive isotope to label red blood cells. Multiple gated radionuclide ventriculograms are obtained using a gamma camera[88] (Fig. 17-10). However, this technique does have limitations, including the need for repeated administration of radioactive material, unavailability, increased cost, and increasing restrictions imposed by the radiation protection authorities.[88] Contrast cineangiography is also widely used in determining left ventricular ejection fraction. This technique, like radionuclide techniques, is invasive and carries its own set of risks.

Fractional Shortening and Velocity of Fiber Shortening

Fractional shortening and velocity of fiber shortening are typically derived from M-mode measure-

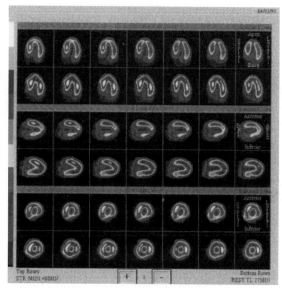

Figure 17-10. Myocardial perfusion SPECT study of left ventricle, indicating a slightly dilated LV with severe and extensive ischemic defect of the interior wall extending to the apex and antero-apical region. (Courtesy Ronald Schwartz, University of Rochester Nuclear Cardiology Department.) (See also Color Plate 58.)

ments. These measurements are based on the angiographic observations that the systolic decrease in ventricular volume is due primarily to minor axis shortening and that the percentage of change in that axis during systole has a linear relationship with the ejection fraction.[57,105] These methods represent simple means of estimating left ventricular performance in a symmetrically contracting left ventricle. The formula for calculating fractional shortening is:

$$\%\Delta D = \frac{LVID_d - LVID_s}{LVID_d} \times 100$$

where ΔD is fractional shortening, $LVID_d$ is left ventricular internal diameter in diastole, and $LVID_s$ is left ventricular internal diameter in systole. The normal value is usually greater than 25%.[105] The formula for velocity of fiber shortening is expressed as

$$Vcf = \frac{LVID_d - LVID_s}{LVID_d} \times ET$$

where ET is ejection time and is calculated from the duration of aortic valve opening. The lower limit of normal for Vcf is 1.1 circumferences per second.[105]

REGIONAL WALL SEGMENTS

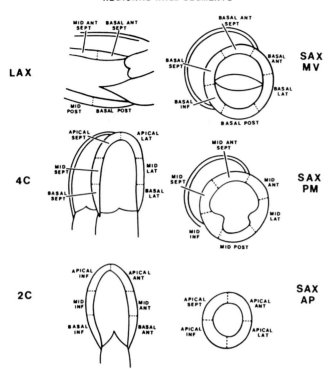

Figure 17-11. Diagram demonstrating the location of the 16-segment approach to dividing the left ventricle. All 16 segments can be identified either with three longitudinal views, long-axis (LAX), four-chamber (4C), two-chamber (2C), three short-axis views at the mitral valve level (SAX MV), the papillary muscle level (SAX PM), or the apical level (SAX AP). (From Feigenbaum H. Echocardiography, 5th ed. Philadelphia, Lea & Febiger; 1994:148, Fig. 3-27. Reprinted with permission.)

Regional Wall Motion Assessment

Echocardiography is ideally suited for evaluating regional function of the left ventricle. The various windows available allow all the segments to be visualized. Assessment and identification of regional wall motion abnormalities is made on a visual view of the various segments. To help describe the findings, the left ventricle is typically divided into 16 segments (Fig. 17-11). The walls are scored on a scale of 1–4, where 1 is normal systolic function, 2 is reduced systolic function or hypokinetic, 3 is no systolic function or akinesis, and 4 is when a segment bulges outward in systole or what is referred to as *dyskinesis*.[85] The visual method is subjective, and no two observers may score a segment the same way. This has caused the development of a number of computer programs to help provide a more scientific approach to wall motion analysis. These computer approaches vary considerably and are not easy to standardize among practitioners. Unlike the visual methods, these programs take into consideration anatomic logic or relationships to the known coronary arterial supply. In addition, poor-quality images and the lack of a well-demarcated endocardial border may lead to erroneous calculations. The American Society of Echocardiography recommends using the visual approach until a widely applicable and practical quantitative method is developed.[85] Regional wall motion analysis is covered in Chapters 7 and 20.

Diastolic Function

Diastole refers to that part of the cardiac cycle between the closing of the aortic valve, or the second heart sound, and the opening of the mitral valve, or the first heart sound. During this period, the heart is said to be in a state of relaxation. To understand diastolic function, it is important to understand the relationships between pressure and volume. During cardiac relaxation, the ventricle is allowed to fill. Pressure within the left ventricle is less than that in the aorta, so the aortic valve remains closed, and pressure in the left atrium is greater, so the mitral valve remains open, allowing blood to enter the ventricle. As volume increases within the chambers, the cardiac muscle needs to expand in order to accommodate the increase in volume. As cardiac muscles or cardiac muscle cells increase in length, a force or pressure develops. The amount of "stretch" allowed by the cells eventually reaches a maximum level or pressure. This pressure then begins to equal the pressure within the left atrium, causing the mitral valve to close. This pressure does not quite exceed the pressure within the aorta, so the aortic valve remains closed during this period. This period of time during which the pressure continues to increase within the left ventricle, but with no increase in volume, is called *isovolumic* (iso = same) *contraction*. Eventually, the pressure within the left ventricle becomes so great that it exceeds the pressure within the aorta and the valve is forced open, allowing the emission of blood into the aorta. This contraction is due in part to the pressure generated by the cardiac cells as a result of the increased volume and subsequent stretch of the cells due to the volume increase.

The diastolic properties of the left ventricle are a function of the left ventricle's compliance. A "stiff" ventricle has decreased compliance and therefore higher diastolic pressure. Another property of diastolic function of the left ventricle is the rate at which it relaxes in later diastole. Measurements of either of these properties can provide information on the diastolic state of the left ventricle. Diastolic function of the left ventricle is extremely complex, and many of the hemodynamic relationships in this phase are poorly understood. It is important to develop quantitative measures of diastolic function of the left ventricle since impairment of this phase produces significant hemodynamic abnormalities. Diastolic dysfunction may be responsible for or may contribute to the pathophysiology of many cardiac diseases.[25,96,103]

Diastolic dysfunction in left ventricular hypertrophy, or in hypertrophic or restrictive cardiomyopathies, may lead to cardiac failure even in the setting of normal systolic function. Diastolic dysfunction in acute myocardial ischemia occurs before systolic dysfunction. Throughout diastole several hemodynamic phases occur. Quantitative measures of any one of these phases can be indicative of diastolic dysfunction.

Direct measures of left ventricular diastolic function, filling patterns, and pressures can be achieved directly and reliably by invasive pressure and volume measurements. However, these methods are impractical for routine clinical use. Noninvasive imaging modalities such as radionuclide angiography, computed tomography, and magnetic resonance imaging can assess diastolic function indirectly by analyzing changes in ventricular volume during diastole.[70]

More recently, echocardiography has been used to determine left ventricular diastolic function using several techniques. Unfortunately, measuring the diastolic function of the left ventricle is a complex process, and many of the techniques used can be misleading or difficult to apply reliably.[35] A thorough understanding of the diastolic properties of the left ventricle, proper echocardiography techniques such as ultrasound beam alignment to flow, an understanding of proper ultrasound machine settings, recognition of various Doppler audio and spectral characteristics across the mitral valve, and internal validation are all important before these measurements can be used to provide diagnostic information.[7]

MITRAL FLOW VELOCITIES

E/A Velocities/Ratios

Changes in the E and A points of the Doppler signal across the mitral valve can indicate diastolic dysfunction. Normally, the E point is higher than the A point during normal filling of the left ventricle. Doppler E velocities are most reflective of relaxation phase or early rapid filling, whereas A velocities are most affected by passive compliance or late filling caused by atrial contraction.[22] The mitral flow patterns are recorded using pulsed wave Doppler, with the sample volume positioned between the tips of the mitral valve leaflets.[7] Patterns that are normally measured include the peak flow velocities and acceleration and deceleration rates of both E and A waves, flow velocity at the end of diastasis—before atrial contraction (E at A)—peak velocity at atrial contraction (A wave), and mitral A wave duration (Fig. 17-12).

To obtain these measurements, the patient is placed in a left lateral position and the transducer is placed in the apical position. The use of color flow Doppler will greatly enhance the operator's appreciation of flow dynamics across the mitral valve. Once the direction of flow is determined, fine adjustments can be made to align the cursor properly. Frequently, the transducer may need to be moved lat-

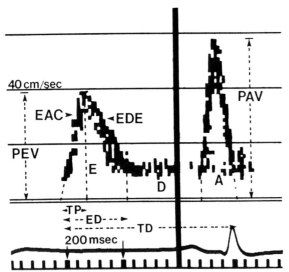

Figure 17-12. Normal spectral Doppler display across the mitral valve. Three stages are noted in this display. The first is the early filling phase, represented by the E wave. The second is diastasis (D), which represents the time just before atrial contraction. Diastasis can be short or completely missing in patients with high heart rates. The third phase is atrial contraction, or the A wave. A number of measurements can be made from a tracing like this, such as the peak E wave velocity (PEV), the peak A wave velocity (PAV), the E wave acceleration time (EAC), the E wave deceleration time (EDE), the E wave duration (ED), the duration of peak transmitral flow—measured from the onset of transmitral flow to the peak of the E wave (TP)—and the total filling time or duration (TD). The peak E and A wave velocities, their ratio, and the E deceleration times are routine diastolic measurements. (From Choong CY, Herrmann HC, Weyman AE, et al. Preload dependence of Doppler-derived indexes of left ventricular diastolic function in humans. J Am Coll Cardiol. 1987;10:800. Reprinted with permission from the American College of Cardiology.)

erally to obtain the best parallel flow position.[7] The mitral flow recordings are made with pulsed wave Doppler and a sample volume of 1 to 2 mm placed between the tips of the mitral valve leaflets.[7] Velocity filters are adjusted as low as possible to optimize the Doppler signal. The operator listens for the clearest, highest-pitched sound. The sweep speed is no higher than 50 mm, and the flow patterns are observed throughout several respiratory cycles to check for any respiratory variations that may indicate constrictive pericarditis or tamponade. Recordings are made with the patient suspending respirations. The spectral display is then frozen, and measurements are made.

The E/A ratio is obtained by measuring the peak velocities of the E and A waves. Once these measurements are made, the ultrasound systems automatically calculates the E/A ratio. Normally, this ratio is between 1 and 2. However, an abnormal ratio can also be seen in patients with restrictive physiology or pseudonormalization of the E/A ratio. Patients with abnormal left ventricular relaxation have a lower E/A ratio. However, once again, a thorough understanding of the patient's clinical history and other echocardiographic findings must be considered. In addition, there are other factors that ultimately affect the E and A wave velocities and the E/A ratio. With age the E and A wave velocities can change dramatically. There is a gradual increase in A wave velocity so that by age 65, A wave velocity nearly equals E wave velocity and by age 70, A wave velocities may exceed E wave velocities, resulting in an E/A ratio of less than 1.[7] Respiratory variation and heart rate can also affect transmitral inflow. The placement of the pulsed wave sample volume has a dramatic effect on the flow profile[72] (Fig. 17-13).

Three separate physiologic states can affect the mitral flow patterns: abnormal left ventricular relaxation (Fig. 17-14), restrictive physiology (different from restrictive cardiomyopathy) (Fig. 17-15), and pseudonormalization[7] (Fig. 17-16).

Changes in left ventricular diastolic function may alter the normal pattern. In the presence of diastolic dysfunction, the cells of the myocardium become less compliant and more resistant to change. Therefore, the diastolic pressures within the left ventricle may remain higher, thereby reducing the amount of filling provided by the left atrium. In turn, the left atrium is unable to empty completely. The A point may be higher than the E point in patients with diastolic dysfunction due to the pressure of atrial systole and the increased initial volume remaining from the incomplete passive filling (Fig. 17-17B).

Isovolumic Relaxation Time

The isovolumic relaxation time (IVRT) is the time between aortic valve closure and mitral valve flow,[6,64] and may be prolonged in patients with diastolic dysfunction. In left ventricular diastolic dysfunction the pressure within the left ventricle remains high, resulting in an increase in the time it takes for the left ventricular pressure to fall in diastole. This results in a delay in mitral valve opening,

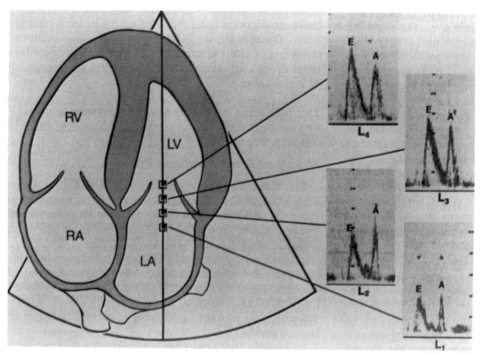

Figure 17-13. Spectral Doppler displays at various positions on the same patient. E and A wave velocities differ considerably with changing sample volume positions. (From Ref. 72, p. 40. Reprinted with permission.)

since pressure in the left ventricle remains higher than in the left atrium. Therefore, this interval is primarily dependent on the timing of mitral valve opening, which is determined by the rate of left ventricular relaxation and left atrial pressures.[6,69] Unlike other transmitral flow measurements, continuous wave Doppler can be used here since pulsed

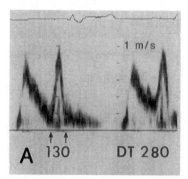

Figure 17-14. Pulsed wave spectral Doppler display of mitral inflow in a patient with an abnormal left ventricular relaxation pattern. (From Ref. 70, p. 253, Fig. 6. Reprinted with permission.)

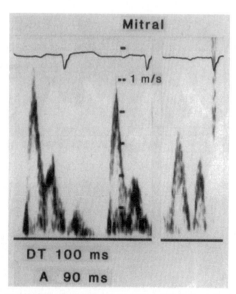

Figure 17-15. Pulsed wave spectral Doppler display of mitral inflow in a patient with a restrictive cardiomyopathy pattern. (From Ref. 70, p. 254, Fig. 7. Reprinted with permission.)

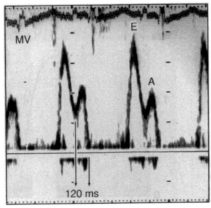

Figure 17-16. Pulsed wave spectral Doppler display of mitral inflow in a patient with a pseudonormalization pattern. (From Ref. 70, p. 255, Fig. 8b. Reprinted with permission.)

wave Doppler may not provide enough information to see both left ventricular inflow and outflow patterns. From an apical position, the cursor is placed between the left ventricular outflow tract and the anterior mitral valve leaflet. With the two-dimensional image frozen, the Doppler signal should demonstrate an aortic valve closure click, which appears both above and below the zero-velocity baseline and the onset of mitral valve flow.[7] The interval between aortic valve closure and mitral valve flow

is then measured. The cursor is placed in the area of the mitral valve tips until mitral flow is visualized. The cursor is then slightly angled toward the left ventricular outflow tract so that the aortic valve closure click is seen. If pulsed wave Doppler is used, a sample size of 3–4 mm is used. With Doppler, isovolumic relaxation times less than 100 m/sec are considered normal, regardless of age, although there are slight variations in IVRT intervals among age groups. IVRTs greater than 120 m/sec are considered to be indicative of diastolic dysfunction (Fig. 17-17A,B).

Four common errors can be made in measuring IVRT. First, wall motion or velocity artifacts can be mistaken for aortic closure clicks. Making sure that the clicks are seen on both sides of the zero-velocity baseline helps reduce the chances of making this error. Second, angling the cursor too far toward the left ventricular outflow tract can cause a delay in the recorded onset of mitral valve opening. This error can be reduced by comparing the time of the start of mitral flow with IVRT with that of mitral valve recordings.[7] Third, the mitral valve opening click may be taken as the start of mitral valve flow. Remember that mitral valve flow starts after the separation of the mitral valve leaflets.[53] Finally, too high a gain setting can result in poor spectral displays, making measurements difficult.

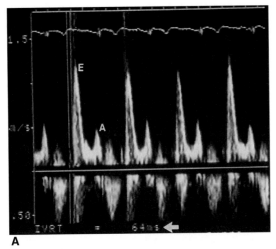

A

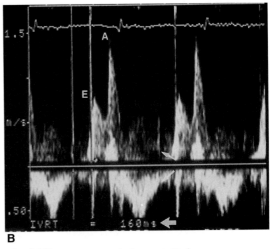

B

Figure 17-17. Spectral Doppler tracings demonstrating the IVRT measurements in a normal patient (**A**) with an IVRT of 64 m/sec (large arrow) and in a patient with diastolic dysfunction (**B**) with an IVRT of 160 m/sec. Aortic clicks can be seen (small arrows), which help identify proper measurement locations. In (**B**) the A wave velocity is much higher than the E wave velocity, which also indicates diastolic dysfunction.

Mitral Deceleration Time

The mitral deceleration time is also used to evaluate for diastolic dysfunction. The deceleration time is measured from the peak of the E velocity to the zero-velocity baseline.[6] In diastolic dysfunction, the deceleration time is prolonged again because diastolic pressures remain higher, requiring more time for passive filling to occur. In a normal, healthy heart, relaxation of the left ventricle is vigorous, resulting in deceleration times of 150–240 m/sec (Fig. 17-18A). Deceleration times greater than 240 m/sec are consistent with diastolic dysfunction (Fig. 17-18B). Deceleration times less than 150 m/sec have been noted in patients with increased filling pressures in the setting of coronary artery disease,[5,33] restrictive cardiomyopathies,[50] and dilated cardiomyopathies.[47,71,91]

To measure these parameters, it is important to ensure proper cursor position. These measurements are best obtained from pulsed wave Doppler. The cursor should be placed at the tips of the mitral valve leaflets. As with measuring E and A wave peak velocities, improper cursor placement across the mitral valve can produce very different absolute values. Careful attention to this issue is important.

PULMONARY VENOUS FLOW

Evaluation of pulmonary venous flow can also be used to evaluate the diastolic function of the left ventricle. Normally, the Doppler patterns exhibit a forward systolic and diastolic component and a reversed atrial component (Fig. 17-19). These patterns may change in patients with diastolic dysfunc-

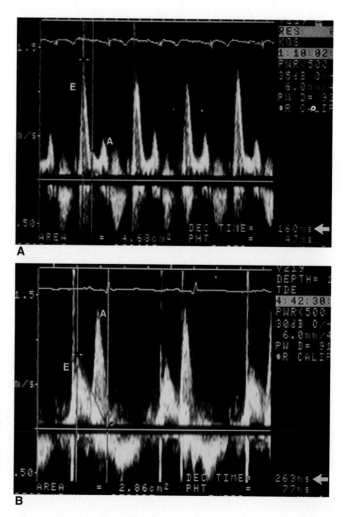

Figure 17-18. Normal and abnormal deceleration times. In (**A**) the deceleration time is 160 m/sec (arrow), indicating normal relaxation and diastolic pressures. In (**B**) the diastolic pressures remain elevated, resulting in a longer deceleration time (arrow). Note the marked differences in the E and A wave velocities between the two patients.

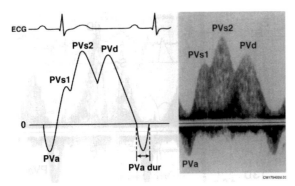

Figure 17-19. Pulsed Doppler of normal pulmonary venous flow. PVs1 and PVs2, systolic flow; PVd, diastolic flow; PVA, reversed atrial component. (From Ref. 70, p. 249, Fig. 3. Reprinted with permission.)

tion. In patients with elevated diastolic pressures there is a discernible decrease in the diastolic component of the Doppler signal and an increase in the atrial component (Fig. 17-20).

Although these measurements can be used to provide some information on the diastolic state of the left ventricle, it is important to note that these findings may not be conclusive due to other factors unrelated to diastolic dysfunction that can cause similar alterations in these Doppler patterns. Doppler patterns typically seen in diastolic dysfunction can also be seen in patients with left ventricular hy-

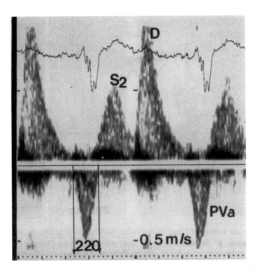

Figure 17-20. Pulsed Doppler of pulmonary veins in a patient with diastolic dysfunction. Note the increase in the atrial component (PVa) and the loss of S_1. S_2, systole; D, diastole. (From Ref. 70, p. 250, Fig. 4. Reprinted with permission.

pertrophy, myocardial ischemia, cardiomyopathies, abnormal heart rate,[73,95] and valvular disease,[90] as well as in older persons. This pattern has also been noted in patients with decreased filling pressures in the left ventricle that result from a decrease in left ventricular volume, such as hypovolemia or dehydration, and in cases where flow to the left heart is decreased as a result of pulmonary hypertension. The placement of the Doppler sample volume is also important, since placement too far into the pulmonary vein can cause degradation of the signal.[15]

Left Atrial Measurements

Assessing left atrial size and contents is an important feature of an echocardiogram. Assessment of the left atrium can also provide insight into the severity of mitral regurgitation. With the advent of transesophageal echocardiography, the left atrial appendage can now be seen and the presence of clot identified. This has led to better management of patients needing cardioversion and invasive procedures. The variety of tomographic planes available makes echocardiography an ideal diagnostic tool for the evaluation of the left atrium.

ECHOCARDIOGRAPHIC VIEWS

Assessment of the left atrium is possible from a number of imaging planes. Essentially all of the standard windows allow an image of the left atrium. The left atrium can be seen from both parasternal and all apical windows, as well as from the subcostal four-chamber view.

LEFT ATRIAL SIZE AND FUNCTION

Left atrial dimensions can be taken from essentially any view where the borders are well defined. The atrium can be measured in an anterior-posterior, superior-inferior, or medial-lateral dimension (Fig. 17-21). The anterior-posterior dimension provides the usual reported measurement.[27,42] It can be made in M-mode or two-dimensional echocardiography and is taken in systole or when the left atrium is at its maximum excursion. Using American Society of Echocardiography guidelines, M-mode measurements are usually recorded from the leading edge to the leading edge, while two-dimensional measurements are recorded from inside to inside borders. The measurement is made from the ante-

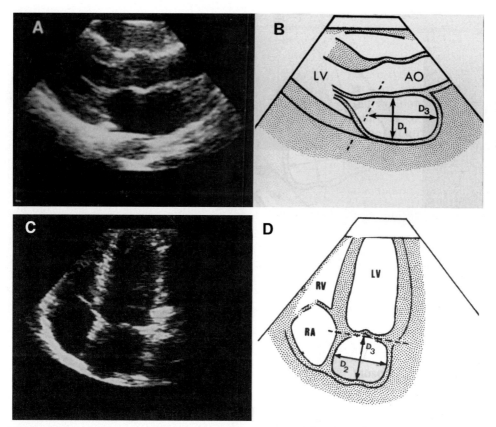

Figure 17-21. Various acoustic windows used to measure left atrial size. The parasternal long-axis, anteroposterior dimensions are most frequently reported. D_1 anterior-posterior dimension; D_2, medial-lateral dimension; D_3, superior-inferior dimension. (From Weyman AE. Principles and Practice of Echocardiography, 2nd ed. Philadelphia, Lea & Febiger; 1994.)

rior wall of the left atrium to the posterior wall. A quick assessment of atrial size can be made by comparing the appearance of the left atrium to that of the left ventricle (the latter should, of course, be larger) or the aortic root. In patients with no abnormalities, the ratio of left atrium to aortic root diameter, taken at the same position in the cardiac cycle, should be less than or equal to $1.1:1$.[12] Left atrial dimension from the anterior-posterior dimension is no more than 4.0 cm.

Errors in this measurement come from several sources. First, in a parasternal long-axis view, the descending thoracic aorta lies posterior to the left atrium (Fig. 17-22). It is important to distinguish these two structures since inclusion of the thoracic aorta in the left atrial measurements will indicate left atrial enlargement. Second, in dilated left atriums, side lobe artifacts can create a linear structure

that resembles the back wall of the left atrium.[27] Third, due to transducer angulation, "cloudy" echoes frequently appear at the posterior wall of the left atrium (Fig. 17-23). Repositioning the transducer usually resolves the last two problems. Evaluation of the left atrium from all views provides a better appreciation of left atrial size and helps resolve some of these difficulties.

The apical views are also frequently used to measure the left atrial size. The left atrium can be measured in its medial-lateral or superior-inferior dimension. The medial-lateral dimension is measured from the lateral wall of the left atrium to the interatrial septum. This measurement can be problematic since the structures used as the borders are parallel to the sound beam. A more accurate measurement is the superior-inferior dimension. This measurement is made in the center of the left atrium

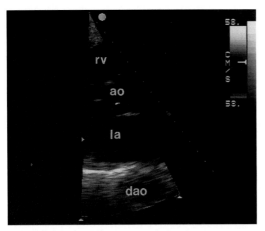

Figure 17-22. Parasternal long-axis view of the left atrium and descending thoracic aorta posteriorly. In making left atrial measurements, the descending thoracic aorta may appear as part of the left atrium. Proper gain settings can help resolve these two structures. rv, right ventricle; ao, aorta; la, left atrium; dao, descending thoracic aorta.

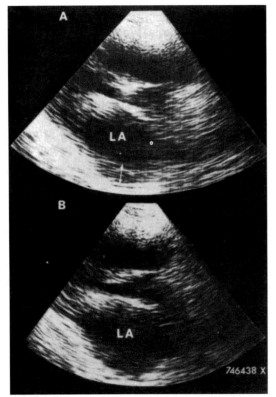

Figure 17-23. (**A**) Parasternal long-axis view of the left atrium with "fuzzy" echoes obscuring the posterior wall. (**B**) Adjusting gain settings and transducer positions can help eliminate some of these artifacts. (From Feigenbaum H. Echocardiography, 5th ed. Philadelphia, Lea & Febiger; 1994.)

from the most superior wall of the left atrium to the mitral annular plane.[111]

Left atrial dilatation results from a number of pathologic states including chronic mitral valve regurgitation, mitral stenosis, left ventricular failure, left-to-right shunts—including patent ductus arteriosus[8,93] and ventricular septal defects[14]—and left atrial fibrillation.[83] The left atrium can also be small, usually as a result of compression from external structures such as a dilated aortic root, masses, or tumors. Defects that divert the flow of blood from the left atrium, such as partial or complete pulmonary venous drainage, will also result in an abnormally small left atrium.[10]

In general, no echocardiographic techniques are accepted as standard methods for calculating left atrial volume. Transthoracic approaches are unable to visualize the left atrial appendage clearly, so this area, as well as the pulmonary veins, is excluded from these calculations. Transesophageal echocardiography, although able to visualize the appendage, cannot image the entire left atrium and the appendage in a single plane. Still, there are several transthoracic measurements that provide reasonable calculations.[111]

One of the simpler formulas for volume calculations is the biplane ellipsoid area-length method:

$$\text{Volume} = 8A_1 \times A_2 \div 3\pi L$$

where A_1 is the left atrial area traced from the apical four-chamber view, A_2 is the left atrial area traced from the apical two-chamber view, and L is the length of the left atrium taken from both views.[31,38,43] This method assumes that the left atrium has the shape of an ellipsoid.

The assessment of left atrial function using echocardiography generally looks at changes in volume. This can be appreciated using M-mode and observing the motion of the left atrial posterior wall and the motion of the posterior aortic wall[3,102] (Fig. 17-24). This motion can also be observed with two-dimensional echocardiography. Transesophageal echocardiography also provides an excellent look at the entire left atrium using a variety of views. Pulsed wave Doppler can be used to help assess the flow dynamics within the left atrial appendage, thereby providing some idea of function. When function is decreased, blood flow is decreased within the appendage and may facilitate thrombus formation (Fig. 17-25). An on-line automatic boundary detec-

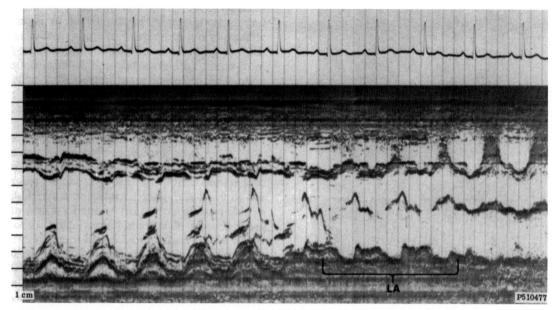

Figure 17-24. M-mode method for determining left atrial function. In the normal functioning left atrium excursion of the posterior wall should be observed (LA). Likewise the posterior wall of the aorta should also demonstrate excursion. (From Feigenbaum H. Echocardiography, 5th ed. Philadelphia, Lea & Febiger; 1994.)

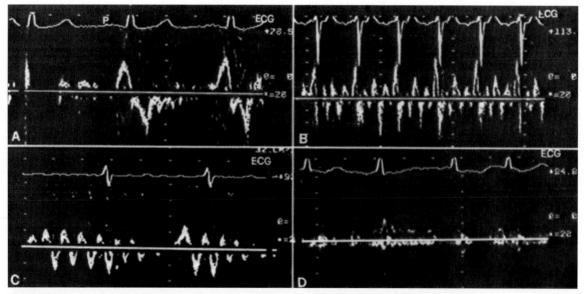

Figure 17-25. Pulsed Doppler recording from the left atrial appendage using transesophageal echocardiography. With sinus rhythm (**A**), one sees fairly tall atrial velocity after the P wave of the electrocardiogram. In (**B**), note atrial flutter with 2:1 block showing forward velocities after each P wave. The second P wave is within the T wave of the electrocardiogram. In (**C**) the patient has flutter fibrillation, and only gross oscillating velocities are noted in the left atrial appendage. With chronic atrial fibrillation (**D**), no organized flow velocity can be recorded within the left atrial appendage. (From Pozzoli M, et al. Left atrial appendage dysfunction: A cause of thrombosis? Evidence by transesophageal echocardiography—Doppler studies. J Am Soc Echocardiogr. 1991;5:436. Reprinted with permission.)

tion technique available on particular ultrasound systems has also been shown to provide a reasonable quantitative analysis of left atrial function. This technique involves the computation of varying chamber cavity areas within a region of interest and instantaneously displaying the changes in area throughout a period of time. The changes in area can be used to assess the overall function of the left atrium.[107]

Summary

Echocardiography is ideal for assessment of the left ventricle and left atrium. The various views available allow a thorough examination of both chambers. The noninvasive assessment of chamber size, area, and function makes echocardiography an ideal diagnostic tool.

REFERENCES

1. Adams T, Yanowitz F, Fisher A, et al. Noninvasive evaluation of exercise training in college-age men. Circulation. 1981;64:958–965.
2. Ahmadpour H, Shah A, Allen J, et al. Mitral E point septal separation: A reliable index of left ventricular performance in coronary artery disease. Am Heart J. 1983;106:21–28.
3. Akgun G, Layton C. Aortic root and left atrial wall motion: An echocardiographic study. Br Heart J. 1977;39:1082.
4. Amico AF, Lichtenberg G, Reisner S, et al. Superiority of visual versus computerized echocardiographic estimation of radionuclide left ventricular fraction. Am Heart J. 1989;118:1259.
5. Appleton CP, Hatle LK. The natural history of left ventricular filling abnormalities: Assessment by two-dimensional and Doppler echocardiography. Echocardiography. 1992;9:437–457.
6. Appleton CP, Hatle LK, Popp RL. Relation of transmitral flow velocity patterns to left ventricular diastolic function: New insights from a combined hemodynamic and Doppler echocardiographic study. J Am Coll Cardiol. 1988;12:426–440.
7. Appleton CP, Jensen JL, Hatle LK, et al. Doppler evaluation of left and right ventricular diastolic function: A technical guide for obtaining optimal flow velocity recordings. J Am Soc Echocardiogr. 1997;10:271–292.
8. Baylen B, Meyer RA, Kaplan S. Echocardiographic assessment of patent ductus arteriosus in prematures with respiratory distress. Circulation. 1974;50(suppl 3):III-16.
9. Bennett D, Rowlands D. Test of reliability of echocardiographic estimation of left ventricular dimensions and volumes. Br Heart J. 1976;38:1133–1136.
10. Bierman FZ, Williams RG. Subxiphoid two-dimensional echocardiographic diagnosis of total anomalous pulmonary venous return in infants (abstract). J Am Coll Cardiol. 1979;43:401.
11. Bommer W, Chun T, Kwan O, et al. Biplane apex echocardiography versus biplane cineangiography in the assessment of left ventricular volume and function: Validation by direct measurements. Am J Cardiol. 1980;45:471.
12. Brown OR, Harrison DC, Popp RL. An improved method for echocardiographic detection of left atrial enlargement. Circulation. 1974;50:58.
13. Byrd BR III, Wahr D, Wang YS, et al. Left ventricular mass and volume/mass ratio determined by two-dimensional echocardiography in normal adults. J Am Coll Cardiol. 1985;6:1021–1025.
14. Carter WH, Bowman CR. Estimation of shunt flow in isolated ventricular septal defect by echocardiogram. Circulation. 1973;48(suppl 4):IV-64.
15. Castello R, Pearson A, Lenzen P, et al. Evaluation of pulmonary venous flow by transesophageal echocardiography in subjects with normal heart: Comparison with transthoracic echocardiography. J Am Cardiol. 1991;18:65.
16. Cohen A, Hagan A, Watkins J, et al. Clinical correlated in hypertensive patients with left ventricular hypertrophy diagnosed with echocardiography. Am J Cardiol. 1981;47:335–341.
17. Collins HW, Kronenberg MW, Byrd BF III. Reproducibility of left ventricular mass measurements by two-dimensional and M-mode echocardiography. J Am Coll Cardiol. 1989;14:672–676.
18. Cooper R, O'Rourke R, Karliner J, et al. Comparison of ultrasound and cineangiographic measurements of the mean rate of circumferential fiber shortening in man. Circulation. 1972;46:904–923.
19. Corya B, Rasmussen S, Phillips J, et al. Forward stroke volume calculated from aortic echograms in normal subjects and patients with mitral regurgitation secondary to left ventricular dysfunction. Am J Cardiol. 1981;47:1215–1222.
20. DeMaria A, Neumann A, Schubart P, et al. Systemic correlation of cardiac chamber size and ventricular performance determined with echocardiography and alterations in heart rate in normal persons. Am J Cardiol. 1979;43:1–9.
21. DeMaria A, Neumann A, Lee G, et al. Alterations in ventricular mass and performance induced by exercise training in man evaluated by echocardiography. Circulation. 1978;57:237–244.

22. Devereux RB. LV diastolic dysfunction: Early diastolic relaxation and late diastolic compliance. J Am Coll Cardiol. 1989;13:337–339.

23. Devereux R, Reichek N. Echocardiographic determination of left ventricular mass in man. Circulation. 1977;55:613–618.

24. Ditchey R, Schuler G, Peterson K. Reliability of echocardiographic and electrocardiographic parameters in assessing serial changes in left ventricular mass. Am J Cardiol. 1981;70:1042–1050.

25. Douherty AH, Naccarelli G, Gray E, et al. Congestive heart failure with normal systolic function. Am J Cardiol. 1984;54:778.

26. Erbel R, Krebs W, Henn G, et al. Comparison of single plane and biplane volume determination by two-dimensional echocardiography. I. Asymmetric heart model. Eur Heart J. 1983;3:469–480.

27. Feigenbaum H. Echocardiography, 2nd ed. Philadelphia, Lea and Febiger; 1976.

28. Felner J, Blumenstein B, Schlant R, et al. Sources of variability in echocardiographic measurements. Am J Cardiol. 1980;45:995–1004.

29. Fisher D, Sahn D, Friedman M, et al. The effect of variations of pulsed Doppler sampling site on calculation of cardiac output: An experimental study in open chest dogs. Circulation. 1983;67: 370–376.

30. Friedman M, Roeske W, Sahn D, et al. Accuracy of M mode echocardiography measurements of the left ventricle. Am J Cardiol. 1982;49:716–723.

31. Gehl LG, Mintz GS, Kotler MN, et al. Left atrial volume overload in mitral regurgitation: A two-dimensional echocardiographic study. Am J Cardiol. 1982;49:33.

32. Gerstenblith G, Frederiksen J, Yin F, et al. Echocardiographic assessment of a normal adult aging population. Circulation. 1977;56:273–278.

33. Giannuzzi P, Imparato A, Temporelli PL, et al. Doppler derived mitral deceleration time of early filling as a strong predictor of pulmonary capillary wedge pressure in postinfarction patients with left ventricular systolic dysfunction. J Am Coll Cardiol. 1994;23:1630–1637.

34. Gopal AS, Keller AM, Zhanqing S, et al. Three dimensional echocardiography: In vitro and in vivo validation of left ventricular mass and comparison with conventional echocardiographic methods. J Am Coll Cardiol. 1994;24:504–513.

35. Grodecki P, Klein A. Pitfalls in the echo-Doppler assessment of diastolic dysfunction. Am J Cardiovasc Ultrasound Allied Tech. 1993;10:213–234.

36. Gueret P, Wyatt H, Meehbaum S, et al. A practical two dimensional echocardiographic model to assess volume in the ischemic left ventricle. Am J Cardiol. 1980;45:471.

37. Gutgesell H, Paquet M, Duff D, et al. Evaluation of left ventricular size and function by echocardiography. Circulation. 1977;56:457–462.

38. Haendchen RV, Povzhitkov M, Meerbaum S, et al. Evaluation of changes in left ventricular end-diastolic pressure by left atrial two-dimensional echocardiography. Am Heart J. 1982;104:740.

39. Hains AD, Khawaja IA, Hinge DA, et al. Radionuclide left ventricular ejection fraction: A comparison of three methods. Br Heart J. 1987;57:232–236.

40. Helak J, Reichek N. Quantitation of human left ventricular mass and volume by two-dimensional echocardiography: In vitro anatomic validation. Circulation. 1981;63:1398–1407.

41. Henry W, Gardin J, Ware J. Echocardiographic measurements in normal subjects from infancy to old age. Circulation. 1980;62:1054–1061.

42. Hirata T, Wolfe S, Popp R, et al. Estimation of left atrial size using ultrasound. Am Heart J. 1969;78: 43.

43. Hofstetter R, Bartz-Bazzanella P, Kentrup H, et al. Determination of left atrial area and volume by cross-sectional echocardiography in healthy infants and children. Am Coll Cardiol. 1991;68:1073.

44. Hood W, Rackley C, Rolett E. Wall stress in the normal and hypertrophied human left ventricle. Am J Cardiol. 1968;22:550–558.

45. Huntsmann L, Stewart D, Barnes S, et al. Noninvasive Doppler determination of cardiac output in man. Circulation. 1983;67:593–602.

46. Ikaheimo M, Palatsi L, Takkunen D. Noninvasive evaluation of the athletic heart: Sprinter versus endurance runners. Am J Cardiol. 1979;44:24–30.

47. Iwase M, Sotobata I, Takagi S, et al. Effects of diltiazem on left ventricular diastolic behavior in patients with hypertrophic cardiomyopathy: Evaluation with exercise pulsed Doppler echocardiography. J Am Coll Cardiol. 1987;9:1099–1105.

48. Katz R, Karliner J, Resinik R. Effects of a natural volume overload state (pregnancy) on left ventricular performance in normal human subjects. Circulation. 1978;58:434–441.

49. King DL, Gopal AS, Keller AM, et al. Three-dimensional echocardiograph: Advances for measurements of ventricular volume and mass. Hypertension. 1994;23:I172–I179.

50. Klein AL, Hatle LK, Taliercio CP, et al. Prognostic significance of Doppler measures of diastolic function in cardiac amyloidosis: A Doppler echocardiographic study. Circulation. 1991;83:808–816.

51. Koren MJ, Devereux RB, Casale PN, et al. Relation of left ventricular mass and geometry to morbidity

and mortality in uncomplicated essential hypertension. Ann Intern Med. 1991;114:335–352.

52. Labovitz A, Buckingham T, Habermehl K, et al. The effect of sampling site on the two-dimensional echo-Doppler determination of cardiac output. Am Heart J. 1984;109:327–332.

53. Lee CH, Bancher IF, Josen MS, et al. Discrepancies in the measurement of isovolumic relaxation time: A study comparing M-mode and Doppler. Br Heart J. 1982;47:253–260.

54. Levy D, Garrison RJ, Savage DD, et al. Prognostic implications of echoradiographically determined left ventricular mass in the Framingham Heart Study. N Engl J Med. 1990;322:1561–1566.

55. Lew W, Henning H, Schelbert H, et al. Assessment of mitral valve E point separation as an index of left ventricular performance in patients with acute and previous myocardial infarction. Am J Cardiol. 1978; 41:836–845.

56. Lewis J, Kuo L, Nelson J, et al. Pulsed Doppler echocardiographic determination of stroke volume and cardiac output: Clinical validation of two new methods using the apical window. Circulation. 1984;70:425–431.

57. Lewis RP, Sandler H. Relationship between changes in left ventricular dimensions and the ejection fraction in man. Circulation. 1971;44: 548–557.

58. Linhart J, Mintz G, Segal B, et al. Left ventricular volume measurement by echocardiography: Fact or fiction? Am J Cardiol. 1975;36:114–118.

59. Loeppky J, Hoekenga D, Greene R, et al. Comparison of noninvasive pulsed Doppler and Fick measurements of stroke volume in cardiac patients. Am Heart J. 1984;107:339–346.

60. Magnin P, Stewart J, Myers S, et al. Combined Doppler and phased-array echocardiographic estimation of cardiac output. Circulation. 1981;63: 388–392.

61. Manyari DE, Kostuk WJ. Left and right ventricular function at rest and during bicycle exercise in the supine and sitting positions in normal subjects and patients with coronary artery disease: Assessment by radionuclide ventriculography. Am J Cardiol. 1983: 51:36–42.

62. Marcomichelakis J, Withers R, Newman G, et al. The relation of age to the thickness of the interventricular septum, the posterior left ventricular wall and their ratio. Int J Cardiol. 1983;4:405–415.

63. Massie B, Schiller N, Ratshin R, et al. Mitral septal separation: New echocardiographic index of left ventricular function. Am J Cardiol. 1977;39: 1008–1016.

64. Matteos M, Shapiro E, Oldershaw PJ, et al. Noninvasive assessment of changes in left ventricular re-

laxation by combined phono-, echo- and mechanocardiography. Br Heart J. 1982;47:253–260.

65. Mercier J, DiSessa T, Jarmakani J, et al. Two dimensional echocardiographic assessment of left ventricular volumes and ejection fraction in children. Circulation. 1982;65:962–969.

66. Moynihan P, Parisi A, Feldman C. Quantitative detection of regional left ventricular contraction abnormalities by two dimensional echocardiography. Circulation. 1981;63:752–760.

67. Naik MM, Diamond GA, Pai T, et al. Correspondence of left ventricular ejection fraction determinations from two-dimensional echocardiography, radionuclide angiography and contrast cineangiography. J Am Coll Cardiol. 1995;25:937–942.

68. Nishimura R, Callahan M, Schaff H, et al. Noninvasive measurement of cardiac output by continuous-wave Doppler echocardiography: Initial experience and review of the literature. Mayo Clin Proc. 1984; 59:484–489.

69. Nishimura R, Housmans PR, Hatle LK, et al. Assessment of diastolic function of the heart: Background and current applications of Doppler echocardiography, part II: Clinical studies. Mayo Clin Proc. 1989;64:181–204.

70. Oh JK, Appleton CP, Hatle LK, et al. The noninvasive assessment of left ventricular diastolic function with two-dimensional and Doppler echocardiography. J Am Soc Echocardiogr. 1997;10:246–270.

71. Oh JK, Ding ZP, Gersh BJ, et al. Restrictive LV diastolic filling identifies patients with heart failure after acute myocardial infarction. J Am Soc Echocardiogr. 1992;5:497–503.

72. Pearson AC, et al. Effect of sample volume location on pulsed Doppler-echocardiographic evaluation of left ventricular filling. Am J Cardiac Imaging. 1988; 2:40.

73. Percy RF, Conetta DA. Comparison of velocity and volumetric indexes of left ventricular filling during increased heart rate with exercise and amyl nitrate. J Am Soc Echocardiogr. 1994;7:388–393.

74. Popp R, Filly K, Brown O, et al. Effect of transducer placement on echocardiographic measurement of left ventricular dimensions. Am J Cardiol. 1975;35: 537–540.

75. Pratt R, Parisi A, Harrington J, et al. The influence of left ventricular stroke volume on aortic root motion. Circulation. 1976;53:947–952.

76. Quinones M, Mokotoff D, Nouri S, et al. Noninvasive quantification of left ventricular wall stress. Am J Cardiol. 1980;45:782–790.

77. Quinones M, Gaasch W, Alexander J. Echocardiographic assessment of left ventricular function. Circulation. 1983;67:348–352.

78. Reichek N, Helak J, Plappert T, et al. Anatomic

validation of left ventricular mass estimates from clinical two-dimensional echocardiography: Initial results. Circulation. 1983;67:348–352.

79. Reichek N, Wilson J, Sutton M, et al. Noninvasive determination of left ventricular end-systolic stress: Validation of the method and initial application. Circulation. 1982;65:99–108.

80. Rein A, Hsieh K, Elixson M, et al. Cardiac output estimates in the pediatric intensive care unit using a continuous-wave Doppler computer: Validation and limitations of the technique. Am Heart J. 1985; 112:97–103.

81. Rose J, Nanna M, Rahimtoola S, et al. Accuracy of determination of changes in cardiac output by transcutaneous continuous-wave Doppler computer. Am J Cardiol. 1984;54:1099–1101.

82. Sahn D, Deely W, Hagan A, et al. Echocardiographic assessment of left ventricular performance in normal newborns. Circulation. 1974;49: 232–236.

83. Sanfilippo AJ, Abascal V, Sheehan M, et al. Atrial enlargement as a consequence of atrial fibrillation: A prospective echocardiographic study. Circulation. 1990;82:792–797.

84. Schiller N, Acquatella H, Portis T, et al. Left ventricular volume from paired biplane two-dimensional echocardiography. Circulation. 1979;60: 547–555.

85. Schiller NB, Shah PM, Crawford M, et al. Recommendations for quantitation of the left ventricle by two-dimensional echocardiography. J Am Soc Echocardiogr. 1989;2:358–367.

86. Schiller NB, Skioldebrand CG, Schiller EJ. Canine left ventricular mass estimation by two-dimensional echocardiography. Circulation. 1983;68:210–216.

87. Schnittger I, Gordon EP, Fitzgerald PJ, et al. Standardized intracardiac measurements of two-dimensional echocardiography. J Am Coll Cardiol. 1983; 2:934–938.

88. Senior R, Sridhara BS, Basu S, et al. Comparison of radionuclide ventriculography and 2D echocardiography for the measurement of left ventricular ejection fraction following acute myocardial infarction. E Heart J. 1994;15:1235–1239.

89. Shah PK, Picher M, Berman DS, et al. Left ventricular ejection fraction determined by radionuclide ventriculography in early stages of first transmural infarction. Am J Cardiol. 1980:45:542–546.

90. Shaikh MA, Lavine SJ. Effect of mitral regurgitation on diastolic filling with left ventricular hypertrophy. Am J Cardiol. 1988;61:590–594.

91. Shen WF, Tribouilloy C, Rey JL, et al. Prognostic significance of Doppler derived left ventricular diastolic variables in dilated cardiomyopathy. Am Heart J. 1992;124:1524–1533.

92. Shub C, Klein AL, Zachariah PK, et al. Determination of left ventricular mass by echocardiography in a normal population; effect of age and sex in addition to body size. Mayo Clin Proc. 1994;69: 205–211.

93. Silverman NH, Lewis AB, Heyman, et al. Echocardiographic assessment of ductus arteriosus in premature infants. Circulation. 1974;50:821–826.

94. Silverman NH, Portis T, Snider R, et al. Determination of left ventricular volume in children: Echocardiographic and angiographic comparisons. Circulation. 1980;62:548–557.

95. Smith SA: Transmitral velocities measured by pulsed Doppler in healthy volunteers. Br Heart J. 1989;61:344–347.

96. Soufer R, Wohlgelernter O, Vita N, et al. Intact left ventricular systolic function in clinical congestive heart failure. Am J Cardiol. 1985;55:1032–1036.

97. Stamm RB, Carabello B, Mayers D, et al. Two-dimensional echocardiographic measurement of left ventricular ejection fraction: Prospective analysis of what constitutes an adequate determination. Am Heart J. 1982;104:136–144.

98. Starling M, Crawford M, Sorensen S, et al. Comparative accuracy of apical biplane cross sectional echocardiography and gated equilibrium radionuclide angiography for estimating left ventricular size and performance. Circulation. 1981;63:1075–1084.

99. Stein P, Sabbah H. Rate of change of ventricular power: An indicator of ventricular performance during ejection. Am Heart J. 1976;91:219–227.

100. Steingart R, Meller J, Barovick J, et al. Pulsed Doppler echocardiographic measurements of beat-to-beat changes in stroke volume in dogs. Circulation. 1980;62:542–548.

101. Strauer B. Myocardial oxygen consumption in chronic heart disease: Role of wall stress, hypertrophy and coronary reserve. Am J Cardiol. 1979;44: 730–740.

102. Strunk BL, Fitzgerald JW, Lipton M, et al. The posterior aortic wall echocardiogram: Its relationship to left atrial volume change. Circulation. 1976; 54:744–756.

103. Topol EJ, Traill TA, Fortuin NJ. Hypertensive hypertrophic cardiomyopathy of the elderly. N Engl J Med. 1985;312:277–283.

104. Tortoledo F, Quinones M, Fernandez G, et al. Quantification of left ventricular volumes by two dimensional echocardiography: A simplified and accurate approach. Circulation. 1983;67:579–584.

105. Vuille C, Weyman AE. *Left ventricular* I: General considerations, assessment of chamber size and function. *In* Weyman AE (ed): Principles and Practice of Echocardiography, 2nd ed. Philadelphia, Lea & Febiger; 1994:599.

106. Wackers FJT, Berger HJ, Johnstone DE, et al. Multiple gated cardiac blood pool imaging for left ventricular ejection fraction: Validation of the technique and assessment of variability. Am J Cardiol. 1979;43:1159–1166.

107. Waggoner AD, Barzilai B, Miller JG, et al. On-line assessment of left atrial area and function by echocardiographic automatic boundary detection. Circulation. 1993;88:1142–1149.

108. Wahr DW, Wang YS, Schiller NB. Left ventricular volumes determined by two-dimensional echocardiography in a normal adult population. J Am Coll Cardiol. 1983;1:863–868.

109. Wallmeyer K, Wann S, Sagar K, et al. The influence of preload heart rate on Doppler echocardiographic indexes of left ventricular performance: Comparison with invasive indexes in an experimental preparation. Circulation. 1986;74:181–186.

110. Weiss J, Eaton L, Kallman C, et al. Accuracy of volume determination by two-dimensional echocardiography: Defining requirements under controlled conditions in the ejecting canine left ventricle. Circulation. 1983;67:889–895.

111. Weyman AE. Principles and Practice of Echocardiography, 2nd ed. Philadelphia, Lea & Febiger; 1994:472.

112. Wilson J, Reichek N. Echocardiographic indices of left ventricular function. Chest. 1979;76:441–447.

113. Wong M, Shah P, Taylor R. Reproducibility of left ventricular internal dimensions with M mode echocardiography: Effects of heart size, body position and transducer angulation. Am J Cardiol. 1981;47:1068–1074.

114. Wyatt H, Heng M, Meehbaum S, et al. Cross sectional echocardiography. Circulation. 1980;61:1119–1125.

18

Echocardiographic Assessment of the Right Chambers

The right ventricle lies on the anteromedial border of the left ventricle. Its medial wall is formed by the muscular interventricular septum, but its free margin is formed by a thinner wall. The inside walls of the right ventricle are irregular in shape, with numerous trabeculations or muscles, including the prominent moderator band, seen on echocardiography in most patients. The right ventricle pumps blood to the lungs. Due to its relatively low resistance and shorter distance, the walls of the right ventricle are not as thick as those of the left ventricle. The pattern of contraction of the right ventricle differs from that of the left ventricle in that its ejection velocity increases more gradually, peaks later, and decreases more slowly.[1]

Echocardiographic Views

Table 18-1 summarizes the various views used to obtain images of the right ventricle. These views include the parasternal long-axis position, which reveals only a small section of the ventricle and so provides little functional information (Fig. 18-1). The parasternal short-axis view provides a look at portions of the anterior lateral and inferior walls of the right ventricle, but again, only a small region of each can be evaluated (Fig. 18-2). The apical four-chamber and subcostal four-chamber views provide the most useful information. The apical four-chamber view provides a good appreciation of chamber size and function (Fig. 18-3). The subcostal four-chamber view is ideal for measuring wall thickness since the right ventricular walls are perpendicular to the sound beam. This position is also ideal for identifying and assessing the degree of right heart collapse in patients with tamponade physiology. Right ventricular wall thickness can also be measured from the parasternal lung axis view (Fig. 18-4).

Dimensions

Right ventricular dimensions can be determined by M-mode or two-dimensional echocardiography. Two-dimensional views are preferable since there are fewer potential errors from incorrect transducer angles. Additionally, the observer can make comparisons with other chambers, which can add to the overall impression. All available views should be used to thoroughly assess the right ventricle. Caution should be exercised in using only one view to assess dimensions. Although the actual measurement may be made in one view, the other views should support the findings. For example, a right ventricle that seems enlarged from an apical four-chamber view should, if truly enlarged, appear so in all other views. As a general comparison, the right ventricle is less than or equal to two-thirds of the left ventricle.[1]

Right ventricular cavity dimensions can be measured from the apical four-chamber view[11] (Fig. 18-5). Typically, the measurements are made from

365

◢◢◢ TABLE 18-1. ECHOCARDIOGRAPHIC VIEWS USED TO EVALUATE THE RIGHT ATRIUM AND VENTRICLE

View	Region Visualized
Parasternal long axis	RV—anterior wall
Parasternal long axis—outflow	RV—anterior wall, outflow region
Parasternal long axis—inflow	RV—anterior wall, inferior wall, inflow regions
Parasternal short axis	
At base	RV—anterior wall, inferior wall, inflow and outflow regions
At mitral valve level	RV—anterior, lateral, and inferior walls
At papillary muscle level	RV—midanterior, lateral, and inferior walls
At apex	RV—apical region of anterior wall, lateral, and inferior walls
Apical four-chamber view	RV—apex, lateral free wall, basal walls
	RA—superior, lateral, and septal walls
Subcostal four-chamber view	RV—diaphragmatic aspects of inferior wall, apex, and basal regions
	RA—septal, superior, and diaphragmatic aspect of the lateral wall
Subcostal short-axis view	
At base	RV—anterior wall, inferior, inflow, and outflow regions
	RA—small segment of the inferior segments
At papillary muscle	RV—anterior, lateral, and inferior walls

RA, right atrium; RV, right ventricle.

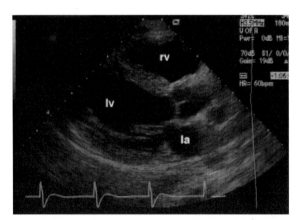

Figure 18-1. Parasternal long-axis view. A small portion of the right ventricle (rv) can be seen. A grossly dilated right ventricle can be identified from this view; however, little information regarding function is available. la, left atrium; lv, left ventricle.

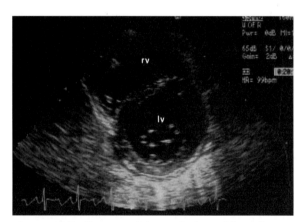

Figure 18-2. Parasternal short-axis view of the right ventricle (rv). Its size can be appreciated from this position. lv, left ventricle.

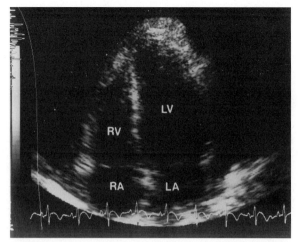

Figure 18-3. Apical four-chamber view. Right ventricular size and function can be seen from this view. A quick comparison of the left ventricle (LV) to the right ventricle (RV) can provide an idea of relative sizes. LA, left atrium; RA, right atrium.

one inside border to the other. Table 18-2 summarizes normal values for right ventricular dimensions.[10] Measurements of the right ventricular walls can be made from a parasternal long-axis, in flow view[11] (Fig. 18-6) or from a subcostal four-chamber view (Fig. 18-7).

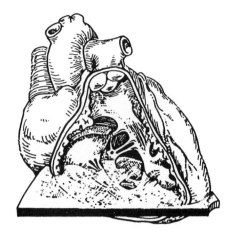

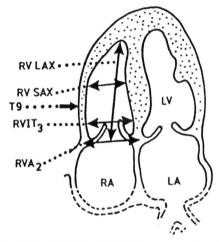

Figure 18-5. Apical four-chamber view demonstrating the various measurements that can be made. RV, right ventricle; LV, left ventricle; RA, right atrium; LA, left atrium; LAX, long axis; SAX, short axis; T, wall thickness, RVIT, right ventricular inflow tract; RVA, right ventricular annulus. (From Ref. 11, p. 36, Fig. 3. Reprinted with permission.)

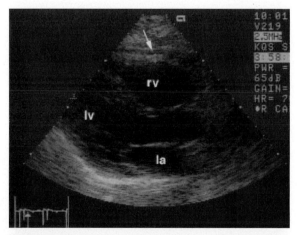

Figure 18-4. Parasternal long-axis view. The lateral free wall is well seen in this view because it is perpendicular to the sound beam. This view makes wall thickness (arrow) measurements ideal. This patient has right ventricular hypertrophy. rv, right ventricle; lv, left ventricle; la, left atrium.

TABLE 18-2. Normal Dimensions of the Right Atrium and Ventricle

	Range (cm)	Mean (cm)	Number
RVD—flat	0.7–2.3	1.5	84
RVD—left lateral	0.9–2.6	1.7	83
RVD/M² —flat	0.4–1.4	0.9	76
RVD/M² —left lateral	0.4–1.4	0.9	79
RV—free wall	.19–.29		
RA—dimensions	3.3–4.1		

RVD, right ventricular cavity dimensions. Measurements reported are made with the patient flat or in the left lateral decubitus position. Measurements are made from the inside to the inside edges. (Source: Ref. 10.)

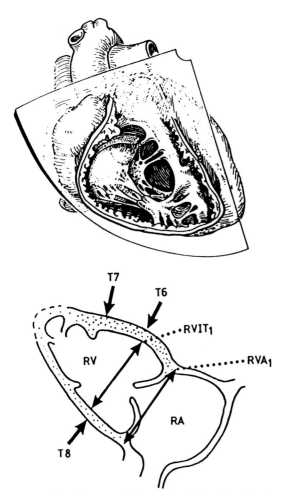

shapes as models for the right ventricle.[6-8] However, all of these methods are rather complex, and the lack of standards makes their use impractical in busy laboratories.

Global right ventricular systolic function can be assessed by measuring the excursion of the tricuspid valve from end-diastole to end-systole from an apical four-chamber view[9] (Fig. 18-8). This method correlates well with right ventricular ejection fractions measured by radionuclide angiography.

Perhaps more widely used is a visual estimation of right ventricular systolic function. Right ventricular systolic function is compared to left ventricle sys-

Figure 18-6. Parasternal long-axis, inflow view. In clear images the cavity and wall thickness can be measured from this view. RVA, right ventricular annulus; T, wall thickness, RVIT, right ventricular inflow tract; RV, right ventricle; RA, right atrium. (From Ref. 11, p. 36, Fig. 1. Reprinted with permission.)

Volume and Function Determinations

Right ventricular volumes and function determinations are much more complicated than left ventricular determinations, primarily because of the complexity of right ventricular shape and the limited number of views. Formulas used to calculate volumes include the single plane and Simpson's rule.[2-5] Additionally, right ventricular volumes have been calculated assuming a variety of geometric

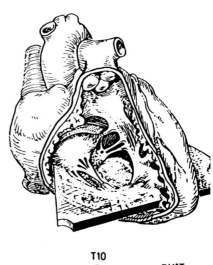

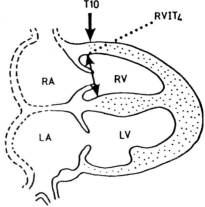

Figure 18-7. Subcostal four-chamber view demonstrating measurements of the right ventricular cavity and wall thickness. RVIT, right ventricular inflow tract; LA, left atrium; RA, right atrium; LV, left ventricle; RV, right ventricle. (From Ref. 11, p. 36, Fig. 4. Reprinted with permission.)

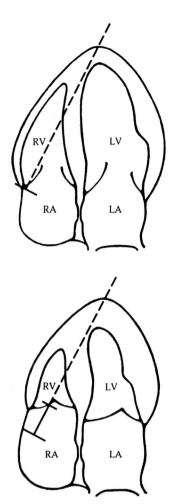

Figure 18-8. Tricuspid valve excursion method of determining right ventricular ejection fraction. A line is drawn from the midpoint of the sector to the junction of the right atrium and ventricle at the attachment of the tricuspid valve in diastole (upper panel). In systole the tricuspid valve moves superiorly, and the distance traveled is equal to the right ventricular ejection fraction. RA, right atrium; RV, right ventricle; LA, left atrium; LV, left ventricle. (From Ref. 9, p. 526, Fig. 1. Reprinted with permission.)

tolic function. Unfortunately, the left ventricle usually receives most of the attention during an echocardiogram, and the right ventricle may be ignored. A dilated right ventricle is usually an indication of poor systolic function. The right ventricle should be evaluated from all available echocardiographic views. The apical four-chamber and subcostal four-chamber views are ideal for the assessment of systolic function. The system's magnification or

"zoom" feature should be used to examine the right ventricle more closely in each exam.

Right Ventricular Volume Overload

Right ventricular volume overload can occur most commonly from (1) tricuspid regurgitation, (2) pulmonic valve regurgitation, (3) atrial septal defects, or (4) partial or total anomalous pulmonary venous connections. Less common causes of right ventricular volume overload are (1) ventricular septal defects with left ventricular-to-right atrial shunts or (2) ruptured sinus of Valsalva or coronary artery fistula with a communication to the right atrium or ventricle.[1] Ventricular septal defects without a communication between the ventricle and atrium do not cause right ventricular volume overload.[7]

The classic echocardiographic signs of right ventricular volume overload include (1) a dilated right ventricle (Fig. 18-9) and (2) a flattened septum or "D" sign[12–14] (Fig. 18-10). Right ventricular dilatation can be observed in a number of echocardiographic planes. In the parasternal short-axis view, the right ventricle appears more oval than its usual crescent shape. In the apical four-chamber view, the ventricle loses its characteristic triangular shape and appears oval. In grossly dilated right ventricles, the right ventricular apex may extend beyond the left ventricular apex (Fig. 18-11).

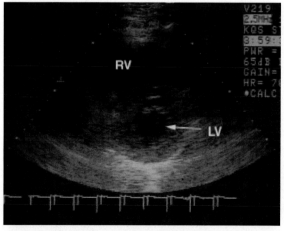

Figure 18-9. Parasternal short-axis view demonstrating a dilated right ventricle. Notice the oval shape of the ventricle. RV, right ventricle; LV, left ventricle.

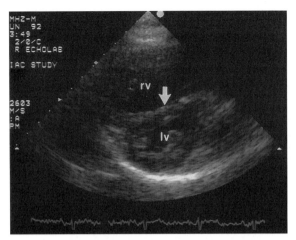

Figure 18-10. Parasternal short-axis view demonstrating right ventricular overload. The interventricular septum flattens (arrow), making the left ventricle resemble a D. rv, right ventricle; lv, left ventricle.

Right Ventricular Hypertrophy and Pressure Overload

Right ventricular hypertrophy may occur under the following conditions: (1) pulmonic valve stenosis or obstructions of the infundibular or supravalvular regions, (2) tetralogy of Fallot, (3) chronic pulmonary hypertension, (4) mitral stenosis, (5) pulmonary emboli, or (6) Eisenmenger's physiology.[1] Right ventricular hypertrophy is generally deter-

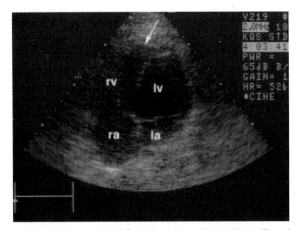

Figure 18-11. Apical four-chamber view with a dilated right ventricle. The left ventricle appears displaced. The right ventricular apex extends beyond the left ventricular apex. rv, right ventricle, ra, right atrium; lv, left ventricle; la, left atrium.

mined by measuring the right ventricular free wall. Normal values for right ventricular walls range from 1.9 to 2.9 mm.[15] Wall thickness is generally measured from the parasternal long-axis or subcostal approach due to the perpendicular orientation of the wall to the sound beam in these views. The brightly reflective nature of the anterior chest wall can make separation of the right ventricular wall from other structures difficult from a parasternal position. Gain settings must be adjusted to optimize wall identification. The subcostal view may provide a better position from which to measure because no such reflective barriers exist in this view. Good correlations exist between echocardiographically derived right ventricular wall thickness measurements and postmortem studies.[18]

The right ventricle may become thickened in the absence of these pathologic processes. Infiltrative diseases such as amyloid and hypertrophic cardiomyopathy involving the right heart may cause right ventricular thickening as well.[16,17]

Right ventricular pressure overload results from an increase in volume to the right ventricle or from an obstruction to right ventricular blood flow. Volume overload results from one of the causes listed above. Obstruction to right ventricular flow results primarily from pulmonary embolism.[1] A pulmonary embolus that obstructs 25% of the pulmonary vasculature results in elevated right heart pressures. The natural course of an acute pressure overload of the right ventricle begins with right ventricular dilatation, followed by the development of tricuspid regurgitation. As volume increases the right ventricle begins to fail, resulting in hypokinesis. As a consequence of these events, the right atrium, inferior vena cava, and main pulmonary artery all begin to dilate.[1] Hypertrophy of the right ventricular walls can also occur. With successful and early thrombolysis or removal of the obstruction, these conditions can be reversed.[23a]

Echocardiography is able to identify all of these signs. In addition, interventricular septal motion becomes erratic or paradoxical as the septum flattens in systole and diastole[19] (Fig. 18-12). This septal motion is different from the diastolic flattening seen in volume overload alone. This abnormal septal pattern is also noted in patients following cardiac surgery. Right-sided pressure can be calculated using Doppler techniques described in Chapter 15. Using continuous wave Doppler to measure the peak trans

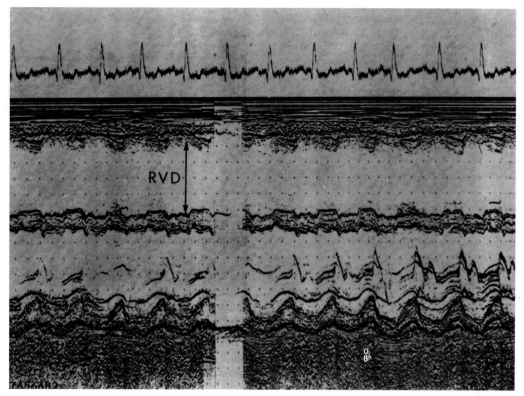

Figure 18-12. M-mode demonstrating paradoxical septal motion in a patient with right-sided pressure overload. RVD, right ventricular cavity dimensions. (From Ref. 10, Fig. 3-48. Reprinted with permission.)

tricuspid regurgitant velocity, the pressure can be calculated using the modified Bernoulli equation: $\Delta P = 4\ V^2$. The pulmonary artery pressure is then calculated by adding the jugular venous pressure, which is normally 10 mm Hg. In the absence of tricuspid regurgitation or a clear tricuspid signal, the acceleration time across the pulmonic valve can be calculated by measuring the time between the onset of pulmonary flow to the maximal velocity. Although this method fails to provide specific quantitative data, it can be used to distinguish mild from moderate and severe pulmonary hypertension.

In right ventricular or pulmonary hypertension, the timing of pulmonic valve opening and closing is altered. With increasing pulmonary pressure, the time required for right ventricular pressure to exceed pulmonary artery pressure increases, which essentially delays the opening of the pulmonic valve. As a consequence, the pulmonary flow patterns take on specific characteristics[20] (Fig. 18-13). A useful measure that correlates well with pulmonary hyper-

DOPPLER PULMONARY ARTERIAL VELOCITY PROFILES

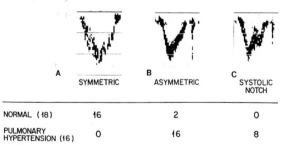

	A SYMMETRIC	B ASYMMETRIC	C SYSTOLIC NOTCH
NORMAL (18)	16	2	0
PULMONARY HYPERTENSION (16)	0	16	8

Figure 18-13. Comparison of pulmonary flow patterns in a group of 18 patients with normal pulmonary artery pressures and in 16 patients with documented pulmonary hypertension. A symmetric flow pattern is generally seen only in patients with normal pulmonary artery pressures. An asymmetric pattern predominates in patients with pulmonary hypertension. A midsystolic notch is highly specific for pulmonary hypertension. (From Weyman AE [ed]. Principles and Practice of Echocardiography, 2nd ed. Philadelphia, Lea & Febiger; 1994:Fig. 27-33. Reprinted with permission.)

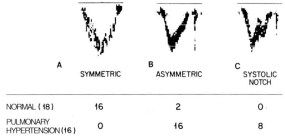

	SYMMETRIC	ASYMMETRIC	SYSTOLIC NOTCH
NORMAL (18)	16	2	0
PULMONARY HYPERTENSION (16)	0	16	8

Figure 18-14. In the absence of tricuspid regurgitation, the pulmonic valve acceleration time can be measured in order to determine the presence of pulmonary hypertension. (From Weyman AE [ed]. Principles and Practice of Echocardiography, 2nd ed. Philadelphia, Lea & Febiger; 1994:Fig. 27-33. Reprinted with permission.)

tension is the pulmonary acceleration time.[21–23] To determine the pulmonary acceleration time, the pulsed wave Doppler cursor is placed across the pulmonic valve, usually in a parasternal short-axis view. The spectral Doppler display is optimized and then frozen. The interval between onset of flow and maximum velocity is measured using the system's on-line calipers (Fig. 18-14).

The acceleration time in patients with normal pulmonary artery pressures ranged from 115 to 145 m/sec in one study,[22] and from 113 to 161 m/sec in another study.[21] Generally speaking, acceleration times of less than 115 m/sec are considered abnormal. The acceleration time of patients with borderline or mild pulmonary hypertension (20 to 39 mm Hg) ranged from 77 to 117 m/sec. In patients with significant pulmonary artery pressure ($\geq$40 mmHg), acceleration time ranged from 51 to 79 m/sec.[21]

Right Ventricular Infarct

Identification of right ventricular infarcts by echocardiography is possible in 20%[24] to 50%[25] of patients. The right ventricle is supplied by the right coronary artery (see Chapter 19), so it is not surprising that right ventricular infarcts are seen in inferior myocardial infarction of the left ventricle. The echocardiographic findings in right ventricular infarcts include (1) akinesis or other degrees of wall motion abnormality of the involved region, (2) right ven-

tricular dilatation, (3) tricuspid regurgitation, and (4) paradoxical septal motion. The most sensitive and specific echocardiographic finding is the presence of right ventricular wall motion abnormalities.[26–28] The other findings are less sensitive and occur more as a consequence of wall motion abnormalities. In addition, they are seen in other disease states.

The shape and contours of the right ventricle make the diagnosis of right ventricular infarct more challenging with echocardiography. Only in the clearest, best-defined images can the diagnosis be made on the basis of echocardiography alone. Wall motion abnormalities should be confirmed from all available acoustic windows.

Right Atrium

The rather complex anatomy of the right atrium is discussed in Chapter 1. The right atrium can be imaged from a number of echocardiographic views (see Table 18-1). The right atrium is assessed with echocardiography primarily to assess size or dimensions and the presence of masses or tumors. Size determination can be made by comparing the right atrium to the left atrium. Linear measurements can also be made. Most measurements are made from an apical four-chamber view in a medial-lateral dimension and a superior-inferior dimension (Fig. 18-15). The medial-lateral measurement is made from the interatrial septum to the free wall. The superior-inferior measurement is made from the most superior wall of the right atrium to the level of the tricuspid valve annulus. Other views such as the subcostal, modified parasternal long-axis, and short-axis views can be used to measure right atrial size, but they are less reliable than the apical four-chamber view. Normal right atrial dimensions range from 3.8 to 4.6 cm in a superior-inferior dimension and from 3.3 to 4.1 cm in a medial-lateral dimension.[29] Right atrial dilatation occurs in right ventricular volume and pressure overload conditions.[30]

Within the right atrium are a number of echogenic structures, most notably the eustachian valve and the Chiari network. It is important to remember that these structures exist and can frequently be seen on an echocardiogram, so that they are not confused with abnormal structures.

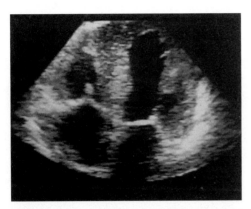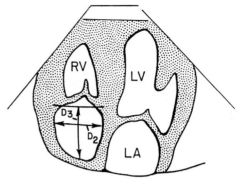

Figure 18-15. Apical four-chamber view demonstrating linear dimensions of the right atrium. The medial-lateral dimension (D_2) is taken from the interatrial septum to the lateral free wall. The superior-inferior dimension is taken from the superior wall of the right atrium to the tricuspid valve annulus (D_3). LA, left atrium; RV, right ventricle; LV, left ventricle. (From Weyman AE [ed]. Principles and Practice of Echocardiography, 2nd ed. Philadelphia, Lea & Febiger; 1994:Fig. 26-35. Reprinted with permission.)

Summary

Echocardiography is well suited to evaluate the right heart. Due to the high-profile status of the left heart and the relative ease of visualizing left-sided structures compared to those of the right heart, it is tempting not to give full attention to the right ventricle and atrium. In the setting of left ventricular inferior wall motion abnormalities, particular attention to right ventricular function is important, since in some autopsy studies right ventricular involvement was observed in as many as 90% of left ventricular inferior wall infarcts.[31] Right atrial masses can easily be missed without careful attention to the cavity. Using all available imaging planes and taking advantage of all of the system's controls, such as its magnification or "zoom" function, provides for a more thorough exam.

REFERENCES

1. Jiang L, Wiegers SE, Weyman AE. Right ventricle. *In* Weyman AE (ed): Principles and Practice of Echocardiography, 2nd ed. Philadelphia, Lea & Febiger; 1994:901–921.
2. Saito A, Ueda K, Nakano H. Right ventricular volume determinations by two-dimensional echocardiography. J Cardiogr. 1981;11:1159.
3. Ninomiya K, Duncan W, Cook D, et al. Right ventricular ejection fraction and volumes after Mustard repair: correlation of two-dimensional echocardiograms and cineangiograms. Am J Cardiol. 1981;48:317–324.
4. Panidis IP, Kottler M, Mintz G, et al. Two-dimensional echocardiographic estimation of right ventricular ejection fraction in patients with coronary artery disease. J Am Coll Cardiol. 1983;2:911–918.
5. Watanabe T, Katsume H, Matsukubo H, et al. Estimation of right ventricular volume with two-dimensional echocardiography. Am J Cardiol. 1982;49:1946–1953.
6. Graham TP, Jarmakani JW, Atwood GF, et al. Right ventricular volume determinations in children. Circulation. 1973;47:144–153.
7. Fisher EA, DuBrow IW, Hastreiter AR. Right ventricular volume in congenital heart disease. Am J Cardiol. 1975;36:67–75.
8. Arcilla RA, Tsai P, Thilenius OG, et al. Angiographic method for volume estimation of right and left ventricles. Chest 1971;60:446–454.
9. Kaul S, Tei C, Hopkins JM, et al. Assessment of right ventricular function using two-dimensional echocardiography. Am Heart J. 1984;107:526–531.
10. Feigenbaum H. Echocardiography, 5th ed. Philadelphia, Lea & Febiger; 1994;658–659.
11. Foal ER, et al. Echocardiographic measurements of normal adult right ventricle. Br Heart J. 1986;56:36–44.
12. Ryan T, Dillon J, Petrovia O, et al. An echocardiographic index for separating right ventricular volume and pressure overload. J Am Coll Cardiol. 1985;5:918.

13. King ME, Brown H, Goldblatt A, et al. Interventricular septal configuration as a predictor of right ventricular systolic hypertension in children: A cross-sectional echocardiographic study. Circulation. 1983; 68:68–75.

14. Feneley M, Garagham T. Paradoxical and pseudoparadoxical interventricular septal motion in patients with right ventricular volume overload. Circulation. 1986;74:230.

15. Tsuda T, Sawayama T, Kawai N, et al. Echocardiographic measurement of right ventricular wall thickness in adults by anterior approach. Br Heart J. 1980; 44:55–61.

16. Child JS, Krivokapich J, Abbasi AS. Increased right ventricular wall thickness on echocardiography in amyloid infiltrative cardiomyopathy. Am J Cardiol. 1979;44:1391–1395.

17. Falk RH, Plehn J, Deering T, et al. Sensitivity and specificity of the echocardiographic features of cardiac amyloidosis. Am J Cardiol. 1987;59:418–422.

18. Prakash R. Determination of right ventricular wall thickness in systole and diastole. Br Heart J. 1978; 40:1257–1261.

19. Kasper W, Meinertz T, Henkel B, et al. Echocardiographic findings in patients with proved pulmonary embolism. Am Heart J. 1986;112:1284–1290.

20. Weyman AE. Right ventricular outflow tract. *In* Weyman AE (ed): Principles and Practice of Echocardiography, 2nd ed. Philadelphia, Lea & Febiger; 1994:878–883.

21. Kitabatake A, Inque M, Asao M, et al. Noninvasive evaluation of pulmonary hypertension by a pulsed Doppler technique. Circulation. 1983;678: 302–309.

22. Isobe M, Yazaki Y, Takaku F, et al. Prediction of pulmonary arterial pressure in adults by pulsed Doppler echocardiography. Am J Cardiol. 1986;57: 316–321.

22a. Beard JT, Newman JH, Loyd JE, et al. Doppler estimation of changes in pulmonary artery pressure during hypoxic breathing. J Am Soc Echocardiogr. 1991;4:121.

23. Martin-Duran R, Larman M, Trugeda A, et al. Comparison of Doppler-determined elevated pulmonary arterial pressure with pressure measured at cardiac catheterization. Am J Cardiol. 1986;57:859–863.

23a. Come PC, Kim D, Parker A, et al. Early reversal of right ventricular dysfunction in patients with acute pulmonary embolism after treatment with intravenous tissue plasminogen activator. J Am Coll Cardiol. 1987;10:971–978.

24. Panidis IP, Kottler M, Mintz G, et al. Right ventricular function in coronary artery disease as assessed by two-dimensional echocardiography. Am Heart J. 1984;107:1187–1194.

25. Dell-Italia LJ, Sterling M, Crawford M, et al. Right ventricular infarction: Identification by hemodynamic measurements before and after volume loading and correlation with noninvasive techniques. J Am Coll Cardiol. 1984;4:931–939.

26. D'Arcy B, Nanda NC. Two-dimensional echocardiographic features of right ventricular infarction. Circulation. 1982;65:167–173.

27. Lopez-Sedon J, Garcia Fernandez A, Coma-Canalla I, et al. Segmental right ventricular function after acute myocardial infarction: Two-dimensional echocardiographic study in 63 patients. Am J Cardiol. 1983;51:390–396.

28. Baigrie RS, Haq A, Morgan C, et al. The spectrum of right ventricular involvement in inferior wall myocardial infarction: A clinical, hemodynamic and noninvasive study. J Am Coll Cardiol. 1983;1: 1396–1404.

29. Triulzi MO, et al. Normal adult cross-sectional echocardiographic values: Linear dimensions and chamber areas. Echocardiography. 1984;1:403.

30. Kushner FG, Lam W, Morganrath J. Apex sector echocardiography in evaluation of the right atrium in patients with mitral stenosis and atrial septal defect. Am J Cardiol. 1978;42:733–737.

31. Anderson HR, Falk E, Nielsen D. Right ventricular infarction: Frequency, size and topography in coronary heart disease. J Am Coll Cardiol. 1987;10: 1223–1232.

Coronary Artery Disease

19

Coronary Arteries

MARK N. ALLEN

The coronary artery anatomy was briefly discussed in Chapter 1. The purpose of this chapter is to provide a more in-depth perspective on coronary artery anatomy as it relates to echocardiography. This chapter begins Part VI, "Coronary Artery Disease," because a thorough understanding of the heart's vasculature is important in interpreting wall motion abnormalities. Advances in technology as well as new techniques may allow echocardiography to see the coronary anatomy in more detail. Today the primary role of echocardiography is to provide identification of wall motion abnormalities. Since specific coronary arteries supply particular regions of the heart, which coronary artery is diseased can be inferred.

Coronary Anatomy

The two main coronary arteries arise from the sinus of Valsalva, located at the proximal segment of the aorta just above the aortic valve. The left main coronary artery arises near the left coronary cusp and varies in length from 2–3 mm to 2–3 cm.[3] Its diameter makes it the larger of the two coronaries. It runs between the pulmonary trunk and the left atrial appendage, where it continues along the atrioventricular sulcus. At the level of the coronary sulcus the artery usually divides into two branches, the left anterior descending (anterior interventricular) artery and the circumflex artery (Fig. 19-1).

The left anterior descending (LAD) artery is a long vessel usually running along the interventricu-

lar sulcus to reach the cardiac apex and running around the apex to the posterior interventricular sulcus. Along its course it provides right and left anterior ventricular arteries, as well as an anterior septal and posterior septal arteries. Several large left anterior ventricular arteries branch from the LAD and run along the anterior aspect of the left ventricle. One of these arteries may be larger than the others and may arise directly from the left main coronary artery. This artery, the left diagonal or first diagonal,[3] is seen in 33–50% of cases. The left anterior ventricular arteries supply the anteroapical wall of the left ventricle, including the anterior papillary muscle.

The right anterior ventricular arteries are small and travel along the anterior surface of the right ventricle. The left septal artery or first septal perforator is a large branch from the LAD, which supplies roughly two-thirds of the interventricular septum, including the bundle of His and bundle branches of the conduction system. It may also supply the anterior papillary muscle of the right ventricle. The posterior septal artery supplies the posterior septal one-third of the septum from the apex.

The circumflex artery curves to the left and runs along the atrioventricular sulcus to the left cardiac border (Fig. 19-1). It is usually overlapped by the left atrial appendage. In the majority of cases, a large branch, the left marginal artery or obtuse marginal artery, originates from the circumflex and runs at a right angle to supply the lateral left ventricular wall

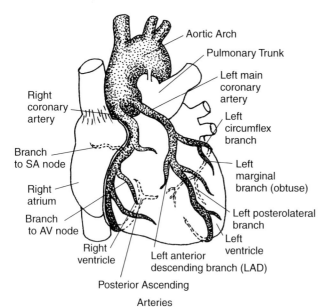

Figure 19-1. Schematic of the coronary arteries viewed from an anterior position.

to the apex. The circumflex also gives rise to anterior and posterior ventricular branches. Other branches of the circumflex supply the left atrium predominantly, and in 35% of cases it may supply the sinoatrial (SA) node and in 20% of cases the atrioventricular (AV) node.[3]

The right coronary artery arises from the right sinus of Valsalva and runs along the right atrioventricular sulcus between the right atrial appendage and the pulmonary trunk (Fig. 19-1). It reaches the crux of the heart, where it divides into numerous branches which supply the bulk of the right ventricle. A large branch, the posterior descending (PDA), descends along the interventricular groove, terminating just before the apex. This branch supplies the posteroinferior one-third of the interventricular septum, as well as the diaphragmatic regions of the right ventricle. This branch may also supply the posteromedial papillary muscle of the left ventricle, which commonly has a dual blood supply. Shortly after the origin of the right coronary artery, the superior vena caval or sinoatrial nodal artery travels along the anterior medial wall of the right atrium. This artery supplies the right atrium, SA node, crista terminalis, and pectinate muscles. Table 19-1 summarizes the coronary distributions and the regions they supply. There are a number of variations that can occur in coronary distributions.

There are four major veins which drain the heart: the great and middle cardiac veins, posterior left ventricular vein, and Marshall's vein (oblique vein of the left atrium or small cardiac vein). These vessels enter into the coronary sinus, which delivers venous blood to the right atrium (Fig. 19-2).

Echocardiographic Views

Echocardiographic imaging of the coronary vessels poses a challenge because of the complex three-dimensional structure of these vessels. Additionally, there are numerous normal variations of the coronary anatomy. Still, echocardiographic imaging of the proximal coronary arteries can be accomplished from various positions. From a left parasternal short-axis orientation with the aorta in the center of the image and at the level of the aortic valve, the left main coronary artery may be seen by rocking the transducer in a superior-inferior arc using the pulmonary artery as the most superior landmark and the superior border of the left ventricle as the most inferior landmark. It is between these two areas that the ostium and proximal left main coronary artery can be visualized.[6] A short course of the left main coronary artery can be followed by rotating the transducer along the course of the vessel. In some

TABLE 19-1. CORONARY ARTERY DISTRIBUTION

LEFT MAIN CORONARY ARTERY

Left Anterior Descending	Left ventricle
	Interventricular septum
Left anterior ventricular (left or first diagonal)	Anterior, apex, anterior papillary muscle
Right anterior branch	Anterior wall of RV
Left septal branch	Two-thirds of IVS bundle of His, bundle branches
	Anterior papillary muscle of RV
Posterior septal	Posterior one-third of septum from apex
Circumflex	
Obtuse marginal	LV lateral wall
Anterior and posterior	Left atrium, SA and AV nodes

RIGHT CORONARY ARTERY

Posterior descending (PDA)	RV, posteroinferior one-third of IVS, posterior medial papillary muscle
Sinoatrial nodal artery	RA, SA node, crista terminalis, pectinate muscle

IVS, interventricular septum; LV, left ventricle; RV, right ventricle; SA, sinoatrial node; AV, atrioventricular

cases, the left main coronary artery can be seen to the level of the bifurcation.

The left main coronary artery can also be seen from the apical views. Once a four-chamber view is acquired, the transducer is angled anteriorly to view the aorta. With minimal rotation of the transducer in a clockwise manner, the ostium and proximal segment of the left main coronary artery can be visualized.[2,5]

The right coronary artery is also visualized from the left parasternal short-axis view, with the transducer angled more superiorly. The aorta is centered in the middle of the screen at the level of the valve cusps. The right coronary artery can be seen between the 10 and 11 o'clock positions on the aorta.[7] The subcostal view can also be used to image the right coronary artery.

Various segments of the coronary arteries may be seen from other standard as well as nonstandard views (Fig. 19-3). Success depends, however, on image quality and may be difficult in many patients.

Transesophageal imaging has enhanced visualization of the coronary arteries. Due to the close proximity of the transducer to the coronary arteries and the increased frequency typical of transesophageal imaging, the coronary arteries can be seen well. Quantification of coronary artery stenosis, though documented by several investigators,[4,7,8] continues to be difficult in routine exams. Cardiac motion, large Doppler-to-flow angles, and inconsistent imaging make quantification of coronary stenosis difficult. Techniques such as myocardial perfusion imaging using contrast agents hold more promise in the quantification of stenosis than does simple imaging.

Transesophageal short-axis views frequently allow visualization of the coronary arteries. The left main coronary artery can be seen by positioning the transesophageal probe superior to the aortic valve cusps, with anterior angulation and slight leftward

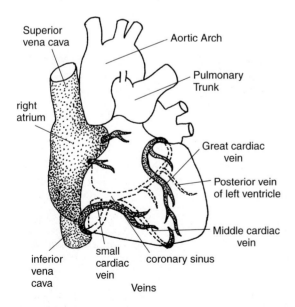

Figure 19-2. Schematic of the coronary veins viewed from an anterior position.

Superior vena cava

Aortic Arch

Pulmonary Trunk

right atrium

Great cardiac vein

Posterior vein of left ventricle

Middle cardiac vein

inferior vena cava

small cardiac vein

coronary sinus

Veins

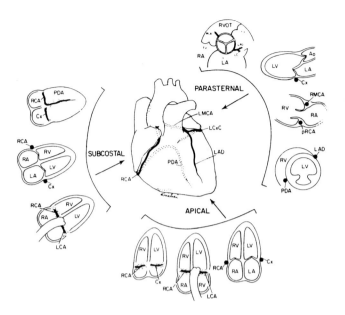

Figure 19-3. Diagram depicting views in which the larger coronary arteries may be seen using a variety of echocardiographic windows. RVOT, right ventricular outflow tract; PV, pulmonic valve; TV, tricuspid valve; LV, left ventricle; LA, left atrium; Ao, aorta; RV, right ventricle; LCA, left coronary artery; Cx, circumflex coronary artery; PDA, posterior descending coronary artery; RMCA, right main coronary artery; RCA, right coronary artery; pRCA, posterior right coronary artery; LC, left circumflex artery. (From Weyman AE. *Principles and Practice of Echocardiography*, 2nd ed. Philadelphia, Lea & Febiger; 1994: Reprinted with permission.)

rotation (Fig. 19-4). Further manipulation of the probe allows the vessel to be followed to its bifurcation. The right coronary artery can be seen by withdrawing the probe 1 to 2 cm (Fig. 19-5). Fine angulations and other manipulations will be required to bring the vessel into view.[5] Color flow Doppler can aid in the identification of these vessels. Pulsed wave recordings can also be obtained; however, large angles will create difficulties in spectral displays.

Wall Segments

INFARCT ZONES

Infarctions of the heart can occur in a variety of places and may involve a single site or multiple sites, depending on the extent of coronary disease. One must keep in mind that there may be considerable overlap of coronary vessels within a given region. Knowing which vessels supply a particular segment allows the echocardiographer to infer which vessel

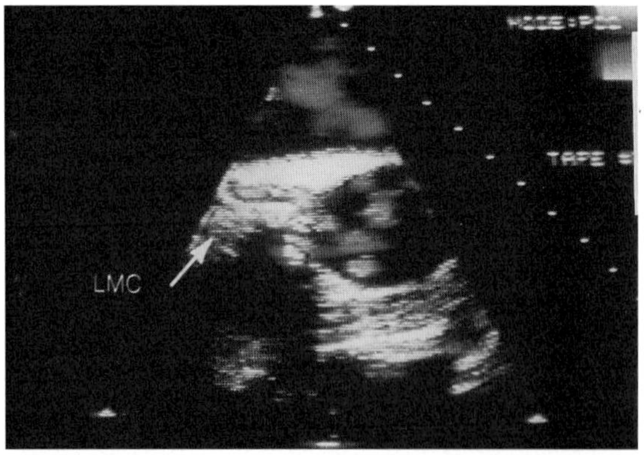

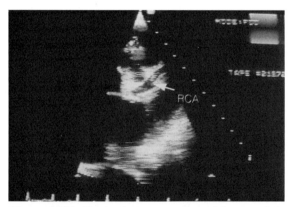

Figure 19-4. Short-axis transesophageal image of the left main coronary artery (arrow). LMC, left main coronary. (From DeBruijn NP, Clements FM. Transesophageal color flow imaging. *In* Kisslo J, Adams DB, Belkin RN (eds.). *Doppler Color Flow Imaging.* New York, Churchill Livingstone; 1988:170. Reprinted with permission.)(See also Color Plate 59.)

Figure 19-5. Short-axis transesophageal image of the right coronary artery (arrow). RCA, right coronary artery. (From DeBruijn NP, Clements FM. Transesophageal color flow imaging. *In* Kisslo J, Adams DB, Belkin RN (eds.). *Doppler Color Flow Imaging.* New York, Churchill Livingstone; 1988:170. Reprinted with permission.)(See also Color Plate 60.)

REGIONAL WALL SEGMENTS

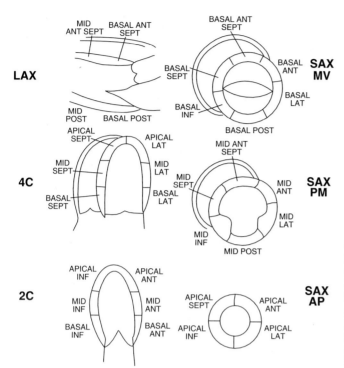

Figure 19-6. *The left ventricle is typically divided into 16 segments which are helpful in identifying and describing regional wall motion abnormalities. Using the longitudinal views (LAX, long axis; 4C, four chamber; 2C, two chamber) or short-axis views (SAX MV, short-axis mitral valve; SAX PM, short-axis papillary muscle; SAX AP, short-axis apex), one can see how the segments complement one another. (From Feigenbaum H.* Echocardiography, *5th ed. Lea & Febiger; 1994: Reprinted with permission.)*

or vessels are diseased. The left ventricle can be divided into 16 segments to help describe specific regions or walls.[1] This classification aids in describing regional wall motion abnormalities (Fig. 19-6).

Knowing which coronary artery supplies which regional segment can provide important information in determining which vessel is diseased. For example, a wall motion abnormality noted in the lateral wall suggests disease of the circumflex coronary artery. A wall motion abnormality noted in the apex suggests disease of the LAD artery. A wall motion abnormality in the basal septum and inferior walls suggests disease of the posterior descending coronary artery. Figure 19-7 shows coronary artery perfusion to the various segments. Each of these segments is assigned to a specific coronary artery. Before attempting to quantify wall motion abnormalities, a thorough understanding of these distributions is essential. There is some overlap of coronary anatomy. For example, the apical lateral wall can be supplied by the LAD artery as well as the circumflex artery. The apical inferior wall can be supplied by the LAD and right coronary arteries.

Each regional segment is given a score of 1 for normal contractility, 2 for hypokinetic contractility, 3 for akinesis or no contractility, or 4 for dyskinesis. Regions not well visualized are scored with an "N" for nonvisualization. The left ventricular score index can then be derived by summing the scores and dividing by the number of segments evaluated. There are a number of computer programs that can generate this index, and many are built into the ultrasound systems.

CORONARY ARTERY STENOSIS

Angiographic images of the coronary anatomy are helpful in illustrating this anatomy. Figure 19-8*A,B* represents the normal coronary anatomy. When dye is passed through the coronary arteries, stenotic regions are seen as areas of low opacification. Infarcts of the midseptum, basal anterior septum, midanterior septum, apical anterior, midanterior and basal anterior walls, and the entire apex (including the septal, inferior, anterior, and lateral apical walls) are caused by stenosis of the LAD. Infarctions of the

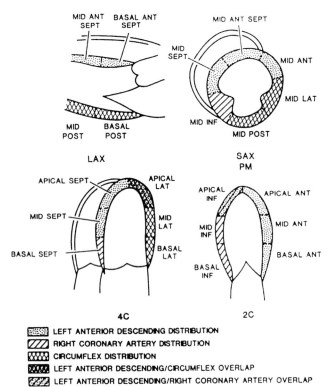

Figure 19-7. Diagram showing how the 16 segments are assigned to specific coronary arteries. The apical lateral and inferior apical segments (crosshatch) are overlap segments. The apical lateral segment may be supplied by either the left anterior descending or circumflex arteries. If the segment is scored as abnormal, then the computer looks at how the apical septal segment is scored. If it too is abnormal, then the apical lateral segment is included in the anterior descending score. If the apical septum is normal and the mid lateral wall is abnormal, then the apical lateral segment is classified as circumflex. An abnormal apical inferior segment will be designated as left anterior descending if the apical septum on the four-chamber view is also abnormal. If the apical septum is normal and the basal inferior wall is abnormal, the apical inferior abnormality is classified as right coronary artery. (From Segar DS, et al. Dobutamine stress echocardiography: Correlation with coronary lesion severity as determined by quantitative angiography. *J Am Coll Cardiol.* 1992;19:1197. Reprinted with permission.)

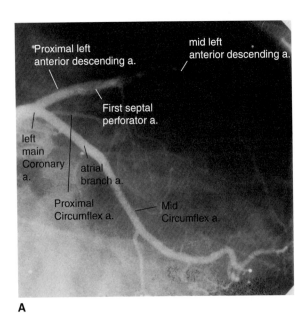

A

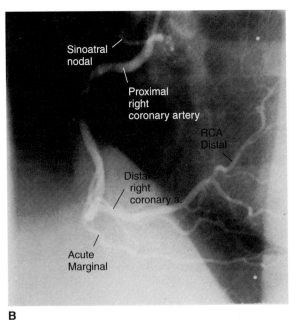

B

Figure 19-8. (**A**) Angiogram of a normal left coronary artery. (**B**) Angiogram of a normal right coronary artery.

lateral segments (including the basal, middle, and apical segments), and of the basal posterior and midposterior walls, are caused by stenosis of the left circumflex artery. Infarcts of the basal and midinferior and basal septums are caused by stenosis of the posterior descending coronary artery (PDA), which is the major branch of the right coronary artery. The two areas where overlap occurs are the apical lateral, which is supplied by both the LAD and left circumflex arteries, and the apical inferior segment, which is supplied by both the LAD and the PDA.

Summary

Echocardiography has developed into a major diagnostic tool in the evaluation of patients with coronary artery disease. The use of exercise and pharmacologic testing to determine left ventricular function and viability in a number of clinical settings continues. New techniques promise to yield even greater information.

Acknowledgment

The author wishes to acknowledge Michael Cunningham, M.D., who helped compile the angiographic images for this chapter.

REFERENCES

1. Bourdillon PDV, Broderick TM, Sawada SG, et al. Regional wall motion index for infarct and noninfarct regions after reperfusion in acute myocardial infarction: Comparison with global wall motion index. *J Am Soc Echocardiol.* 1989;2:398.
2. Chen CC, et al. Differential density and luminal irregularities as criteria to detect disease in the left main coronary artery by apex phased array cross-sectional echocardiography. *Am J Cardiol.* 1979;43:386.
3. Gabella G. Cardiovascular. *In Gray's Anatomy.* New York, Churchill Livingstone; 1995:1509.
4. Kyo S, Takamoto S, Matsumura M, et al. Transesophageal 2-dimensional echo-Doppler visualization of left main coronary arterial anatomy and flow (abstract). *J Am Coll Cardiol.* 1987;9(Suppl):179A.
5. Ogawa S, et al. A new approach to visualize the left main coronary artery using apical cross-sectional echocardiography. *Am J Cardiol.* 1980;45:301.
6. Weyman AE, et al. Noninvasive visualization of the left main coronary artery by cross-sectional echocardiography. *Circulation.* 1976;54:169.
7. Yamagishi M, Miyatake K, Beppo S, et al. Assessment of coronary blood flow by transesophageal two-dimensional pulsed Doppler echocardiography. *Am J Cardiol.* 1988;62:304.
8. Zwicky P, Daniel WG, Mügge A, et al. Imaging of coronary arteries by color coded transesophageal Doppler echocardiography. *Am J Cardiol.* 1988;62:639.

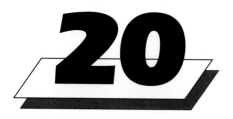

Echocardiography in the Patient with Coronary Artery Disease

ALAN D. WAGGONER and BENICO BARZILAI

Introduction

Two-dimensional Doppler echocardiography with color flow imaging plays a key role in evaluating the patient with coronary artery disease. Its unique advantages as a noninvasive imaging technique include the fact that it can be performed immediately at the bedside or in the emergency room to determine the location and extent of left ventricular wall motion abnormalities and provide diagnostic information such as an estimation of systolic and diastolic performance. Serial studies can be obtained, when necessary, to assess changes in left ventricular function or wall motion after infarction or reperfusion therapy. Complications of myocardial infarction can be readily detected with transthoracic or transesophageal echocardiographic (TEE) methods. As new myocardial contrast agents are employed, better delineation of infarct size is possible and identification of viable myocardium using ultrasonic tissue characterization represents the future applications of two-dimensional imaging.[1-161]

Consequences of Acute Myocardial Ischemia

Sonographers should understand the cascade of events that occur following coronary artery occlusion (Table 20-1). Immediately following coronary artery occlusion, diastolic dysfunction occurs first, with impaired left ventricle (LV) relaxation and reduction in early diastolic filling. LV diastolic compliance is reduced, and end-diastolic pressure increases above normal levels.[136] When infarction is transmural (involving the endocardial and epicardial layers of the myocardium), impaired systolic thickening, reduction in endocardial motion, and dyssynchronous contraction of myocardial segment(s) are immediately evident.[106] Depending on the extent of myocardial ischemia, LV chamber dilatation may also occur, with concomitant reduction in global systolic performance. In large infarctions LV diastolic pressure increases further and congestive heart failure (CHF) develops. The heart rate increases as a compensatory mechanism to maintain adequate cardiac output.

ELECTROCARDIOGRAPHIC/CLINICAL/ LABORATORY FINDINGS

The classic finding of ST-segment elevation with Q waves is associated with transmural infarction. Absence of Q waves but electrocardiographic (ECG) evidence of ST-T-wave changes with elevation in CK enzyme level are typical of nontransmural infarctions confined to the subendocardial layer. Chest pain, shortness of breath, nausea, and vomiting are usually the well-described symptoms but are

385

▟▟ TABLE 20-1. THE CASCADE OF EVENTS IN MYOCARDIAL ISCHEMIA IN DESCENDING ORDER

(LV diastolic dysfunction)
↓
Impaired relaxation and decreased compliance
↓
Increased LVEDP
↓
(LV systolic dysfunction)
↓
Regional wall motion abnormalities (transmural)
↓
Decreased LV ejection fraction*
↓
ECG ST-T-wave changes, Q waves
↓
Patient symptoms (chest pain)
↓

* Dependent on extent of ischemic myocardium.

the last events to occur (Table 20-1). It is important to understand that not all patients experience symptoms of myocardial ischemia, particularly the elderly or those with diabetes, who may not have chest pain; the physical examination may be normal in a patient with uncomplicated myocardial infarction (MI).[123] Enzymatic measurements are crucial for diagnosis. Elevations in serum creatinine kinase (CK) levels (>300 units) and the MB fraction of CK (>5%) are observed in all patients with larger values often seen in extensive infarcts. The first ECG-detectable abnormalities are hyperacute T waves followed by ST-segment elevation and then the development of Q waves (Fig. 20-1). It should

be noted that ECG changes often develop after the diastolic or systolic abnormalities described previously.

TWO-DIMENSIONAL DOPPLER EXAMINATION

Table 20-2 summarizes a two-dimensional and Doppler echocardiographic imaging approach in patients with coronary artery disease. The sonographer must be familiar with the clinical history of the patient, particularly if there were prior cardiac events. The findings of the physical examination, such as cardiac murmurs, evidence of CHF, and systolic blood pressure, are important to document. In patients in the coronary care unit, hemodynamic information may be available from pulmonary artery catheterization that can be used to correlate with the results of two-dimensional echocardiography. Twelve-lead ECG will often disclose the location of the presumed infarct and is helpful in guiding the two-dimensional and Doppler echocardiographic examination. The standard two-dimensional echocardiography approach should include multiple views for assessment of LV and right ventricle (RV) chamber sizes, the presence and extent of wall motion abnormalities, and evidence of valvular integrity, particularly in the mitral and aortic valves. Pulsed and continuous wave Doppler with color flow imaging should be used for detection of valvular regurgitation (mitral and tricuspid) and for assessment of LV diastolic filling parameters. This includes the mitral early (E) and atrial filling (A) wave

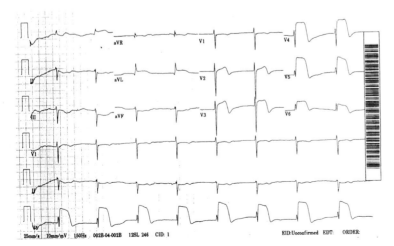

Figure 20-1. Twelve-lead ECG of a patient with an acute anterolateral MI. There is ST-segment elevation in leads I, AVL, and V3 to V6, with reciprocal ST-segment depression in leads II, III, and AVF.

TABLE 20-2. IMAGING APPROACH TO THE PATIENT WITH CORONARY ARTERY DISEASE

I. Review Clinical History, Physical Examination, 12-Lead Electrocardiogram
II. Parasternal Long Axis View
   A. Basal and midseptal wall motion
   B. Basal and midposterior wall motion
   C. Fractional shortening of the base of the LV
   D. Mitral valve apparatus
      1. Leaflet coaptation
      2. Color flow imaging: MR
   E. RV inflow view
      1. Color flow: TR
      2. Wall motion
III. Parasternal Short Axis View
   A. Papillary muscle level: segmental LV analysis
      1. Anterior, medial, posterior septum
      2. Anterior wall
      3. Lateral wall
      4. Posterior wall
      5. Inferior wall
   B. Color flow imaging if suspected ventricular septal rupture
   C. RV wall motion
      1. Inferior
      2. Free wall
      3. Anterior
   D. Chordal level
   E. Mitral valve level
      1. Color flow imaging: MR jet direction
IV. Apical Four-Chamber View
   A. Mid-, apical-septal wall motion
      1. Color flow imaging for ventricular septal rupture
      2. Basal septum (supplied by right coronary postdescending)
   B. Apex
   C. Basal, mid-, apical-lateral wall motion
   D. Mitral valve
      1. Color flow imaging: MR
      2. Pulsed Doppler (leaflet tips): E, A, E/A, DT
   E. Tricuspid valve
      1. Color flow imaging: TR
      2. Pulsed Doppler (leaflet tips): E, A, E/A, DT
   F. LV outflow
      1. Pulsed or continuous wave Doppler: isovolumic relaxation time (IVRT)
      2. Pulsed Doppler: Velocity time integral
   G. Pulmonary vein (right)
      1. Pulsed Doppler in orifice: Systolic, diastolic, and atrial reversal
         Note: Inferior angulation to visualize posterior septal and lateral walls and apex.
V. Apical Two-Chamber View
   A. Basal, mid-, apical, anterior wall motion
   B. Apex
   C. Basal, mid, apical, inferior wall motion
      1. Note papillary muscle (posteroinferior)
   D. Mitral valve apparatus
      1. Color flow imaging: MR
VI. Apical Long Axis View (Three-Chamber)
   A. Anteroseptal wall motion
   B. Inferior posterior wall motion
   C. Color flow imaging: MR, AR
VII. Subcostal View
   A. Four-chamber plane
      1. RV free wall motion
      2. Pericardial effusion
   B. Cross-sectional plane
      1. RV and LV wall motion
   C. Inferior vena cava (long axis)
      1. Size, collapsibility

velocities, deceleration, and isovolumic relaxation times. Right pulmonary venous flow velocities (systolic, diastolic, and atrial reversal) are also useful.

TWO-DIMENSIONAL WALL MOTION ANALYSIS

Regional wall motion abnormalities identified with two-dimensional echocardiography, even in patients with nondiagnostic ECG findings, correspond to the occluded coronary artery perfusion bed.[35,41,48,50,51,76,85,108,111,145,148] If subtotal occlusion exists (i.e., 75–90% stenosis), regional wall motion may not appear abnormal unless accompanied by hemodynamic alterations such as increased afterload or decreased aortic diastolic pressure.[106] Proximal location of coronary artery obstruction leads to a greater amount of ischemic or jeopardized myocardium (the "watershed" phenomenon) unless extensive collateral circulation exists or spontaneous reperfusion occurs.[133] Proximal left anterior descending (LAD) occlusion will lead to middle and basal septum, anterior wall, and apical wall motion abnormalities. Mid-distal LAD occlusion (after the septal perforators or diagonal branches) may affect only the distal septum or anterior wall in addition to the apex (Fig. 20-2). Left circumflex occlusion results in lateral and posterior wall abnormalities

(Fig. 20-3), while right coronary occlusion affects the inferior wall and the inferior septum, as well as the posterior wall in some patients (Fig. 20-4). When the right coronary artery is occluded in the middle or proximal portion, right ventricular free wall motion may also be abnormal.

ECHOCARDIOGRAPHIC FINDINGS

Two-dimensional evidence of wall motion abnormalities is always seen in Q-wave or transmural infarction but may or may not be present in non-Q-wave infarcts where ischemia occurs in the subendocardial myocardium. Non-Q-wave infarctions comprise about 6–44% of acute MI and are more often seen in older patients and women.[34] Although the anterior wall is thought to be commonly involved, the posterolateral segment is more often found to be abnormal in non-Q-wave MI.[88] However, many patients have normal wall motion unless prior MI is evident. Generally, non-Q-wave infarcts are smaller and short-term mortality is lower compared to that of patients with transmural infarctions.[42] The origin of non-Q-wave MI is not always clear. One hypothesis is that these patients present with myocardial ischemia, perhaps due to coronary spasm, but have spontaneous reperfusion, which prevents transmural necrosis.[43] This type of infarc-

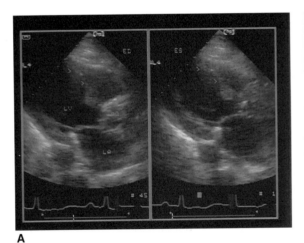

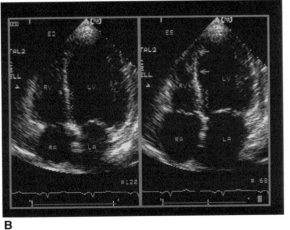

A   **B**

Figure 20-2. (**A**) Parasternal long axis view at end diastole (ED) and end systole (ES) in a patient with a septal infarct. The arrows indicate the lack of motion in the midseptum. AO, aorta; LA, left atrium; LV, left ventricle (**B**) Apical four-chamber view in another patient with an anteroseptal MI and akinesis of the mid and apical septum (large arrows) with preserved basal septum thickening (small arrows). RA, right atrium; RV, right ventricle.

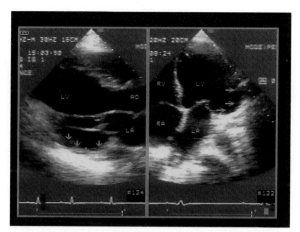

Figure 20-3. Parasternal long axis view at end diastole (left panel) and apical four-chamber view (right panel) in a patient with a posterolateral basal infarct (arrows) due to left circumflex occlusion. LV, left ventricle; RV, right ventricle; LA, left atrium; RA, right atrium; AO, aorta.

tion often is an unstable process, and the long-term prognosis of these patients, particularly for reinfarction, is two times that of patients with Q-wave MI.[43,102]

TWO-DIMENSIONAL EVALUATION OF THE EXTENT OF MI

Quantification of the extent of MI requires visualization of all myocardial segments in the six standard views (parasternal, long and short axis, apical four-

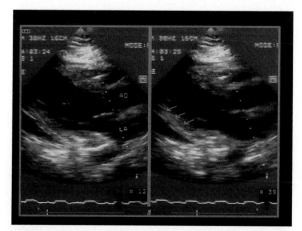

Figure 20-4. Parasternal long axis view of a patient with a posterior LV hypokinesis due to right coronary artery disease. LV, left ventricle; LA, left atrium; AO, aorta.

and two-chamber, apical long or three-chamber, and subcostal) (Table 20-2). This is possible in only 70%–80% of patients. Methods to quantitate wall motion involve a sophisticated analysis using a center point in the LV cavity in a series of short axis views, with calculation of radial or chordal shortening or regional area change.[33] Visual scoring of segments in each view is more commonly employed. The American Society of Echocardiography has recommended a scoring method that divides the LV into 16 segments. Normal motion is assigned a value of 1, hypokinesis 2, akinesis 3, and dyskinesis 4. The higher the sum of the values obtained in each of the segments seen, the greater the amount of ischemic myocardium. Transmural infarction results in akinesis or dyskinesis of the affected segment in nearly all cases. Hypokinesis may be the only abnormality detected, such as in non-Q-wave MI, but it is difficult to recognize unless significantly impaired segmental thickening or diminished excursion is evident.

The wall motion abnormalities detected with two-dimensional echocardiography in patients with acute MI often overestimate the actual size of the infarct.[32,133,156] This can occur because segments adjacent to the infarct region (where akinesis or dyskinesis is present) may be hypokinetic due to "stunned" myocardium or are tethered and not ischemic. Stunned myocardium results from periods of ischemia (<20 min) too brief for necrosis and can occur in the setting of a subtotal occlusion with reduced blood flow.[12] When ischemia is recurrent over several hours (e.g., in a patient with unstable angina), regional dysfunction will occur and may persist for days. This condition is distinguished from hibernating myocardium resulting from chronic decreases in myocardial perfusion over months or years, such as in a patient with multivessel coronary artery disease.[118]

Patients with "stunning" may not exhibit chest pain or ECG changes.[12] Stunned myocardial segments often show recovery of normal function, particularly when reperfusion to the ischemic segment is restored in a timely fashion.[12] Recovery is variable and is generally dependent on the duration of the occlusion and the extent of ischemia. The greater the interval between coronary occlusion and the reestablishment of vessel patency by angioplasty or thrombolytic agents, the longer for recovery of wall motion abnormalities in both jeopardized regions and ischemic segments, where it may not be reversible.

Recovery of myocardial function may occur in a few days, after 4–6 weeks, or even after several months.[11,17,105,109] Inferior or non-Q-wave infarcts will usually show improvement by 3 months, while anterior infarcts may require a longer recovery period.[119] Serial evaluation by two-dimensional echocardiography can be useful but may be deferred because of the associated costs,[69] and the difficulty in establishing the optimal time period for performing serial studies. An important two-dimensional echocardiographic finding in a patient with acute MI is evidence of remote asynergy or segmental dysfunction observed at a site not involved in the acute event. These observations indicate that multivessel coronary artery disease is present.[137]

Global LV systolic function is the most important prognostic variable in patients with ischemic heart disease. Both ejection fraction and end-diastolic volume are key determinants of morbidity (i.e., heart failure), as well as short- and long-term mortality.[123] As might be expected, the lower the ejection fraction (i.e., <40%) and the greater the LV end-diastolic volume, the poorer the clinical outcome. Two-dimensional echocardiography can be extremely valuable in measuring ejection fraction and cardiac volumes, as shown in several studies.[41,50,100,145] Generally, patients with anterior MI have lower ejection fractions and larger end-diastolic volumes than those with inferior or non-Q-wave MI. The critical determinant is often the size of the infarct, as measured by the extent of wall motion abnormality, which in turn affects global LV performance.

Infarct expansion may occur after acute coronary occlusion as a consequence of intramural rupture of the myocardium and can be identified with two-dimensional echocardiography.[53] This complication is associated with regional dilatation and thinning of the involved LV segments. Patients with anterior infarcts are more likely to develop expansion than those with non-Q-wave or inferior infarctions, and this condition is often evident within 5–7 days of the initial MI.[29,32,53,111,113] LV dilatation occurs, and CHF may develop.[111] It is more often seen in patients with their first MI who have no further ECG changes or enzyme elevations after the initial event. In contrast to expansion, infarct extension can occur at any time following the acute event and is accompanied by ECG and enzyme changes.[53] Usually only a small amount of myocardium is involved in the process, but it is an unstable clinical state and is likely due to continued hypoperfusion of the segment. Two-dimensional echocardiography in these patients may not reveal any changes in regional wall motion.

Two-dimensional echocardiography can also be useful in the recovery phase after myocardial infarction when the process of "remodeling" occurs in the LV.[111,113] Remodeling results in increased LV volumes and wall thickness in the noninfarcted myocardium despite improved hemodynamics with lower LV diastolic pressures. This mechanism is different from the one in infarcted segments, which may expand with thinning of the wall and dilation in the infarct region. Establishing patency of the coronary artery perfusion bed by thrombolytic agents or angioplasty may limit infarct expansion.[99] Further LV dilatation with resultant CHF may thus be prevented in many patients. LV dilatation with remodeling may still occur despite successful establishment of coronary blood flow and is more often observed in anterior MI.[154] Remodeling can also be enhanced by decreasing afterload using angiotension converting enzyme (ACE) inhibitors.[111]

DIASTOLIC FILLING AND THE ROLE OF DOPPLER

Diastolic dysfunction occurs prior to systolic dysfunction in acute myocardial ischemia. Studies during coronary angioplasty have confirmed that alterations in LV filling patterns consistent with impaired relaxation occur immediately with coronary occlusion during balloon inflation (30–90 sec) but normalize soon after deflation.[73] ECG evidence of ST-segment elevation occurs in most, but not all, patients. Chest pain may or may not be present, but it occurs after the diastolic and systolic dysfunction. With diastolic dysfunction, pulsed Doppler provides evidence of prolonged isovolumic relaxation and deceleration times, with reduction in early filling velocities that is demonstrable in patients with acute MI (Fig. 20-5). However, alterations in LV diastolic volumes or end-diastolic pressure may influence Doppler recordings of mitral inflow velocities in the individual patient. When increases occur in LV end-diastolic chamber volumes accompanied by in-

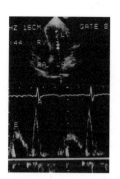 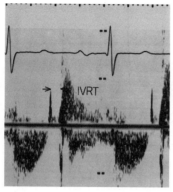

A

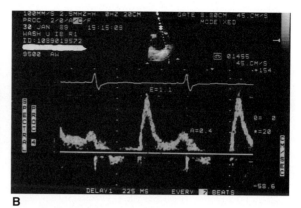

B

Figure 20-5. (**A**) Pulsed Doppler recordings (left panel) of the mitral inflow early (E) and atrial (A) velocities. The E/A ratio is 0.5 and the deceleration time is prolonged (310 m/sec). The right panel was obtained with continuous wave Doppler, demonstrating simultaneous aortic and mitral inflow velocities. Measurement of the isovolumic relaxation time (IVRT) is 110 m/sec. Both findings are consistent with impaired LV relaxation due to ischemia with normal left atrial pressure. (**B**) Pulsed Doppler recording of mitral inflow with high E and low A velocities; the E/A ratio is 2.8 and the deceleration time of early LV filling is 100 m/sec. This is consistent with high left atrial pressure in a patient with a large MI.

creased LV end-diastolic pressure (such as in a large MI), the patient will have a different mitral inflow pattern characterized by a high E velocity, small A wave, and shortened deceleration and isovolumic relaxation times, as seen in Figure 20-5. This is different from the pattern in the patient with a small MI, normal LV diastolic volumes, and minimally elevated LV diastolic pressures, where mitral inflow has reduced or normal E velocity, preserved A wave, and normal deceleration and isovolumic relation times. The sonographer should be aware of how loading conditions influence diastolic mitral inflow velocities.

Recent studies have shown that pulsed Doppler patterns of mitral inflow have predictive value in patients with coronary artery disease and MI.[19,115] Patients with increased E/A ratios and shortened deceleration and isovolumic relaxation times had a greater incidence of CHF than those with normal or reduced mitral E/A ratios and normal deceleration times.[19] When left ventricular end diastolic pressure (LVEDP) was elevated, the E and E/A were increased compared to those of normal controls. If LVEDP was normal, the mitral inflow velocity pattern was consistent with impaired relaxation (low E, E/A). Another confounding variable is age, since many patients with MI are older, and reduced E/A with prolonged isovolumic relaxation and decelera-

tion times are common in elderly patients. Table 20-2 summarizes the application of Doppler and color flow imaging for the evaluation of the patient with coronary artery disease.

COMPLICATIONS OF MYOCARDIAL INFARCTION

Table 20-3 lists the complications of acute MI, including pericarditis and right ventricular extension of inferior MI. Mechanical complications such as mitral regurgitation, LV aneurysm formation (with or without thrombus), ventricular septal rupture, or free wall rupture are adverse prognostic events. These complications are associated with high mortality, particularly when accompanied by cardiogenic shock.[16] Two-dimensional echocardiogra-

▰▰▰ TABLE 20-3. COMPLICATIONS OF ACUTE MI

Pericarditis
RV infarction
Mitral regurgitation
   Ruptured papillary muscle
LV aneurysm
  LV thrombi
  Pseudoaneurysm
Ventricular septal rupture
Ventricular free wall rupture

phy[122] and Doppler echocardiography with color flow imaging or TEE are particularly valuable.

POST-MI PERICARDITIS

Pericardial inflammation can occur with transmural infarction since the visceral pericardium is adjacent to the epicardium. Typically, a friction rub is heard, and the patient may have fever, chest pain, and diffuse ST-T-wave changes evident on ECG. Two-dimensional echocardiography may reveal an echo-free space consistent with a significant pericardial effusion in a minority of patients. When pericardial effusion is evident, however, it is usually small and does not lead to hemodynamic derangement.[16] A large pericardial effusion is inconsistent with post-MI pericarditis, and other causes should be sought in these patients.

RV INFARCTION

RV infarction is recognized as a frequent complication of inferior MI. Clinical signs include hypotension and hemodynamic evidence of increased right atrial pressure exceeding or equal to pulmonary capillary wedge pressure; complete heart block is often present.[20] RV infarction is rare in patients with anterior infarctions.[54] If the posterior septum is not involved (supplied by the posterior descending branch of the right coronary artery), RV infarction is not observed. As many as one-third of patients with fatal MI have evidence of RV infarction.

The antemortem diagnosis of RV infarction is well defined by ECG, hemodynamic, and echocardiographic observations. The ECG can be valuable in evaluating RV infarction by employing right-sided chest leads. ST-segment elevation in lead V4R has high sensitivity and reasonable specificity in patients with hemodynamic evidence of RV infarction.[13,83] ST-segment elevation in leads V1 and V2 may also be seen in RV infarction that is not due to anteroseptal MI.[40] It is important to note that the ST-segment elevation seen in the right-sided chest leads may be subtle in magnitude compared to that seen in the standard ECG leads.

Hemodynamic signs of RV infarction often resemble those of cardiac tamponade.[55] Equilibration of right atrial, pulmonary diastolic, and wedge pressure is noted in many patients, but without evidence of tamponade by M-mode echocardiography.[84] RV pressure tracings may demonstrate a dip and pla-

teau, and the right atrial pressure recordings may have a steep "y" descent. In contrast, constrictive pericarditis or cardiac tamponade usually results in a small, vigorously contracting RV. Patients with RV infarction usually have elevated right atrial mean pressures, but exceptions do occur.[82] Right atrial pressure will increase after volume expansion, resulting in equalization with pulmonary capillary wedge pressure. The specificity of this criterion (right atrial pressure equal to pulmonary capillary wedge) is excellent (>97%), but the sensitivity is reduced (45–73%). The accuracy of this criterion is also not related to the anatomic extent of the infarction.[55]

Two-dimensional echocardiography can be extremely useful for the diagnosis of RV infarction. The echocardiographic features were first described by D'Arcy and Nanda in 10 patients with clinical evidence of RV infarction.[23] Akinesis and dyskinesis of the RV diaphragmatic wall are noted in most patients from cross-sectional or subcostal views, the free wall is involved less often. RV enlargement is present in nearly all patients and paradoxical septal motion in most. Contrast two-dimensional echocardiography with agitated 5% dextrose reveals tricuspid regurgitation in nearly all patients. Akinesis of the RV free wall may also occur in the apical four-chamber view, but without RV enlargement or paradoxical septal motion.[15] Patients with elevated right atrial pressure frequently have RV wall motion abnormalities, but these abnormalities occur less often in patients with normal right atrial (RA) pressure. When paradoxical septal motion is observed, patients may also have elevated RA pressure equal to or greater than pulmonary capillary wedge pressure. Pulsed Doppler or color flow imaging will disclose tricuspid regurgitation in the majority of patients, but the tricuspid regurgitant jet velocity obtained by continuous wave Doppler is usually less than 3.0 m/sec due to the inability of the ischemic RV to generate sufficient force to elevate pulmonary artery pressures.

The extent of LV asynergy in patients with inferior MI and RV infarction may not be as great as in the RV when expressed circumferentially as percent involvement.[58] RV ejection fraction and end-diastolic volumes may not differ significantly in survivors and nonsurvivors. Improvement in RV systolic performance can often be observed after RV infarction. It has been shown that the percent surface area of RV asynergy decreases from day 2 to day 10 and later at 6 months.[160] Several factors appear to influence the improvement of the RV after MI.[160] The timing of the initial study (if after 48 hr, maximum improvement may have occurred), triple-vessel coronary disease, poor LV ejection fraction, or massive RV infarction will have an adverse impact on the functional recovery of the RV.

Another echocardiographic method that may be useful in the future is quantitative two-dimensional integrated backscatter imaging. A further description of this specialized mode of echocardiographic imaging is provided later in this chapter. While integrated backscatter decreases normally from diastole to systole in normal RV segments in control patients, the cyclic reduction in integrated backscatter is reduced in patients with RV infarction.[152]

The sonographer should be attentive to the presence of RV infarction in a patient who presents with inferior MI, particularly with accompanying ECG evidence of ST-segment elevation in right precordial leads and hypotension. RV infarction results in abnormal RV wall motion, which is best detected in short axis, four-chamber, or subcostal views (Figure 20-6). It is usually confined to the posterior or free wall of the RV and may be accompanied by RV dilatation, depending on the extent of intravascular volume loading. Tricuspid regurgitation is often present.

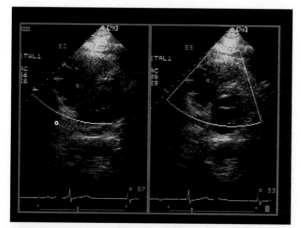

Figure 20-6. Cross-sectional views with attention to right ventricular (RV) wall motion of end diastole (ED) and end systole (ES). The arrows indicate the lack of systolic motion of the inferior and free walls with dilatation of the RV chamber. LV, left ventricle.

Mitral Regurgitation

Mitral regurgitation (MR) is a common complication of acute or recent MI, although the mechanisms may be different in individual patients. The hemodynamic findings are characterized by V waves in the pulmonary capillary wedge pressure tracings when a pulmonary artery catheter has been placed in the patient.[16] However, this is not specific to MR and can be seen in patients with ventricular septal rupture or significant LV dysfunction. Rupture of the papillary muscle can occur, although it is a rare complication (1%). The head of the posteromedial papillary muscle is more commonly involved than the trunk. Since coronary perfusion to the posteromedial papillary muscle occurs from only the right coronary artery, patients with posteroinferior MI are more at risk. Rupture of the anterolateral papillary muscle, which has a blood supply from both the circumflex and anterior descending branches, is unusual. Two-dimensional echocardiography, and particularly TEE, are valuable in detecting this complication.[7,21,96,101] Disruption of the papillary muscle and a mass attached to the chordae or flail mitral leaflets are evident in cross-sectional or apical views, as seen in Figure 20-7. Patients may develop this complication within 24 hr or up to 7 days after the acute event. The clinical picture is typically characterized as new-onset pulmonary edema accompanied by hypotension and a new holosystolic murmur.

MR may occur because of papillary muscle dysfunction due to localized ischemia, with a concomitant underlying wall motion abnormality. This mechanism is responsible for a majority of the cases of ischemic MR. Marked ventricular enlargement with a spherical change in LV shape can result in abnormal coaptation of the mitral leaflets due to this change in LV geometry, causing MR.[72] Generally, patients with MR have a higher incidence of CHF, are older, are female, and have had a prior MI.[6] Of importance, mortality is higher in these patients despite the fact that MR may be transient or decrease in severity over time.

The diagnosis and qualitative assessment of MR due to ischemic heart disease is usually performed with two-dimensional-Doppler echocardiography with color flow imaging.[6,57,78] Recent work by several groups of investigators, however, has focused on the quantitative analysis of MR jets by combined

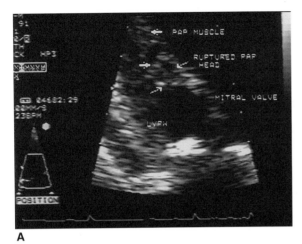
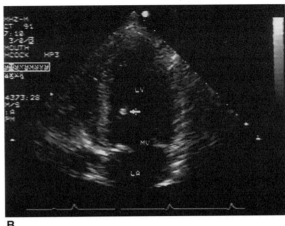

A   **B**

Figure 20-7. (**A**) Apical four-chamber view of a patient with mitral regurgitation and a bright echo density (arrow) that was attached to the chordae tendinae. PAP muscle, papillary muscle; LVFW, left ventricular free wall. (**B**) Apical two-chamber expanded view of the mitral apparatus demonstrating a ruptured papillary muscle head. (**A** and **B** courtesy of Dr. Kevin Harris.)

color flow imaging and continuous wave Doppler using the proximal isovelocity surface area (PISA) method.[5,18,44,144] Measurements of the radius of the convergence zone of aliased flow (defined by color flow imaging) on the ventricular side of the mitral leaflet tips, the velocity at the distance where the radius is measured (Nyquist limit), and the orifice velocity (from continuous wave Doppler) provide an accurate quantitation of regurgitant orifice area. However, this technique has not been widely used in patients with MI. It should be noted that the severity of MR detected by Doppler color flow imaging can be influenced by hemodynamic factors including preload, afterload, chamber compliance, and contractility. Technical factors such as attenuation, receiver gain, wall filter, and transducer frequency also affect Doppler sensitivity.

The use of two-dimensional Doppler echocardiographic techniques has revealed that MR occurs more often than previously established by auscultation. Studies demonstrate that more than 40% of patients with acute MI have MR.[6,78] The locus of infarction appears to be equally distributed between inferior and anterior walls in these patients with Doppler-detected MR. These patients have larger ventricular volumes, a history of prior infarctions, and a lower LV ejection fraction. All of these factors may contribute to higher mortality in patients with MR compared to those without it. Figure 20-8 shows a patient with MR in the setting of inferior MI.

The sonographer should incorporate all of the standard two-dimensional views and employ color flow imaging to detect the systolic flow disturbance of MR. Particular attention to structural abnormalities of the MV leaflets, chordae tendinae, and papillary muscles is critical, in addition to abnormal LV and left atrial (LA) size. Pulsed Doppler flow velocity recording of mitral inflow and pulmonary venous flow are helpful in assessing diastolic filling abnormalities and providing evidence of increased LA pressure.

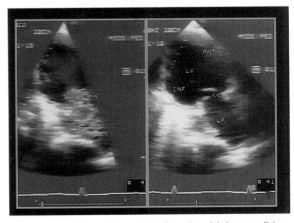

Figure 20-8. Apical two-chamber view (right panel) in a patient with an extensive inferior MI and flail mitral leaflets (arrows) resulting in severe mitral regurgitation (left panel) detected by color flow imaging. LV, left ventricle; LA, left atrium; INF, inferior; ANT, anterior. (See also Color Plate 61.)

LV ANEURYSM

Following acute MI, an aneurysm may form at the site of the infarction in up to 30% of patients.[16] Most commonly involved are the anterior wall and apex, followed by the inferior or posterolateral walls. LV aneurysms are characterized by a distortion of the LV contour at both end diastole and end systole, with dyskinesis seen in the acute stage. In the later stage there is akinesis of the wall of the aneurysm, which becomes fibrotic and calcified. Thrombus frequently form within the aneurysm due to stasis of flow. Clinically, patients with LV aneurysm may have CHF, ventricular arrhythmias, or systemic embolization.[16]

Two-dimensional echocardiography is a more sensitive and specific method for detecting aneurysmal formation, regardless of the site, than LV angiography.[7,90,149,150,157] Early studies revealed that LV thrombi can be observed in patients who are asymptomatic and many have had previous MI.[149] The formation of an LV aneurysm after anterior MI occurs by day 3 in 50% of patients and is concomitant with infarct expansion.[90] Inferior LV aneurysm tends to develop later than anterior MI, but by 3 months nearly all patients have developed an LV aneurysm, regardless of the site.[150] Mortality in patients with an LV aneurysm is significantly higher than in those with MI, but no aneurysm and early aneurysm formation are also associated with higher mortality. Nearly all patients have had a prior anterior MI.

Typical two-dimensional features include LV dilatation and a "hinge point" demarcating the infarct zone and aneurysm formation from normal myocardium (Fig. 20-9). Apical views are extremely useful in detecting anterior and inferior MI (when located at the base), while parasternal views are best suited for posterior aneurysms. Thrombus formation should be assessed within the aneurysm, which requires the use of high-frequency transducers (3.5 or 5.0 MHz). Many sonographers have found that LV aneurysm, and particularly LV thrombi, occur less frequently with changes in the medical management of patients with acute MI, such as increased use of thrombolytic agents to reduce infarct size or the use of heparin therapy.

LV THROMBUS AFTER MI

The two-dimensional echocardiographic detection of LV thrombi has been investigated for over 10 years and is established as a reasonably accurate

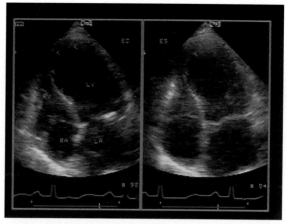

Figure 20-9. Apical four-chamber view at end diastole (ED) and end systole (ES) in a patient with an LV aneurysm following an anterior MI. Note the loss of the normal end-diastolic LV contour (compare with Figure 20-2*B*) and akinesis of the septum during systole. LV, left ventricle; LA, left atrium; RV, right ventricle; RA, right atrium.

technique.[1,2,24,26,28,37,47,59,64,65,92,94,138,139,151,155] Specific two-dimensional features must be present to make the diagnosis, including a mass of echoes with well-defined borders in the LV cavity located in a dyssynergistic myocardial segment (usually at the apex) and evident in more than one tomographic plane (Fig. 20-10). Several studies have shown that the sensitivity of two-dimensional echocardiography ranges from 77% to 95%, with a speci-

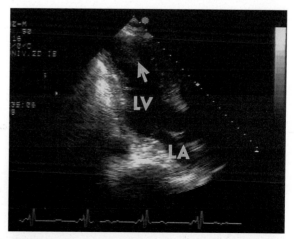

Figure 20-10. Apical long axis view of a large, pedunculated apical thrombus (arrow) in a patient with an apical infarction. LV, left ventricle; LA, left atrium.

ficity of 86% to 93%.[1,28,138] Limitations of two-dimensional echocardiography include poor visualization of the segment with suspected thrombus and near-field artifacts caused by reverberations from the chest wall or beam width. A high-frequency transducer (5 MHz) may be necessary to provide improved resolution of the cardiac apex from apical views.

The incidence of embolization in patients with an MI and an LV thrombus has been reported by numerous groups.[2,24,26,37,47,59,64,65,94,139,151,155] DeMaria et al. first reported 5 patients (from a group of 25 nonconsecutive patients) with evidence of systemic embolization, all of whom had echocardiographic evidence of LV thrombus.[24] Larger patient studies, including those by Asinger et al. and Visser et al., noted apical thrombi in one-third of patients with anterior infarction.[2,151] Systemic embolization, however, occurred in none of these patients. All had been treated with low-dose prophylactic heparin as part of standard medical therapy for acute MI. In each of these studies, LV mural thrombi rarely occurred in patients with inferior MI.

In other studies in which patients had been treated with anticoagulant agents, LV thrombi still occurred but embolic events were rare.[37] In a study of patients with LV thrombi, some treated with anticoagulation and others not treated, embolic events occurred only in the latter group; no anticoagulated patient had events during a 3-month follow-up period.[64] A separate investigation in patients with anterior MI, who manifested early thrombi development (<48 hr), had higher mortality, but the rate of embolization was less than 10%.[139]

Some investigators have attempted to define more precisely those patients who are at high risk for embolization and have looked at the characteristics of the thrombus. One factor is that embolization occurs more often in thrombi exhibiting vigorous motion and protrusion into the LV cavity.[47] A second factor is that thrombi detected early after infarction are more likely to embolize than those detected more than 3 weeks after infarction.[94] Recent evidence suggests that protruding thrombi are uncommon and that in some patients the thrombus may resolve with anticoagulation. Thrombus mobility rather than type (layered versus protruding) and the absence of anticoagulant therapy correlate with a higher probability of embolization.[59,155] Importantly, thrombi tend to decrease in size or resolve by 2 years in most patients treated with anticoagulant therapy. Patients with LV thrombus also tend to have poorer LV wall motion scores than those without thrombus.

Institution of thrombolytic therapy during the acute infarction does not influence thrombus occurrence.[65] Although patients may have no thrombus at the time of discharge, some may develop LV thrombi during the follow-up period. Many have associated in-hospital heart failure, MI, aneurysm formation, and deterioration in LV function. Anticoagulant therapy (coumadin) and apical akinesis (rather than dyskinesis) are the factors likely responsible for thrombus resolution in patients with evidence of thrombi before hospital discharge. However, other studies have reported that thrombolytic therapy in patients with protruding thrombus may result in systemic embolization.[65]

The presence of an anterior MI, particularly with LV dysfunction and apical akinesis/dyskinesis, warrants anticoagulant therapy. Contraindications to anticoagulation include active gastrointestinal bleeding and recent stroke; in patients scheduled for any kind of surgery, anticoagulation is also ruled out. The sonographer should carefully evaluate the patient with an acute MI (particularly anterior) for the development of LV thrombus. The probability of thrombus formation is higher if significant LV dysfunction exists and an aneurysm is recognized by two-dimensional echocardiography. The characteristics of the thrombus, particularly if it is mobile and protrudes into the LV chamber, need to be documented. Anticoagulant therapy will decrease the risk of embolization but may not necessarily influence mortality. Resolution or a decrease in thrombus size may occur either spontaneously or due to anticoagulant therapy and may be followed with two-dimensional echocardiography.

LV PSEUDOANEURYSM

LV pseudoaneurysms are an unusual complication of ischemic heart disease and represent myocardial rupture contained by the parietal pericardium. Although more commonly seen in the setting of recent MI, pseudoaneurysms may also occur following cardiac trauma, myocarditis, infective endocarditis, and cardiac surgery.[125,141] Clinical features are nonspecific and include abnormal apical impulse, chest pain, CHF, systemic embolization, or ECG evidence of MI. The distinction between a true LV aneurysm and pseudoaneurysm is based on the composition of the walls of the aneurysm. Fibrous pericardial tissue forms the wall of the pseudoaneurysm, while the true LV aneurysm is composed of myocardium. The opening or neck of the pseudoaneurysm is usually narrow compared to the size of the aneurysm. Blood flow from the LV chamber into the pseudoaneurysm results in systolic expansion of the aneurysm, while the LV cavity decreases in size. Surgical intervention is recommended in the patient with an LV pseudoaneurysm since rupture may occur due to the inability of the pericardium to withstand intra-aneurysmal pressure.[125,141]

Diagnosis of LV pseudoaneurysm can be made with a chest x-ray, radionuclide ventriculography, and cardiac catheterization.[10] However, the location of the pseudoaneurysm may render these techniques nondiagnostic in some patients. Two-dimensional echocardiography has been also employed for the diagnosis of LV pseudoaneurysm, with numerous case studies reporting locations both posterior or posterolateral (the most common sites of formation) and anterior or anteroapical.[14,39,61,62,67,74,126,129,131] Catherwood and coworkers first described a series of five patients with LV pseudoaneurysm at catheterization; four were successfully detected by two-dimensional echocardiography, and three had thrombus visualized within the false chamber.[14] Two-dimensional measurements of the ratio of the neck orifice to the aneurysmal sac diameter were less than 0.45, while in 22 patients with true LV aneurysm this ratio was greater than 0.78. Others have reported similar findings, confirmed with inconclusive LV angiography.[39,129] Most pseudoaneurysms are located posteriorly and are best detected with modified apical four-chamber views. Other conditions that may simulate a pseudoaneurysm include loculated pericardial effusion, pericardial cyst, and left ventricular diverticulum.

Doppler echocardiography with color flow imaging may also provide information complementary to that of two-dimensional imaging and is useful for identification of the pattern of flow both within the LV chamber and into the pseudoaneurysm.[38,45,79] Systolic flow can be detected by pulsed Doppler in the pseudoaneurysm and reverses during diastole, or there may be systolic and diastolic turbulence in the neck of a posterior LV pseudoaneurysm.[127,135,153] The instantaneous pressure differences can be measured by continuous wave Doppler between a posterolateral pseudoaneurysm and the LV chamber.[140] For example, if the pressure in the pseudoaneurysm during systole is calculated as the LV systolic pressure minus the pressure drop, this yields the intra-aneurysmal pressure. A low pulse pressure and an increased gradient are typically due to the noncompliant nature of a pseudoaneurysm and the small size of the neck. If there is impaired diastolic emptying of the pseudoaneurysm, thrombus may extend into the neck and increase the size of the pseudoaneurysm. The increased pressure within the pseudoaneurysm might explain the likelihood of rupture that commonly occurs in these patients. Figure 20-11 is an example of two patients with LV pseudoaneurysms.

VENTRICULAR SEPTAL RUPTURE

The development of a new systolic murmur accompanied by signs of hypoperfusion after acute MI stems from either ventricular septal rupture or severe MR. Clinical differentiation between these two complications is often difficult and unreliable.[16] Combining two-dimensional and Doppler echocardiography with color flow imaging can be extremely valuable in this setting, quickly establishing the diagnosis. A complete two-dimensional Doppler echocardiographic examination should attempt to answer the following questions: (1) what is the etiology of the systolic murmur? (2) what is the status of the ventricular septum and mitral apparatus? (3) what is the extent of wall motion abnormalities involving the LV and RV? and (4) what is the overall LV function?

Two-dimensional echocardiography, alone or with peripheral venous contrast, may reveal an echo-free area or akinesis/dyskinesis, with thinning in the involved area of the septum, but these findings are not always specific to rupture.[9,25,30,96,130] Small, even multiple defects or a serpiginous tunnel between the LV and RV may also preclude two-dimensional visualization of the LV-RV communication.[22,25] The addition of a peripheral venous contrast injection can improve detection by demonstrating evidence of either a negative contrast effect in the RV or a positive contrast appearance in the LV.

The addition of Doppler color flow imaging to two-dimensional echocardiography has improved

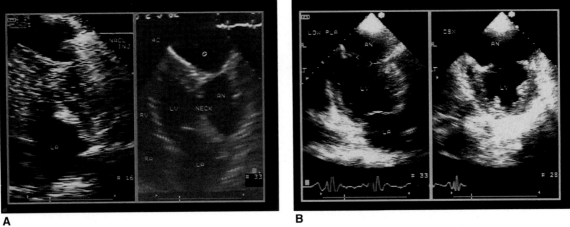

A   **B**

Figure 20-11. **(A)** Apical four-chamber view of an LV pseudoaneurysm located in the lateral wall (right panel). The patient was sent for cardiac catheterization in which two-dimensional echocardiography was performed simultaneously with injection of agitated saline (NACL INJ) into a catheter positioned in the LV. Note the microbubbles in the pseudoaneurysm. LV, left ventricle; LA, left atrium; RV, right ventricle; AN, aneurysm; NECK, neck of pseudoaneurysm. (See also Color Plate.) **(B)** Apical two-chamber view (right) and parasternal cross-sectional view of another patient with an apical LV pseudoaneurysm (AN). Arrows delineate the neck. LV, left ventricle; LA, left atrium; CSX, cross-sectional; LOW PLA, low parasternal levy axis.

detection of ventricular septal rupture, eliminating the need for peripheral venous injections.[4,8,22,27,36,46,49,66,91,97,107,121,161] The presence of a systolic flow disturbance along the right side of the ventricular septum is diagnostic of the left-to-right shunt of ventricular septal rupture even in cases where two-dimensional echocardiography fails to visualize the defect. Importantly, two-dimensional Doppler echocardiography can distinguish MR from ventricular septal rupture due to acute MI. Furthermore, the authors and others report concomitant severe MR and ventricular septal rupture that have been documented by Doppler echocardiography.[22,27,97] When assessing patients with new systolic murmurs and hypotension in the presence of acute MI, it is essential to perform two-dimensional Doppler echocardiography in multiple parasternal, apical, and subcostal views. Most often, the cross-sectional and apical four-chamber views prove to be the most useful for denoting the site of rupture with Doppler interrogation (Figure 20-12). Cross-sectional views at the papillary muscle level are best for detecting posterior septal rupture due to inferior MI. Attention should also be directed to RV wall motion since RV infarction is not infrequent in ventricular septal rupture. The apical four-

chamber view is best for mid- or apical septal rupture in the setting of anterior MI.

Color flow imaging has been reported to be very sensitive in detecting ventricular septal rupture due to acute MI.[4,46,91,97,161] The high-velocity systolic jet resulting from the large gradient between the LV and RV produces disturbed systolic flow and a mosaic of color signals through the ventricular septal defect into the RV. This finding usually eliminates the need for tedious interrogation of the flow on the right side of the septum by pulsed Doppler. The superiority of color flow imaging over other echocardiographic techniques is due to the fact that the site of rupture can be defined even when it is not clearly evident on two-dimensional echocardiography. Color flow imaging also provides good estimation of the size and relative magnitude of left-to-right shunt flow across the rupture site.[49] Flow acceleration can be seen proximal to the defect on the LV side of septum in nearly all patients. Continuous wave Doppler can be useful in estimating RV pressure. Several groups have reported the use of continuous wave Doppler to estimate RV pressure in adults with ventricular septal rupture.[4,49] The systolic gradient between the LV and RV determined by Doppler correlates with the hemodynamics ob-

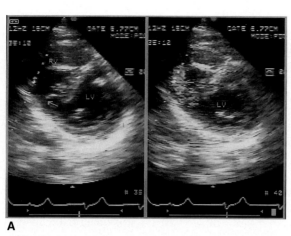
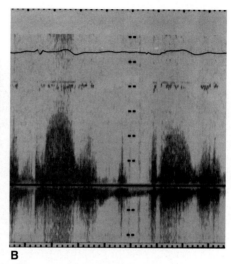

Figure 20-12. **(A)** Parasternal short axis view of the LV demonstrating thinning of the inferior septum (left panel) and a systolic flow disturbance evident by color flow imaging in a patient with ventricular septal rupture due to an acute inferior MI. (See also Color Plate 62.) **(B)** Continuous wave Doppler examination of the systolic jet of a ventricular septal rupture obtained with use of a nonimaging transducer. The velocity (3 m/sec) indicates a 36 mm Hg pressure difference between the LV and RV due to the patient's low systemic pressure of 70 mm Hg. The estimated RV pressure of 34 mm Hg closely correlated with pressures in the pulmonary artery obtained by right heart catheterization.

tained at cardiac catheterization. Since it is sometimes difficult to detect the maximal velocity with continuous wave Doppler, color flow imaging may be useful in directing the continuous wave Doppler cursor through the ventricular septal defect. TEE is also useful in patients with suspected septal rupture, particularly when transthoracic two-dimensional Doppler scanning is technically difficult.[71] Ballal et al. reported five patients with septal rupture detected by TEE and confirmed at surgery; in one patient, the rupture was missed by transthoracic echocardiography.[3] Interestingly, two of the five patients had dissection of the septum, and one had complex rupture within the dissection.

Studies in the echocardiographic literature emphasize the importance of assessing LV and RV function in these patients.[9,98] Ventricular septal rupture was reported by Moore et al. in 25 of 1264 (2%) consecutive patients with acute MI.[98] These investigators found that mortality was higher in those with inferior versus anterior infarcts, presumably due to extensive RV involvement (as documented on two-dimensional echocardiography). Others, utilizing two-dimensional echocardiography in patients with ventricular septal rupture, re-

ported that the extent of LV asynergy was twice as great in nonsurvivors than in survivors.[9]

The long-term outcome of ventricular septal ruptures is dismal, and patient management is difficult. Ventricular septal rupture tends to occur in patients during the first infarction when collateral circulation in the infarct region is limited.[52] Operative repair of acute ventricular septal defect carries a high mortality, but with medical therapy alone, death occurs in more than 80% of patients within 2 months of diagnosis. The mortality of patients who undergo early repair (<21 days after MI) of the ventricular septal rupture is high due to the poor physiologic status of the patient rather than to the timing of surgery.[98] Most clinicians advocate early closure to avoid further multisystemic deterioration, even though the extensive and recent myocardial necrosis may make the repair of the ventricular septal defect technically difficult.

LV FREE WALL RUPTURE

The occurrence of a large MI (lateral or posterolateral) in an elderly patient with post-MI hypertension and no prior coronary artery disease are predisposing factors in LV rupture.[104,116] LV ruptures can be seen within 48 hr of the acute MI, often accompanied by persistent ECG evidence of ST-segment elevation, chest pain, agitation, and repetitive emesis.[104] The site of rupture is often in the zone between necrotic and normal myocardial tissue, with leakage of blood (over hours) into the pericardium and resultant hemopericardium.[104] Hypotension and bradycardia due to cardiac tamponade become evident, and death follows unless surgical repair is attempted; even with this intervention, survival is rare. It is important to note that LV rupture is not always acute.

Two-dimensional echocardiography can demonstrate highly suspicious signs of myocardial rupture. Studies suggest that in patients with echocardiographically diagnosed ruptures there is a higher survival rate.[119] Reported features include pericardial effusion or intrapericardial clot localized at the site of infarction (with or without cardiac tamponade) and decreased LV wall thickness with regional dilatation. The sensitivity of pericardial effusion with clot formation at the site of rupture appears to be extremely high, but the specificity is lower. If pericardial tamponade is included as a criterion, specificity improves but sensitivity decreases.[81]

FUTURE DIRECTIONS: MYOCARDIAL CONTRAST AGENTS AND TISSUE CHARACTERIZATION WITH ULTRASOUND

For assessing myocardial perfusion and coronary flow reserve with contrast agents, two-dimensional echocardiography and TEE are a promising area of application.[56,60,63,68,75,104,116,117,124,128,132,147,158] Early studies used sonicated renografin, which has a large bubble size (20 μm), with adverse hemodynamic effects reported with injections. The injection of sonicated albumin, with a smaller microbubble size (4–6 μm), has been reported to have no hemodynamic effects.[104,117,128] The potential value of myocardial contrast echocardiography is in the identification of regional perfusion of the myocardium, since it may not be predictable from the coronary anatomy as visualized with coronary arteriography.[63] The extent of collateral circulation, commonly seen in patients with coronary artery disease, may be better defined with contrast echocardiography because coronary arteriography only defines vessels large than 100 μm in size.[56] Work with myocardial contrast echocardiography suggests that regional function is better in these collateralized beds, particularly when thrombolytic therapy is employed during acute MI, and results in less residual asynergy.[75] There are several factors, however, that must be considered before myocardial contrast echocardiography is widely accepted.

Microbubbles are scatterers rather than reflectors of ultrasound, with bubble concentration and size influencing the scatter energy. The rate of injection is critical, particularly when assessing transit times of perfusion and the "washout effect."[128] Bubbles are pressure sensitive and at high pressure will break down.[63,68] It is also known that coronary blood flow (CBF) is not quantifiable in regard to transmural distribution, with differences evident in the epicardium compared to the endocardium.[63] Measurements of CBF will be influenced by timing the appearance of the bubbles in relation to the cardiac cycle, myocardial mass, and LV filling pressures. Moreover, coronary flow reserve (ratio of hyperemic/baseline flow) needs to be determined with the injection of vasodilators to assess the difference in perfusion to regions supplied by critically stenotic arteries.[117] Current ultrasound instruments have certain limitations. The narrow dynamic range of image processing (30–70 dB) and the nonlinearity of postprocessing curves influence the signal intensity of the myocardial contrast effect and may not reflect the amount of agent delivered to the perfusion bed.[158] Acoustic power levels, if too high, will affect pixel intensity relative to bubble concentration.[159] Depth and attenuation may be additional factors. The problem of perfusion beds distal to the site of contrast effect (i.e., septum versus posterior wall) or at the apex are other obstacles. Digital subtraction techniques and color encoding have been used in some studies, but they require careful alignment of pre- and postcontrast images.[63]

Sonographer issues that need clarification include who inserts the intravenous line and performs the injection and what rates and dosages are necessary. Imaging views and transducer position/stability are concerns, as well as instrument settings (overall gain, transmit power). The cost of the agents is a matter of concern, as well as the time for quantification and other off-line equipment (i.e., for digital storage and videodensitometry) that will be needed. The reproducibility of myocardial contrast echocardiography also is not well established.[68] Another important issue remains unresolved: current applications of contrast opacification of the myocardium require that a catheter be positioned in the aortic root or left atrium. Consequently, two-dimensional echocardiography will need to be performed in the catheterization lab (where the patient is supine and imaging views are often suboptimal) or the operating room.

MYOCARDIAL TISSUE CHARACTERIZATION

Myocardial tissue characterization using analysis of backscattered radiofrequency signals is being employed in patients with coronary artery disease.[31,77,86,87,89,95,110,134,142,143,146,152] This technique remains promising, although widespread application has been limited to a few centers. The fundamental difference between quantitative myocardial tissue characterization and conventional echocardiography resides in the type of acoustic interface. In conventional imaging, specular reflections (i.e., the acoustic interface between endocardium and blood) are used for assessment of ventricular wall motion and thickness. Reflections occur because the incident ultrasonic wavelength is smaller than the dimensions of the boundary. Tissue characterization employing analysis of integrated backscatter radiofrequency (rf) signals also provides information regarding specular reflections, but imaging is directed to the intramyocardial echoes. The ultrasonic wavelength used is larger than the dimensions of the interfaces or boundaries among the different structural components. Instead of being reflected, as is the case in specular echoes, the incident waveforms are scattered in multiple directions, including a component that is redirected at 180 degrees to the transmitting transducer (i.e., backscattered). These backscattered radiofrequency waves result from the interactions of ultrasound and differences in the intramural and tissue structures. The amount of backscatter from a segment of tissue, expressed in decibels (i.e., integrated backscatter), is a descriptive parameter of tissue structure, and in principle it should be useful for characterization of the tissue in quantitative terms.

Although ultrasonic waveforms can be analyzed in different ways, one approach uses analysis of the radiofrequency signals backscattered from the myo-

cardium segment of interest in the time domain.[31,77,87,89,95,134,142,143,152] This method of estimating the backscatter uses a 3-μsec integration time, resulting in individual data points (typically 100) along each radiofrequency (A or scan) line in the composite two-dimensional view. The resulting average power from each radiofrequency line is compared with a reference power within the imaging system to express the integrated backscatter in decibels. There is no postprocessing of the radiofrequency acoustic data in this modified system, and the displayed real-time image is fully quantitated in decibels. Regional myocardial values of integrated backscatter can be obtained by placing a region of interest within the mural myocardium (avoiding the bright specular echoes of the endocardium–blood interfaces) in the real-time two-dimensional image or via an approach that uses M-mode, in which only a single line is directed to the segment of interest[31,77] (Figure 20-13).

Integrated backscatter of normal myocardium exhibits a cardiac cycle–dependent variation, with higher values (higher intensity) in late diastole and lower values in systole.[87] The diastolic-to-systolic cyclic variation in the myocardial integrated backscatter represents the principal parameter obtained currently in patients. Clinical studies carried out in patients with normal ventricular function demonstrate that the cyclic variation of myocardial integrated backscatter averages approximately 4–6 dB.[77] Qualitatively, intramyocardial echoes are relatively echo-dense during diastole compared to the intensity displayed in systole (i.e., the relative echo density of the intramyocardial echoes decreases). A correlative measurement is the delay, or phase, defined as the time from the onset of ventricular systole, denoted by the ECG R wave, to the nadir of the backscatter waveform from a segment divided by the duration of systole (approximated by the ECG QT interval). A value less than 1.0 can be seen in patients with normal regional myocardial characteristics.

Several factors may influence the cyclic variation of myocardial backscatter, including age and, importantly, the angle between beam direction and the myocardium where insonification must be as perpendicular as possible.[89,142] The most accurate values are obtained from the septum and posterior wall using parasternal long axis or short axis views. Posteroseptal, lateral, anterior, or apical regions do

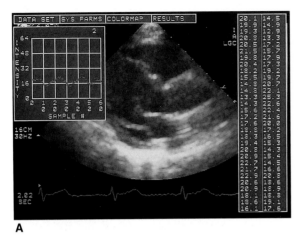 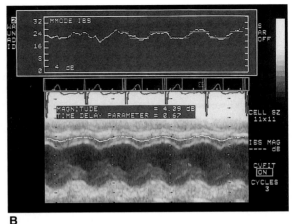

A   **B**

Figure 20-13. (**A**) Parasternal long axis view of the LV employing integrated backscatter imaging. A circular region of interest is positioned in the posterior wall. The graph on the left is the intensity (in decibels) display of the cyclic variation of backscatter, and the graph on the right shows the individual values of backscatter in decibels for 60 samples. (See also Color Plate 63.) (**B**) M-mode echocardiogram of the septum and left ventricular posterior wall employing integrated backscatter imaging. A region of interest has been traced through the midseptal myocardium with the graphic display of backscatter over time. The average magnitude of cyclic variation was normal (4:1 dB), as was the delay of 0.67 (normal, <1.0). (See also Color Plate 64.)

not exhibit cyclic variation of backscatter due to the angle between transducer position and the myocardium.[130] An M-mode approach to measuring the cyclic variation of backscatter of normal RV myocardium has been attempted, with limited success[152] due to the relative thinness of the RV myocardium. The magnitude of the cyclic variation of backscatter and the delay obtained from RV myocardium are comparable to those previously measured from the LV septum and posterior wall in normal patients.

ISCHEMIC OR INFARCTED MYOCARDIUM

Vered et al. studied 15 patients with prior MI and noted that segments with normal wall motion exhibited cyclic variation values of approximately 3.2 dB, whereas infarcted segments had significantly blunted values (mean, 1.1 dB).[146] The average delay is 0.87 in normal segments and 1.47 in those with remote infarction. Vandenberg et al. studied 18 patients after recent MI and reported that ischemic or infarcted regions exhibit lower values of cyclic variation than normal regions.[143] A subsequent study by Milunski et al. used integrated backscatter imaging (M-mode method) in 21 patients with acute MI, all of whom underwent coronary thrombolysis.[95] Patients who have reestab-

lished coronary flow in a previously occluded coronary vessel have partial recovery of cyclic variation in the affected myocardial segment, while patients with occluded vessels (i.e., no vessel patency) continue to exhibit blunted cyclic variation in the affected myocardial segments at follow-up. Independent analysis of the conventional two-dimensional images reveals no significant changes in wall motion or thickening between the time of the two studies in all patients. Therefore, these results suggest that tissue characterization may have a role in identifying viable but stunned myocardium in the setting of acute ischemia.

The observed reductions in the amplitude of the cyclic variation in integrated backscatter from ischemic and infarcted myocardium are probably related to edema in ischemic tissue or collagen deposition that replaces normal myocardium in the infarcted segment. Cardiac specimens removed at necropsy from patients with myocardial fibrosis revealed that the collagen content correlates strongly with the level of myocardial integrated backscatter.[110] Therefore, blunted or absent cyclic variation in clinical studies of patients with remote infarction is probably due to collagen deposition, associated loss of segmental contractile function, or a combination of these factors.[86] It is likely that collagen accumulation in the infarcted segment is responsible for the increased echo density representing the "scar" seen in patients late after MI.

REFERENCES

1. Asinger RW, Mikell F, Elsperger J, et al. Incidence of left ventricular thrombosis after acute transmural myocardial infarction: Serial evaluation by two dimensional echocardiography. N Engl J Med. 1981; 305:297–302.
2. Asinger RW, Mikell F, Sharma B, et al. Observations on detecting left ventricular thrombus with two dimensional echocardiography: Emphasis on avoidance of false positive diagnosis. Am J Cardiol. 1981;47:145–156.
3. Ballal RS, Sanyal RS, Nanda NC, et al. Usefulness of transesophageal echocardiography in the diagnosis of ventricular septal rupture secondary to acute myocardial infarction. Am J Cardiol. 1993;71: 367–369.
4. Bansal RS, Eng AK, Skakudo M. Role of two dimensional echocardiography, pulsed continuous wave and color flow Doppler techniques in the assessment of ventricular septal rupture after acute myocardial infarction. Am J Cardiol. 1990;65: 852–860.
5. Bargiggia GS, Tronconi L, Sahn DJ, et al. A new method for quantitation of mitral regurgitation based on color flow Doppler imaging of flow convergence proximal to regurgitant orifice. Circulation. 1991;84:1481–1489.
6. Barzilai B, Gessler C, Perez JE, et al. Significance of Doppler detected mitral regurgitation in acute myocardial infarction. Am J Cardiol. 1988;61: 220–223.
7. Baur HR, Daniel JA, Nelson RR. Detection of left ventricular aneurysm on two dimensional echocardiography. Am J Cardiol. 1982;50:191–196.
8. Bhatia S, Plappert T, Theard M, et al. Transseptal Doppler flow velocity profile in acquired ventricular septal defect in acute myocardial infarction. Am J Cardiol. 1987;60:372–373.
9. Bishop HL, Gibson RS, Stamm RB, et al. Role of two dimensional echocardiography in the evaluation of patients with ventricular septal rupture post myocardial infarction. Am Heart J. 1981;102: 965–971.
10. Botvinick EH, Shames D, Hutchinson JC, et al. Non-invasive diagnosis of a false left ventricular aneurysm with radioisotope gated cardiac blood pool imaging. Am J Cardiol. 1976;37:1089–1093.
11. Bourdillon PDV, Broderick TM, Williams ES, et al. Early recovery of regional left ventricular function after reperfusion in acute myocardial infarction assessed by serial two dimensional echocardiography. Am J Cardiol. 1989;63:641–646.
12. Braunwald E, Rutherford JD. Reversible ischemic left ventricular dysfunction: Evidence for the hibernating myocardium. J Am Coll Cardiol. 1986;8: 1467–1470.
13. Candell-Riera J, Figueras J, Valle V, et al. Right ventricular infarction: Relationships between ST segment elevation in V4R and hemodynamic, scintigraphic and echocardiographic findings in patients with acute inferior myocardial infarction. Am Heart J. 1981;101:281–287.
14. Catherwood E, Mintz GS, Kotler MN, et al. Two dimensional echocardiographic recognition of left ventricular pseudoaneurysm. Circulation. 1980;62: 294–302.
15. Cecchi F, Zuppiroli A, Di Bari M, et al. Echocardiographic features of right ventricular infarction. Clin Cardiol. 1984;7:405–412.
16. Charuzi Y, Beeder C, Marshall LA, et al. Improvement in regional and global left ventricular function after intracoronary thrombolysis: Assessment with two dimensional echocardiography. Am J Cardiol. 1984;53:662–665.
17. Chatterjee K. Complications of acute myocardial infarction. Curr Probl Cardiol. 1993;18(1):7–79.
18. Chen C, Koschyk D, Brockhoff C, et al. Noninvasive estimation of regurgitant flow rate and volume in patients with mitral regurgitation by Doppler color flow imaging of accelerating flow field. J Am Coll Cardiol. 1993;21:374–383.
19. Chenzbraun A, Keren A, Stern S. Doppler echocardiographic patterns of left ventricular filling in patients early after acute myocardial infarction. Am J Cardiol. 1992;70:711–714.
20. Cohn JN, Guiha NH, Broder MI, et al. Right ventricular infarction. Am J Cardiol. 1974;33: 209–214.
21. Come P. Doppler detection of acquired ventricular septal defect. Am J Cardiol. 1985;55:586–588.
22. Come PL, Riley MF, Weintraub R, et al. Echocardiographic detection of complete and partial papillary muscle rupture during acute myocardial infarction. Am J Cardiol. 1985;56:787–789.
23. D'Arcy B, Nanda NC. Two dimensional echocardiographic features of right ventricular infarction. Circulation. 1982;65:167–173.
24. DeMaria AN, Bommer W, Neumann A, et al. Left ventricular thrombi identified by cross-sectional echocardiography. Ann Intern Med. 1979;90: 14–18.
25. Drobac M, Gilbert B, Howard R, et al. Ventricular septal defect after myocardial infarction: Diagnosis

by two dimensional contrast echocardiography. Circulation. 1983;67:335–341.

26. Eigler N, Maurer G, Shah PK. Effect of early systemic thrombolytic therapy on left ventricular mural thrombus formation in acute anterior myocardial infarction. Am J Cardiol. 1984;54: 261–263.

27. Eisenberg P, Barzilai B, Perez J. Noninvasive detection by Doppler echocardiography of combined ventricular septal rupture and mitral regurgitation in acute myocardial infarction. J Am Coll Cardiol. 1984;4:617–620.

28. Ekekowitz MD, Wilson DA, Smith DO, et al. Comparison of Indium-111 platelet scintigraphy and two dimensional echocardiography in the diagnosis of left ventricular thrombi. N Engl J Med. 1987; 306:1509–1513.

29. Erlebacher JA, Weiss JL, Eaton LW, et al. Late effects of acute infarct dilatation on heart size: A two dimensional echocardiographic study. Am J Cardiol. 1982;49:1120–1126.

30. Farcot JC, Boisante L, Rigand M, et al. Two dimensional echocardiographic visualization of ventricular septal rupture after acute anterior myocardial infarction. Am J Cardiol. 1980;45:370–377.

31. Feinberg MS, Gussak HM, D'Sa AP, et al. Ultrasonic tissue characterization based on 2D integrated backscatter images: Quantitative scattering of normal, hypertrophic, and asynergic myocardial segments (abstract). J Am Soc Echocardiogr. 1994; 7:S45.

32. Force T, Kemper A, Perkins L, et al. Over-estimation of infarct size by quantitative two dimensional echocardiography: The role of tethering and of analytic procedures. Circulation. 1986;73: 1360–1368.

33. Force T, Parisi AF. Quantitative methods for analyzing regional systolic function with two dimensional echocardiography. Echocardiography. 1986; 3:319–331.

34. Fouet X, Pillot M, Leizorovicz A, et al. "Non Q-wave," alias "non transmural," myocardial infarction: A specific entity. Am Heart J. 1989;117: 892–902.

35. Freeman AP, Giles RW, Walsh WF, et al. Regional left ventricular wall motion assessment: Comparison of two dimensional echocardiography and radionuclide angiography with contrast angiography in healed myocardial infarction. Am J Cardiol. 1985;56:8–12.

36. Freeman WK, Miller FA, Oh JK, et al. Postinfarct ventricular septal rupture: Diagnosis and management facilitated by two dimensional and Doppler echocardiography. Echocardiography. 1987;4: 75–81.

37. Friedman MJ, Carlson K, Marcus FI, et al. Clinical correlations in patients with acute myocardial infarction and left ventricular thrombus detected by two dimensional echocardiography. Am J Med. 1982;72:894–898.

38. Garrahy PJ, Kwan OL, Booth DC, et al. Assessment of abnormal systolic intraventricular flow patterns by Doppler imaging in patients with left ventricular dyssynergy. Circulation. 1990;82:95–104.

39. Gatewood RP, Nanda NC. Differentiation of left ventricular pseudoaneurysm from true aneurysm with two dimensional echocardiography. Am J Cardiol. 1980;46:869–878.

40. Geft IL, Shah PK, Rodriguez L, et al. ST elevations in leads V1 and V5 may be caused by right coronary artery occlusion and acute right ventricular infarction. Am J Cardiol. 1984;53:991–996.

41. Gibson RS, Bishop HL, Stamm RB, et al. Value of early two dimensional echocardiography in patients with acute myocardial infarction. Am J Cardiol. 1982;49:1110–1119.

42. Gibson RS. Non Q wave myocardial infarction: Diagnosis, prognosis and management. Curr Probl Cardiol. 1988;13:1–72.

43. Gibson RS. Non Q wave myocardial infarction: Prognosis, changing incidence and management. *In* Gersh BJ, Rahimtoola SH (ed): Acute Myocardial Infarction. Current Topics in Cardiology. New York, Elsevier; 1991:284–307.

44. Giesler M, Grossmann G, Schmidt A, et al. Color Doppler echocardiographic determination of mitral regurgitant flow from the proximal velocity profile of the flow convergence region. Am J Cardiol. 1993;71:217–224.

45. Grube E, Redel D, Janson R. Noninvasive diagnosis of a false left ventricular aneurysm by echocardiography and pulsed Doppler echocardiography. Br Heart J. 1980;43:232–236.

46. Harrison MR, MacPhail B, Gurley JC, et al. Usefulness of color Doppler flow imaging to distinguish ventricular septal defect from acute mitral regurgitation complicating acute myocardial infarction. Am J Cardiol. 1989;64:697–701.

47. Haugland JM, Asinger RW, Mikell FL, et al. Embolic potential of left ventricular thrombi detected by two dimensional echocardiography. Circulation. 1984;70:588–598.

48. Heger JJ, Weyman AE, Wann LS, et al. Cross-sectional echocardiographic analysis of the extent of left ventricular asynergy in acute myocardial infarction. Circulation. 1980;61:113–118.

49. Helmcke F, Mahan EF, Nanda NC, et al. Two dimensional echocardiography and Doppler color flow mapping in the diagnosis and prognosis of ven-

tricular septal rupture. Circulation. 1990;81: 1775–1783.

50. Horowitz RS, Morganroth J, Parrott C, et al. Immediate diagnosis of acute myocardial infarction by two dimensional echocardiography. Circulation. 1982;65:323–329.

51. Horowitz RS, Morganroth J. Immediate detection of early high risk patients with acute myocardial infarction using two dimensional echocardiographic evaluation of left ventricular regional wall motion abnormalities. Am Heart J. 1982;103:814–822.

52. Hutchins GM, Bulkley BH. Infarct expansion versus extension: Two different complications of acute myocardial infarction. Am J Cardiol. 1978;41: 1127–1132.

53. Hutchins GM. Rupture of the interventricular septum complicating myocardial infarction: Pathologic analysis of 10 patients with clinically diagnosed perforations. Am Heart J. 1979;97:165–173.

54. Isner JM, Mosseri M. Right ventricular myocardial infarction: Clinical aspects. Coronary Artery Dis. 1990;1:287–297.

55. Isner JM, Roberts WC. Right ventricular infarction complicating left ventricular infarction secondary to coronary heart disease. Am J Cardiol. 1978;42: 885–894.

56. Ito H, Tomooka T, Sakai N, et al. Lack of myocardial perfusion immediately after successful thrombolysis: A predictor of poor recovery of left ventricular function in anterior myocardial infarction. Circulation. 1992;85:1699–1705.

57. Izumi S, Miyatake K, Beppu S, et al. Mechanisms of mitral regurgitation in patients with myocardial infarction: A study using real two dimensional Doppler flow imaging and echocardiography. Circulation. 1986;76:777–785.

58. Jugdutt BI, Sivaram CA, Wortman C, et al. Prospective two-dimensional echocardiographic evaluation of left ventricular thrombus and embolism after acute myocardial infarction. J Am Coll Cardiol. 1989;13:554–564.

59. Jugdutt BI, Sussex BA, Sivaram CA, et al. Right ventricular infarction: Two dimensional echocardiographic evaluation. Am Heart J. 1984;107: 505–518.

60. Kabas JS, Kisslo J, Flick CL, et al. Intraoperative perfusion contrast echocardiography: Initial experience during coronary artery bypass grafting. J Thorac Cardiovasc Surg. 1990;99:536–542.

61. Katz RJ, Simpson A, Dibianco R, et al. Noninvasive diagnosis of left ventricular pseudo-aneurysm. Role of two dimensional echocardiography and radionuclide gated pool imaging. Am J Cardiol. 1979;44: 372–376.

62. Kaul S, Josephson MA, Tei C, et al. A typical echocardiographic and angiographic presentation of a postoperative pseudoaneurysm of the left ventricle after repair of a true aneurysm. J Am Coll Cardiol. 1983;2:780–784.

63. Kaul S. Clinical applications of myocardial contrast echocardiography. Am J Cardiol. 1992;69: 46H–55H.

64. Keating EC, Gross SA, Schlamowitz RA, et al. Mural thrombi in myocardial infarctions: Prospective evaluation by two dimensional echocardiography. Am J Med. 1983;74:989–995.

65. Keren A, Goldberg S, Gottlieb S, et al. Natural history of left ventricular thrombi: Their appearance and resolution in the posthospitalization period of acute myocardial infarction. J Am Coll Cardiol. 1990;15:790–800.

66. Keren G, Sherez J, Roth A, et al. Diagnosis of ventricular septal rupture from acute myocardial infarction by combined two dimensional and pulsed Doppler echocardiography. Am J Cardiol. 1984; 53:1202–1203.

67. Kessler KM, Kieval J, Saksena S, et al. Echocardiographic features of posterior left ventricular wall pseudoaneurysm due to *Escherichia coli* endocarditis. Am Heart J. 1982;103:139–142.

68. Klein AL, Bailey AS, Moura A, et al. Reliability of echocardiographic measurements of myocardial perfusion using commercially produced sonicated serium albumin (Albunex). J Am Coll Cardiol. 1993;22:1983–1993.

69. Klone RA, Parisi AF. Acute myocardial infarctions: Diagnostic and prognostic applications of two dimensional echocardiography. Circulation. 1987; 75:521–524.

70. Koenig K, Kasper W, Hofman T, et al. Transesophageal echocardiography for diagnosis of rupture of the ventricular septum or left ventricular papillary muscle during acute myocardial infarction. Am J Cardiol. 1987;59:362.

71. Koenig K, Kasper W, Hofmann T, et al. Transesophageal echocardiography for diagnosis of rupture of the ventricular septum or left ventricular papillary muscle during acute myocardial infarction. Am J Cardiol. 1987;59:362–365.

72. Kono T, Sabbah HN, Stein PD, et al. Left ventricular shape as a determinant of functional mitral regurgitation in patients with severe heart failure secondary to either coronary artery disease or idiopathic dilated cardiomyopathy. Am J Cardiol. 1991;68:355–359.

73. Labovitz AJ, Lewen MK, Kern M, et al. Evaluation of left ventricular systolic and diastolic dysfunction during transient myocardial ischemia produced by

angioplasty. J Am Coll Cardiol. 1987;10:748–755.

74. Levy R, Rozanski A, Chanuzi Y, et al. Complementary roles of two dimensional echocardiography and radionuclide ventriculography in ventricular pseudoaneurysm diagnosis. Am Heart J. 1981;102:1066–1069.

75. Lim Y, Nanto S, Masuyama T, et al. Coronary collaterals assessed with myocardial contrast echocardiography in healed myocardial infarction. Am J Cardiol. 1990;66:556–561.

76. Loh IK, Charnzi Y, Beeder C, et al. Early diagnosis of nontransmural myocardial infarction by two dimensional echocardiography. Am Heart J. 1982;104:963–968.

77. Loomis JF, Waggoner AD, Schechtman KB, et al. Ultrasonic integrated backscatter two-dimensional imaging: Evaluation of M-mode guided acquisition and immediate analysis in 55 consecutive patients. J Am Soc Echocardiogr. 1990;3:255–265.

78. Loperfido F, Biasucci LM, Pennestri F, et al. Pulsed Doppler echocardiographic analysis of mitral regurgitation after myocardial infarction. Am J Cardiol. 1986;58:692–697.

79. Loperfido F, Pennestri F, Mazzari M, et al. Diagnosis of left ventricular pseudoaneurysm by pulsed Doppler echocardiography. Am Heart J. 1985;110:1291–1298.

80. Lopez-Sendon J, Coma-Canella I, Ascasena S, et al. Electrocardiographic findings in acute right ventricular infarction: Sensitivity and specificity of electrocardiographic alterations in right precordial leads V4R, V3R, V1, V2, and V3. J Am Coll Cardiol. 1985;6:1273–1279.

81. Lopez-Sendon J, Coma-Canella I, Gamall C. Sensitivity and specificity of hemodynamic criteria in the diagnosis of acute right ventricular infarction. Circulation. 1981;64:515–525.

82. Lopez-Sendon J, Garcia-Fernandez MA, Coma-Canella I, et al. Segmental right ventricular function after acute myocardial infarction: Two dimensional echocardiographic study in 63 patients. Am J Cardiol. 1983;51:390–396.

83. Lopez-Sendon J, Gonzalez A, Lopez De Sae, et al. Diagnosis of subacute ventricular wall rupture after acute myocardial infarction: Sensitivity and specificity of clinical, hemodynamic and echocardiographic criteria. J Am Coll Cardiol. 1992;19:1145–1153.

84. Lorrell B, Leinbach RC, Pohost GM, et al. Right ventricular infarction. Clinical diagnosis and differentiation from cardiac tamponade and pericardial constriction. Am J Cardiol. 1979;43:464–471.

85. Lundgren C, Bourdillon PDV, Dillon JC, et al. Comparison of contrast angiography and two dimensional echocardiography for the evaluation of left ventricular regional wall motion abnormalities after acute myocardial infarction. Am J Cardiol. 1990;65:1071–1073.

86. Lythall DA, Logan-Sinclair RB, Ilsley CJD, et al. Relation between cyclic variation in echo amplitude and segmental contraction in normal and abnormal hearts. Br Heart J. 1991;66:268–276.

87. Madaras EI, Barzilai B, Perez JE, et al. Changes in myocardial backscatter throughout the cardiac cycle. Ultrasonic Imaging. 1983;5:229–239.

88. Marshall SA, Picard MH, Ray PA, et al. Ventricular morphology and function in acute non Q wave myocardial infarction (abstract). Circulation. 1990;82(suppl III):III–73.

89. Masuyama T, Nellessen U, Schnittger I, et al. Ultrasonic tissue characterization with real time integrated backscatter imaging system in normal and aging human hearts. J Am Coll Cardiol. 1989;14:1702–1708.

90. Matsumoto M, Watanbe F, Goto A, et al. Left ventricular aneurysm and the prediction of left ventricular enlargement studied by two dimensional echocardiography: Quantitative assessment of aneurysm size in relation to clinical course. Circulation. 1985;72:280–286.

91. Maurer G, Czer LSC, Shah PK, et al. Assessment by Doppler color flow mapping of ventricular septal defect after acute myocardial infarction. Am J Cardiol. 1989;64:668–670.

92. Maze SS, Kotler MN, Parry W. Flow characteristics in the dilated left ventricle with thrombus: Qualitative and quantitative Doppler analysis. J Am Coll Cardiol. 1989;13:873–881.

93. McKay RG, Pfeffer MA, Pasternak RC, et al. Left ventricular remodeling after myocardial infarction: A corollary to infarct expansion. Circulation. 1986;74:693–702.

94. Meltzer RS, Visser CA, Kan G, et al. Two dimensional echocardiographic appearance of left ventricular thrombi with systemic emboli after myocardial infarction. Am J Cardiol. 1984;53:1511–1513.

95. Milunski MR, Mohr GA, Perez JE, et al. Ultrasonic tissue characterization with integrated backscatter: Acute myocardial ischemia, reperfusion, and stunned myocardium in patients. Circulation. 1989;80:491–503.

96. Mintz GS, Victor MF, Kotler MN, et al. Two dimensional echocardiographic identification of surgically correctable complications of acute myocardial infarction. Circulation. 1981;64:91–96.

97. Miyatake K, Okamoto M, Kinoshita N, et al. Doppler echocardiographic features of ventricular septal

defect in myocardial infarction. J Am Coll Cardiol. 1985;5:182–187.

98. Moore CA, Nygaard TW, Kaiser DL, et al. The importance of location of infarction and right ventricular function in determining survival. Circulation. 1986;74:45–55.

99. Nidorf SM, Siu SC, Galambos G, et al. Benefit of late coronary reperfusion on ventricular morphology and function after myocardial infarction. J Am Coll Cardiol. 1993;21:683–691.

100. Nishimura RA, Schaff HV, Shub C, et al. Papillary muscle rupture complicating acute myocardial infarction: Analysis of 17 patients. Am J Cardiol. 1983;51:373–377.

101. Nishmura RA, Tajik AJ, Shub C, et al. Role of two dimensional echocardiography in the prediction of in hospital complications after acute myocardial infarction. J Am Coll Cardiol. 1984;6:1080–1087.

102. Ogawa H, Hiramori K, Haze K, et al. Comparison of clinical features of non Q wave and Q wave infarctions. Am Heart J. 1986;111:513–518.

103. Oh JK, Ding ZP, Gersh BJ, et al. Restrictive left ventricular diastolic filling identifies patients with heart failure after acute myocardial infarction. J Am Soc Echocardiogr. 1992;5:497–503.

104. Oliva PB, Hammill SC, Edwards WD. Cardiac rupture, a clinically predictable complication of acute myocardial infarction: Report of 70 cases with clinicopathologic correlations. J Am Coll Cardiol. 1993;22:720–726.

105. Otto CM, Stratton JR, Maynard C, et al. Echocardiographic evaluation of segmental wall motion early and late after thrombolytic therapy in acute myocardial infarction: The Western Washington Tissue Plasminogen Activator Emergency Room Trial. Am J Cardiol. 1990;65:132–138.

106. Pandian NG, Kieso RA, Kerber RE. Two dimensional echocardiography in experimental coronary stenosis. II: Relationship between systolic wall thinning and regional myocardial perfusion in severe coronary stenosis. Circulation. 1982;66:603–611.

107. Panidis IP, Mintz GS, Goel I, et al. Acquired ventricular septal defect after myocardial infarction: Detection by combined two dimensional and Doppler echocardiography. Am Heart J. 1986;111:427–429.

108. Peels CH, Visser CA, Funke Kupper AJ, et al. Usefulness of two dimensional echocardiography for immediate detection of myocardial ischemia in the emergency room. Am J Cardiol. 1990;65:687–691.

109. Penco M, Romano S, Angati L, et al. Influence of reperfusion induced by thrombolytic treatment on natural history of left ventricular regional wall motion abnormality in acute myocardial infarction. Am J Cardiol. 1993;71:1015–1020.

110. Perez JE, McGill JB, Santiago JV, et al. Abnormal myocardial acoustic properties in diabetic patients and their correlation with the severity of disease. J Am Coll Cardiol. 1992;19:1154–1162.

111. Pfeffer MA, Braunwald E. Ventricular remodeling after myocardial infarction: Experimental observations and clinical implications. Circulation. 1990; 81:1161–1172.

112. Picard MH, Ray P, Weyman AE. Left ventricular size and function during the year following acute myocardial infarction (abstract). J Am Coll Cardiol. 1991;17:2A.

113. Picard MH, Wilkins GT, Ray PA, et al. Natural history of left ventricular size and function after acute myocardial infarction. Assessment and prediction by echocardiographic endocardial surface mapping. Circulation. 1990;82:484–494.

114. Picard MH, Wilkins GT, Ray PA, et al. Progressive changes in ventricular structure and function during the year after acute myocardial infarction. Am Heart J. 1992;124:24–31.

115. Pipilis A, Meyer TE, Ormerod O, et al. Early and late changes in left ventricular filling after acute myocardial infarction and the effect of infarct size. Am J Cardiol. 1992;70:1397–1401.

116. Pohoja-Sintonen S, Muller JE, Stone PH, et al. Ventricular septal and free wall rupture complicating acute myocardial infarction: Experience in the multicenter investigation of limitation of infarct size. Am Heart J. 1989;117:809–818.

117. Quinones MA, Cheirif J. New perspectives for perfusion imaging in echocardiography. Circulation. 1991;83(suppl III):I104–I110.

118. Rahimtoola SH. The hibernating myocardium. Am Heart J. 1989;117:211–221.

119. Raitt MH, Kraft CD, Gardner CJ, et al. Subacute ventricular free wall rupture complicating acute myocardial infarction. Am Heart J. 1993;126:946–955.

120. Ratliff NB, Hackel DB. Combined right and left ventricular infarction: Pathogenesis and clinicopathologic correlations. Am J Cardiol. 1980;45:217–221.

121. Recusani F, Raisaro A, Sgalambro A, et al. Ventricular septal defect after myocardial infarction: Diagnosis by two dimensional and pulsed Doppler echocardiography. Am J Cardiol. 1984;54:277–281.

122. Reeder GS, Gersh BJ. Modern management of acute myocardial infarction. Curr Probl Cardiol. 1993;18:81–156.

123. Reeder GS, Seward JB, Tajik AS. The role of two dimensional echocardiography in coronary artery

disease. A critical appraisal. Mayo Clin Proc. 1982; 57:247–258.

124. Reisner SA, Ong LS, Lictenberg GS, et al. Quantitative assessment of the immediate results of coronary angioplasty by myocardial contrast echocardiography. J Am Coll Cardiol. 1989;13:852–856.

125. Roberts WC, Morrow AG. Pseudoaneurysm of the left ventricle. An unusual sequel of myocardial infarction and rupture of the heart. Am J Med. 1967; 43:639–644.

126. Roelandt J, Vanden Brand M, Vietter WB, et al. Echocardiographic diagnosis of pseudoaneurysm of the left ventricle. Circulation. 1975;52:466–472.

127. Roelandt JT, Sutherland GR, Yoshida K, et al. Improved diagnosis and characterization of left ventricular pseudoaneurysm by Doppler color flow imaging. J Am Coll Cardiol. 1988;12:807–811.

128. Rovai D, Lombardi M, Distante A, et al. Myocardial perfusion by contrast echocardiography. From off-line processing to radiofrequency analysis. Circulation. 1991;83(suppl III):97–103.

129. Saner HE, Asinger RW, Daniel JA, et al. Two dimensional echocardiographic identification of left ventricular pseudoaneurysm. Am Heart J. 1986; 112:977–985.

130. Scanlan JG, Seward JB, Tajik AJ. Visualization of ventricular septal rupture utilizing wide angle two dimensional echocardiography. Mayo Clin Proc 1979;54:381–384.

131. Sears TD, Ong YS, Starke H, et al. Left ventricular pseudoaneurysm identified by cross-sectional echocardiography. Ann Intern Med. 1979;90:936–939.

132. Shapiro JR, Reisner SA, Amico AF, et al. Reproducibility of quantitative myocardial contrast echocardiography. J Am Coll Cardiol. 1990;15:602–609.

133. Shen W, Khandheria BK, Edwards WD, et al. Values and limitations of two dimensional echocardiography in predicting myocardial infarct size. Am J Cardiol. 1991;68:1143–1149.

134. Skorton DJ, Miller JG, Wickline S, et al. Ultrasonic characterization of cardiovascular tissue. *In* Marcus ML, Schelbert HR, Skorton DJ, et al. (eds): Cardiac Imaging—A Companion to Braunwald's Heart Disease. Philadelphia, WB Saunders; 1991: 538–556.

135. Smeal WE, Dianzumba SB, Joyner CR. Evaluation of pseudoaneurysm of the left ventricle by echocardiography and pulsed Doppler. Am Heart J. 1987; 113:1508–1510.

136. Smith M, Ratshin RA, Harrell FE, et al. Early sequential changes in left ventricular dimension and filling pressures in patients after acute myocardial infarction. Am J Cardiol. 1974;33:363–369.

137. Spirito P, Bellotti P, Chiarella F, et al. Prognostic significance and natural history of left ventricular thrombi in patients with acute anterior myocardial infarction: A two dimensional echocardiographic study. Circulation. 1985;72:774–780.

138. Stamm RB, Gibson RS, Bishop HL, et al. Echocardiographic detection of infarct-localized asynergy and remote asynergy during acute myocardial infarction: Correlation with the extent of angiographic coronary disease. Circulation. 1983;67: 233–244.

139. Stratton JR, Lighty GW, Pearlman AS, et al. Detection of left ventricular thrombus by two dimensional echocardiography sensitivity, specificity, and causes of uncertainty. Circulation. 1982;66: 156–166.

140. Tunick PA, Slater W, Kronzon I. The hemodynamics of left ventricular pseudoaneurysm: Color Doppler echocardiographic study. Am Heart J. 1989;117:1161–1164.

141. Van Brabandt H, Piessens J, Stalpaert J, et al. Pseudoaneurysm of the left ventricle following cardiac surgery: Report of 3 cases and review of the literature. Thorac Cardiovasc Surg. 1985;33:118–124.

142. Van Reet RE, Quinones MA, Poliner LR, et al. Comparison of two dimensional echocardiography with gated radionuclide ventriculography in the evaluation of global and regional left ventricular function in acute myocardial infarction. J Am Coll Cardiol. 1984;3:243–252.

143. Vandenberg BF, Rath L, Shoup TA, et al. Cyclic variation of ultrasound backscatter in normal myocardium is view dependent: Clinical studies with real-time backscatter imaging system. J Am Soc Echocardiogr. 1989;2:308–314.

144. Vandenberg BF, Stuhlmuller JE, Rath L, et al. Diagnosis of recent myocardial infarction with quantitative backscatter imaging: Preliminary results. J Am Soc Echocardiogr. 1991;4:10–18.

145. Vandervoort PM, Rivera JM, Mele D, et al. Application of Doppler color flow mapping to calculate effective regurgitant orifice area. An in-vitro study and initial clinical observations. Circulation. 1993; 88:1150–1156.

146. Vered Z, Mohr GA, Barzilai B, et al. Ultrasonic integrated backscatter tissue characterization of remote myocardial infarction in human subjects. J Am Coll Cardiol. 1989;13:84–91.

147. Villanueva FS, Glasheen WP, Sklenar J, et al. Characterization of spatial patterns of flow within the reperfused myocardium by myocardial contrast echocardiography. Implications in determining extent of myocardial salvage. Circulation. 1993;88: 2595–2606.

148. Visser CA, Kan G, David GK, et al. Echocardiographic–cineangiographic correlation in detecting left ventricular aneurysm: A prospective study of 422 patients. Am J Cardiol. 1982;50:337–341.

149. Visser CA, Kan G, Meltzer RS, et al. Incidence, timing and prognostic value of left ventricular aneurysm formation after myocardial infarction: A prospective, serial echocardiographic study of 158 patients. Am J Cardiol. 1986;57:729–732.

150. Visser CA, Kan G, Meltzer RS, et al. Long term follow-up of left ventricular thrombus after acute myocardial infarction: Two dimensional echocardiographic study in 96 patients. Chest. 1984;86:532–536.

151. Visser CA, Lie KI, Kan G, et al. Detection and quantification of acute, isolated myocardial infarction by two dimensional echocardiography. Am J Cardiol. 1981;47:1020–1025.

152. Waggoner AD, Perez JE, Miller JG, et al. Differentiation of normal and ischemic right ventricular myocardium with quantitative two dimensional integrated backscatter imaging. Ultrasound Med Biol. 1992;18:249–253.

153. Wang R, DeSantola JR, Reichek N, et al. An unusual case of postoperative pseudoaneurysm of the left ventricle: Doppler echocardiographic findings. J Am Coll Cardiol. 1986;8:699–702.

154. Warren SE, Royal HD, Markis JE, et al. Time course of left ventricular dilation after myocardial infarction: Influence of infarct-related artery and success of coronary thrombolysis. J Am Coll Cardiol. 1988;11:12–19.

155. Weinrich DJ, Burke JF, Pamletto FJ. Left ventricular mural thrombi complicating acute myocardial infarction: Long term follow up with serial echocardiography. Ann Intern Med. 1984;100:789–794.

156. Weiss JL, Bulkley BH, Hutchins GM, et al. Two dimensional echocardiographic recognition of myocardial injury in man: Comparison with post-mortem studies. Circulation. 1981;63:401–407.

157. Weyman AE, Peskoe SM, Williams ES, et al. Detection of left ventricular aneurysms by cross-sectional echocardiography. Circulation. 1976;54:936–944.

158. Wiencek JG, Feinstein SB, Walker R, et al. Pitfalls in quantitative contrast echocardiography: The steps to quantitation of perfusion. J Am Soc Echocardiogr. 1993;6:395–416.

159. Wray RA, Quinones MA, Zoghbi WA, et al. Relation of mean pixel intensity to concentration of sonicated albumin microspheres: Effects of ultrasound system settings. Clin Cardiol 1991(suppl V);14:V23–V28.

160. Yasuda T, Okada RD, Leinbach RL, et al. Serial evaluation of right ventricular dysfunction associated with acute inferior myocardial infarction. Am Heart J. 1990;199:816–822.

161. Zachariah ZP, Hsiung MC, Nanda NL, et al. Diagnosis of rupture of the ventricular septum during acute myocardial infarction by Doppler color flow mapping. Am J Cardiol. 1987;59:162–163.

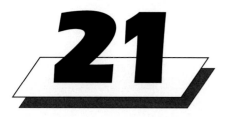

Stress Echocardiography in Coronary Artery Disease

MARK N. ALLEN

In coronary artery disease, left ventricular function may be normal, wall motion abnormalities are not always present, and a routine echocardiogram will not reveal any abnormality. A stress test, either exercise or pharmacologically induced, combined with echocardiography helps identify patients with stress-induced ischemia. Newer technologies make stress echocardiography one of the diagnostic methods of choice for evaluating ischemia. Practical applications and techniques for stress echocardiography are covered in Chapters 7 and 12.

In the United States, treadmill exercise is the most common form of stress echocardiography. The major disadvantage of exercise echocardiography is the inability to obtain images during the exercise portion. Images are obtained after the patient stops exercising, walks back to the exam bed, and gets into the left lateral decubitus position. During this time, heart rate and left ventricular contractility begin to return to normal. Recovery depends on how vigorous the exercise is.[1] Patients should be encouraged to exercise as much as possible to make the test more diagnostic. Digital equipment is essential, and allows capture of resting and postexercise images with side-by-side display of the same views. The cardiac cycle with no respiratory interference also can be captured.

Pharmacological versus Exercise Stress Echocardiography

The forms of stress echocardiography (Table 21-1) range from exercise using a treadmill or stationary bike to drug inducing agents. For patients who are unable to perform an adequate exercise type of exam, a form of nonexercise stress testing must be used. These exams essentially have the same effect as exercise echocardiography: they increase myocardial oxygen demand and alter myocardial blood flow. Dobutamine is an ideal agent because it increases myocardial oxygen demand by increasing heart rate, blood pressure, and contractility,[3,5,6,9,11] which simulates exercise without actually exerting the patient. Agents such as dipyridamole and adenosine are potent coronary vasodilators and provoke myocardial ischemia by creating a supply and demand mismatch.[2]

Pharmacologic agents are used instead of exercise in patients with peripheral vascular disease, amputations, or any inability to ambulate. Patients in whom adequate exercise would not be achieved should be considered for pharmacologic stress echocardiography. The results with dobutamine are good (sensitivity, 76%–90%; specificity, 70%–90%).[3,5,6,9,11] Sensitivity is highest for multivessel disease. Dobutamine is most widely used in the United States.

The endpoints for dobutamine infusion include: infusion of maximal dose; detection of new wall motion abnormalities; electrocardiogram changes indicative of ischemia; ventricular arrhythmia; a drop in systolic or diastolic blood pressure; or intolerable symptoms. Most patients tolerate the procedure well, achieve one of the endpoints, and therefore have a diagnostic test.[3,11] Imaging can be performed throughout the exam and image quality is not degraded or otherwise influenced by patient

▨◢ **TABLE 21-1.** MOST COMMONLY USED
STRESS ECHOCARDIOGRAPHY METHODS

Exercise	Post treadmill
	Supine bicycle
	Upright bicycle
Pacing	Esophageal, atrial
	Direct atrial
	Post ventricular
Pharmacological	Dobutamine
	Adenosine
	Dipyridamole

▨◢ **TABLE 21-2.** REGIONAL WALL MOTION
RESPONSES NOTED IN STRESS
ECHOCARDIOGRAPHY

Description	Normal	Stress
Normal	Normal	Hyperkinetic
	Hypokinetic	Hyperkinetic
Abnormal	Normal	HK, AK, DK
	Hypokinetic	HK, AK, DK
	Akinetic/dyskinetic	same

HK, hypokinetic; AK, akinetic; DK, dyskinetic.

motion or respiratory variations.[3,11] The viability of the myocardium may also be determined by dobutamine echocardiography.

Endpoints for exercise echocardiography include a routine treadmill endpoint (80%–100% of maximal age-determined heart rate), heart rate response, symptoms, and ECG analysis. Since imaging is not performed with the patient on the treadmill, detection of wall motion abnormalities cannot be used as an endpoint as it is with dobutamine.

Regional Wall Motion Abnormalities

The identification of a regional wall motion abnormality following exercise is considered a positive finding for ischemia, and is the most sensitive finding for the presence of coronary artery disease. Severity of the abnormality is directly related to severity of the coronary stenosis.

The wall motion analysis is performed by identifying the walls as normal, hyperdynamic, hypokinetic, akinetic, or dyskinetic. Each wall segment is examined and scored, as previously discussed. In patients with no prior cardiac events, the only normal response to exercise is a hyperdynamic one. New wall motion abnormalities are identified as any segment that remains the same or worsens with exercise.

A hyperdynamic response includes increased myocardial thickening and increased endocardial excursion. The LV cavity becomes smaller in systole with an overall increase in regional contractility with increasing levels of stress. An abnormal response is defined by regional wall motion abnormalities in one or more segments with decreased overall LV systolic function. Worsened mitral and tricuspid regurgitation and increased pulmonary artery pressures as assessed by tricuspid regurgitation velocity also indicate ischemia.

The development of hypokinesis in a region can be difficult to assess, particularly if subtle. The patient's level of stress must be accounted for in the assessments. Hypokinesis after maximal exercise or

pharmacologic stress implies ischemia. Hypokinesis after submaximal exercise is less specific, and more difficult to assess.[2] Akinesis or dyskinesis of a segment is more obvious and open to less interpretative discord. Table 21-2 represents typical normal and abnormal responses.

The interpretation of post stress wall motion abnormalities from a normal resting heart is more straightforward than interpreting the stress results from an abnormal baseline echocardiogram. Segments that are akinetic or dyskinetic at rest indicate the effects of myocardial infarction. Changes in contractility with stress in these regions may represent a passive change rather than a change due to improved contractility or worsening due to ischemia.[2] On the other hand, hypokinesis of a region at rest may be due to myocardial stunning or hibernation, prior nontransmural myocardial infarction, imaging accuracy, or patient age.[2] A resting segment described as hypokinetic at rest can have a variety of responses with exercise, ranging from hyperkinesis to dyskinesis. Figure 21-1 demonstrates a resting

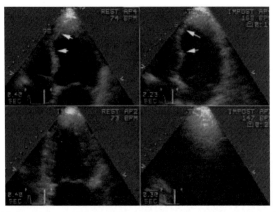

Figure 21-1. Quad screen of the apical four- (*top*) and apical two-chamber (*bottom*) views with resting images on the left and post exercise images on the right of the image. Arrows denote area of hypokinesis noted at rest (*left*), which worsens with exercise (*right*).

hypokinetic region in the apical septum, which worsened with exercise. At rest, this region was hypokinetic, but became dyskinetic with immediate post treadmill exercise.

Wall Motion Scoring

Segmental wall scoring is described on a numeric scale from 1 to 4: 1, normal contractility; 2, hypokinesis; 3, akinesis; and 4, dyskinesis. Occasionally, some echocardiography labs use the number 5 or 6 to indicate aneurysms. However, for calculating a wall motion score index, 1 through 4 are typically used. The wall motion score index is derived by adding the total score assigned to each segment and dividing by the total number of segments visualized. A wall motion score index of 1 is normal, and progressively higher wall motion score indices indicate greater degrees of LV dysfunction. Variations of these scoring systems exist. For example, wall segments are assigned half scores (1.5 or 2.5) to indicate more subtle degrees of dysfunction. Whatever system is used, consistency within the lab is essential.

Ventricular Geometry

Ventricular geometry can be an important indicator of LV dysfunction. Although regional wall motion abnormalities may be the most important indicator of ischemia, secondary changes can help confirm the diagnosis. The normal left ventricle is conical or bullet shaped in the absence of disease. Recognition of the LV shape at rest and its deviations following exercise should be apparent to the experienced echocardiographer.[2] Commonly observed shape deformities include a rounding of the apex or scooping of the apical septum or inferior walls (Fig. 21-2), the result of myocardial ischemia. These observations are useful in identifying both the presence of myocardial ischemia and the diseased vessel.

   Shape deformities of the apex (Fig. 21-2*A*, top and bottom) are usually associated with disease of the left anterior descending coronary artery (LAD). Shape deformities of the basal septum (Fig. 21-2*A*, lower right) and inferior basal walls (Fig. 21-2*B*, top right) are associated with disease of the posterior descending coronary artery (PDA). Shape deformities of the lateral wall are associated with disease of the circumflex coronary artery.

Size Changes

Another change frequently noted with stress-induced ischemia is dilatation of the left ventricle (Fig. 21-3). Normal left ventricular response to exercise includes hyperkinesis of the regional segments and

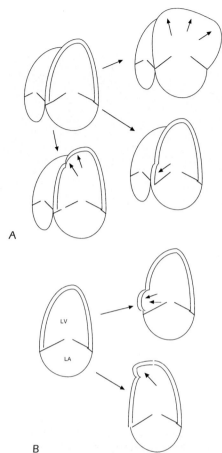

Figure 21-2. Geometric changes often noted with stress-induced ischemia. Apical four-chamber view (**A**) demonstrating rounding of the apex (*top right*) or scooping of the apical septum (*bottom left*) as would be seen in left anterior descending coronary artery (LAD) distribution disease. Ischemia of the posterior descending coronary artery (PDA) may demonstrate scooping of the basal septum (*bottom left*). Apical two-chamber view (**B**) demonstrating scooping of the inferior basal wall indicating PDA disease (*top right*). Scooping of the inferior apex (*bottom right*) indicates LAD disease. LA, left atrium; LV, left ventricle. (Modified from Ref. 11.)

a decrease in cavity size. Dilatation of the LV with exercise may indicate global or regional dysfunction. It can be observed in all standard views and comparison with resting images is important. The parasternal short axis view may be ideal for this observation, as it shows a cross-section of the left ventricle.

Global Left Ventricular Function

A decrease in overall systolic function is the least sensitive predictor of coronary artery disease, but indicates significant stenosis. In one study, an ab-

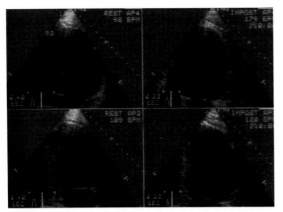

Figure 21-3. Usually readily apparent, dilatation of the left ventricle following stress indicates ischemia. These apical views demonstrate an increased left ventricular size following exercise. The apical two-chamber view (*bottom right*) demonstrates this.

normal ejection fraction response was observed in only 70% of patients with coronary artery obstruction.[8] There is a disparity in the ejection fraction in patients with single-vessel disease. The most dramatic decreases in overall ejection fraction are observed in patients with a depressed resting ejection fraction or in patients with multivessel disease.[4,7]

Advantages and Disadvantages of Stress Echocardiography

In today's changing health care environment, the need for low-cost, yet accurate, diagnostic testing is increasingly important. Stress echocardiography has distinct advantages and disadvantages. The advantages are its relative low cost and versatility. Compared to other imaging modalities, the equipment is less expensive and requires less space and no special environmental conditions. Stress echocardiography is also more versatile. The entire heart can be imaged and a full baseline echocardiogram is typically always performed before the stress component, providing a tremendous amount of structural and functional information. Contraindications as well as cardiac abnormalities that exist concurrently with, or that may mimic or mask, coronary artery disease can be ascertained. In addition, echocardiography is ideally suited when ECG is problematic, as in patients with left ventricular hypertrophy, conduction abnormalities, and other baseline ECG changes. Middle-aged females, patients with hypertension, and patients taking cardiac medications also pose a problem for ECG interpretation only.

A disadvantage of stress echocardiography is the degree of technical expertise required. Sonographers must possess exceptional scanning skills and a sound knowledge of cardiac anatomy, physiology, and pathology. The physician interpreting the studies must have additional training in stress echocardiography and must routinely interpret these exams. In addition, some patients have difficult windows so that image quality may be poor, in that all segments may not be imaged. Although a problem in the past, new technology such as harmonic imaging and the use of contrast agents should significantly improve, if not totally eliminate, this problem. Finally, special equipment is required for the digital acquisition of images. Newer ultrasound equipment now provides integrated, digital acquisition and storage of images.

REFERENCES

1. Aboul-Enein H, et al. Effect of the degree of effort on exercise echocardiography for the detection of restenosis after coronary artery angiography. Am Heart J 1991;122:430–437.
2. Armstrong WF. Stress echocardiography: Introduction, history and methods. Prog Cardiovasc Dis 1997;39:499–522.
3. Berthe C, et al. Predicting the extent and location of coronary artery disease in acute myocardial infarction by echocardiography during dobutamine infusion. Am J Cardiol 1986;58:1167–1172.
4. Bryg RJ, et al. Effect of coronary artery disease on Doppler-derived parameters of aortic flow during upright exercise. Am J Cardiol 1986;58:14–19.
5. Cohen JL, et al. Dobutamine digital echocardiography for detecting coronary artery disease. Am J Cardiol 1991;67:1311–1318.
6. Fung AY, Gallaghar KP, Buda AJ. The physiologic basis of dobutamine as compared with dipyridamole stress interventions in the assessment of critical coronary stenosis. Circulation 1987;76:943–951.
7. Harison MR, et al. Uses and limitations of exercise Doppler echocardiography in the diagnosis of ischemic heart disease. J Am Col Cardiol 1987;10:809–817.
8. Limacher MC, et al. Detection of coronary artery disease with exercise two-dimensional echocardiography. Circulation 1983;67:1211–1218.
9. Mannering D, et al. The dobutamine stress test as an alternative to exercise testing after acute myocardial infarction. Br Heart J 1988;59:521–526.
10. Martin TW, et al. Comparison of adenosine, dipyridamole and dobutamine in stress echocardiography. Ann Intern Med 1992;116:190–196.
11. Sawada SG, et al. Echocardiographic detection of coronary artery disease during dobutamine infusion. Circulation 1991;83:1605–1614.

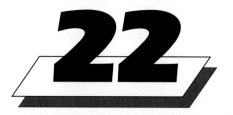

22

Contrast Echocardiography in the Assessment of the Coronary Artery

MARK N. ALLEN

Contrast echocardiography was first reported to be potentially valuable in enhancing left ventricular myocardium in 1980, when CO_2 bubbles injected into the left main coronary artery of a dog enhanced the ultrasound signals in that area.[9] Since then, the use of contrast echocardiography to facilitate the assessment of coronary artery disease in humans has expanded into several clinical arenas.[1–4,7, 14–18,20–24,26–31,33–35,37,38,44,45,48] *Myocardial contrast echocardiography* is a term used to describe the use of echocardiography to image the heart when a contrast agent is injected into the coronary arteries. When these sonicated contrast agents containing microbubbles are injected into coronary arteries, a brisk homogeneous enhancement of myocardial echogenicity can be seen on the echocardiogram. This contrast effect may last for several minutes, allowing clear delineation of normally perfused myocardium.[15] Myocardial contrast echocardiography provides information about coronary artery distribution, as well as the degree of damage of the coronary microvasculature. In patients with normal coronary arteries, the introduction of a contrast agent into the coronary arteries creates an increase in reflectivity of the myocardium, which is seen on echocardiography as opacification of the infused area(s). In the presence of coronary artery disease such as an occlusion, the microbubbles are unable to pass through the diseased territory, so no opacification is detected by echocardiography (Fig. 22-1).

Acute Myocardial Infarction

In acute myocardial infarction, the size of the infarct is the major determinant of functional damage.[40] Reperfusion and adequate collateral circulation favor blood flow to the myocardium during prolonged ischemia, thereby decreasing the potential for irreversible myocardial damage.[18] Restoring blood flow in the area of infarction has been shown to be beneficial in the subacute phase of myocardial infarction. Using myocardial contrast echocardiography, no contrast effect is noted in the area at risk of necrosis during the acute phase of infarction. After reperfusion, the amount of salvageable myocardium within the area at risk may be enhanced with contrast, indicating that this area may recover functionally if reperfused sufficiently.[18,23,37] In other words, it would be helpful to determine myocardial viability following acute infarction.

During coronary artery occlusion, if residual flow continues to be low, the cells in the region of infarction will necrose or die. By contrast, if residual flow is high, the cells in that region may continue to be viable. Residual flow usually involves a network of collaterals. Myocardial contrast echocardi-

415

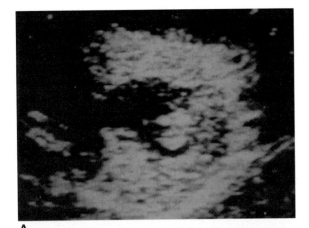

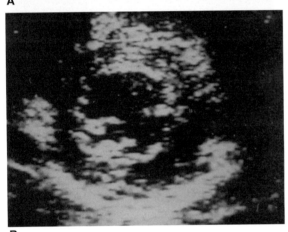

Figure 22-1. (**A**) Injection of contrast into the left main coronary artery in an animal model. (**B**) Injection into the left main coronary artery in the same model with coronary occlusion. Note the absence of opacification with the occluded vessel.

ography helps to define the region where residual flow may be present following infarction.[12] If contrast is noted in this region, this usually indicates that some residual flow is present and that cellular viability is likely.[19,29,32]

The role of myocardial contrast echocardiography in this setting appears promising since it may provide several important bits of information in regard to viable myocardium and the degree of perfusion (Fig. 22-2). Studies have shown that myocardial salvage is unlikely if there is no contrast effect (absence of contrast) immediately after reperfusion if adequate collaterals are not present.[36] Further, myocardial contrast may provide information re-

garding the acute protective effects of coronary collaterals during coronary occlusion.[37]

In one study,[23] 28 patients with acute myocardial infarction demonstrated evidence of contrast defect (no opacification seen by echocardiography following coronary injection of contrast agents) before reperfusion. Following reperfusion, contrast was seen in the infarct region in 20 patients (71%), indicating revascularization in that region. The remaining eight patients (28%) demonstrated a persistent absence of perfusion, indicating no reperfusion to the infarct region. In the chronic stage of myocardial infarction (roughly 4 weeks), myocardial contrast echocardiography was again performed. The eight patients with no contrast effect following reperfusion continued to show no contrast effect, indicating that contrast enhancement in the risk area will not occur later if the area failed to reperfuse at the acute stage of infarction. Of the 20 patients with contrast enhancement following reperfusion, 16

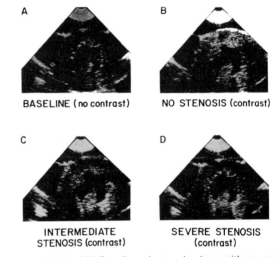

Figure 22-2. (**A**) Baseline short-axis view with no contrast injection. (**B**) Short-axis view with contrast injection in a patient without coronary artery stenosis. (**C**) Short-axis view of a patient with intermediate left anterior descending coronary artery stenosis with contrast injection. (**D**) Short-axis view of a patient with severe left anterior descending coronary artery stenosis with contrast injection. With no stenosis, the contrast effect is dramatic and decreases with increasing severity of stenosis. (From Keller MW, et al: Intraoperative assessment of myocardial perfusion using quantitative myocardial contrast echocardiography: An experimental evaluation. J Am Coll Cardiol. 1990;16:1267. Reprinted with permission from the American College of Cardiology.)

continued to demonstrate the contrast enhancement but the remaining 4 did not. This indicates that contrast enhancement in the acute stage with reperfusion does not necessarily guarantee myocardial salvage in the chronic stage. The mechanisms of this late contrast defect are unclear and further research is necessary, but they probably have something to do with the adequacy of the collateral vessels.

The use of myocardial contrast echocardiography in assessing myocardial viability in the setting of acute myocardial infarction appears to be valuable. Serial myocardial contrast echocardiograms of these patients may allow a more precise prediction of myocardial viability.[38] With advances in technique and with the development of newer agents, myocardial contrast echocardiography may become widely utilized for the assessment of postinfarction myocardial viability.

Myocardial Contrast and Stress Echocardiography

Two of the challenges faced by echocardiographers are the assessment of regional wall motion abnormalities and the identification of patients at risk for myocardial infarction. Several techniques have been developed in an effort to provide clinicians with this information. Stress echocardiography has proven to be a safe, accurate, noninvasive method for the evaluation of suspected or known coronary artery disease. The visualization of endocardial borders both before and after stress echocardiography allows assessment of regional wall motion changes that may indicate the presence of ischemia. However, visualization of all endocardial borders is not always possible in roughly 10–20% of cases because of poor acoustic windows, chest wall configuration, body habitus, and other technical factors.[13] The use of contrast agents through IV administration has been demonstrated to enhance endocardial border detection of the left ventricle during exercise and dobutamine echocardiography.[5,6,10,11,48]

Administration of a contrast agent into a peripheral vein during stress procedures enhances or opacifies the left ventricular cavity. A contrast agent capable of crossing the pulmonary vasculature is required so that it may reach the left ventricle. In this process, the delineation of the wall from the blood pool is enhanced, allowing the operator to differentiate the real endocardial border (Fig. 22-3).

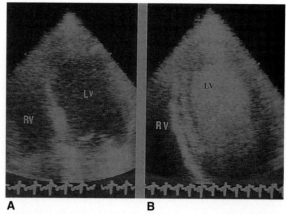

A   **B**

Figure 22-3. (**A**) Four-chamber view of a patient during dobutamine echocardiography with poorly delineated endocardial borders. (**B**) With contrast injection during the dobutamine in the same patient, the endocardial borders are better appreciated. Before the contrast injection, the exam was uninterpretable. LV-left ventricle, RV-right ventricle. (From Nanda NC, Schlief R, Goldberg BB (eds): Advances in Echo Imaging Using Contrast Enhancement, 2nd ed. Dordrecht, the Netherlands, Kluwer; 1993:365. Reprinted with permission.)

In a study by Crouse et al.,[6] 175 patients underwent IV administration of contrast; in 145 of these patients, an improvement in endocardial border delineation was demonstrated after one dose of Albunex. The use of contrast agents to enhance the endocardial borders also improved the interpreters' confidence in assessing regional wall motion in 67 (77%) of the 87 patients in whom the interpreters were not confident in assessing the baseline images. The use of contrast agents to enhance right ventricular endocardial borders has also been reported to improve the accuracy of right ventricular ejection fraction calculations.[42] Other studies have demonstrated improved assessment of lateral and apical endocardial border resolution, ventricular function, and regional wall motion; increased speed of interpretation; improved confidence of interpretation in scans of patients undergoing dobutamine stress echocardiography combined with contrast enhancement.[11] The use of contrast agents during exercise echocardiography has also been reported. In one study,[48] the use of IV Albunex increased the endocardial border visualization from 86% to 91%.

The use of contrast agents to facilitate the visualization of endocardial borders in exercise and pharmacologic stress echocardiography appears to hold great promise. This technique is cost effective since the number of limited conclusions is reduced.[41] It is a safe and noninvasive method that provides significant improvements in endocardial border detection.

Contrast enhancement has also been used in conjunction with stress echocardiography.[1,35] The purpose of these studies was to examine whether myocardial contrast echocardiography can be used to study regional myocardial blood flow distribution during dipyridamole-induced coronary dilatation (hyperemia) in regions of known coronary artery stenosis. In these studies, contrast agents were injected into the coronary arteries before and after dipyridamole infusion. The presence and intensity of the contrast material in these regions provided information on the integrity of the microvasculature. This information may be useful in determining the viability of these infarcted or stenotic areas.[35]

Harmonic Imaging and Contrast Echocardiography

Harmonic ultrasound imaging improves the signal-to-noise ratio in the myocardium and the left ventricular cavity by taking advantage of the nonlinear scattering properties of ultrasound contrast media.[30] Recall from previous chapters that bubbles, when struck with sound waves, oscillate, creating a resonant frequency as well as multiples of this frequency, or harmonics.[8] This essentially allows the sound waves to be transmitted at a lower, less attenuating frequency and to be received at a higher frequency, which improves the signal-to-noise ratio.[8,39] This resonant frequency of the microbubbles utilized in contrast agents coincides with the range of ultrasound used in transthoracic echocardiography. Transmission of ultrasound at or near the resonant frequency of the contrast microbubbles enhances the harmonic signals and improves detection of the contrast agent (Fig. 22-4).[46]

Microbubbles, however, are susceptible to collapse from pressures exerted on them by the sound waves.[25,43,47] This is particularly true of microbubbles in certain contrast agents. The use of intermittently triggered acquisition or *transient-response imaging (TRI)* may reduce the amount of microbubble destruction.[28,30] In this technique, instead of continuous imaging, the pulses are transmitted at one point in the cardiac cycle. This may

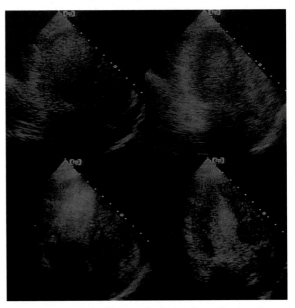

Figure 22-4. Apical long-axis views of a patient undergoing a dobutamine stress echocardiogram (30 μg/kg/min) and 10 ml intravenous Albunex infusion. End-diastolic views in the left panels with (top) fundamental imaging and with (bottom) second harmonic imaging. End-systolic views on the right side with fundamental imaging (top) and second harmonic imaging (bottom). Notice the marked improvement in image quality between the fundamental contrast images (top panels) and the second harmonic contrast images (bottom panels). (From Nanda NC, Schlief R, Goldberg BB [eds]: Advances in Echo Imaging Using Contrast Enhancement, 2nd ed. Dordrecht, the Netherlands, Kluwer; 1993:441. Reprinted with permission.)

reduce the destruction of microbubbles and enhance their detection.[46] Second harmonic imaging clearly allows better visualization of left ventricular endocardial borders, and with the development of newer agents, particularly those capable of passing through the pulmonary vasculature, contrast-harmonic imaging will have great clinical utility in echocardiography.

Limitation of Myocardial Contrast Echocardiography

Despite the promising data, there are several obstacles that need to be overcome. For myocardial imaging, the contrast agent needs to be injected into or near the coronary arteries; this procedure is not easily performed at the patient's bedside. Newer agents capable of being injected intravenously, passing through the pulmonary vasculature and reaching the myocardium via the coronary arteries, hold great potential but require further investigation. In addition, lateral dropout and shadowing pose a problem in imaging all the regional segments. Just as the contrast effect can enhance images, it can also mask or hide areas of interest. The contrast effect can be too strong in some settings. Further, because bubble size and concentration may vary within a given area, the intensity of the signals will be heterogeneous, making the distinction between the physiologic effect, an effect of the interaction of sound with the agent, and effects of signal processing difficult.

REFERENCES

1. Agati L, Voci P, Bilotta F, et al. Dipyridamole myocardial contrast echocardiography in patients with single vessel coronary artery disease: Perfusion, anatomic, and functional correlates. Am Heart J. 1994; 128:28–35.

2. Bach D, Muller D, Cheirif J, et al. Regional heterogeneity on myocardial contrast echocardiography without severe obstructive coronary artery disease. Am J Cardiol. 1995;75:982–986.

3. Bolognese L, Antoniucci D, Rovai D, et al. Myocardial contrast echocardiography versus dobutamine echocardiography for predicting functional recovery after acute myocardial infarction treated with primary coronary angioplasty. J Am Coll Cardiol. 1996;28: 1677–1683.

4. Camarano G, Ragosta M, Gimple L, et al. Identification of viable myocardium with contrast echocardiography in patients with poor left ventricular systolic function caused by recent or remote myocardial infarction. Am J Cardiol. 1995;75:215–219.

5. Crouse L. Sonicated serum albumin in contrast echocardiography: Improved segmental wall motion depiction and implications for stress echocardiography. Am J Cardiol. 1992;69:42H–45H.

6. Crouse L, Cheirif J, Hanley D, et al. Opacification and border delineation improvement in patients with suboptimal endocardial border definition in routine echocardiography: Results of the Phase III Albunex Multicenter Trial. J Am Coll Cardiol. 1993;22: 1494–1500.

7. De Filippi C, Willett D, Irani W, et al. Comparison of myocardial contrast echocardiography and low dose dobutamine stress echocardiography in predicting recovery of left ventricular function after coronary revascularization in chronic ischemic heart disease. Circulation. 1995;92:2863–2868.

8. De Jong N, Ten Cate F, Lancee CT, et al. Principles and recent developments in ultrasound contrast agents. Ultrasonics. 1991;29:324–330.

9. DeMaria AN, Bonner WS, Riggs K, et al. Echocardiographic visualization of myocardial perfusion by left heart intracoronary injection of echo contrast agents (abstract). Circulation. 1980;60(suppl 3):III-143.

10. Falcone R, Marcovitz P, Perez J, et al. Intravenous Albunex during dobutamine stress echocardiography: Enhanced localization of left ventricular endocardial borders. Am Heart J. 1995;130:254–258.

11. Feinstein SB, Cheirif J, Ten Cate FJ, et al. Safety and efficacy of a new transpulmonary ultrasound contrast agent: Initial multicenter clinical results. J Am Coll Cardiol. 1990;16:316–324.

12. Firschke C, Kaul S. Assessment of myocardial viability post-infarction with myocardial contrast echocardiography. In Nanda NC, Schlief R, Goldberg BB (eds): Advances in Echo Imaging Using Contrast Enhancement, 2nd ed. Dordrecht, the Netherlands, Kluwer; 1997:401–414.

13. Freeman AP, Giles RW, Walsh WF, et al. Regional left ventricular wall motion assessment: Comparison of two-dimensional echocardiography and radionuclide angiography with contrast angiography in healed myocardial infarction. Am J Cardiol. 1985; 56:8–12.

14. Groundstroem K, Tarkka M, Kirklin J, et al. Single right coronary artery assessed by contrast angiography and transesophageal echocardiography. Eur Heart J. 1995;16:1739–1741.

15. Himbert D, Seknadji P, Karila-Cohen D, et al. Myocardial contrast echocardiography to assess spontaneous reperfusion during myocardial infarction. Lancet. 1997;349:617–619.

16. Hirata N, Shimazaki Y, Nakano S, et al. Evaluation of regional myocardial perfusion in areas of old myocardial infarction after revascularization by means of intraoperative myocardial contrast echocardiography. J Thorac Cardiovasc Surg. 1994;108: 1119–1124.

17. Iliceto S, Galiuto L, Marchese A, et al. Analysis of microvascular integrity, contractile reserve, and myocardial visibility after acute myocardial infarction by dobutamine echocardiography and myocardial contrast echocardiography. Am J Cardiol. 1996;77: 441–445.

18. Iliceto S, Marangelli V, Marchese A, et al. Myocardial contrast echocardiography in acute myocardial infarction. Pathophysiological background and clinical applications. Eur Heart J. 1996;17:344–353.

19. Jugdutt BI, Hutchins GM, Bulkley BM, et al. Myocardial infarction in the conscious dog: Three-dimensional mapping of infarct, collateral flow and region at risk. Circulation. 1979;60:1141–1150.

20. Kaul S. Myocardial contrast echocardiography in coronary artery disease: Potential applications using venous injections of contrast. Am J Cardiol. 1995;71: 61D–68D.

21. Kaul S, Jayaweera A. Myocardial contrast echocardiography has the potential for the assessment of coronary microvascular reserve. J Am Coll Cardiol. 1993; 21:356–358.

22. Lim Y, Masuyama T, Nanto S, et al. Left ventricular papillary muscle perfusion assessed with myocardial contrast echocardiography. Am J Cardiol. 196;78: 955–958.

23. Lim Y, Nanto S, Masuyama T, et al. Myocardial salvage: Its assessment and prediction by the analysis of serial myocardial contrast echocardiograms in patients with acute myocardial infarction. Am Heart J. 1994;128:649–656.

24. Meza M, Mobarek S, Sonnemaker R, et al. Myocardial contrast echocardiography in human beings: Correlation of resting perfusion defects to sestamibi single photon emission computed tomography. Am Heart J. 1996;132:528–535.

25. Mor-Avi V, Robinson K, Shroff S, et al. Stability of Albunex microspheres under ultrasonic irradiation: An in vitro study. J Am Soc Echocardiogr. 1994;7: S29.

26. Perkins A, Frier M, Hindle A, et al. Human biodistribution of an ultrasound contrast agent (Quantison) by radiolabeling and gamma scintigraphy. Br J Radiol. 1997;70:603–611.

27. Porter T, D'sa A, Pesko L, et al. Usefulness of myocardial contrast echocardiography in detecting the immediate changes in antegrade blood flow reserve after coronary angioplasty. Am J Cardiol. 1993;71: 893–896.

28. Porter T, D'Sa A, Turner C, et al. Myocardial contrast echocardiography for the assessment of coronary blood flow reserve: Validation in humans. J Am Coll Cardiol. 1993;21:349–355.

29. Porter T, Li S, Kricsfeld D, et al. Detection of myocardial perfusion in multiple echocardiographic windows with one intravenous injection of microbubbles using transient response second harmonic imaging. J Am Coll Cardiol. 1997;29:791–799.

30. Porter T, Xie F, Kricsfeld D, et al. Improved myocardial contrast with second harmonic transient ultrasound response imaging in humans using intravenous perfluorocarbon-exposed sonicated dextrose albumin. J Am Coll Cardiol. 1996;27:1479–1501.

31. Redberg RF. Coronary flow by transesophageal Doppler echocardiography: Do saccharide-based contrast agents sweeten the pot? J Am Coll Cardiol. 1994;23:191–193.

32. Reimer KA, Jennings RB. The "wavefront phenomenon" of myocardial ischemic cell death. II. Transmural progression of necrosis within the framework of ischemic bed size (myocaradium at risk) and collateral flow. Lab Invest. 1979;40:633–644.

33. Rovai D, DeMaria A, L'Abbate A. Myocardial contrast echo effect: The dilemma of coronary blood flow and volume. J Am Coll Cardiol. 1995;26: 12–17.

34. Rovai D, Ferdeghini E, Mazzarisi A, et al. Quantitative aspects in myocardial contrast echocardiography. Eur Heart J. 1995;16(suppl J):42–45.

35. Rovai D, Zanchi M, Lombardi M, et al. Residual myocardial perfusion in reversibly damaged myocardium by dipyridamole contrast echocardiography. Eur Heart J. 1996;17:296–301.

36. Sabia PJ, Powers ER, Ragosta M, et al. An association between collateral blood flow and myocardial viability in patients with recent myocardial infarction. N Engl J Med. 1992;327:1825–1831.

37. Sakata Y, Kodama K, Adachi T, et al. Comparison of myocardial contrast echocardiography and coronary angiography for assessing the acute protective effects of collateral recruitment during occlusion of the left anterior descending coronary artery at the time of elective angioplasty. Am J Cardiol. 1997;79: 1329–1333.

38. Sakuma T, Hayashi Y, Shimohara A, et al. Usefulness of myocardial contrast echocardiography for the assessment of serial changes in risk areas in patients with acute myocardial infarction. Am J Cardiol. 1996;78:1273–1277.

39. Scrope BA, Newhouse VL. Second harmonic ultrasonic blood perfusion measurement. Ultrasound Med Biol. 1993;19:567.

40. Sharper W, Frenzel H, Hort W. Experimental coronary artery occlusion. I. Measurement of infarct size. Basic Res Cardiol. 1979;74:46–53.

41. Tejpal Y, Block R, Sagireddy B, et al. Cost-effectiveness in patients undergoing dobutamine stress echocardiography with and without ultrasound contrast. J Am Soc Echocardiogr. 1996;9:402 (abstract A801F).

42. Tokgözoglu SL, Caner B, Kabakci G, et al. Measurement of right ventricular ejection fraction by contrast echocardiography. Int J Cardiol. 1997;59:71–74.

43. Vandenberg BF, Melton HE. Acoustic liability of albumin microspheres. J Am Soc Echocardiogr. 1994; 7:582–589.

44. Vernon S, Camarano G, Kaul S, et al. Myocardial contrast echocardiography demonstrates that collateral flow can perserve myocardial function beyond a chronically occluded coronary artery. Am J Cardiol. 1996;78:958–960.

45. Villanueva F, Jankowski R, Manaugh C, et al. Albumin microbubble adherence to human coronary endothelium: Implications for assessment of endothelial function using myocardial contrast echocardiography. J Am Coll Cardiol. 1997;30:689–693.

46. Villarraga HR, Foley DA, Chung SM, et al. Harmonic imaging during contrast echocardiography: Basic principles and potential clinical value. *In* Nanda NC, Schlief R, Goldberg BB (eds): Advances in Echo Imaging Using Contrast Enhancement, 2nd ed. Dordrecht, the Netherlands, Kluwer; 1997: 433–450.

47. Wray RA, Zoghbi WA, Quinones MA, et al. Contrast echocardiography: Relation of acoustic power and time gain compensation to contrast intensity duration. J Am Soc Echocardiogr. 1992;4:286.

48. Yvorchuk K, Sochowski R, Chan K, et al. Sonicated albumin in exercise echocardiography: Technique and feasibility to enhance endocardial visualization. J Am Soc Echocardiogr. 1996;9:462–469.

PART VII

Diseases of the Myocardium

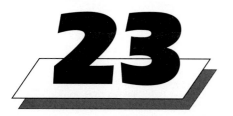

23

Hypertrophic Cardiomyopathy

J. CHARLES POPE

A primary cardiomyopathy is a disease of the cardiac muscle of unknown cause. There are three distinct classes of cardiomyopathy—hypertrophic, dilated (congestive), and restrictive (infiltrative). Secondary cardiomyopathies—other systemic diseases that affect the myocardium in a similar manner—are caused by viruses, ischemia, metabolic abnormalities, endocrinopathies, hypertension, and toxic reactions. The definition and classification of the cardiomyopathies as reported by the World Health Organization (WHO) task force are shown in Table 23-1. This chapter will discuss the subjective and objective findings of patients with hypertrophic cardiomyopathy and review the echocardiographic criteria for establishing the diagnosis.

Hypertrophic Cardiomyopathy

Hypertrophic cardiomyopathy (HCM) is a condition classically characterized by the presence of asymmetrical septal hypertrophy of the left ventricle and systolic anterior motion (SAM) of the mitral valve. Occasionally the right ventricle may also be involved. The finding of asymmetrical septal hypertrophy is more common than concentric left ventricular hypertrophy or apical hypertrophy. Typically, the size and volume of the left ventricular cavity are normal or reduced. Systolic pressure gradients across the left ventricular outflow tract (LVOT) are common. HCM is transmitted by an autosomal dominant gene, but partial characteris-

tics of the disorder may be noted in incomplete gene penetrance. Characteristic morphologic changes of muscle fiber disarray and disorganization usually are most severe in the interventricular septum.[2] Idiopathic hypertrophic subaortic stenosis (IHSS) and hypertrophic obstructive cardiomyopathy (HOCM) may be used synonymously. IHSS may be subcategorized into obstructive (with a subaortic gradient) and nonobstructive (without a subaortic gradient).

CLINICAL PRESENTATION

The three major symptoms of HCM are dyspnea, angina, and syncope.[17] Symptoms usually develop in the second or third decade of life. Approximately 90% of patients with HCM experience dyspnea, but it is poorly correlated with the underlying dynamic outflow tract gradient. The proposed pathophysiologic cause of dyspnea is elevated left ventricular end-diastolic filling pressure and subsequent alteration of volume–pressure relationships in that chamber. This increases left atrial pressure and pulmonary venous pressure, which, in turn, may cause dyspnea. Approximately 70% of HCM patients experience angina, but only 25% of patients with HCM over 45 years of age have evidence of significant coronary artery disease on coronary arteriography.[29] The remainder of patients experience angina even though their extramural coronary arteries are normal. The pathophysiologic alterations proposed for producing angina are small-vessel coronary ar-

◢▬◢ **TABLE 23-1. PRIMARY CARDIOMYOPATHIES**

Definition	Heart muscle diseases of unknown cause
Classification	Dilated cardiomyopathy
	Hypertrophic cardiomyopathy
	Restrictive cardiomyopathy

SPECIFIC HEART MUSCLE DISEASE

Definition	Heart muscle disease of known cause or associated with disorders of other systems. Disorders of the myocardium due to systemic or pulmonary hypertension, coronary artery disease, valvular heart disease, or congenital cardiac anomalies have been excluded.
Classification	**INFECTIVE**
	METABOLIC
	Endocrine
	Familial storage and infiltration
	Deficiency
	Amyloid
	SYSTEMIC DISEASES
	Systemic lupus erythematosus
	Sarcoidosis
	Muscular dystrophies
	Friedreich's ataxia
	TOXIC
	Ethanol
	Radiation
	Doxorubicin

Source: Report of the WHO/ISFC task force on the definition and classification of cardiomyopathies. Br Heart J. 1980;44:672–673.

tery stenosis, intramyocardial compression of small arteries by the massive muscle hypertrophy, and abnormal diastolic filling dynamics resulting in an imbalance between oxygen supply and demand (MVO_2).[31]

Presyncope or syncope occurs in approximately 50% of patients with HCM.[28] The most common cause of syncope is cardiac arrhythmia. Ventricular tachycardia has been seen in as many as 40% of these patients.[15] Congestive heart failure is rare in HCM. The physical examination of patients with HCM may be completely normal if there is no underlying outflow tract gradient. In contrast, physical findings are variable if a systolic gradient is present across the LVOT. Classic physical findings in patients with HCM with an LVOT gradient include a brisk carotid upstroke with a bifid contour (pulsus biferiens) in a large majority of patients. This is related to exaggerated early systolic contraction and rapid early emptying of the left ventricle followed by a midsystolic premature closure of the aortic valve that coincides with systolic anterior motion of the mitral valve. The presence of a bifid pulse contour with a brisk upstroke is helpful in differentiating HCM from aortic stenosis in which there is a slow rate of rise of the carotid upstroke and a decrease in the amplitude of the carotid pulse. On palpation of the chest, the apical cardiac impulse is usually prominent because of significant left ventricular hypertrophy. A presystolic apical impulse (palpable S_4) is common, whereas a pathognomonic triple impulse is noted in a small number of patients. Provocations that decrease the left ventricular volume and reduce the outflow tract diameter, such as Valsalva's maneuver, amyl nitrite inhalation, and sudden assumption of an upright position from a lying or sitting position, increase the subaortic gradient and thus increase the intensity of the heart murmur (Fig. 23-1). In contrast, maneuvers that increase left ventricular volume, such as sudden squatting, leg raising in a supine position, or phenylephrine infusion, decrease the subaortic gradient and produce a low-intensity murmur. It is important to note that the only other cardiac abnormality that responds simi-

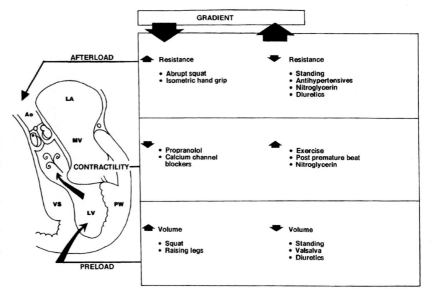

Figure 23-1. Various maneuvers and interventions that alter the LVOT gradient. LA, left atrium; Ao, aorta; MV, mitral valve; VS, ventricular septum; LV, left ventricle; PW, posterior wall. (Reprinted with permission of the American Society of Echocardiography. Nomenclature and Standards: Identification of Myocardial/Wall Segments, November 1992.)

larly to these maneuvers is mitral valve prolapse, but this should be distinguishable by the presence of a late systolic click and by the location and quality of the murmur. In the majority of patients with HCM the electrocardiogram (ECG) is abnormal. The most common resting ECG abnormalities are left ventricular hypertrophy, left atrial enlargement, and prominent Q waves in the inferior and lateral leads that may simulate the presence of a myocardial infarction.[7,26] Twenty-four-hour Holter monitor recordings have shown a high incidence of supraventricular arrhythmias (50%), multiform premature ventricular contractions (45%), and ventricular tachycardia (40%). Atrial fibrillation is also seen in a minority of patients, which may be associated with the patient's clinical deterioration because of the loss of atrial contribution to cardiac output. The patient's chest x-ray may be perfectly normal, but if there is an abnormality, it usually displays mild to moderate enlargement of the cardiac silhouette. The left atrium may also be enlarged (Fig. 23-2).

ECHOCARDIOGRAPHIC FEATURES (TWO-DIMENSIONAL AND M-MODE)

Patients with HCM classically demonstrate three hallmarks of the disease: (1) asymmetrical septal hypertrophy (ASH), (2) disorganization or disarray of the septal myocardial cells, and (3) SAM of the mi-

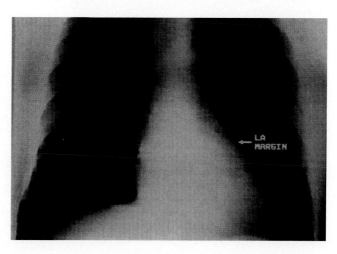

Figure 23-2. Posteroanterior chest film depicts cardiomegaly and left atrial (LA) enlargement (arrow).

tral valve apparatus.[18] Figure 23-3 is an anatomic photograph that corresponds to a two-dimensional (2-D) echocardiographic parasternal long axis view in a patient with an HCM. Note the significant abnormal thickness of the interventricular septum. In addition, the posterior wall of the ventricle is thickened and the papillary muscle is hypertrophied. The LVOT diameter is narrowed.

Normally, the anterior and posterior mitral valve leaflets remain together during systole and do not move forward to impinge on the interventricular septum. Figure 23-4 demonstrates SAM of the mitral valve. This patient had evidence of ASH with a narrow LVOT in a small left ventricular cavity. The mitral valve apparatus is noted to coapt with the interventricular septum. Figure 24-5 is an M-mode echocardiogram through the area of SAM of the mitral valve demonstrated on the 2-D examination. This shows evidence of SAM of the anterior mitral valve leaflet. The anterior mitral valve leaflet moves anteriorly to contact the interventricular septum, which produces an obstruction in the LVOT and a subsequent gradient. The patient also has evidence of a ratio of interventricular septal thickness to posterior lateral wall thickness greater than 1.3 to 1.0. This is an additional echocardiographic criterion for HCM. Reduction in contractility of the interventricular septum has been described and may

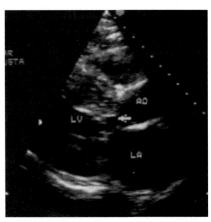

Figure 23-4. Parasternal long axis view demonstrates ASH and SAM of the mitral valve. Note obstruction to the LVOT (arrow). LA, left atrium; PW, posterior wall; AO, aorta; S, septum.

be secondary to muscle fiber disarray seen histologically in hypertrophic septum.[32] It should be noted that this finding is not exclusive to HCM. Investigators using 2-D echocardiography have pointed out that septal hypertrophy may extend uniformly or may be localized or exaggerated at various loci within the ventricle (e.g., in the basement portion of the ventricle or lateral wall and the apex).[19] Although M-mode echocardiography is useful, it may produce an erroneous diagnosis of HCM if the M-mode cursor is misaligned at an oblique angle to the interventricular septum, making it appear

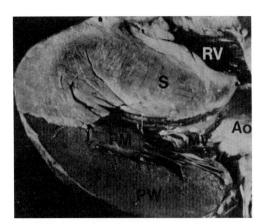

Figure 23-3. Anatomic view of a sectioned left ventricle shows abnormal thickness of the septum (S). The posterior wall (PW) is also hypertrophic. Note the narrow LVOT (arrow). PM, papillary muscle; MV, mitral valve; Ao, aorta. (From Hagan AD, DiSessa TG, Bloor CM, et al. Two-Dimensional Echocardiography: Clinical–Pathological Correlations in Adult and Congential Heart Disease. Boston: Little, Brown; 1983;298. Reprinted with permission.)

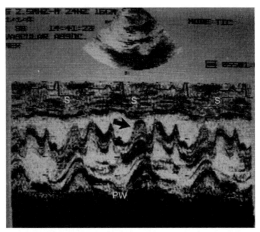

Figure 23-5. M-mode panel shows SAM of the mitral valve (arrow). The septum (S) is thick, and the posterior wall (PW) is normal in thickness.

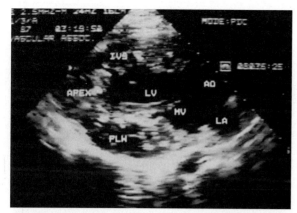

Figure 23-6. Parasternal long axis 2-D echocardiogram of abnormal bright echoes (arrow) in the myocardium. IVS, interventricular septum; PLW, posterior lateral wall; LV, left ventricle; AO, aorta; MV, mitral valve; LA, left atrium.

thicker than its true diameter. This alters the ratio of septal thickness to posterior wall thickness and produces a false appearance of ASH. In addition, ASH may occur in a variety of conditions that are not related to HCM. Such conditions can be seen in athletes with physiologic cardiac hypertrophy,[14] right ventricular volume overload, as in patients with tetralogy of Fallot,[14] primary pulmonary hypertension,[8] hypertension,[1] aortic stenosis,[13] and aortic atresia.[13] Also, patients with a history of inferior wall myocardial infarction or posterior wall infarction may present with asymmetrical hypertrophy

due to thinning of the posterior inferior wall segment in relation to normal septal thickness.[12] ASH is a normal feature of embryonic life,[22] and a subset of infants born to diabetic mothers have benign ASH, which resolves in approximately 6 months.[10] ASH has also been reported in patients undergoing hemodialysis in association with mural thrombus and with lymphoma.[4,25] An additional feature of HCM on 2-D echocardiography is a change in the acoustic property of the interventricular septal echoes.[23] This finding is more prominent in the intramyocardial echoes of the interventricular septum noted proximally and has been labeled *speckling* (Fig. 23-6).

SAM of the mitral valve is said to be present when the mitral valve apparatus moves anteriorly toward the interventricular septum shortly after the onset of systole and then returns to its normal position just prior to the onset of ventricular diastole. This has been associated with systolic pressure gradients or obstructions across the LVOT[9] (Fig. 23-7). True SAM should return to the baseline on M-mode recordings prior to the onset of ventricular diastole. This can be sensitively illustrated with an M-mode echocardiogram (Fig. 23-8). SAM of the mitral valve is not specific for the diagnosis of HCM and may be seen in other conditions such as transposition of the great vessels,[24] aortic regurgitation,[6] hypovolumic shock,[3] Pompe's disease,[27] and hypertension. The basic physiology of SAM is produced by the Venturi effect as blood velocity increases in

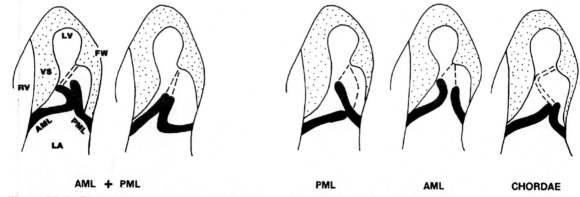

Figure 23-7. Diagram demonstrates the various parts of the mitral valve apparatus that can encroach on the LVOT and possibly produce obstruction. AML, anterior mitral leaflet; PML, posterior mitral leaflet; LV, left ventricular free wall; LA, left atrium; RV, right ventricle; VS, ventricular septum; PW, posterior wall. (From Spirito R, Baron, BJ. Patterns of systolic anterior motion of the mitral valve in hypertrophic cardiomyopathy; Assessment by two-dimensional echocardiography. Am J Cardiol. 1984;54:1039. Reprinted with permission.)

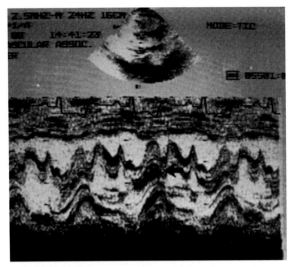

Figure 23-8. M-mode tracing of SAM of the mitral valve. Note the complete return to the baseline segment prior to the opening of the mitral valve (arrow).

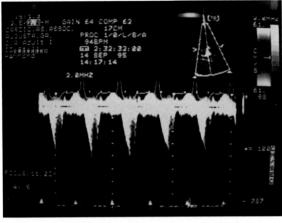

Figure 23-9. Dynamic LVOT gradients. CW Doppler from the apex shows a jet velocity of 2.0 m/sec (gradient = 16 mm Hg). The patient became dehydrated, and subsequent CW Doppler shows a gradient of 4.0 m/sec (gradient = 64 mm Hg). IVRT, isovolumic relaxation time; LVOT, left ventricular outflow tract.

the narrowed LVOT. The LVOT obstruction is dynamic and depends on the loading conditions and contractility of the LV. When aortic flow is interrupted because of the development of LVOT obstruction, the aortic valve develops premature midsystolic closure. The distorted mitral valve results in mitral regurgitation; therefore, varying degrees of mitral regurgitation accompany the obstructive form of HCM (Fig. 23-9). Pseudosystolic anterior motion of the mitral valve or false SAM is seen in the presence of hyperdynamic left ventricular posterior walls, which produce parallel anterior motion of the mitral valve. This can be seen in atrial septal defects,[30] pericardial effusions,[11] and mitral valve prolapse.[20] Further, 2-D echocardiographic examination has proven that if the M-mode beam is directed into the area of the mitral valve cords, and not the valve, the SAM or buckling that is noted is not true SAM. This condition may be seen in nonobstructive cardiomyopathy, hypertension, mitral valve prolapse, and normal hearts. Other classic M-mode features associated with HCM include early systolic aortic valve closure and a decreased rate of septal thickening.

Two dimensional echocardiography has become *the diagnostic tool of choice* for patients suspected of having HCM. The primary technical advantage of the 2-D echocardiographic scan is the multiple windows for interrogation of the heart. It is imperative to use both parasternal long and short axis views to allow accurate measurement of interventricular septum and posterior wall thickening, as well as the chamber size. The problem with abnormal tangential cuts of the interventricular septum with M-mode examination is eliminated because the entire interventricular septum may be visualized by the 2-D echocardiographic examination. Two-dimensional apical four- and two-chamber views are also very important for the identification of left ventricular eccentric areas of hypertrophy and left ventricular ejection fraction. Therefore, the 2-D examination may identify sites of proposed or prior myectomy.[28] Two-dimensional echocardiography has also identified a subset of patients who have pronounced concentric hypertrophy located at the left ventricular apex labeled *apical hypertrophy cardiomyopathy.*[16] Figure 23-10 presents such a patient. It should be noted that the patient has evidence of massive apical hypertrophy and no LVOT obstruction. The absence of LVOT obstruction is common in this presentation. Most reports of this type of patient have been documented by Yamaguchi and associates.[33] This type of apical hypertrophic cardiomyopathy is not commonly seen in the United States and is more endemic in the Japanese population.

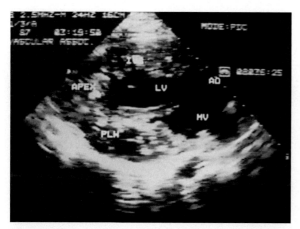

Figure 23-10. Parasternal long axis 2-D echocardiogram of a patient with apical hypertrophic cardiomyopathy. Note the apical hypertrophy. IVS, interventricular septum; PLW, posterior lateral wall; LV, left ventricle; AO, aorta; MV, mitral valve.

DOPPLER (PULSED WAVE, CONTINUOUS WAVE) AND COLOR FLOW IMAGING

Doppler echocardiography also provides valuable information in patients with HCM. The primary hemodynamic problems with HCM are subaortic obstruction and left ventricular diastolic dysfunction due to abnormal thickness of this chamber. Management of such a patient with HCM depends on which hemodynamic abnormality predominates in the patient's presentation. The subaortic obstruction of HCM is dynamic, and a continuous wave (CW) Doppler sample produces a unique spectral tracing (Fig. 23-11). Flow velocity increases gradu-

ally during early systole and peaks in late systole, creating a dagger-shaped Doppler display. Changes in flow velocity may be measured with a simplified version of Bernoulli's equation ($DP = 4(V_2)^2$), where V_2 is the velocity distal to an obstruction in centimeters per second and P equals the pressure in millimeters of mercury. This peak velocity can be converted into a subaortic pressure gradient. Pulsed wave (PW) Doppler is useful in assessing diastolic function in HCM. A noncompliant, hypertrophied ventricle has a prolonged relaxation time compromising early ventricular filling, and the pressure in the left atrium slowly drops. This may be measured by prolongation of the isovolumic relaxation time (IVRT).[18] The IVRT is defined as the amount of time required for left ventricular pressure to drop below left atrial pressure, allowing the mitral valve to open. This is measured by the aortic value (A_2) closure to mitral valve opening (MVO) (normal, 70 ± 15). The mitral valve velocity pattern by PW reflects the diastolic filling abnormality. The peak E wave is less than the peak A wave, and the mitral valve deceleration time is prolonged (Fig. 23-12). However, not all patients with HCM have this pattern. The diastolic filling may become pseudonormalized or a restrictive pattern may develop when the left atrial pressure becomes elevated. Color flow imaging is also physiologically useful in timing the flow associated with HCM. In addition, it aids in identifying mitral valve regurgitation, which may occur in as

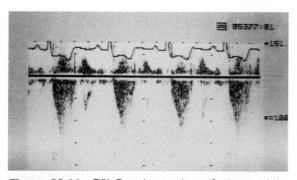

Figure 23-11. CW Doppler tracing of abnormal increased velocity at 2.5 m/sec in a patient with a subaortic gradient.

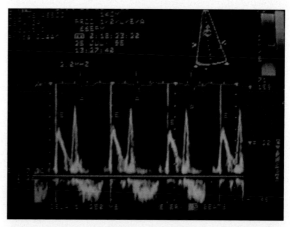

Figure 23-12. PW Doppler tracing of a patient with MCM. Note the reduction in early diastolic filling (E) and the increased velocity following atrial systole (A). The deceleration time is increased.

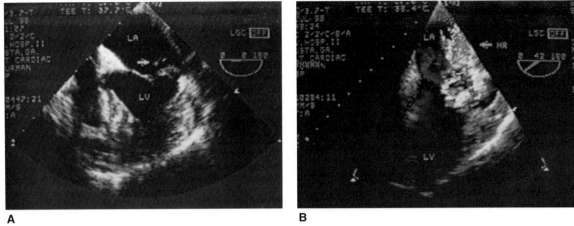

Figure 23-13. (**A,B**) This TEE examination reveals the presence of severe mitral valve regurgitation in a patient with ruptured mitral valve leaflet. MV, mitral valve; LV, left ventricle; LA, left atrium. (See also Color Plate 65.)

many as 90% of patients with HCM. The classic sequence in patients with HCM is increased left ventricular ejection time, obstruction, and mitral regurgitation. Regurgitation is variable but usually correlates directly with the severity of obstruction to the LVOT. Differential diagnosis of HCM includes patients with long-standing moderate to severe hypertension whose echocardiogram may suggest HCM and patients with infiltrative diseases such as amyloidosis and hypereosinophilic syndrome, whose markedly thickened ventricles resemble those of HCM. Patients with other conditions such as chronic renal disease, Friedreich's ataxia, cardiac sarcoma, and lymphoma have been reported to develop disproportional septal thickening that simulates HCM. HCM may occasionally cause obstruction to the right ventricular outflow tract. The echocardiogram shows evidence of right ventricular hypertrophy with increased anterior right ventricular wall thickness. There is systolic anterior motion of the tricuspid valve, and midsystolic closure of the pulmonic valve may occur.[5]

TRANSESOPHAGEAL ECHOCARDIOGRAPHY (TEE)

TEE is useful in patients with HCM—first, to assist and investigate intraoperatively the site of septal myectomy and, second, to evaluate the mitral valve apparatus in patients who may suddenly develop acute congestive heart failure. A small group of patients with HCM develop chordal rupture resulting in severe mitral valve regurgitation (Fig. 23-13*A,B*). These patients require urgent mitral valve repair or replacement. TEE is also indicated to evaluate interventricular septal thickness with suboptimal surface echo studies.

THERAPY

Therapy for patients with HCM consists of either medical or surgical intervention. Medical management may include β-adrenergic receptor blocking drugs, calcium channel blocking drugs, antiarrhythmic agents, insertion of dual-chamber cardiac pacemakers, and prophylaxis for infective endocarditis. Surgical intervention consists of myectomy.[21]

Display 23-1 Quick Reference Guide: Hypertrophic Cardiomyopathy

VENTRICULAR FUNCTION

VS-EDD	>11 mm	End-diastolic diameter of the interventricular septum
LVPW-EDD	≥11 mm	End-diastolic diameter of the left ventricular posterior wall
LAD(max)	41 mm	Maximum diameter of the left atrium
LVEDD	<56 mm	Left ventricular end-diastolic diameter
LVESD	<30 mm	Left ventricular end-systolic diameter
LVFS	>35	Left ventricular fractional shortening
LVEF	>65	Left ventricular ejection fraction

VALVE MORPHOLOGY AND DYNAMICS

SAM of the mitral valve	Redundant cords
Early systolic closure of the aortic valve?	

PRESSURE–FLOW RELATIONSHIPS (DOPPLER ECHOCARDIOGRAPHY)

Parameters of diastolic function
E wave ↓
A wave ↑
E/A ratio ↑
E-(DT) (deceleration time) ↑
DPIDT ↑ normal to increased
Regurgitation
   Qualitative visual proof and semiquantitation of regurgitation (detection, velocity measurement, mapping, and follow-up of mitral and tricuspid regurgitation; graphic display of regurgitation)
Determination of peak systolic pulmonary artery pressure
Determination of mean pulmonary artery pressure
Determination of cardiac output

Tubulent or laminar flow signal in the LVOT? (PW and CW Doppler)
Measurement of intracavitary pressure gradients (CW Doppler)
Measurement of left ventricular ejection time (PW and CW Doppler) ↑
Measurement of isovolumic relaxation time (PW and CW Doppler) ↑

REFERENCES

1. Ballas M, Zoneraich S, Unis M, et al. Non-invasive cardiac evaluation in chronic alcoholic patients with alcohol withdrawal syndrome. Chest. 1982;82:148–153.
2. Brandenburg RO, Chazov E, Cherian G, et al. Report of WHO/ISFC task force on definition and classification of cardiomyopathies. Circulation. 1981;64:437A–438A.
3. Bulkley BH, Fortuin NJ. Systolic anterior motion of the mitral valve without asymmetrical septal hypertrophy. Chest. 1976;69:694–696.
4. Cabin HS, Costello RM, Vasudevan C, et al. Cardiac lymphoma mimicking hypertrophic cardiomyopathy. Am Heart J. 1981;104:466–468.
5. Cardiel EA, Alonso M, Delcon JL, et al. Echocardiographic sign of right-sided hypertrophic obstructive cardiomyopathy. Br Heart J. 1978;40:1321–1325.
6. Feigenbaum H. Echocardiography, 3d ed. Philadelphia, Lea & Febiger; 1981:462.
7. Frank S, Braunwald E. Idiopathic hypertrophic subaortic stenosis: Clinical analysis of 126 patients with emphasis on the natural history. Circulation. 1968;37:759–788.
8. Goodman DJ, Harrison DC, Popp DC. Echocardiographic features of primary pulmonary hypertension. Am J Cardiol. 1974;33:438–443.
9. Gustavson A, Liedholm H, Tylen U. Hypertrophic cardiomyopathy: A correlation between echocardiography, angiographic and hemodynamic findings. Ann Radiol (Paris). 1977;20:419–430.
10. Gutgesell HP, Speer ME, Rosenberg HS. Characterization of the cardiomyopathy in infants of diabetic mothers. Circulation. 1980;64:441–450.
11. Hearne MJ, Sherber HS, deLeon AD. Asymmetric septal hypertrophy in acromegaly: An echocardio-

graphic study (abstract 130). Circulation. 1975; 52(suppl 2):II-35.

12. Henning H, O'Rourke RA, Crawford MH, et al. Inferior myocardial infarction as a cause of asymmetric septal hypertrophy: An echocardiographic study. Am J Cardiol. 1978;41:817–822.

13. Kansac S, Roitman D, Sheffield LT. Interventricular septal thickness and left ventricular hypertrophy: An echocardiographic study. Circulation. 1979;60: 1058–1065.

14. Larter WE, Allen HD, Sahn DJ, et al. The asymmetrically hypertrophied septum: Further differentiation of its causes. Circulation. 1976;53:19–27.

15. McKenna WJ, England D, Doi YL, et al. Arrhythmias in hypertrophic cardiomyopathy: I. Influence on prognosis. Br Heart J. 1981;46:168–172.

16. Maron BJ, Bonow RO, Seshagiri TNR, et al. Hypertrophic cardiomyopathy with ventricular septal hypertrophy localized to the apical region of the left ventricle (apical hypertrophic cardiomyopathy). Am J Cardiol. 1982;49:1838–1848.

17. Maron BJ, Epstein SE. Clinical course of patients with hypertrophic cardiomyopathy. Cardiovasc Clin. 1971;10(1)L253–L265.

18. Maron BJ, Epstein SE. Hypertrophic cardiomyopathy. Recent observations regarding the specificity of three hallmarks of the disease: Asymmetric septal hypertrophy, septal disorganization and systolic anterior motion of the anterior mitral leaflet. Am J Cardiol. 1980;45:141–154.

19. Maron BJ, Gottdiener JS, Epstein SE. Patterns and significance of distribution of left ventricular hypertrophy in hypertrophic cardiomyopathy: A wide-angle, two-dimensional echocardiographic study of 125 patients. Am J Cardiol. 1981;48:418–428.

20. Maron BJ, Gottdiener JS, Perry LW. Specificity of systolic anterior motion of anterior mitral leaflet for hypertrophic cardiomyopathy. Br Heart J. 1981;45: 206–216.

21. Maron BJ, Merrill WH, Freier PA, et al. Long-term clinical course and symptomatic status of patients after operation for hypertrophic subaortic stenosis. Circulation. 1978;57:1205–1213.

22. Maron BJ, Verter J, Kapur S. Disproportionate ventricular septal thickening in the developing normal human heart. Circulation. 1978;57:520–526.

23. Martin RP, Rakowski H, French J, et al. Idiopathic hypertrophic subaortic stenosis viewed by wide-angle, phased-array echocardiography. Circulation. 1979;59:1206–1217.

24. Nanda NC, Gramiak R, Manning JA, et al. Echocardiographic features of subpulmonic obstruction in dextrotransposition of the great vessels. Circulation. 1975;51:515–521.

25. Pollick C, Koilpillai C, Howard R, et al. Left ventricular thrombus demonstrating canalization and mimicking asymmetrical septal hypertrophy on echocardiographic study. Am Heart J. 1982;104:641–643.

26. Prescott R, Quinn JS, Littmann D. Electrocardiographic changes in hypertrophic subaortic stenosis which simulate myocardial infarction. Am Heart J. 1963;66:42–48.

27. Rees A, Eibl F, Minhas K, et al. Echocardiographic evidence of outflow tract obstruction in Pompe's disease (glycogen storage disease of heart). Am J Cardiol. 1976;27:1103–1106.

28. Spirito P, Maron BJ, Rosing DR. Morphologic determinants of hemodynamic state after ventricular septal myotomy-myectomy in patients with obstructive hypertrophic cardiomyopathy: M-mode and two-dimensional echocardiographic assessment. Circulation. 1984;70:984–995.

29. Stewart S, Schreiner B. Co-existing idiopathic hypertrophic subaortic stenosis and coronary artery disease: Clinical implication and operative management. J Thorac Cardiovasc Surg. 1981;82:278–280.

30. Tajik AJ, Gau GT, Schattenberg TT. Echocardiographic "pseudo IHSS" pattern in atrial septal defect. Chest. 1972;62:324–325.

31. TenCate FJ, Balakumaran K, McGhie J, et al. Angina pectoris in hypertrophic cardiomyopathy (HCM): Cause or consequence of disturbed relaxation? (abstract). Circulation. 1980;62(suppl 3):317.

32. TenCate FJ, Hugenholtz PG, VanDorp WG, et al. Prevalence of diagnostic abnormalities in patients with genetically transmitted asymmetric septal hypertrophy. Am J Cardiol. 1979;43:731–737.

33. Yamaguchi H, Ishimura T, Nishyama S, et al. Hypertrophic non-obstructive cardiomyopathy with giant negative T waves (apical hypertrophy): Ventriculographic and echocardiographic features in 30 patients. Am J Cardiol. 1979;44:401–412.

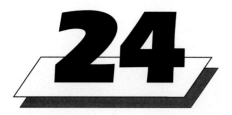

Dilated and Restrictive Cardiomyopathies

J. CHARLES POPE

Dilated Cardiomyopathy

Dilated cardiomyopathy (DCMP) is recognized by dilatation of unknown cause of one or both ventricles. Dilatation often becomes severe, and it is invariably accompanied by hypertrophy. Systolic ventricular function is impaired, and congestive heart failure may or may not supervene. Presentations with disturbances of ventricular or atrial rhythm are common, and death may occur at any stage.[4]

Clinical Presentation

A careful history is of paramount importance in patients suspected of having DCMP. Patients should be questioned about their consumption of alcohol, possible exposure to toxic substances, and any history of infection, hypertension, or systemic illnesses, including rheumatic fever. It may be difficult to separate DCMP from ischemic cardiomyopathy. Clues may be derived from a history of chest pain or heart attack, from electrocardiographic (ECG) or radionuclide imaging, and from echocardiographic studies.[7,8,25] Patients with DCMP may have no symptoms, and cardiomegaly on the chest x-ray may be the only clinical finding. They may have symptoms of subjective arrhythmias and exertional dyspnea, orthopnea, paroxysmal nocturnal dyspnea, periph-

eral edema, or abdominal pain due to hepatic congestion. Less frequently, chest discomfort typical of angina pectoris or atypical chest discomfort may occur.[26]

Physical examination usually reveals an arterial pulse of small volume and increased venous pressures. Blood pressure is usually normal or low. Palpation of the precordium often detects a diffuse lateral and inferiorly displaced left ventricular apex. There may also be a left parasternal lift or left ventricular heave. Auscultation reveals muffled heart sounds with an accentuated pulmonic component of S_2. An S_4, S_3 gallop or a summation gallop may be present. Murmurs of tricuspid and mitral regurgitation are heard when there is atrioventricular valve annular dilatation. The chest film shows generalized cardiomegaly without calcification of the valves or coronary arteries. There may be a large globular cardiac silhouette, in which case pericardial effusion should be expected. The pulmonary vasculature may suggest increased pulmonary venous pressure. The ECG reveals nonspecific ST- and T-wave changes. There may be Q waves suggestive of infarction, and any type of dysrhythmia may be present. Atrial fibrillation is seen in approximately 20% of these patients.[16] Ventricular arrhythmias are also common. On 24-hr Holter monitoring, ventricular tachycardia has been reported in approximately 60% of patients.[11]

Echocardiographic Features (Two-Dimensional and M-Mode)

M-mode echocardiography (Fig. 24-1) reveals left and right ventricular enlargement with abnormal indices of left ventricular function (i.e., decreased ejection fraction and fractional shortening). The amplitude of separation of the mitral valve leaflets may be decreased, and the mitral apparatus may be located posteriorly. So-called miniaturization of the mitral valve may be present, related to decreased cardiac output and decreased volumes flowing through the mitral valve during diastole. Abnormal closure of the mitral valve, as noted by a B notch, may signify elevated left ventricular end-diastolic filling pressure.[14] Pericardial effusion is usually seen, and mural thrombi are common.[8] The two-dimensional examination usually demonstrates a dilated left ventricle with evidence of poor left ventricular ejection fraction and mitral and tricuspid valve regurgitation due to annular dilatation. There is usually multiple cardiac chamber enlargement. In addition, the two-dimensional echocardiographic examination provides increased sensitivity in identifying mural thrombus and evaluating for segmental wall motion abnormalities, as seen in patients with ischemic cardiomyopathies (Fig. 24-2).

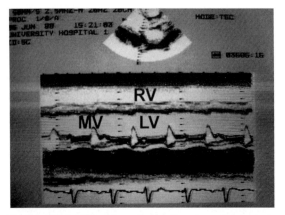

Figure 24-1. M-mode echocardiogram demonstrates right and left ventricular enlargement and poor contractility of both ventricles. Increased E-point to septal separation (EPSS). RV, right ventricle; LV, left ventricle; MV, mitral valve.

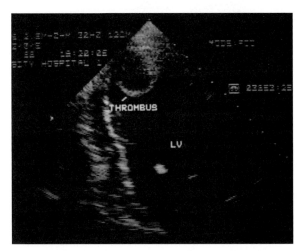

Figure 24-2. This two-dimensional apical view shows a large apical thrombus in a dysfunctional left ventricle (LV).

Doppler (Pulsed Wave, Continuous Wave) and Color Flow Imaging

The Doppler examination reveals abnormal diastolic function. There is evidence on pulsed wave Doppler of diminished flow velocities through the mitral and tricuspid valves. There may be a reversed E to A ratio; however, pseudonormalization or restrictive diastolic patterns may be present. In addition, multiple-valve regurgitation is common, affecting the mitral and tricuspid valves. The color-flow Doppler pattern, interrogated from the cardiac apex, reveals a series of "puffs of smoke" during diastole (Fig. 24-3). This is related to the low cardiac output state. Most patients with DCMP have associated atrioventricular valvular regurgitation of varying degrees. Color flow Doppler imaging demonstrates mitral regurgitation as a bright blue or mosaic jet entering the left atrium (Fig. 24-4). Meese and colleagues demonstrated a very high incidence of atrioventricular valvular regurgitation in patients with DCMP.[18] Mitral regurgitation was noted in all patients, and tricuspid regurgitation was present in 91%. Valvular regurgitation is usually mild to moderate. Semilunar valve regurgitation is less common. Studies have shown that approximately 23% of patients with DCMP had aortic regurgitation, and 58% had pulmonic regurgitation.[18]

Right ventricular pressures may be calculated with pulsed or continuous wave Doppler informa-

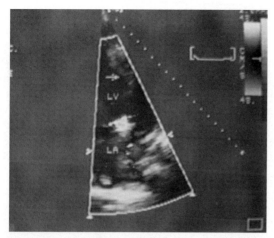

Figure 24-3. Color flow Doppler tracing of a patient with congestive cardiomyopathy. Note the low-velocity flow in the middle to distal left ventricle (LV). See arrow. LA, left atrium. Black-and-white image with spontaneous contrast noted in a patient with DCMP and a low flow state. (See also Color Plate 66.)

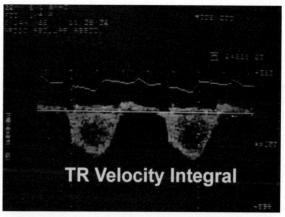

Figure 24-5. Calculation of right ventricular (RV) or pulmonary artery (PA) (without pulmonic stenosis) systolic pressure from a continuous wave Doppler tracing: Maximum tricuspid regurgitation velocity (MAX TR VEL) = 4.5 m/sec.
Transvalvular pressure gradient = $4(4.5)^2$ = mm Hg.
PA systolic pressure = $4 \times (4.5)^2$ + right atrial pressure = 81 mm Hg + 20 mm Hg (approximately) = 101 mm Hg.
Numerical assignment of right atrial pressure (in millimeters of mercury) is subjective and based on the sizes of the right ventricle and right atrium and/or the presence of dilated inferior vena cava or jugular venous distention.

tion by observing the peak tricuspid regurgitant velocity on a color flow–guided examination. This calculation may be made by adding the determined transtricuspid valve systolic gradient to the calculated or assumed right atrial pressure. This is performed by observing the inferior vena cava and its inspiratory decrease. The velocity shift through the tricuspid valve is calculated by the Bernoulli equation ($DP = 4 (V_2)^2$) (Fig. 24-5). Similarly, the peak end-diastolic pulmonary regurgitant velocity can be

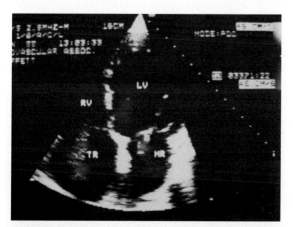

Figure 24-4. Apical four-chamber two-dimensional echocardiogram with color flow Doppler mapping. The patient has mitral (MR) and tricuspid (TR) valve regurgitation. RV, right ventricle; LV, left ventricle. (See also Color Plate 67.)

used to determine the pulmonary artery diastolic pressure[12] (Fig. 24-6). Values for cardiac output calculated by Doppler method sampling of the pulmonary artery or the left ventricular outflow tract (LVOT) are usually decreased.

Doppler-derived mitral flow velocities have proven useful in characterizing left ventricular filling patterns in patients with congestive cardiomyopathy. An analysis of the mitral flow velocity waveforms in patients with congestive cardiomyopathy found a significantly lower peak velocity during rapid diastolic filling and reduced ratios of peak velocity during atrial systole to peak velocity during rapid diastolic filling.[28] These findings suggest that atrial systole is responsible for the majority of cases of diastolic filling of the ventricles. In the same study, peak velocities of patients with DCMP and mitral regurgitation during rapid diastolic filling were similar to those of normal subjects. This observation probably reflects the increased flow from left atrium to left ventricle in diastole secondary to mitral valve regurgitation. Therefore the presence of mitral regurgitation may falsely alter the ratio of peak E and A velocities in diastole.

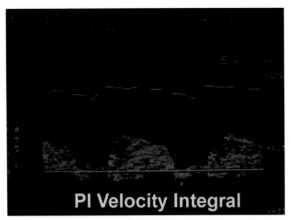

Figure 24-6. Calculating pulmonary artery (PA) diastolic pressure from continuous wave Doppler tracing. Maximum pulmonary artery velocity at end diastole (MAX PA VEL) = 2.5 m/sec.
Transvalvular pressure gradient = 4 $(2.5)^2$ = 25 mm Hg.
PA diastolic pressure = 25 mm Hg + right atrial pressure = 25 mm Hg + 10 mm Hg = 35 mm Hg.
Numerical values of pressure (in millimeters of mercury) within the right atrium are subjective, based on the size of the right ventricle and right atrium and the presence of jugular venous or inferior vena cava distention.

Additional Doppler information may include mitral valve inflow filling patterns. In general, the abnormal left ventricular relaxation is noted by a decreased E/A ratio, a prolonged deceleration time (DT), and an increased isovolumic relaxation time (IVRT). This pattern is seen in patients with normal to mildly elevated filling pressures. These patients have minimal symptoms. As the disease progresses, a restrictive pattern of filling is seen, including increased E wave, decreased A wave, increased E/A ratio, shortened DT, and decreased IVRT. This corresponds to significant increases in left ventricular end-diastolic pressures, left atrial pressures, and symptoms of congestive heart failure.

DCMP of Known Cause

Myocarditis should be considered in patients with a relatively short history of congestive heart failure, particularly if there was a prior febrile illness, in which case endomyocardial biopsy should be considered.[21] In addition, long-standing valvular heart disease may precipitate global left ventricular dysfunction. Color flow Doppler imaging is important in the assessment of the severity of valvular lesions; thereafter cardiac catheterization may be necessary to determine the appropriateness of surgical treatment of valvular regurgitation instead of DCMP. Clinically, severe aortic stenosis with low-output states may masquerade as DCMP. Again, Doppler examination is extremely important in evaluating this condition. The Doppler examination is sensitive enough to accurately assess the severity of the patient's aortic valve disease so that appropriate management can be instituted.

Familial DCMP has been reported with approximately a 20% incidence of inheritance. Such patients should have immediate family members screened with an echocardiogram.

Additionally, arrhythmogenic right ventricular dysplasia (ARVD or UHLS) anomaly has a genetic inheritance. This is a right ventricular cardiomyopathy caused by a fatty infiltrative process involving the right ventricular free wall. The echocardiogram reveals a dilated, poorly contracting right ventricle proportionally more severe than left ventricular findings. Low right ventricular pressure is generated; therefore tricuspid regurgitation velocities are low, usually less than 2 m/sec. Patients with ARVD have a high incidence of malignant ventricular arrhythmias.

Peripartum cardiomyopathy is typically considered an idiopathic primary congestive cardiomyopathy. This event may develop late in the third trimester or in the first 3 postpartum months, with echocardiographic features of a DCMP. The clinical course varies, but approximately 50% of patients show complete or near-complete recovery of cardiac function within the first 6 months postpartum. The remaining 50% demonstrate persistent left ventricular dysfunction and chronic congestive heart failure with a high incidence of morbidity and mortality.

Transesophageal Echocardiography

Transesophageal echocardiography (TEE) may also provide additional information in patients with DCMP. The presence of left atrial thrombi may be sensitively investigated with TEE, particularly the area of the left atrial appendage, which is not seen well from the surface echo (Fig. 24-7). In patients with difficult surface echocardiographic studies, TEE provides clear windows of left and right ven-

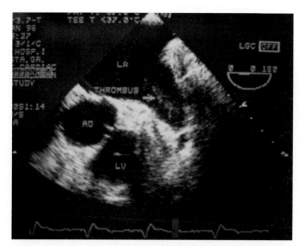

Figure 24-7. *This TEE examination reveals a dilated left atrium with spontaneous contrast within the left atrial chamber. A formed thrombus is noted in the left atrial appendage (arrow). LA, left atrium; LV, left ventricle.*

tricular function and Doppler information on the amount of regurgitation through the atrioventricular valves. Both left and right ventricular thrombi may also be visualized with TEE in patients with suboptimal surface examinations.

Therapy

Treatment of patients with DCMP consists of weight reduction, sodium restriction, and abstinence from alcohol and tobacco. Diuretics, positive inotrophic agents, vasodilators, anticoagulants, and antiarrhythmics all are indicated at various points in the natural history of the disease. In addition, immunosuppressants have been used to treat a subset of patients determined by endomyocardial biopsy to have myocarditis. "Physiologic" dual-chamber pacing and cardiac transplantation may decrease the morbidity and mortality associated with congestive cardiomyopathies.

Other Congestive Cardiomyopathies

Other disorders associated with a clinical picture resembling DCMP are abnormalities of the autoimmune system such as those seen in patients whose body has rejected a heart transplant. IVRTs are highly sensitive and specific in identifying patients who reject cardiac transplants. There is a significant decrease in the IVRT during the acute process compared to nonrejection phases.[22] Cardiac abnormalities have also been noted in patients with acquired immunodeficiency syndrome (AIDS); they usually include pericardial effusion, hypokinetic left ventricle, and secondary myocarditis.[9] Additional reported findings are segmental wall motion abnormalities, left ventricular enlargement, and abnormal left ventricular systolic function.

Chagas' disease is endemic to South America. It results from chronic parasitic infections caused by the protozoan *Trypanosoma cruzi* and produces severe left ventricular dysfunction and apical aneurysms, with evidence of multiple segmental wall motion abnormalities.[19] Some drugs may cause cardiac toxicity—doxorubicin, cyclophosphamides, antiparasitic drugs, chloroquine, and psychotrophic drugs such as phenothiazines, tricyclic antidepressants, and lithium. Hypersensitivity myocarditis has been reported secondary to therapy with sulfonamides and methyldopa.[29] Cardiac toxicity has also been induced by chemicals such as hydrocarbons, carbon monoxide, arsenic, lead, phosphorus, mercury, and cobalt.[29] Physical agents such as radiation may precipitate congestive heart failure or pericardial disease. Connective tissue diseases such as systemic lupus erythematosus, Kawaski's disease, periarteritis nodosa, and systemic giant cell arteritis have all been implicated in producing depressed left ventricular cardiac function. Hemochromatosis and sarcoidosis also may produce dilated cardiomyopathies, (Table 24-1). Additionally, patients who have chronic alcoholism may develop dilated cardiomyopathy.[3]

Restrictive Cardiomyopathy

Restrictive cardiomyopathy is a condition that may exist with or without obliteration of the left ventricle and right ventricular cavity. Restrictive cardiomyopathies include myocardial fibrosis and Löeffler's cardiomyopathy. Endomyocardial scarring usually affects either one or both ventricles and restricts ventricular filling. Involvement of the atrioventricular valves is common, but the outflow tracts are spared. Cavity obliteration of the left ventricle is characteristic of advanced cases.[4] Another class of disease similar to restrictive cardiomyopathy, and

TABLE 24-1. Congestive Cardiomyopathies and Associated Echocardiographic Findings

	LV Dimension	LVWT	FS%	Wall Motion	Doppler	Other Findings
Friedreich's Ataxia	Normal, dilated	Thick	Normal, decreased	Normal, globally decreased	Reversed E/A	Similar to hypertrophic myopathy without LVOT obstruction
Hemochromatosis	Dilated	Normal, diminished	Decreased	Globally decreased	↑ E/A ratio with short DT (advanced stages)	Multiple valvular regurgitation, atrial enlargement
Sarcoidosis	Normal, dilated	Normal, diminished	Decreased	Regional abnormalities, posterior basilar aneurysm	↑ E/A ratio with short DT (advanced stages)	
Systemic Lupus Erythematous (SLE)	Normal	Normal, thick	Normal, decreased	Normal, globally decreased	Possible constrictive pathology	Pericardial effusion, Libman-Sachs endocarditis
Peripartum Cardiomyopathy	Normal, dilated	Normal	Decreased	Globally decreased	Reversed E/A or E/A ratio (advanced stages)	Pericardial effusion

usually included with it, is infiltrative cardiomyopathy. The pathophysiology of these conditions is essentially the same as that of restrictive cardiomyopathies of known origin (Table 24-2).

Clinical Presentation

The most common clinical presentation in patients with restrictive cardiomyopathy is congestive heart failure. Other symptoms may be arrhythmia, atypical chest discomfort, syncope, or sudden death. The examination may reveal evidence of biventricular failure or elevated jugular venous pressure with prominent jugular vein distention. The chest radiograph may be normal, but more frequently it shows an enlarged cardiac silhouette. The ECG may demonstrate rhythm disturbances consisting of sinus node dysfunction with evidence of sick sinus syndrome, various degrees of atrioventricular disease, or complete heart block. Sudden death has been reported in approximately 30% of patients with restrictive cardiomyopathy, and is presumed to be related to disturbances in conduction and rhythm.

Echocardiographic Features (Two-Dimensional and M-Mode)

All restrictive cardiomyopathies (primary restrictive cardiomyopathy, Löeffler's endocarditis, and endomyocardial fibrosis) have similar pathophysiologic findings, typically atrial enlargement out of proportion to the ventricular internal dimensions. This is primarily the result of reduced left ventricular compliance and resultant atrial dilatation. Figure 24-8 is an apical four-chamber view of a patient with classic features of restrictive cardiomyopathy. There is evidence of normal left and right ventricular wall thickness and interventricular septal thickness, but there is also evidence of biatrial enlargement and abnormal elevated atrial pressures. Hemodynamic data from cardiac catheterization are consistent with abrupt elevation of early diastolic pressures at rest and with exercise, and usually can be differentiated from that seen in constrictive pericardial disease.[17] Recent studies using Doppler interrogation provide evidence that restrictive cardiomyopathy and constrictive pericarditis may be separated by the evaluation of Doppler inflow through the atrioventricular

TABLE 24-2. RESTRICTIVE CARDIOMYOPATHIES AND ASSOCIATED ECHOCARDIOGRAPHIC FINDINGS

	LV Dimension	LVWT	FS%	Wall Motion	Doppler (PW, CW)	Valve	Other
AMYLOIDOSIS	Normal	Increased, granular myocardium	Normal, diminished (advanced)	Normal, globally depressed (advanced)	Reversed E/A ratio or ↑ E/A ratio, short DT (advanced)	Multiple thickening and regurgitation	Pericardial effusion atrial enlargement
CARCINOID	Normal	Normal	Normal	Normal	↑ E/A	Right-sided valves, thickened multiple regurgitation PS, TS	May involve left side with patent foramen ovale; right ventricular enlargement
HYPEREOSINOPHILIC SYNDROME	Normal, dilated	Increased (apex)	Normal, diminished	Normal, globally depressed	↑ E/A, short DT	MV leaflet thickening, regurgitation	Apical thrombus; apical obliteration
HEMOCHROMAIOSIS (INFILTRATIVE DILATED PROPERTIES)	Normal, dilated	Normal	Decreased	Globally depressed	↑ E/A, short DT	MV leaflet thickening	Multiple regurgitation
SARCOIDOSIS (INFILTRATIVE WITH DILATED PROPERTIES)	Normal, dilated	Normal, diminished	Decreased	Regional abnormalities	↑ E/A, short DT (advanced)	MV leaflet thickening	

valves.[1,10] In the presence of constrictive pericarditis, significant respiratory variation in E and A velocities through the mitral and tricuspid valves is noted during the first beat of inspiration and expiration. This feature separates constrictive pericarditis from

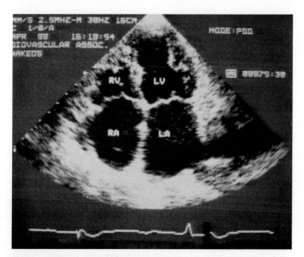

Figure 24-8. *Apical four-chamber two-dimensional echocardiogram in a patient with severe biatrial enlargement and normal-sized ventricles. RV, right ventricle; LV, left ventricle; RA, right atrium; LA, left atrium.*

restrictive cardiomyopathy in that there is a static Doppler abnormality in diastolic filling with restrictive cardiomyopathy not dependent on variations in loading conditions related to respiration. Endomyocardial biopsies have not been helpful in defining the cause of restrictive cardiomyopathy except in patients with amyloid heart disease.

The most commonly reviewed restrictive (infiltrative) cardiomyopathy is that secondary to amyloidosis (extracellular deposition of the fibrous protein amyloid in one or more sites).[15] The primary form of amyloid has a predilection for mesenchymal structures, including the heart. In advanced forms, the two-dimensional echocardiographic examination identifies abnormal myocardial tissue characteristics, notably a hyperrefractile granular appearance of the myocardium.[27] Figure 24-9 is a two-dimensional parasternal long axis view of a patient with classic features of restrictive cardiomyopathy. There is evidence of hypertrophy of the left and right ventricular walls and the interventricular septum and evidence of a small left ventricular cavity with hypokinesia of all cardiac walls. There is also evidence of multiple valvular thickenings and pericardial effusion.

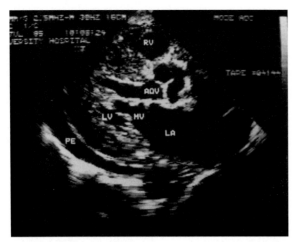

Figure 24-9. Parasternal long axis two-dimensional echocardiogram shows severe left ventricular hypertrophy with a granular, sparkling appearance consistent with infiltrative cardiomyopathy. The valves are thickened, and there is a pericardial effusion (PE). Severe left atrial enlargement is present. LA, left atrium; RV, right ventricle; LV, left ventricle; MV, mitral valve; AOV, aortic valve.

The primary hemodynamic abnormality seen in these patients is ventricular diastolic dysfunction. The unifying hemodynamic changes include rapid completion of early diastolic filling into a nonelastic ventricle, resulting in completion of ventricular filling early in diastole, with very little

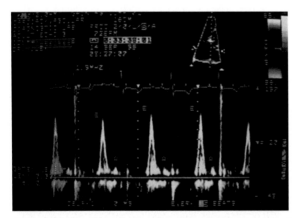

Figure 24-10. Pulsed wave Doppler echocardiogram of a patient with abnormal diastolic filling. The deceleration time is significantly shortened. E, early rapid filling velocity; A, filling velocity following atrial systole.

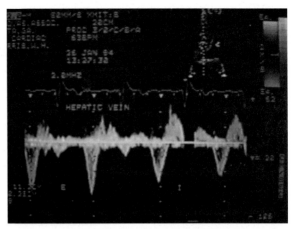

Figure 24-11. Pulsed wave Doppler tracing in the hepatic vein illustrating a restrictive myopathic pattern of flow. Note the increase in diastolic filling and reversed flow during atrial systole. (See also Color Plate 68.)

late diastolic flow.[13] A sensitive diagnostic Doppler echocardiographic feature is represented by a shortened deceleration time of the mitral and tricuspid velocity envelopes and diminished IVRTs.[2] Figure 24-10 demonstrates the restrictive Doppler flow pattern seen on pulsed wave examination.[6] The mitral inflow velocity pattern in restrictive cardiomyopathy typically produces increased E velocity ($\geq$1.0 m/sec), decreased A velocity ($\leq$0.5 m/sec), increased E/A ratio ($\geq$2.0), decreased DT ($\leq$150 msec), and decreased IVRT ($\leq$70 msec). Pulmonary or hepatic vein flow in restrictive cardiomyopathy produces systolic forward flow that is less than diastolic forward flow and increased diastolic (atrial) flow reversals with inspiration in the hepatic vein (Fig. 24-11).

Other Infiltrative Cardiomyopathies of Known Cause

Additional infiltrative cardiomyopathies include sarcoidosis, hemochromatosis, and hypereosinophilic syndrome. Sarcoidosis is a multisystemic granulomatous disease that may involve the heart.[24] The incidence of heart involvement with sarcoidosis is low. Approximately 5% of patients may present with conduction system abnormalities, including complete heart block, ventricular dysrhythmias, progres-

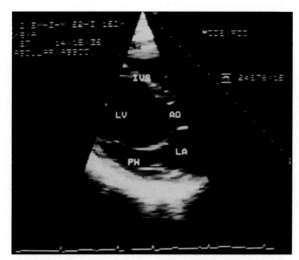

Figure 24-12. Parasternal long axis view shows thinning of the basilar posterior wall in this patient with sarcoidosis. IVS, interventricular septum; AO, aorta; LV, left ventricle; PW, posterior wall; LA, left atrium.

phils per cubic millimeter and evidence of organ involvement. Cardiac involvement is common. Typically, both right and left cardiac chambers are involved, with thickening of the inflow areas and thrombotic-fibrotic obliteration of the ventricular apices. Echocardiographic features include reduced motion of the posterior mitral leaflet, in addition to thickening of the inferobasal left ventricular wall, with biapical obliteration resulting from thrombotic-fibrotic infiltration. The resultant pathophysiology is that of restrictive ventricular diastolic filling, as noted on pulse wave Doppler interrogation (Fig. 24-13). A rare event of ventricular cavity dilatation and marked decrease in systolic function is seen in acute hypereosinophilic crisis. These patients die from severe heart failure and ventricular arrhythmias.

Other chemical storage disorders, such as those of glycogen and lipid, have been identified, al-

sive heart failure, and recurrent pericardial effusions, sudden death may occur. These findings are most common in young or middle-aged adult patients. Echocardiographic features include abnormal ventricular wall thickness, pericardial effusions, and right ventricular dysfunction secondary to cor pulmonale (which is caused by the pulmonary sarcoidosis) (Fig. 24-12).

Hemochromatosis is an iron-storage disease that affects multiple organs and tissue systems. There are primary and secondary forms.[5] Echocardiographic features (principally in the early stages) include nondilated, thickened left ventricular walls with preserved systolic function and diminished compliance. In later stages of hemochromatosis the ventricular cavities become dilated, with impaired systolic function and left atrial enlargement. Doppler assessment reveals a restrictive abnormal relaxation pattern. The mortality rate of these patients is approximately 50%.[20] Secondary hemochromatosis has been identified in patients with anemia who require multiple transfusions. Their echocardiographic features have been described by Valdes-Cruz and co-workers.[30]

Hypereosinophilic syndrome is defined as a persistent eosinophilia with more than 1500 eosino-

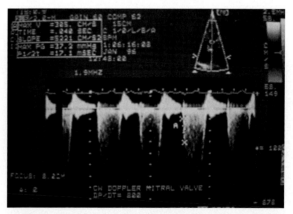

Figure 24-13. This continuous wave Doppler tracing of mitral regurgitation is used to calculate the DP/DT, which is reduced at 800 mm Hg/sec, indicating failing left ventricular systolic function. The DP/DT represents the isovolumic phase index of LV pressure rise (DP/DT) can be estimated. Left atrial pressure does not change significantly during the isovolumic contraction period. Therefore, the MR velocity changes during this period reflect DP/DT. The time interval between 1 and 3 m/sec on the MR velocity integral is measured. The DP/DT is calculated by 32 mm Hg/time (sec). Normal is greater than 1200 mm Hg/sec. The right ventricular DP/DT is derived from the TR jet velocity integral. The time interval between 1 and 2 m/sec is used for the right side. The DP/DT is calculated by 12 mm Hg/time (sec). (See also Color Plate 69.)

though few echocardiographic studies have been performed in these patients.[23]

Therapy

The treatment and prognosis of patients with restrictive cardiomyopathy are currently unsatisfactory. To date, no mode of treatment has proved safe and effective in reversing or even slowing the progress of amyloid deposition. Mean survival among patients with primary amyloidosis, with or without heart disease, averages approximately 1 year from the time of diagnosis; survival beyond 2 years is unusual.

Display 24-1. Quick Reference Guide: DCMP

VENTRICULAR FUNCTION

RVEDD	>35 mm	Right ventricular end-diastolic diameter
LAD (max)	>41 mm	Maximum diameter of the left atrium
LVEDD	>56 mm	Left ventricular end-diastolic diameter
LVESD	>35 mm	Left ventricular end-systolic diameter
LVFS	<25	Left ventricular fractional shortening
LVEF	<50	Left ventricular ejection fraction
Wall motion analysis	Globally ↓	Qualitative

VALVE MORPHOLOGY AND DYNAMICS

Reduced aortic root excursion
Premature mitral valve closure
Reduced mitral and aortic valve opening amplitude
Shoulder in the A-C slope—"B" notch ↑ LVEDP

PRESSURE–FLOW RELATIONSHIPS (DOPPLER)

Regurgitations:
Qualitative, semiquantitation findings
   Detection, velocity measurement, and mapping of regurgitation
   Follow-up of mitral and tricuspid regurgitation
   Graphic display of regurgitation
Determination of peak systolic pulmonary artery pressures
Determination of mean pulmonary artery pressure
Determination of cardiac output
Reduced DP/DT

TRANSESOPHAGEAL ECHOCARDIOGRAPHY

Detection of intracardiac thrombi
Image quality superior to that of transthoracic echocardiography

---

Display 24-2.   Quick Reference Guide: Restrictive Cardiomyopathy

VENTRICULAR FUNCTION

IVS-EDD	≥ 11 mm	End-diastolic diameter of the interventricular septum
LVPW-EDD	≥ 11 mm	End-diastolic diameter of the left ventricular posterior wall
LAD (max)	41 mm	Maximum diameter of the left atrium
LVEDD	Variable	Left ventricular end-diastolic diameter
LVESD	Variable	Left ventricular end-systolic diameter
LVFS	Variable	Left ventricular fractional shortening
LVEF	Variable	Left ventricular ejection fraction

VALVE MORPHOLOGY AND DYNAMICS

Multiple valvular thickening
Reduced valvular excursions, multiple valvular regurgitation

PRESSURE–FLOW RELATIONSHIPS (DOPPLER ECHOCARDIOGRAPHY)

Doppler echocardiography criteria in different stages of restrictive cardiomyopathy

Early Stage	**Advanced Stage**
v_{max} E, mitral valve ↓	v_{max} E, mitral valve ↔ ↑
v_{max} A, mitral valve ↑	v_{max} A, mitral valve ↓
E/A ratio ↓	E/A ratio ↑
Deceleration time ↑ (>240 msec)	Deceleration time ↓ (<160 msec)
Isovolumic relaxation ↑ (>70 msec)	Isovolumic relaxation ↔ (↓)(≤70 msec)
v_{max} systolic, hepatic vein ↑	v_{max} systolic, hepatic vein ↓
v_{max} diastolic, hepatic vein ↓	v_{max} diastolic, hepatic vein ↑
Mild valvular incompetence possible	Mild valvular incompetence possible

REFERENCES

1. Appleton CP, Hatle LK, Popp RL. Central venous flow velocity patterns can differentiate constrictive pericarditis from restrictive cardiomyopathy (abstract). J Am Coll Cardiol. 1987;9:119.

2. Appleton CP, Hatle LK, Popp RL. Demonstration of restrictive ventricular physiology by Doppler echocardiography. J Am Coll Cardiol. 1988;2(4):757–768.

3. Ballas M, Zoneraich S, Unis M, et al. Non-invasive cardiac evaluation in chronic alcoholic patients with alcohol withdrawal syndrome. Chest. 1982;82:148–153.

4. Brandenburg RO, Chazov E, Cherian G, et al. Report of WHO/ISFC task force on definition and classification of cardiomyopathies. Circulation. 1981;64:437A–438A.

5. Buja LM, Roberts NC. Iron in the heart: Etiology and clinical significance. Am J Med. 1971;51:209–221.

6. Chen C, Rodriguez L, Guerrero L, et al. Non-invasive estimation of the instantaneous first derivative of left ventricular pressure using continuous wave Doppler echocardiography. Circulation. 1991;83:2101–2110.

7. Curtius JM, Freimuth M, Kuhn H, et al. Exercise echocardiography in dilated cardiomyopathy. Ztschr Kardiol. 1982;71:727–730.

8. Demaria AN, Bommer W, Lee G, et al. Value and limitations of two-dimensional echocardiography in assessment of cardiomyopathy. Am J Cardiol. 1980;46:1224–1231.

9. Fink L, Reichele N, Sutton MGSJ. Cardiac abnormalities in acquired immune deficiency syndrome. Am J Cardiol. 1984;54:1161–1163.

10. Hatle LK, Appleton CP, Popp RL. Constrictive pericarditis and restrictive cardiomyopathy differentiation by Doppler according to atrioventricular flow velocities (abstract). J Am Coll Cardiol. 1987;9:178.

11. Huang SK, Messer JV, Denes P. Significance of ventricular tachycardia in idiopathic dilated cardiomyopathy: Observations in 35 patients. Am J Cardiol. 1983;51:507–512.

12. Kitabatake A, Kodama K, Masuyama T, et al. Continuous wave Doppler echocardiographic detection of pulmonary regurgitation and its application to non-

invasive estimation of pulmonary artery pressure. Circulation. 1986;74:484–492.

13. Klein AL, Luscher TF, Hatle LK, et al. Spectrum of diastolic function abnormalities in cardiac amyloidosis (abstract 499). Circulation. 1987;76(suppl 4): 4–126.

14. Konecke LL, Feigenbaum H, Chang S, et al. Abnormal mitral valve motion in patients with elevated left ventricular diastolic pressures. Circulation. 1973;47: 989–996.

15. Kyle RA, Greipp PR. Amyloidosis (AL): Clinical and laboratory features in 229 cases. Mayo Clin Proc. 1983;58:665–683.

16. Mann B, Ray R, Goldberger AL, et al. Atrial fibrillation in congestive cardiomyopathy: Echocardiographic and hemodynamic correlates. Cathet Cardiovasc Diagn. 1981;7:387–395.

17. Meaney E, Shabetai R, Bhargava V, et al. Cardiac amyloidosis, constrictive pericarditis and restrictive cardiomyopathy. Am J Cardiol. 1976;38:547–556.

18. Meese R, Adams D, Kisslo J. Assessment of valvular regurgitation by conventional and color-flow Doppler in dilated cardiomyopathy. Echocardiography. 1987;3(6):505–511.

19. de Oliveira JAM, Frederigue U, Filho EC. Apical aneurysm of Chagas' heart disease. Br Heart J. 1981; 46:432–437.

20. Olson LJ, Baldus WP, Tajik AJ. Cardiac involvement in idiopathic hemochromatosis: Echocardiographic and clinical correlations. Am J Cardiol. 1987;60(10): 885–889.

21. Parrillo JE, Aretz HT, Palacios I, et al. The results of transvenous endomyocardial biopsy can frequently be used to diagnose myocardial disease in patients with idiopathic heart failure: Endomyocardial biopsies in 100 consecutive patients revealed a substantial incidence of myocarditis. Circulation. 1984;69: 93–101.

22. Pope JC, Zumbro GL, Battey LL, et al. Isovolumic relaxation period as an indicator of cardiac allograft rejection (abstract). J Heart Transplant. 1986;5(5): 380.

23. Rees A, Eibl F, Minhas K, et al. Echocardiographic evidence of outflow tract obstruction in Pompe's disease (glycogen storage disease of heart). Am J Cardiol. 1976;27:1103–1106.

24. Roberts WC, Ferrans VJ. Pathologic anatomy of the cardiomyopathies: Idiopathic, dilated and hypertrophic types, infiltrative types and endomyocardial disease with and without eosinophilia. Hum Pathol. 1975;6:287–342.

25. Saltissi A, Hockings B, Croft DN, et al. Thallium 209 myocardial imaging in patients with dilated and ischemic cardiomyopathy. Br Heart J. 1981;46: 209–295.

26. Segal JP, Stapleton JF, McClellan JR, et al. Idiopathic cardiomyopathy: Clinical features, prognosis and therapy. Curr Prob Cardiol. 1978;3:1–48.

27. Sigueira-Filho AG, Cunha CL, Tajik AJ, et al. M-mode and two-dimensional echocardiographic features in cardiac amyloidosis. Circulation. 1981;63: 188–196.

28. Takenaka K, Dabestani A, Gardin JM, et al. Pulsed Doppler echocardiographic study of left ventricular filling in dilated cardiomyopathy. Am J Cardiol. 1986;58:143–147.

29. Taliereio CP, Olney BA, Lie JT. Myocarditis related to drug hypersensitivity. Mayo Clin Proc. 1985;60: 463–468.

30. Valdes-Cruz LM, Reinecke C, Rutkowski M, et al. Preclinical abnormal segmental cardiac manifestations of thalassemia major in children on transfusion-chelation therapy: Echocardiographic alterations of left ventricular posterior wall contraction and relaxation patterns. Am Heart J. 1982;103:505–525.

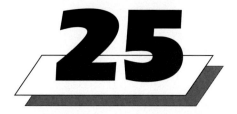

Cardiac Trauma

HENNY J. RUDANSKY, ALVIN GREENGART, and JUDAH A. CHARNOFF

Chest trauma has become increasingly common in the past few decades, mainly due to the increased incidence of high-speed motor vehicle accidents[63] and violent crime.[2] Cardiac injury resulting from chest trauma may initially go unnoticed as attention is directed to more visible injuries.[4] Recognition of cardiac injury is crucial, as it may alter the management of patients with chest injuries.[17]

The large constellation of possible cardiac abnormalities that can result from trauma makes detection of cardiac injury a challenge. Diagnosis is usually based on clinical findings and on the results of procedures such as radiography, electrocardiography, and cardiac enzyme studies.[4] Echocardiography can contribute important diagnostic information, though the transthoracic echocardiography (TTE) examination may be hampered by the serious physical condition of the patient or by bandages or other injuries.[52] The advent of transesophageal echocardiography (TEE) has greatly expanded the workup of these patients, as it bypasses external wounds and provides enhanced imaging of the cardiac structures as well as the thoracic aorta. TEE can also be utilized intraoperatively to assess cardiac function during repair of traumatic injuries.

The incidence of iatrogenic cardiac injuries is rising as a result of the increasing use of invasive cardiac diagnostic and therapeutic procedures (penetrating injury) and of cardiopulmonary resuscitation (blunt injury).[10] Blunt thoracic injuries are more common than penetrating injuries.[4] The two major life-threatening consequences of cardiac trauma are hemorrhage and cardiac tamponade. Effective treatment has resulted in an increased number of immediate survivors, and later sequelae—including myocardial infarction, aneurysm, ventricular septal defects, valve damage or injury, recurrent pericarditis, and constrictive pericarditis—are becoming far more common.[10] In this chapter, the common injuries resulting from cardiac trauma are discussed and the role of echocardiography in their diagnosis and management is described.

Nonpenetrating Chest Trauma

Blunt chest trauma accounts for one-fourth of all traumatic deaths annually in the United States.[39] The most common cause of blunt chest injury is motor vehicle accidents; damage to the heart most often results from steering wheel contusion. The violent decelerative force of impact can damage the heart and great vessels even if the chest wall is not punctured (Fig. 25-1). Other causes include sports injuries, falls from heights, blows from blunt objects, and closed chest massage during cardiopulmonary resuscitation.[10,63]

Cardiac damage can result from direct compression of the sternum against the heart or from increased intrathoracic pressure transmitted from a blow to the chest or abdomen.[63]

Cardiac injury due to trauma covers a wide spectrum of anatomic and physiologic abnormalities. Injury can occur immediately or develop gradually. Table 25-1 lists the different forms of injury that blunt chest trauma produces.[10] It is important to obtain the details of the traumatic events, as a steering wheel injury sustained in a high-speed motor vehicle accident has different effects on the heart than does striking one's chest during a minor fall.[8]

Fractures of the ribs, clavicle, or sternum are the hallmarks of chest trauma. The associated pain often masks underlying cardiac injury and may make diagnosis difficult. Cardiac trauma may be present even in the absence of fractures and may be more severe in this setting if the heart absorbs most of the energy of impact.[6,55,63]

With severe or massive cardiac injury, death can occur. If damage is less severe, patients may survive to reach an emergency room, where prompt diagnosis and treatment is necessary. The myocardium may be injured by fragments of bone driven into the heart or from compression of the heart between the sternum and the spine or against the chest wall.[8] When time and the patient's condition permit, echocardiography is a valuable screening tool for

TABLE 25-1. TYPES OF CARDIAC INJURY FROM BLUNT TRAUMA

Myocardium
  Contusion
  Laceration
  Rupture
  Septal perforation
  Aneurysm, pseudoaneurysm
  Hemopericardium, tamponade
  Thrombosis, systemic embolism
Pericardium
  Pericarditis
  Postpericardiotomy syndrome
  Constrictive pericarditis
  Pericardial laceration
  Hemorrhage
  Cardiac herniation
Endocardial structures
  Rupture of papillary muscle
  Rupture of chordae tendineae
  Rupture of atrioventricular and semilunar valves
Coronary artery
  Thrombosis
  Laceration
  Fistula

Source: Jackson DH, Murphy GW. Nonpenetrating cardiac trauma. Mod Conc Cardiovas Dis. 1976;45:123. Reprinted with permission of the American Heart Association, Inc.

the evaluation of cardiac involvement following blunt chest trauma.

In patients who are considered clinically brain dead following trauma, echocardiography can assess if the heart is suitable for organ donation. The echocardiographic examination includes a determination of valvular and left ventricular function, as well as ruling out the presence of cardiac injury.[47]

Pericardial Effusion

Pericardial effusion often follows blunt chest trauma and usually indicates that the heart has been injured. Pericardial effusion rarely appears as a solitary lesion; usually it is found in association with cardiac contusion or great vessel or myocardial tears. Effusions due to trauma frequently are bloody; they may accumulate rapidly or take a week or more to develop. The major sequela of pericardial effusion due to trauma—cardiac tamponade—can develop immediately or several days or weeks after the traumatic event.[1] A possible long-term complication of a

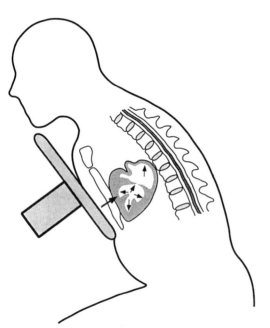

Figure 25-1. Decelerative impact forces of steering wheel injury. (Illustration by Greg Lawrence. Reprinted with permission.)

bloody pericardial effusion is constrictive pericarditis.[9,10,17]

Echocardiography is the method of choice for detecting pericardial effusion. Bloody effusions and clots usually are more echogenic than serous effusions.[18] Traumatic effusions may be loculated if pericardial adhesions develop following cardiac injury. Multiple echocardiographic views may be needed to delineate a loculated effusion.[35] An apical or subcostal four-chamber view is necessary to make the diagnosis. Tamponade can be detected on the two-dimensional examination by noting small right-sided chambers with respiratory variation and diastolic collapse of the right ventricular or right atrial wall. The role of echocardiographic diagnosis is more important if the patient's hemodynamics are stable. With unstable patients suspected of having cardiac tamponade, emergency chest surgery and exploration are usually performed. In addition to the initial echocardiographic workup, patients with pericardial effusion should have follow-up studies to determine whether the effusion is resolving and to detect complications such as pericardial constriction.[52]

Pneumothorax (air within the pleural space) is a frequent complication of rib fractures due to trauma[54] and is usually recognizable on routine chest x-ray. A pneumothorax may cause the heart to shift its position and can make routine echocardiographic scanning difficult.

Cardiac Contusion

Cardiac contusion can be conceptualized as a bruise to the myocardium. Histologic examination reveals cellular injury, hemorrhage, and resulting necrosis of myocardial fibers. Cardiac contusion may be similar to myocardial infarction, except that the damage is usually patchy instead of discrete and cardiac contusion rarely leads to severe heart failure unless other complications arise.[10,60,63] In addition, patients with contusion may be young, with normal coronary arteries and no evidence of underlying heart disease.[10] The most common cause of this injury is compression of the sternum against the steering wheel in vehicular accidents.

The extent of myocardial injury varies greatly, depending on the degree of trauma. In severe cases the myocardium may rupture. Because the right ventricle is the most anterior cardiac structure, it is the one most susceptible to injury. The interventricular septum is also vulnerable. It tends to rupture near the apex. Myocardial contusion or rupture can also result from closed-chest massage during cardiopulmonary resuscitation.[10,63]

Complications of contusion include atrial and ventricular arrhythmias, hemopericardium with the possibility of tamponade, and thrombus formation.[40] Ventricular aneurysms and pseudoaneurysms may occur as late sequelae.[63]

Clinical manifestations in patients with contusion are variable, depending on the degree of injury and the presence of associated injuries. The most common complaint is angina-type chest pain that is not relieved by the usual therapy.

Until recently, the clinical diagnosis of cardiac contusion was based primarily on serial electrocardiographic changes, but these are often nonspecific and unreliable.[40] Most contusions occur on the right side of the heart, and a standard electrocardiogram is relatively insensitive to right ventricular abnormalities.[63] Electrocardiography can be useful in detecting conduction defects and arrhythmias, both of which are common following cardiac contusion.[4]

Chest radiography is generally of little value in detecting cardiac contusion, although associated findings such as rib fractures can alert the physician to the possibility of its presence.[34] More recently, the presence of contusion has been determined by noting an elevated level of creatine phosphokinase isoenzyme (CPK-MB) in the blood following trauma.[37,40] Although the CPK-MB level appears to be a fairly sensitive test for the diagnosis of myocardial contusion, it is relatively nonspecific and a normal CPK-MB level does not rule out contusion.[63]

The current consensus appears to be that echocardiography coupled with serial electrocardiographic and CPK-MB determinations offers the best chance of detecting cardiac contusion.[4,20,52,62,63]

Myocardial contusion produced in animal models demonstrated characteristic echo patterns: increased echogenicity of the contused area, sonolucencies where intramural hematomas were present (Fig. 25-2), increased wall thickness at end-diastole, and impaired regional systolic function.[45,57]

Several clinical studies have reported the usefulness of two-dimensional echocardiography in the diagnosis of cardiac contusion. Characteristic find-

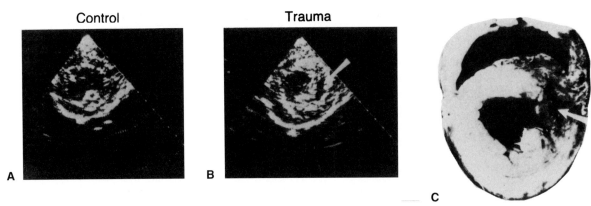

Figure 25-2. Short axis two-dimensional echocardiographic recordings from a dog at the level of the papillary muscles before (**A**) and 15 min after (**B**) left-sided chest trauma. Wall thickness is increased in the contused area. Within the bright sonodense area, a discrete, linear, sonolucent zone is seen, representing an intramural hematoma (arrow). (**C**) A transverse cut section of the pathologic specimen of the same dog shows the contusion (*dark area*) and the hematoma (arrow). (From Pandian NC, Skorton PJ, Doty DB, et al. Immediate diagnosis of acute myocardial contusion by two-dimensional echocardiography. J Am Coll Cardiol. 1983;2:488–496.)

ings include chamber enlargement (usually the right ventricle), mural thrombi, wall motion abnormalities ranging from hypokinesis to aneurysm formation, echodense myocardial areas, and pericardial effusion.[4,16,34] Added advantages of echocardiography are its ability to distinguish between right and left ventricular contusion and to differentiate right ventricular contusion from pericardial effusion, a distinction that has important therapeutic implications.[40,63] TEE is considered by many to be superior to TTE in the evaluation of contusion but its suggested use is only when the TTE is suboptimal. The spectrum of myocardial injury noted on echocardiography is presented in Figure 25-2.

Valve Injury

The prevalence of valve injury in patients with blunt chest injury is in the range of 9%.[10] The aortic and mitral valves appear to be more susceptible to damage than the right-sided valves due to the higher pressures on the left side of the heart.[63] Preexisting valve disease and the presence of a prosthetic valve[9] both tend to predispose to injury during trauma.[52] Valve injury is usually associated with other cardiac abnormalities, as any trauma severe enough to cause valve injury tends to affect other areas of the heart as well.[13,15] Patients with valve injury generally de-

velop new, loud, musical murmurs and varying degrees of congestive heart failure.[10,13] Echocardiography is very useful for assessing valve injury, as it allows visualization of the valves and supporting structures, and for determining the severity of regurgitation and the degree of cardiac function. Severe regurgitation may be seen acutely following trauma or may take several weeks to months to develop. Because a small laceration may develop into a larger tear due to hemodynamic stress on the valve, patients with suspected valve disruption should be followed with serial echocardiography.[21]

AORTIC VALVE

Because most aortic injuries due to blunt trauma result from rapid deceleration with shearing stress at points of relative fixation, tears usually are found near the insertion of the valve to the annulus.[9]

There appears to be a relationship between the timing of the chest wall trauma and the cardiac cycle. The aortic valve is probably most vulnerable to damage early in diastole, when the ventricle and aorta are nearly full.[10]

In a case report of a young child who fell from a tree, the echocardiogram detected rupture of the left coronary aortic valve cusp. The echocardiographic findings included dilatation of the left ventricle, diastolic aortic flutter, posterior motion of the left coronary cusp in diastole, and unusually wide excursion of the valve in systole. The absence of valve thickening and dilatation of the aortic root indicated that other causes of aortic insufficiency were not present.[21] Doppler color-flow mapping would have aided further in the diagnosis of aortic insufficiency in this patient or in any patient with suspected aortic insufficiency.

MITRAL VALVE

Traumatic disruption of the mitral valve can occur at the level of the annulus, leaflets, chordae tendineae, or papillary muscle; the latter two are more common.[13,15] Damage is most likely to develop if trauma occurs during diastole, when left ventricular outflow is obstructed.[10,13] Papillary muscle dysfunction may occur acutely as a result of direct laceration at the moment of impact, or it may develop as a sequela to myocardial contusion.[13]

Two-dimensional echocardiography allows detailed analysis of the mitral valve apparatus. A flail mitral leaflet can be identified by the presence of the tip of the leaflet or chordae in the left atrium during diastole. Pulsed wave and color flow Doppler studies are instrumental in determining the presence and degree of mitral insufficiency. Scarring of the injured valve can lead to stenosis, in which case the continuous wave Doppler technique may be utilized as well.[13] Recent reports suggest the superiority of TEE over TTE for evaluating the mitral valve. TEE can define and localize more precisely the mechanism of disruption.[11,49,54] Figure 25-3 demonstrates a rupture at the base of the mitral valve in a patient who had sustained a five-story fall.[49]

TRICUSPID VALVE

Nonpenetrating traumatic injury to the tricuspid valve is often found in association with rupture of the right ventricular free wall.[15] As with the mitral valve, disruption can occur at the various levels of the tricuspid valve apparatus.[17]

M-mode findings of ruptured tricuspid valve chordae tendineae have included wide diastolic excursion with coarse, erratic diastolic fluttering and paradoxical septal motion.[28] Two-dimensional findings have included motion of the flail tricuspid leaflet into the right atrium during systole and loss of the normal coaptation point.[66] Doppler investigation allows further assessment of ensuing regurgita-

tion. In three rare cases of tricuspid regurgitation in combination with herniation of the heart through a pericardial tear (luxation), echocardiography demonstrated a small left atrium and ruptured papillary muscle of the tricuspid valve with severe tricuspid regurgitation. These patients underwent surgery, and postoperative TEE was used to look for the presence of residual tricuspid regurgitation.[50]

Great Vessel Injury

Aortic laceration, a common complication of blunt chest trauma,[10] unfortunately is usually fatal. Approximately 20% of patients with aortic rupture survived for more than an hour after trauma.[48] Pulmonary artery laceration is less common but is also usually fatal.[27] If the patient survives, great vessel injury can be detected on a chest radiograph by noting a widened mediastinum. Aortography historically was the test of choice for detecting great vessel injury, but it appears that TEE has emerged as the procedure of choice.[32,33,64,65] Advances in TEE technology, specifically multiplane transducers, have eliminated most of the ascending aortic "blind zone" noted with earlier single-plane TEE exams, except for a 3- to 5-cm portion of the upper ascending aorta.[58] The protocol in many centers is to perform aortography only in those patients in whom TEE is contraindicated and for patients with equivocal TEE results. The typical echocardiographic finding in aortic disruption is the presence of mobile intraluminal flaps or intraluminal masses resembling thrombi[32] (Fig. 25-4).

The aortic isthmus (the area between the relatively mobile aortic arch and the tethered descending aorta) is especially vulnerable to rupture.[14] TEE provides a very clear picture of this region. Diagnosis of a tear appears to be based on noting a linear flap, thicker than that seen with dissections, containing a large hole. Color Doppler findings include systolic turbulence near the hole and diastolic flow from the false aneurysm into the aorta. The borders of the surrounding hematoma may be difficult to delineate.[5,32]

Penetrating Trauma

Most penetrating cardiac trauma results from injury due to knives, bullets, or other projectiles; ballistics cause more extensive cell destruction. Penetrating wounds to the heart most often are associated with

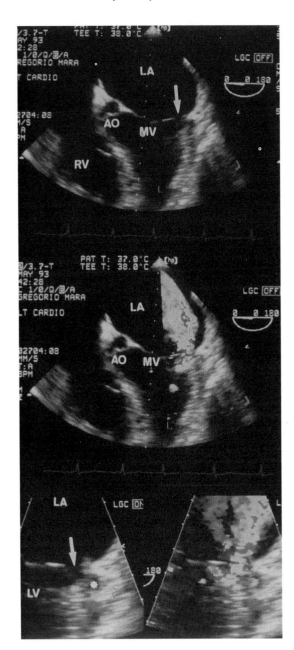

Figure 25-3. (**Top**) Transesophageal echocardiogram in four-chamber view at 0° (multiplane); rupture at the base of the mitral leaflet is discovered (arrow). (**Middle**) Same plane, color Doppler. Eccentric jet of severe mitral regurgitation is detected. (**Bottom**) Magnification of top and middle images. Involvement of mitral annulus can be seen (asterisk); color flow fills this defect. LA, left atrium; MV, mitral valve; LV, left ventricle; AO, aorta; RV, right ventricle; RA, right atrium. (From de Prado, et al. Isolated mitral valve rupture caused by nonpenetrating trauma: Recognition by transesophageal echocardiography. *In* American Heart Journal. St. Louis, Mosby Year Book, 1995.)

injury to the precordium, but they may be seen in conjunction with wounds elsewhere in the chest, neck, or upper abdomen. The frequency of injury to the various cardiac structures correlates with the area of exposure on the anterior chest wall. Thus, the cardiac chamber most often injured is the right ventricle, followed in decreasing order of frequency by the left ventricle, right atrium, and left atrium.[60] Perforation of one or more chambers of the heart, the cardiac valves and their support structures, and the interventricular and interatrial septa may occur.[21,34,56]

The management of suspected acute cardiac trauma depends on the clinical condition of the patient. Most patients with penetrating cardiac wounds die shortly after the injury as a result of cardiac tamponade or massive bleeding. Rarely is there time for diagnostic procedures. The management of those who survive consists primarily of thoracotomy and surgical exploration. First, however, the patient's condition must be stabilized by administering fluids or blood and by placing a chest tube, if indicated. Pericardiocentesis for evaluation and stabilization of patients with suspected cardiac tamponade prior to arrangements for thoracotomy is somewhat controversial.[10]

Most of the literature on echocardiography and penetrating injury to the heart discusses its role after initial repair of the injury and stabilization of the patient's condition. Patients with penetrating cardiac wounds may have multiple cardiac defects, but only the most superficial wounds are usually recognized upon initial evaluation as requiring surgical repair. Several studies address the utility of echocardiography in evaluating patients postoperatively for the presence of residual injury.[23,24,30,42,56] The abnormalities noted on two-dimensional echocardiography included pericardial effusion, abnormal wall motion, chamber enlargement, and an intracardiac retained missile fragment. Doppler examination reveals ventricular septal defects, tricuspid insufficiency, and arteriovenous fistulas. One study concluded that patients who had an abnormal electrocardiogram, chest radiograph, or auscultory find-

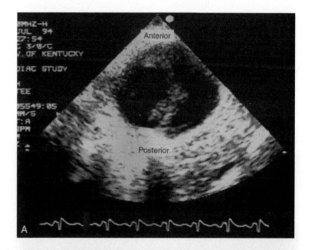

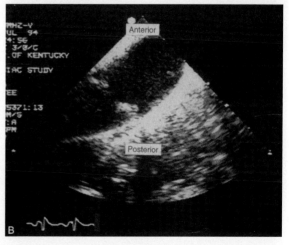

Figure 25-4. (**A**) Characteristic "intimal flap" associated with traumatic aortic disruption. Flap extends from anterior to posterior positions in the horizontal imaging plane. (**B**) Characteristic "intimal flap" as seen on vertical TEE imaging plane. The flap is noted on anterior and posterior surfaces suggestive of a circumference disruption. The superior descending aorta is to the right of the image. (From Johnson SB, Kearney PA, Smith MD. Echocardiography in the evaluation of thoracic trauma. Horizons Trauma Surg. 1995;75: 200.)

ing postoperatively should undergo two-dimensional and Doppler echocardiography.[38]

The echocardiographic findings in this setting can be quite dramatic. Figure 25-5 illustrates a large ventricular septal defect with ragged edges, the result of an icepick wound to the heart. The patient originally underwent emergency surgical repair of a hole in the anterior wall of the right ventricle. Several weeks later, the symptoms of congestive heart failure developed and a systolic murmur was detected. Echocardiographic demonstration of the residual ventricular septal defect led to reoperation and repair of the defect.

Cardiac defects caused by penetrating injury usually are more irregular and complex than congenital or naturally acquired lesions. They are often multiple and may be situated in unusual locations. A cursory two-dimensional echocardiographic examination may miss some of these lesions, so Doppler echocardiography has become important for detecting them. Doppler examination can detect even small lesions and can prompt the echocardiographer to obtain nonstandard two-dimensional views to better demonstrate the abnormalities.[30] Color flow Doppler mapping, in particular, should provide rapid detection of shunts and valvular lesions, resulting in more prompt repair of these defects.

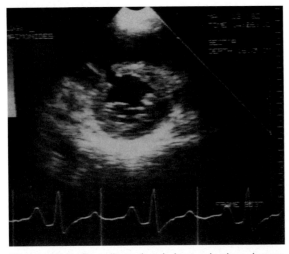

Figure 25-5. Two-dimensional short axis view demonstrates a ventricular septal defect in the anterior septum acquired due to ice pick injury.

Localization of Foreign Bodies with Sonography

Echocardiography has been used extensively in the management of patients with penetrating missile wounds of the heart.[26,53] The dangers of fragments retained in the myocardium are migration, embolization, and erosion into adjacent structures. They also may serve as a locus for endocarditis. Some studies suggest that foreign objects should be surgically removed only if they protrude into the ventricular cavity.[61] Fragments embedded in the myocardium tend to become encased in fibrin and generally do not pose a threat to the patient.[60] Although chest radiography and cardiac fluoroscopy may reveal the metal fragments in the heart, echocardiography is the most effective tool for identifying the exact location of such retained fragments and may be useful in guiding surgical intervention.[26]

Echocardiography may be used to diagnose retained missile fragments in patients with penetrating missile wounds of the heart.[26] Retained fragments are defined echocardiographically as bright targets with multiple reverberations seen in at least two views. Low gain and minimal reject settings are used to distinguish the metallic particles from cardiac tissue. In some studies, patients who required surgery for removal of the missile particles were evaluated during the operation by echocardiography. Intraoperative echocardiograms were found to be very useful, as they provided immediate localization of the fragments and thus shortened the operative procedure and minimized potential tissue damage.

Intraoperative TEE and epicardial echocardiography can be used to localize and assist in removal of fragments, such as the drilling bit fragment lodged in the left atrium[19] in Figure 25-6. Intraoperative echocardiography can be considered standard procedure in the removal of foreign bodies from the heart.

Iatrogenic Injury

An increasingly common source of cardiac trauma is invasive diagnostic and therapeutic procedures. Techniques such as cardiac catheterization, pericardiocentesis, pacemaker implantation, and the administration of cardiopulmonary resuscitation are not without risk, and prompt recognition of compli-

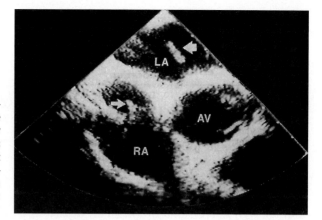

Figure 25-6. Two-dimensional transesophageal echo-cardiogram in a short axis view (partially oblique) at the level of the aortic valve shows a metallic foreign body in the left atrium (large arrow). The small arrow points to a central venous catheter. AV, aortic valve; LA, left atrium; RA, right atrium. (From Font VE, Gill CC, Lammermeier DE: Echocardiographically guided removal of an intracardiac foreign body. Cleve Clin J Med. 1994;61: 229.)

cations is imperative.[29] The role of echocardiography in most cases of suspected iatrogenic injury is to evaluate for the presence of pericardial effusion. Occasionally, however, echocardiography can also be useful in locating intracardiac or pericardial catheters.

Catheterization

Major advances in the application of cardiac catheterization have recently been made. Cardiac catheterization and angiography have been useful diagnostic tools for assessing the extent of coronary artery disease, for determining cardiac hemodynamics, and for evaluating wall motion and valve function. With the advent of interventional cardiology, including angioplasty, atherectomy, laser, stent placement, and valvuloplasty, cardiac catheterization has become a therapeutic tool as well. The manipulation of wires within the heart and great vessels can lead to complications, among them perforation of the coronary arteries, dissection of the aorta, perforation of the cardiac chambers, and injury to the cardiac valves. Many of these complications are recognized during the catheterization procedure and are attended to immediately. Echocardiography is useful in detecting pericardial effusions and possible signs of tamponade when perforation is suspected. In the rare event of aortic dissection due to the passage of catheters within the aorta, TTE and/or TEE can be useful in identifying an intimal flap.[29]

During coronary angiography or angioplasty, perforation or dissection of a coronary artery can cause ischemia in the area of the myocardium normally supplied by the vessel, and wall motion abnormalities may ensue. Visualization of the coronary arteries currently is not reliable with conventional echocardiographic techniques, but it can be used to evaluate changes in regional wall motion that may occur with ischemia.

Both right-sided and left-sided heart catheterization can lead to atrial or ventricular perforation, but right-sided catheterization is more likely to cause perforation because the walls of the right atrium and right ventricle are thinner. Stiffer catheters, such as those used for cardiac catheterization, pose more of a problem than the soft, flexible Swan-Ganz catheters used for hemodynamic monitoring in critically ill patients. Perforation can cause the formation of a pericardial effusion, and occasionally pericardial tamponade, which can be evaluated rapidly and noninvasively by echocardiography.

The technique of percutaneous balloon valvuloplasty involves multiple guidewires and catheters of fairly large diameter; as a consequence, the incidence of associated complications is higher. Valvuloplasty increases the size of the valve orifice but may also cause regurgitation. Echocardiography is used routinely to monitor the improvement in valve function of these patients and to determine the presence and degree of valvular insufficiency. Mitral valvuloplasty is achieved by passing the catheter through the interatrial septum to gain entry into the left atrium and mitral valve orifice. This technique causes a small defect in the interatrial septum, which usually has no clinical significance. Such atrial septal defects were thought to disappear with time, but Doppler color-flow evaluation has shown that they may persist several months after the procedure.[43] Another complication of mitral valvuloplasty is rupture of the chordae tendineae.[44] Two-dimensional and Doppler echocardiography allow careful analysis of this region. As valvuloplasty becomes more commonly used, the need to recognize potential complications will also increase. Echocardiography is certainly suitable for this purpose, as it provides immediate information.[29] Another potential complication of percutaneous balloon valvuloplasty is embolic events. The result of the Duke series[25] of 170 patients undergoing percutaneous balloon valvuloplasty suggests that instituting a preprocedure TEE significantly decreases the chance of an embolic event occurring. TEE can identify thrombi in the left atrium, as well as in the left atrial appendage. Patients with left atrial thrombi that persist should be referred for surgery rather than percutaneous balloon valvuloplasty.

Another complication of intravenous or right-sided heart catheterization occurs when the catheter fractures and a piece migrates into the right atrium, right ventricle, or pulmonary artery. Such fragments most often are detected with fluoroscopy because they are composed of radiopaque material. Echocardiography can also be used to locate such fragments and to guide their removal.

Pericardiocentesis

Pericardiocentesis is a procedure used to drain pericardial effusions for diagnostic or therapeutic purposes. The needle can puncture the heart and damage the myocardium. During the procedure, an echocardiogram can be performed to help guide the needle.

The pericardiocentesis needle is usually inserted in the subxyphoid region under sterile technique. The echocardiographic transducer is then placed at the cardiac apex, outside the sterile field. If an apical approach is chosen for pericardiocentesis, the subcostal echocardiographic view can be used. The echocardiographic plane may have to be modified so that the beam is aligned parallel to the needle to allow better visualization during the procedure.[51] Also, the site of puncture can be preselected by echocardiography to show the location of the effusion. Alternatively, there are sterile needle and transducer holders that can be used for echo-guided pericardiocentesis.

Cardiac Pacemakers and Implantable Defibrillators

When the cardiac conduction system fails to supply impulses at the proper intervals to ensure regular myocardial contraction, an electrical device is often implanted to provide this stimulus. A pacemaker may be required on a temporary or permanent basis. In either case, a transvenous pacing electrode is inserted into the right ventricle and/or the right atrium. With a temporary pacemaker, the electrode is attached to an external battery source; with a permanent pacemaker, the battery is implanted subcutaneously in the chest wall.

The transvenous pacemaker electrode is usually placed into the apex of the right ventricle for ventricular pacing. If sequential activation of the atrium and ventricle is required, two pacemaker electrodes are placed, one in the right atrial appendage and one in the right ventricular apex. Again, atrial or ventricular perforation is a potential problem because of the relatively thin right atrial and right ventricular walls. If the free wall of these chambers is perforated, a bloody pericardial effusion (hemopericardium) will result, with possible cardiac tamponade. In addition to perforation of the right ventricular or right atrial wall, perforation can occur through the interatrial or interventricular septum.[12,56] Echocardiography can be used to guide lead placement and to check for possible misplacement of leads. The exact location of the electrode may be difficult to determine fluoroscopically; the two-dimensional echocardiographic technique can better trace the course of the pacing catheter. Echocardiographically, a catheter generally appears as a bright linear echo coursing through the right side of the heart. Figure 25-7 shows a subcostal echocardiographic view obtained when a change in the QRS configuration was noted on the electrocardiogram after a temporary pacemaker was inserted. The catheter is clearly seen crossing the interventricular septum, with the tip touching the lateral left ventricular wall.

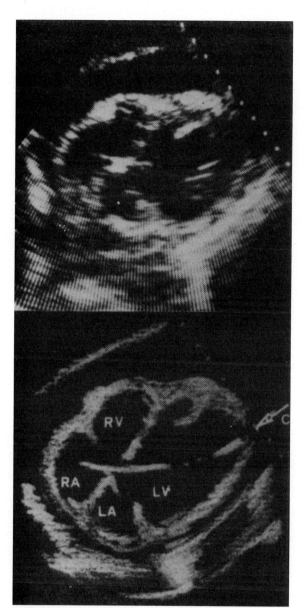

Figure 25-7. Two-dimensional echocardiogram from the subcostal approach. The catheter (c), imaged as a bright band of echoes, is seen entering the left ventricle (LV) through the ventricular septum. LA, left atrium; RA, right atrium; RV, right ventricle. (From Iliceto S, Gianfranco A, Sorino M, et al. Two-dimensional echocardiographic recognition of complications of cardiac invasive procedures. Am J Coll Cardiol. 1984;53:847. Reprinted with permission from the American College of Cardiology.)

Myocardial Biopsy

Occasionally, an exact cardiac diagnosis cannot be made with the usual clinical, electrocardiographic, and imaging techniques that are currently available, and a histologic diagnosis, requiring a sample of tissue from the heart, is necessary. This biopsy technique has been developed mainly to evaluate heart transplant recipients for signs of rejection, to follow patients undergoing chemotherapy with cardiotoxic drugs, and to check for possible inflammatory and infiltrative diseases of the heart. The biopsy is performed with a bioptome, a stiff catheter with steel jaws attached to its end. The bioptome is usually guided via the internal jugular vein into the right ventricle, where a sample of myocardial tissue is obtained. The catheter is most often localized by fluoroscopy, but it can be confirmed with echocardiography. Because this technique involves removal of a piece of tissue, there is a risk of perforation of the right ventricular wall. In the event of such a mishap, echocardiography may be used to detect the presence of hemopericardium.

Cardiac Surgery

Cardiac surgery is a form of cardiac trauma. Echocardiographically, it is not unusual to note some degree of pericardial effusion or pneumomediastinum in patients who have undergone uncomplicated open-heart surgery. Pericardial effusions are frequently loculated because of the adhesions in the pericardium that often occur postoperatively. Occasionally, uncontrolled bleeding following cardiac surgery may result in cardiac tamponade. Large blood clots compressing the right side of the heart can also cause tamponade. Figure 25-8 demonstrates a large clot compressing the right atrium in a 64-year-old male 1 day after coronary artery bypass surgery who exhibited signs of hemodynamic compromise. The echocardiographic examination should therefore include a thorough investigation of the area adjacent to the heart, including subcostal views to evaluate the right atrial and right ventricular borders.

The surgical placement of prosthetic cardiac valves can occasionally lead to unusual complications. Echocardiographic detection of pseudoaneurysm formation following mitral valve replacement

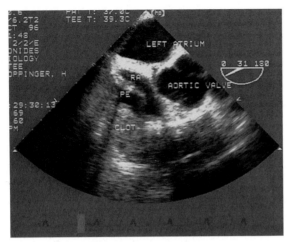

Figure 25-8. Transesophageal echocardiogram in short axis view at 31 degrees (multiplane) demonstrating a large blood clot and hemorrhagic pericardial effusion (PE) compressing the right atrium (RA).

has been reported. The diagnosis was made by noting myocardial discontinuity and a sonolucent space posteriorly adjacent to the prosthetic valve.[36]

Cardiac Resuscitation

The technique of external cardiac massage for cardiopulmonary resuscitation has become widespread. The procedure itself can cause serious complications. Fracture of the sternum or ribs during compression can cause laceration of the heart. Right ventricular papillary muscle rupture, as well as rupture of the atria and aorta, have been reported following closed chest massage.[3,22,59] If the patient survives the resuscitative efforts, and if signs or symptoms of cardiac injury are present, echocardiography may be employed to assess the extent of the cardiac damage.

Summary

For patients who survive the initial event, echocardiography can be a useful technique for the investigation of cardiac trauma. Compared to magnetic resonance imaging and computed tomography, which are time-consuming and require the patient to remain still for prolonged periods with limited life support monitoring, echocardiography can be performed relatively quickly at the patient's bedside.

The most common echocardiographic finding after trauma is pericardial effusion, which indicates that some degree of cardiac injury has occurred. A full echocardiographic workup is then indicated to determine the extent of cardiac injury.

While echocardiography can be used in the immediate care of trauma patients, its most important role appears to be in the evaluation of the long-term sequelae in patients who survive the initial insult.

REFERENCES

1. Allen MN, Nanna M, Lichtenberg GS, et al. Blunt trauma causing delayed cardiac tamponade: Echocardiographic diagnosis. J Diagn Med Sonogr. 1988;4: 269–273.
2. Baillot R, Dontigny L, Verdant A, et al. Penetrating chest trauma: A 20-year experience. J Trauma. 1987; 27:994–997.
3. Baker PB, Keyhani-Rofagha S, Graham RL, et al. Dissecting hematoma (aneurysm) of coronary arteries. Am J Med. 1986;80:317–319.
4. Beggs CW, Helling TS, Evans LL, et al. Early evaluation of cardiac injury by two-dimensional echocardiography in patients suffering blunt chest trauma. Ann Emerg Med. 1987;16:542–545.
5. Berenfeld A, Barraud P, Lusson JR, et al. Traumatic aortic ruptures diagnosed by transesophageal echocardiography. J Am Soc Echocardiogr. 1996;9: 657–662.
6. Beresky R, Klinger R, Peake J. Myocardial contusion: When does it have clinical significance? J Trauma. 1988;28:64–68.
7. Berkery W, Hare C, Warner RA, et al. Nonpenetrating traumatic rupture of the tricuspid valve. Chest. 1987;91:778–780.
8. Boyd AD. Nonpenetrating thoracic injuries. Hosp Med. 1988;24:25–28.
9. Brady PW, Deal CW. An unusual cause of mitral incompetence: Post-traumatic paraprosthetic mitral incompetence. J Trauma. 1988;28:259–261.
10. Cohn PF, Braunwald E. Traumatic heart disease. *In* Braunwald E (ed): Heart Disease: A Textbook of Cardiovascular Medicine, 3rd ed. Philadelphia, WB Saunders; 1988.
11. Coleman DM, Cox PN, Dyck J, et al. Pediatric transesophageal echocardiography in the evaluation of acute disruption of the mitral valve following blunt thoracic trauma: Case report. J Trauma. 1994;36(1): 135–136.
12. Cooper JP, Swanton RH. Complications of transvenous temporary pacemaker insertion. Br J Hosp Med. 1995;53(4):155–161.

13. Cuadros LC, Hutchinson JE III, Mograder AH. Laceration of a mitral papillary muscle and the aortic root as a result of blunt trauma to the chest. J Thorac Cardiovasc Surg. 1984;88:134–140.

14. Dee PM. The radiology of chest trauma. Radiol Clin North Am. 1992;30(2):291–306.

15. Dodd DA, John JA, Graham TP Jr. Transient severe mitral and tricuspid regurgitation following blunt chest trauma. Am Heart J. 1987;114:652–654.

16. Eisenach JC, Nugent M, Miller FA Jr, et al. Echocardiographic evaluation of patients with blunt chest injury: Correlation with perioperative hypotension. Anesthesiology. 1986;64:364–366.

17. Fabian TC, Mangiante EC, Patterson RC, et al. Myocardial contusion in blunt trauma: Clinical characteristics, means of diagnosis, and implications for patient management. J Trauma. 1988;28:50–58.

18. Feigenbaum H. Pericardial disease. *In* Feigenbaum H (ed): Echocardiography, 4th ed. Philadelphia, Lea & Febiger; 1986.

19. Font VE, Gill CC, Lammermeier DE. Echocardiographically guided removal of an intracardiac foreign body. Cleve Clin J Med. 1994;61(3):228–331.

20. Frazee RC, Mucha P, Farnell MB, et al. Objective evaluation of blunt cardiac trauma. J Trauma. 1986;26:510–518.

21. Gay JA, Gottdiener JS, Gomes MN, et al. Echocardiographic features of traumatic disruption of the aortic valve. Chest. 1983;1:150–151.

22. Gerry JL, Buckley BH, Hutchins GM. Rupture of the papillary muscle of the tricuspid valve: A complication of cardiopulmonary resuscitation and a rare cause of tricuspid regurgitation. Am J Cardiol. 1977;40:825–828.

23. Goldberg SE, Parameswaran R, Nakhjavan FK, et al. Echocardiographic diagnosis of traumatic ventricular septal defect. Am Heart J. 1984;107:416–417.

24. Goldman AP, Kotler MN, Goldberg SE, et al. The uses of two-dimensional Doppler echocardiographic techniques preoperatively and postoperatively in a ventricular septal defect caused by penetrating trauma. Ann Thorac Surg. 1985;40:625–627.

25. Harrison JK, Wilson JS, Hearne SE, et al. Complications related to percutaneous transvenous mitral commissurotomy. Cathet Cardiovasc Diagn. 1994;2:52–60.

26. Hassett A, Moran J, Sabiston DC, et al. Utility of echocardiography in the management of patients with penetrating missile wounds of the heart. J Am Coll Cardiol. 1986;7:1151–1156.

27. Hawkins ML, Carraway RP, Ross SE, et al. Pulmonary artery disruption from blunt thoracic trauma. Am Surg. 1988;54:148–152.

28. Ichikawa T, Okudaira S, Yoshioka J, et al. A case of isolated tricuspid insufficiency. J Cardiogr. 1977;6:635.

29. Iliceto S, Antonelli G, Sorino M, et al. Two-dimensional echocardiographic recognition of complications of cardiac invasive procedures. Am J Cardiol. 1984;53:846–848.

30. Jacoby SS, Gilliam LD, Pandian NG, et al. Two-dimensional and Doppler echocardiography in the evaluation of penetrating cardiac injury. Chest. 1985;88:922–924.

31. Jenson BP, Hoffman I, Follis FM, et al. Surgical repair of atrial septal rupture due to blunt trauma. Ann Thorac Surg. 1993;56(5):1172–1174.

32. Johnson SB, Kearney PA, Smith MD. Echocardiography in the evaluation of thoracic trauma. Surg Clin North Am. 1995;75(2):193–205.

33. Karalis D, Victor M, Davis G, et al. The role of echocardiography in blunt chest trauma: A transthoracic and transesophageal echocardiographic study. J Trauma. 1994;36(1):53–58.

34. King MR, Mucha P, Seward JB, et al. Cardiac contusion: A new diagnostic approach utilizing two-dimensional echocardiography. J Trauma. 1983;23:614–620.

35. Kronzon I, Cohen ML, Winer HE. Cardiac tamponade loculated pericardial hematoma: Limitations of M-mode echocardiography. J Am Coll Cardiol. 1983;1:913–915.

36. Lichtenberg GS, Greengart A, Wasser H, et al. Echocardiographic demonstration of pseudoaneurysm after mitral valve replacement. Am Heart J. 1986;112(a):417.

37. Lindsey D, Navin R, Finley PR. Transient elevation of serum activity of MB isoenzyme of creatine phosphokinase drivers involved in automobile accidents. Chest. 1978;74:15–18.

38. Mattox KL, Limacher MC, Feliciano DV, et al. Cardiac evaluation following heart injury. J Trauma. 1985;25:758–765.

39. Mayfield W, Hurley EJ. Blunt cardiac trauma. Am J Surg. 1984;148:162–167.

40. Miller FA Jr, Seward JB, Gersh BJ, et al. Two-dimensional echocardiographic findings in cardiac trauma. Am J Cardiol. 1982;50:1022–1027.

41. Miller JT, Richards KL, Miller JF, et al. Doppler echocardiographic determination of the cause of a systolic murmur following penetrating chest trauma. Am Heart J. 1985;111:988–990.

42. Missri J, Sverrisson J. Doppler echocardiographic detection of traumatic ventricular septal defect: A case report. Angiology 1987;38:785–787.

43. O'Shea JP, Abascal VM, Marshall JE, et al. Long-term persistence of atrial septal defect following percutaneous mitral valvuloplasty: A Doppler-echocar-

diographic follow-up study. Circulation. 1988: 78(suppl II):II-I.

44. O'Shea JP, Abascal WM, Wilkins GT, et al. Unusual sequelae of percutaneous mitral valve valvuloplasty: A Doppler-echocardiographic study. Circulation. 1988;78(suppl II):II-32.

45. Pandian NG, Skotton DJ, Doty DB, et al. Immediate diagnosis of acute myocardial contusion by two-dimensional echocardiography: Studies in a canine model of blunt chest trauma. J Am Coll Cardiol. 1983;2:488–493.

46. Parmley LF. Non-penetrating traumatic injury to the aorta. Circulation. 1958;17:1086.

47. Perlroth MG, Reitz BA, Braunwald E. Heart and heart-lung transplantation. *In* Braunwald E (ed): Heart Disease: Textbook of Cardiovascular Medicine, 5th ed. Philadelphia, WB Saunders; 1997: 515–533.

48. Perez de Prado A, Garcia-Fernandez MA, Barambio M, et al. Isolated mitral valve rupture caused by nonpenetrating trauma: Recognition by transesophageal echocardiography. Am Heart J. 1995;129(5): 1032–1034.

49. Preis HK, Taylor GJ, Martin RP. Two-dimensional echocardiographic visualization of an unfortunate event. Arch Intern Med. 1982;142:2327–2329.

50. Prenger KB, Ophius TO, Van Dantzig JM. Traumatic tricuspid valve rupture with luxation of the heart. Ann Thorac Surg. 1995;59:1524–1527.

51. Reid CL, Kawanishi DT, Rahimtoola SH. Chest trauma: Evaluation by two-dimensional echocardiography. Am Heart J. 1987;113:971–976.

52. Roehm EF, Eilen SD, Crawford MH. Two-dimensional echocardiographic demonstration of a bullet in the heart. Am Heart J. 1985;110:910–912.

53. Shammas NW, Kaul S, Stuhlmuller JE, et al. Traumatic mitral insufficiency complicating blunt chest trauma treated medically: A case report and review. Crit Care Med. 1992;20(7):1064–1068.

54. Shorr RM, Crittenden M, Indeck M, et al. Blunt thoracic trauma. Ann Surg. 1987;206:200–205.

55. Sklar J, Clarke D, Campbell D, et al. Traumatic ventricular septal defect and lacerated mitral leaflet. Chest. 1982;2:247–249.

56. Skotton DJ, Collins SM, Nichols J, et al. Qualitative texture analysis of two-dimensional echocardiography: Application to the diagnosis of experimental myocardial contusion. Circulation. 1983;6: 211–223.

57. Smith MD, Cassidy JM, Souther S, et al. Transesophageal echocardiography in the diagnosis of traumatic rupture of the aorta (see comments). N Engl J Med. 1995;332(6):356–362.

58. Sommers MS. Potential for injury: Trauma after cardiopulmonary resuscitation. Heart Lung. 1991; 20(3):287–293.

59. Symbas PN. Traumatic heart disease. *In* Harvey WP O'Rourke RA (eds): Current Problems in Cardiology. Chicago Year Book Medical; 1982.

60. Symbas PB, DiOrio DA, Tyras DH, et al. Penetrating cardiac wounds: Significant residual and delayed sequelae. Thorac Cardiovasc Surg. 1973;66:526–532.

61. Sweeney MS, Lewis CTP, Murphy MC, et al. Cardiac surgical emergencies. Crit Care Clin. 1989;5(3): 659–677.

62. Tenzer ML. The spectrum of myocardial contusion: A review. J Trauma. 1985;25:620–627.

63. Turturro MA. Emergency echocardiography. Emerg Clin North Am. 1992;10(1):47–57.

64. Vignon P, Lagrange P, Boncoeur MP, et al. Routine transesophageal echocardiography for the diagnosis of aortic disruption in trauma patients without enlarged mediastinum. J Trauma. 1996;40(3): 442–447.

65. Villanueva FS, Heinsimer JA, Burksman MH, et al. Echocardiographic detection of perforation of the cardiac ventricular septum by a permanent pacemaker lead. J Am Coll Cardiol. 1987;59:370–371.

66. Watanabe T, Katsume H, Matsukubo H, et al. Ruptured chordae tendineae of the tricuspid valve due to nonpenetrating trauma. Chest. 1981;80:751–753.

PART VIII

Cardiac Tumors and Masses

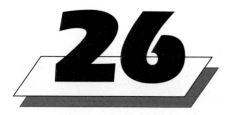

26

Cardiac Tumors and Masses

RAYMOND J. CARLSON and CHRISTOPHER L. HARE

Cardiac masses come from a variety of sources and represent varying degrees of concern to the patient's health. These masses can represent vegetations on infected valves, thrombi formed in dilated chambers with poor ventricular function, or tumors of the heart. Manufactured foreign bodies are commonly identified. Pacemaker and internal cardiac defibrillator lead wires, Swan-Ganz catheters, and Hickman catheters in the right atrium and ventricle need to be identified correctly. Migrated Kimray-Greenfield filters, bullets, and other traumatically introduced objects may also be diagnosed.

Primary Tumors of the Heart

Cardiac tumors are a rare occurrence. Metastatic tumors occur more frequently than primary tumors. Metastatic neoplasms of the heart are reported to occur between 13 and 39 times more frequently than primary tumors.[33] Primary tumors have an incidence on autopsy of between 0.0017% and 0.8%.[33,101] Prior to echocardiography, cardiac tumors were diagnosed by angiography, at surgery, and at autopsy. M-mode echocardiography proved to be the first noninvasive method to diagnose these masses definitively. While M-mode is limited to one dimension, it can demonstrate the presence of some cardiac masses such as left atrial myxoma. The presence of the myxoma, as well as its impact on blood flow, can be clearly shown. Echocardiography has improved the ability to demonstrate cardiac masses with each advance in technology. At its present level

of sophistication, echocardiography provides an excellent tool for diagnosing the presence of masses and showing their impact on heart function.

It is important to understand that echocardiography, at present, cannot determine the exact composition of any cardiac mass. It can, however, provide valuable insight into the anatomic shape, location, and mobility of a mass. These descriptions, coupled with signs, symptoms, clinical history, and blood test results, can aid the physician in diagnosing the mass and determining the subsequent course of treatment.

MYXOMA

Myxoma is the most common primary tumor of the heart. Nearly 75% of all primary cardiac tumors are benign, and myxoma accounts for almost half of this group.[85] Myxomas can occur in all age groups, but some studies suggest that it is more commonly found in middle-aged women.[34,67] These tumors are found sporadically in the population, although rare cases of multiple family members with myxomas have been reported. The familial presentation may in some cases demonstrate a "complex" or "syndrome" that has two or more of the following conditions in addition to cardiac myxoma: skin myxomas, cutaneous lentiginosis, pituitary adenomas, primary nodular adrenal cortical disease with or without Cushing's syndrome, testicular tumors, and myxoid fibroadenoma of the breast. If complex myxoma is diagnosed, screening by echocardiography of immediate family members is recommended. Surgical removal soon after diagnosis is the recommended course of treatment to minimize the possibility of emboli, as well as to spare the atrioventricular valves from mechanical abuse from the tumor. The tumors are easily removed at surgery. The attachment site is excised along with the tumor, and if the tumor is located on the interatrial septum, the hole is repaired with a pericardial or synthetic patch. Recurrence has been reported in up to 14% of cases.[29,61]

Myxomas are neoplasms that arise from the endocardial tissues. Typically, these tumors originate from the left atrium, often arising from the interatrial septum in the region of the fossa ovalis. In only 20% of cases does this tumor arise from another chamber or multiple chambers. The right atrium is the second most common site. Ventricular myxomas account for only 3–6% of all myxomas. There have been a few reports of myxomas occurring on the heart valves or in the atrial appendage.

The size of a myxoma can range from less than 1 cm to 12 cm in length, with the mean size being approximately 6 cm in diameter.[14] The majority of tumors are pedunculated and have a distinct fibrovascular stalk. Figure 26-1 demonstrates a myxoma arising from the posterior aspect of the secundum region of the interatrial septum. This tumor measures 1.7 cm in diameter and has a distinct stalk. Sessile tumors and tumors with a broad-based stalk are uncommon presentations. Figure 26-2 demon-

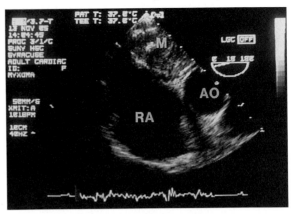

Figure 26-2. In this transesophageal view, the myxoma (M) can be seen nearly filling the left atrium. The right atrium (RA) and aorta (AO) can also be noted.

strates a large myxoma that has a broad base and appears to consume the left atrium. The surface of the tumor is typically smooth and gelatinous, but it can have irregular and lobulated surfaces. Figure 26-3 demonstrates a large, pedunculated myxoma within the left atrium on a transesophageal study. This tumor has a smooth surface and is attached to the interatrial septum. Figure 26-4 shows the tumor in the same patient extending through the mitral valve orifice in a diastolic frame. These tumors are friable, with embolism being a common complication. In Figures 26-5 and 26-6, the myxoma has a smooth surface but with distinct lobes. The tumor prolapses profoundly through the mitral orifice.

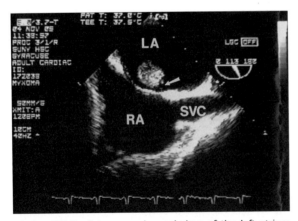

Figure 26-1. A transesophageal view of the left atrium (LA) and right atrium (RA). The myxoma can be seen within the left atrium, with a fibrovascular (arrow) stalk attached to the region of the fossa ovalis. The superior vena cava (SVC) can also be seen.

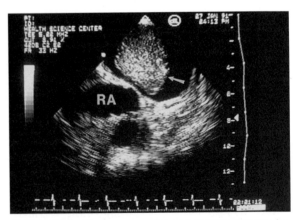

Figure 26-3. The myxoma (arrow) in this transesophageal view is round and can be seen within the left atrium. Note the homogeneous composition of the tumor. The surface has the classic smooth appearance often found with myxoma. RA, right atrium.

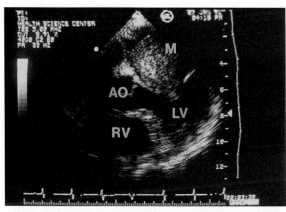

Figure 26-4. *This is a diastolic frame of the same patient shown in Figure 26-3. Note that the myxoma (M) has changed shape from round to a more elongated form as it prolapses through the mitral valve. AO, aortic valve; RV, right ventricle; LV, left ventricle.*

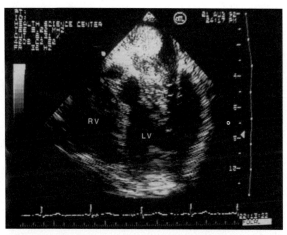

Figure 26-6. *This a diastolic frame in the same patient shown in Figure 26-5. The tumor prolapses through the mitral valve and partially into the left ventricle (LV). RV, right ventricle.*

Patients can present with different symptoms, depending on the origin, as well as the size, of the tumor. Small tumors may be asymptomatic, while large tumors can cause flow disturbances and valve obstruction. Patients with left-sided myxomas can present with signs and symptoms including dyspnea, orthopnea, paroxysmal nocturnal dyspnea, chest pain, cough, hemoptysis, acute pulmonary edema, and syncope. Right-sided myxomas can produce symptoms of right heart failure with peripheral

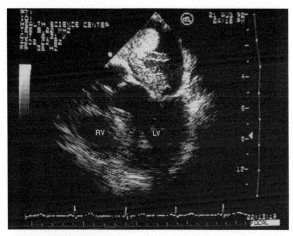

Figure 26-5. *This is a systolic frame from a transesophageal study. A large left atrial myxoma can be seen. Note the multiple lobes of the tumor. LV, left ventricle; RV, right ventricle.*

edema, distended jugular veins, ascites, and hepatomegaly. Rarely, sudden death can occur from acute rupture of the tumor and subsequent pulmonary or systemic obstruction of the cardiac valve or embolization of tumor fragments and adhered thrombus.[12]

If the myxoma is large enough to prolapse into the mitral or tricuspid valve orifice, flow will be reduced (Fig. 26-4). Damage to the valve apparatus, with thickening of the leaflets and rupture of the mitral chordae, has been noted. Symptoms may be limited to specific body positions causing sudden onset.

The first echocardiographic report of a myxoma in the literature was from 1959, describing an M-mode recording.[31] The typical presentation on M-mode of a large left atrial myxoma is of a mass filling the mitral valve opening in diastole. M-mode recordings of the left atrium in systole demonstrate the mass within the atrial cavity. In diastole the tumor can be seen moving toward or prolapsing into the mitral valve orifice. The M-mode recordings of the mitral valve demonstrates a normal early diastolic opening pattern followed by the tumor emerging in the image, with a reduction of the E-F slope as it creates an obstruction to mitral inflow. With a smaller myxoma, particularly on the right side, the M-mode recording may fail to image the tumor. Also, if the tumor has a short stalk or is not highly mobile, the M-mode recording may be of limited assistance in making a diagnosis.

Two-dimensional echocardiography is more suited to the task of imaging myxomas, regardless of their location in the heart. Their precise tumor size, location, mobility, and attachment can be diagnosed. The echocardiographic appearance of the myxoma is typically round or oval, with a smooth, well-defined border, as seen in Figures 26-2 and 26-3. The body of the tumor is echogenic, giving it a solid, homogeneous appearance. The shape of the tumor may change, especially if it prolapses through the mitral or tricuspid valve. The motion of the myxoma is dependent on the stalk, as well as on its location. Many large tumors move freely from the atrium well into the ventricle, becoming elongated as they pass through the atrioventricular valve. If the tumor has a broader base, less motion may be noted. Ventricular myxomas can obstruct flow in the aortic and pulmonic valves.

Myxomas can be demonstrated from the long axis, short axis, four-chamber, and subcostal views. Transesophageal echocardiography is the best ultrasound method for imaging myxomas, though typically it is not required to make the diagnosis. The precise location of the stalk can be defined in 95% of patients on transesophageal echocardiography compared with 65% of those using the transthoracic approach.[34] The entire interatrial septum and surrounding walls can be imaged to determine if more than one tumor is present. Regions of hemorrhage within the tumor, if present, can be noted, thereby helping to distinguish myxoma from vegetation or thrombus. Thrombus formation on the surface of the tumor can occur. Color flow imaging is helpful in demonstrating the impact of the tumor on blood flow. Pulsed and continuous wave Doppler can be used to quantitate the degree of obstruction, if present.

LIPOMA

Lipoma is a neoplasm consisting mainly of mature fat cells. Fibrolipomas contain fibrous connective tissue in addition to mature fat cells, and myolipomas have a component of muscular tissue.[84] Cardiac lipomas are most often found in the left ventricle, right atrium, and interatrial septum. These tumors invade the subendocardial and intermyocardial tissues and can be found in the pericardium. They can occur at any age and are found in both males and females without bias. The symptoms created de-

pend on the tumor's size and location. Their size can range from 1 cm to as much as 15 cm.[26] Figure 26-7 is an example of a lipoma that measured 5 by 6.8 cm. This tumor is located in the interatrial septum and was found incidentally on echocardiography. It created no obstruction to flow, and the patient had no symptoms that could be directly related to the tumor. Subendocardial tumors with intracavitary extension, however, can create flow obstructions. Intermyocardial and subepicardial lipomas, when they become large, may impede cardiac contraction and cause compression of the cardiac chambers. Conduction disturbances and arrhythmias can also occur. Most, however, create no symptoms and are found incidentally on echocardiograms, on chest x-rays, and at autopsy. The echocardiographic appearance of lipoma is of a well-defined, homogeneous, dense mass within the myocardium or extending from the endocardial or epicardial region.

Lipomatous hypertrophy of the interatrial septum is a collection of fat cells within the septum. This is not a true neoplasm. The entire interatrial septum is hypertrophied, with the exception of the region of the fossa ovalis. On the echocardiogram the classic dumbbell shape can be imaged. Figure 26-8 is an example of lipomatous hypertrophy of the septum in a transesophageal study. Note the thickness of the primum and secundum regions of the interatrial septum, with the normal thin appearance of the foramen region. These lesions may range from 1 to 7 cm and are homogeneous and echo-

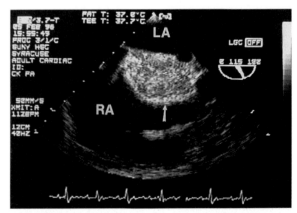

Figure 26-7. This transesophageal view demonstrates a lipoma (arrow) in the interatrial septum. The lipoma is significantly brighter than the surrounding cardiac structures and is homogeneous. There is no obstruction to flow in either the right atrium (RA) or left atrium (LA).

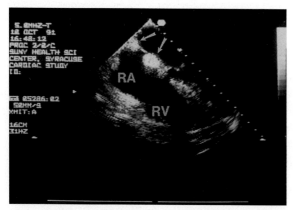

Figure 26-8. With lipomatous hypertrophy, the interatrial septum has a classic dumbbell shape (arrows). This transesophageal view demonstrates the increased thickening of the septum, with sparing of the region of the fossa ovalis. RA, right atrium; RV, right ventricle.

dense.[97] Figure 26-9 is a transthoracic apical four-chamber view. In this patient, only the thickening of the primum region is noted. Some cases of atrial arrhythmia have been reported.

PAPILLARY FIBROELASTOMA

Papillary fibroelastomas account for less than 10% of all primary cardiac tumors but are the most common tumor of the cardiac valves and valve apparatus.[12,57] These tumors have a frond-like appearance and typically are less than 1 cm but can be as large as 4 cm in diameter.[89] They are attached by a single stalk and can arise from any endocardial surface. These tumors

are highly mobile and can be difficult to differentiate from vegetations. There is debate over the significance of these tumors, but their ability to be an embolic source is evident in the literature.

Echocardiographically, papillary fibroelastoma, also known as *papilloma*, appears as a small, round, dense, highly mobile mass extending from the endocardial surface. It typically moves rapidly as the valve leaflets open and close. The tricuspid valve is most commonly involved in children, while the mitral and aortic valves are the most typical sites in adults.[67] An example is shown in Figure 26-10. The patient is an adult whose only complaint was a bounding pulse. In this figure, a 1-cm papillary fibroelastoma is noted on the cusp of the aortic valve.

ANGIOSARCOMA

Angiosarcoma is the fourth most common primary cardiac tumor but the most common malignant cardiac tumor. Angiosarcomas are soft tissue tumors of the blood vessels (hemangiosarcoma) and lymphatic endothelium (lymphangiosarcoma) and most commonly affect the head and face, liver, chest, and heart.[12] When present in the heart, these vascular tumors reside in the right atrium 80% of the time.[12,20] They occur twice as often in males as in females. Patients present with chest pain, cough, and dyspnea.[12] These tumors infiltrate into the surrounding tissues and can rupture into the pericardium, followed by tamponade.[44,73,83] They can obstruct blood flow by external compression of the cardiac chamber or they may consume the chamber

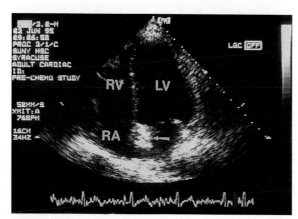

Figure 26-9. This apical four-chamber view demonstrates lipomatous hypertrophy of the primum portion of the interatrial septum (arrow). RV, right ventricle; RA, right atrium; LV, left ventricle.

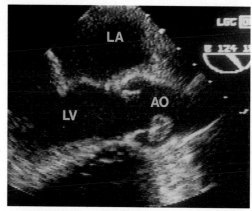

Figure 26-10. This is a transesophageal long axis view at 115 degrees. The aortic valve (AO) appears normal in thickness and excursion. A prominent papillary fibroelastoma measuring 1 cm in diameter is attached to the right coronary cusp. LA, left atrium; LV, left ventricle.

cavity. Approximately 88% of these tumors metastasize to other regions of the body.

The tumors are highly vascular, with poorly defined anastomotic channels that can grow large. Their echocardiographic presentation is of a poorly defined mass with regions of increased echodensity. The tumor can invade the surrounding tissues and is often found in the pericardium. Care should be taken to image any pericardial effusion, if present.

RHABDOMYOMA

Rhabdomyomas are the most common benign tumor of children, with the majority occurring in children under 1 year of age.[39] Multiple rhabdomyomas are found in 70–90% of patients diagnosed with this disease and have a strong association with tuberous sclerosis. The right and left ventricles are the most common sites, and 50% of the tumors are large enough to cause hemodynamic obstruction of the outflow tract or the atrioventricular valves.[39,47] There is a high rate of mortality in infants associated with obstruction and sudden death.[12] Atrial attachments of rhabdomyomas are uncommon.

Echocardiographically, the tumor appears as a solid, echodense mass extending into the ventricular cavity. Some tumors can be intramural and expand into the chamber cavity. They typically impede blood flow, which can be demonstrated on Doppler imaging. Figures 26-11, 26-12, and 26-13 are from a 4-day-old infant diagnosed with multiple rhabdo-

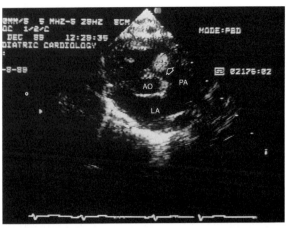

Figure 26-12. In this short axis view of the same patient shown in Figure 26-11, the tumor on the pulmonic valve can be seen (arrow). This is the same tumor that can be seen prolapsing into the right ventricular outflow tract in Figure 26-11. LA, left atrium; AO, aorta; PA, pulmonic valve.

myomas and tuberous sclerosis. Figure 26-11 is a long axis view with three lesions—one on the mitral valve, one in the right ventricle, and one prolapsing into the right ventricular outflow tract from the pulmonic valve. In Figure 26-12 the pulmonic valve tumor is seen from the short axis view. Three lesions can be seen in the four-chamber view in Figure 26-13. There have been reports of these tumors receding over time, though most are considered for surgical removal if obstruction of flow is severe.

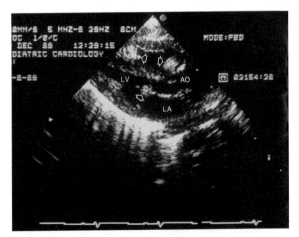

Figure 26-11. This is a long axis view of a rhabdomyoma. Three distinct tumors can be seen (arrows): one in the right ventricle, one on the pulmonic valve that is prolapsing into the right ventricular outflow tract, and one on the mitral valve. LV, left ventricle; AO, aortic valve; LA, left atrium.

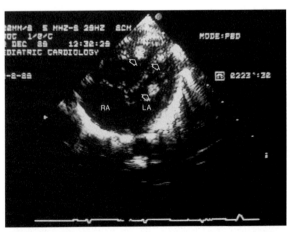

Figure 26-13. An apical four-chamber view in the patient shown in Figure 26-12 demonstrates the lesions on the mitral valve, right ventricle, and septum (arrows). LA, left atrium; RA, right atrium.

RHABDOMYOSARCOMA

These tumors arise from striated muscle fibers that diffusely infiltrate the muscle of the heart. Rhabdomyosarcomas are the most common soft tissue sarcoma in children.[12] They are often found in multiple sites within the heart and can be located in any chamber. Rhabdomyosarcoma invades the tissues that are adjacent to its myocardial origin. It can be found in the pericardium and has been noted to replace valvular tissue. Distal metastatic sites include the lungs, liver, and skeleton.[77] These tumors appear on echocardiography as solid, echodense masses with irregular borders. They can occur at multiple sites.[4,48,77]

FIBROMA

Cardiac fibromas are unencapsulated, well-circumscribed, benign tumors. They are intramural and most often arise from the free wall of the left ventricle or the intraventricular septum.[52,72] They can extend into the cardiac chamber as they enlarge and cause mechanical obstruction to the inflow or outflow tracts. These isolated, slow-growing tumors can cause cardiomegaly, arrhythmias, outflow tract obstruction, congestive heart failure, and even sudden death.[12,79] A fibroma's appearance on echocardiography is typically that of a large mass within the interventricular septum.

FIBROSARCOMA

Fibrosarcomas arise from the right and left ventricles with equal frequency. In half of the cases, the tumor is large enough to protrude into the chamber and cause some degree of obstruction.[10,62,95] Cases of vena caval or pulmonary vein obstruction as well as valvular obstruction have been reported. Thrombus formation due to obstruction has occurred.[94,96] These tumors have a "fish flesh" appearance, with areas of hemorrhage and necrosis. In a third of the cases, the pericardium is involved. Fibrosarcoma can be differentiated from fibroma in that the former invades the surrounding tissues, particularly the pericardium.

HEMANGIOMA

Hemangiomas are vascular tumors and can be located in any cardiac chamber.[93] They can be intramyocardial or intracavitary and are most often found on the right side of the heart. They are typically discrete masses that are smaller than 3–4 cm in diameter. Some can become large and impede cardiac function. Hemangiomas may have lakes or channels within them or may present as highly vascular masses. There have been reports of spontaneous resolution of these tumors. Hemangiomas are the most likely of all benign tumors to be accompanied by a pericardial effusion.[103] Echocardiographically, the tumor typically appears as a single sessile mass that is nonhomogeneous. The presence of a pericardial effusion can be helpful in differentiating this tumor from a rhabdomyoma.

TERATOMA

Teratomas contain all three germ cell layers. These tumors may contain cells from skeletal, nerve, and connective tissues, as well as others.[7,16,78] They occur most often in children and are likely to be found in the right atrium or right ventricle and septum. Upon surgical removal, teeth, hair, and skeletal components can be identified within the tumor mass. Because of the various types of cells that make up the teratoma, the echocardiographic presentation is one of a well-defined mass of varying echodensities.

Secondary Tumors of the Heart

Secondary or metastatic tumors of the heart are far more common than primary tumors. Reports of metastases on autopsy reveal that 5% of the time they involve the heart and 13% of the time they involve the pericardium.[25] The most common tumors to metastasize to the heart are lung and breast tumors, lymphoma, leukemia, and malignant melanoma.[33] The survival rate of patients with metastatic tumors of the heart is poor—7% over 5 years.[33]

Metastases to the heart can occur from either direct extension from adjacent tissue, such as lung carcinomas, or via the lymphatic system or circulatory flow. Melanoma, lymphoma, and leukemia spread through either hematogenous or lymphatic flow.[19,87,88] There have been reports of ovarian and testicular cancers extending directly up the venous system, along the inferior vena cava, and into the right atrium.

When secondary tumors metastasize, they generally invade multiple locations, which may include the heart. Clinical manifestations of cardiac involvement can center on the pericardium, myocardium, or external cardiac compression. The most common clinical manifestations of metastasis to the heart are pericardial effusion and, often, cardiac tamponade.[12] Other manifestations include tachyarrhythmias, atrioventricular block, thromboembolism, hemodynamic obstruction, and congestive heart failure.[33] Pericardial metastatic tumors and effusions are most common with breast and lung cancer. On echocardiography, malignant involvement of the pericardium may present as a mass on either the parietal or visceral surfaces, with or without an effusion. In some cases, the tumor may be large and invasive enough to encircle the heart and obliterate the pericardial space. Care should be taken to differentiate pericardial masses from fibrin strands and regions of thickened, consolidated effusions or thrombus formation, which can be seen in chronic pericardial effusions. It should also be noted that previous radiation therapy to the chest can cause radiation-induced pericarditis. These manifestations, if present, usually occur within the first year after the completion of treatment, but they can develop several years afterward.[64]

Metastatic tumors arising from the endocardium and intramyocardial regions can be difficult to differentiate echocardiographically from primary tumors of the heart. Tumors that extend into the cardiac chambers from the inferior or superior vena cava or the pulmonary veins can help provide some insight into the mass's origin. Often, however, the mass can be clearly demonstrated but difficult to classify. These tumors need to be evaluated for their effect on impedance of blood flow, valve function, and obstruction. They may also result in arrhythmias.

Extracardiac masses can arise from the mediastinum or the pleura. These masses may be from many sources. Lung cancer, hematomas, thymomas, cysts, and metastases from other sites are just a few examples of extracardiac masses. These masses can be echolucent or echodense and can be of any size. They can appear anterior or posterior to the heart. Figure 26-14 is from a 24-year-old male experiencing shortness of breath, cough, and peripheral edema. Echocardiographically, a mass was noted to compress the right ventricle. At surgery this mass was diagnosed as a fibrosarcoma of the mediastinum. Again, echocardiography may be able to

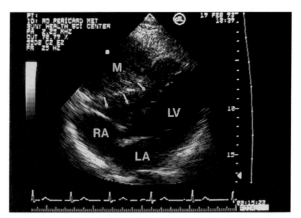

Figure 26-14. An extracardiac mass (M) can be noted compressing the right ventricle (arrows) in this apical four-chamber view. This patient was diagnosed at surgery with a fibrosarcoma of the mediastinum. LV, left ventricle; LA, left atrium; RA, right atrium.

image these masses well, but it is limited in providing an accurate diagnosis of the mass. All masses need to be evaluated for their effects on cardiac function, whether compression of the chambers or more peripherally, such as superior vena caval obstruction or pulmonary vein compression, since cardiac function can be compromised.

PERICARDIAL CYSTS

Pericardial cysts make up 7% of all mediastinal masses. They are benign intrathoracic lesions that are usually located along the right costophrenic angle (70%) and are less commonly found along the left costophrenic angle (10%).[64,102,114] These cysts usually do not cause symptoms, but when they are present, the patient may experience dyspnea, tachycardia, arrhythmias, and chest pain.

On echocardiography, the cyst will appear as a well-circumscribed, echolucent lesion extending from the pericardium. It can be several centimeters in diameter. Care should be taken to differentiate this mass from pericardial diverticulum, an outpouching of pericardium creating a fold that can fill with fluid. Pericardial diverticulum typically moves or swings with changes in body position. Pericardial cysts do not shift significantly with changes in body position and do not change in size.

If symptoms are present or if a more specific differential diagnosis is needed, the pericardial cysts can be drained. Thoracoscopy is a minimally invasive method of draining these cysts without requiring thoracotomy and general anesthesia. No cases of malignant pericardial cyst have been reported, and removal of the cysts is generally not required.[54,74]

Thrombus

The diagnosis of cardiac thrombi may be difficult but critical to the care of the patient. Although the incidence of cardiac thrombi may decrease in the thrombolytic era, the importance of echocardiography in this clinical setting appears to be emerging. Echocardiography remains the standard for the diagnosis of atrial and ventricular thrombus. Its use has been expanded to improve the diagnosis and management of cardiac thrombi related to blunt chest trauma, pulmonary emboli, congenital heart disease, cardiac transplantation, atrial fibrillation or atrial flutter, prosthetic valve dysfunction, and catheter placement.[113] With the increasing use of multiplane transesophageal echocardiography, the standard continues to improve. A significant amount of forthcoming research will determine how transthoracic and transesophageal echocardiography are to be used in the diagnosis of common problems involving cardiac thrombi such as atrial fibrillation, stroke, and myocardial infarction.

VENTRICULAR THROMBI

Most ventricular thrombi are found in association with underlying cardiac disease. The vast majority of patients with thrombi have myocardial ischemia with subsequent wall motion abnormalities. Indeed, it is rare to discover a ventricular thrombus without some underlying wall motion abnormality, although rare cases have been described.[113] Thrombi can be found in dilated cardiomyopathy from any cause, within ventricular aneurysms, associated with various devices such as pacemaker wires (Fig. 26-15) or artificial heart valves, and associated with myocardial trauma.[81] A high level of suspicion is critical to making the diagnosis of ventricular thrombus. Left ventricular thrombi are much more frequently identified than right ventricular thrombi. By far the most common location of left ventricular thrombi is at the apex (Fig. 26-16). Frequently, pa-

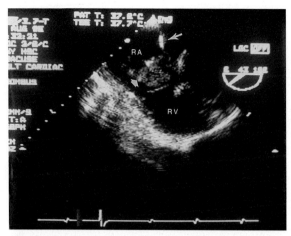

Figure 26-15. This illustration of a transesophageal view depicts a lead wire (long arrow) in the right atrium (RA). Note the 2- to 3-cm mass (short arrow) attached to the lead wire. This is a large, mobile thrombus that has seeded on the pacemaker lead wire. RV, right ventricle.

tients with apical thrombi have a history of a large anterior wall myocardial infarction. It has been estimated than 90% of all left ventricular thrombi are found in this clinical situation.[12] Some apical thrombi can be part of a left ventricular pseudoaneurysm (Fig. 26-17). Ventricular thrombi can form within hours of the time of infarction but usually are identified 1–10 days after myocardial infarction.[113] Although the size of the infarction also influences the likelihood of thrombus formation, approximately 30–35% of all anterior myocardial infarctions

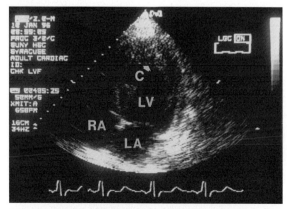

Figure 26-16. This is an apical four-chamber view. Note the dilated left ventricle (LV) with a laminated thrombus at the apex (**C**). LA, left atrium; RA, right atrium.

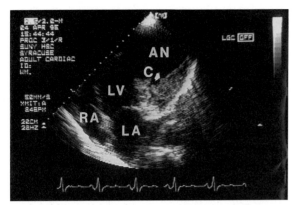

Figure 26-17. An apical four-chamber view of a large pseudoaneurysm (AN) is noted. A large amount of thrombus (C) fills the pseudoaneurysm. LA, left atrium; LV, left ventricle; RA, right atrium.

have associated thrombi compared to less than 5% of inferior myocardial infarctions.[113] Several theories have been put forth to explain this finding: (1) the lack of a buttress, such as the septum or diaphragm, allows excessive ballooning of the apex and promotes clot formation; (2) the thrombi are more accessible to echocardiographic interrogation; (3) the mitral inflow patterns tend to swirl the blood after an anterior infarct near the apex, producing a stagnant flow pattern and promoting clot formation.[66] However, ventricular thrombi may be seen in association with inferoposterior infarctions, particularly if they are associated with aneurysm formation (Fig. 26-18). Such thrombi may be easily missed if the

sonographer is not careful to obtain both short axis and two-chamber views. Frequently, an off-axis short axis view will better define the inferoposterior aneurysm and thus the presence of a thrombus. Despite the higher incidence of apical thrombi with anterior myocardial infarction, there seems to be no relation between stroke and the site of the myocardial infarction.[11] The use of thrombolytics in patients with acute myocardial infarction does not appear to significantly reduce the incidence of ventricular thrombi. It is the degree of left ventricular wall motion abnormality and the lack of postinfarction heparin that appear to account for the similar incidence of ventricular thrombi in patients treated or not treated with thrombolytics.[55]

Right ventricular thrombi are infrequently identified antemorteum. This may be due to the lack of a clinical event such as provided in left ventricular thrombi by ischemic coronary syndromes. Patients with right ventricular thrombi often have subtle symptoms and may not come to medical attention as easily as those with left ventricular thrombi. Often the patient with right ventricular thrombus is referred to the echocardiographic laboratory to assess the degree of pulmonary hypertension and right-sided chamber enlargement, only to have a right ventricular thrombus identified (Fig. 26-19). The development of new techniques such as pulmonary artery endarterectomy, thrombolytic therapy, and prostaglandin infusion may result in an increase in the use of echocardiography as a screening test for chronic pulmonary emboli.[17,86]

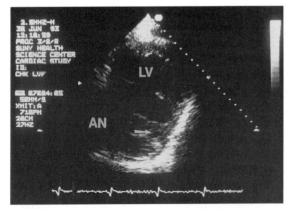

Figure 26-18. A parasternal short axis view of the left ventricle (LV). A pseudoanuerysm (AN) of the inferoposterior wall is noted, with thrombus formation (arrow) along the lateral aspect.

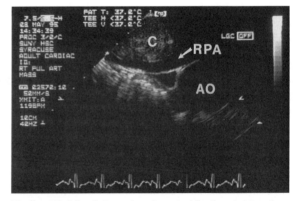

Figure 26-19. A thrombus is noted in the right pulmonary artery on this transesophageal view. AO, aorta; RPA, right pulmonary artery; C, thrombus.

Right ventricular thrombi can be found in patients with right ventricular infarction, cor pulmonale, dilated cardiomyopathy, Löeffler's syndrome, blunt chest trauma, Beçhet's disease, and endomyocardial fibrosis.[63,80] Most right ventricular thrombi arise from emboli originating in the peripheral venous system.

Regardless of the cause of thrombus, an accurate diagnosis is essential to the welfare of the patient. Transthoracic two-dimensional imaging has been the standard in the diagnosis of ventricular thrombus for almost two decades. The sensitivity of transthoracic echocardiography is 75–80%, with a specificity of 90–95% in the detection of left ventricular thrombus.[113] Transthoracic echocardiography is superior to radionuclide imaging or cardiac angiography in the detection of left ventricular thrombi. Apical thrombi can fill in the apical aneurysm and cause a false-negative radionuclide study, while this study may allow superior imaging in patients with poor echocardiographic windows.[82] Most clinicians therefore consider these modalities to be complementary. Several potential pitfalls in the echocardiographic diagnosis of ventricular thrombus can be avoided by following some simple rules. First, all modalities available, including transesophageal echocardiography and Doppler, should be used. Although classically used for atrial thrombi, the high-resolution multiplane images of modern transesophageal equipment may often aid in the diagnosis of ventricular thrombi.[18] Doppler interrogation, particularly with color Doppler, often provides a clue to the diagnosis.[108] Careful Doppler interrogation of the left ventricular velocities can reveal an apical rotating flow or vortex ring flow.[40,108] Second, use of the highest-frequency transducer, such as a 5.0- or even 7.5-MHz probe, aids in visualizing the left ventricular apex. Studies have shown that the diagnosis of ventricular thrombi is enhanced by these transducers.[113] Third, off-axis views help create a mental three-dimensional image of the left ventricular apex. Fourth, near-field artifact should be minimized by carefully adjusting gain and depth settings. Lastly, the diagnosis of thrombus should be made only if the presence of thrombus is certain. More errors are made by identifying suspicious shadows as clot as opposed to undercalling thrombus. Other structures, such as left ventricular false tendons, the moderator band, calcified papillary muscles or mitral annulus (Fig. 26-20), or various catheters that might be mistaken

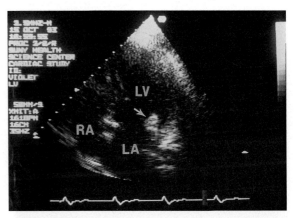

Figure 26-20. In this apical four-chamber view there is a bright, echodense mass (arrow) in the region of the mitral valve. This is a heavily calcified mitral annulus. LV, left ventricle; LA, left atrium; RA, right atrium.

for thrombi, should be considered as differential diagnoses. Artifacts can be distinguished from thrombi by considering several facts. Thrombi are often more echodense than the adjacent myocardial wall, and ventricular thrombi move in synchrony with the underlying myocardium. Thrombus rarely occurs in the presence of normal myocardial wall motion, and artifact frequently occurs with normal wall motion.

The shape and nature of ventricular thrombi may be quite variable. Ventricular thrombi can be laminated, pedunculated, shaggy, or isodense with the surrounding blood pool. Various attempts have been made to identify the echocardiographic characteristics of thrombi likely to embolize. Although the correlation is imperfect, large, shaggy, mobile thrombi that protrude into the left ventricular cavity seem to have an increased embolization rate (Fig. 26-21). Thrombi found in patients with idiopathic dilated cardiomyopathy or ventricular aneurysm also have higher rates of embolization. The overall rate of systemic embolization is 5–10%. Most embolic events occur within the first 6 months of thrombus formation. Echocardiography can be used to follow these patients to ensure that the thrombus has not changed in size or nature. It has not been demonstrated that this is a cost-effective approach to the management of these patients, as the thrombus will endothelialize within 3–6 months regardless of its echocardiographic appearance.

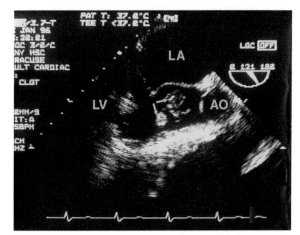

Figure 26-21. *This is a transesophageal long axis view at 121 degrees. A mobile thrombus (arrows) can be seen in the left ventricular outflow tract near the aortic valve (AO). LV, left ventricle; LA, left atrium.*

ATRIAL THROMBI

Left atrial thrombi have generated a significant amount of interest in the last several years. These thrombi are associated with blood stasis within the left atrium. If blood stasis is present, a thrombus can form in 3 days, although some information indicates that the time of thrombus formation can be significantly shorter.[100] Thus nonanticoagulated patients in atrial fibrillation may be at risk of thrombus formation while awaiting transesophageal echo-guided cardioversion. The majority of left atrial thrombi are found within the left atrial appendage—up to 90% in recent studies.[113] It may be that local blood velocities within the left atrial appendage are a key factor in the formation of thrombus in that location.[69] These left atrial appendage velocities are largely dependent on left ventricular systolic function.[46] Poor left ventricular systolic function results in low-velocity left atrial appendage flow and favors thrombus formation. Left atrial appendage function is better during atrial flutter or fib-flutter than during atrial fibrillation.[91] Therefore, it is not surprising that patients with atrial flutter have a lower but still significantly higher incidence of atrial thrombi than normal persons.[8] Because of the increasing use of transesophageal echocardiography, the sensitivity of detection has increased from 30–50% with transthoracic echocardiography to over 95% with multiplane transesophageal imaging.[5,60] Thrombi appear as round or oval structures that can be broad-

based or pedunculated. Risk factors for the development of left atrial thrombi include mitral stenosis, poor left ventricular systolic function, enlarged left atrial chamber, atrial fibrillation, and the presence of a prosthetic mitral valve (Figs. 26-22 to 26-24). Tilting disk valves have a higher incidence of left atrial thrombus formation than ball-cage, bileaflet, or bioprosthetic valves.[113] Heart transplant patients have an increased risk of left atrial thrombus formation.[27] In patients with no significant risk factors, the likelihood of finding a left atrial thrombus is reduced 10-fold.[13]

The association of spontaneous contrast (so-called smoke) makes the diagnosis of left atrial thrombus significantly more likely and increases the possibility of embolization.[37,49] Spontaneous contrast is the echocardiographic finding of clouds of weakly echodense particles within cardiac chambers during times of stasis. Their appearance resembles smoke, and this term has been loosely applied to any pattern of visibly static blood flow. The cause of spontaneous contrast has not been absolutely determined but appears to be related to the formation of stacks of red blood cells called *rouleaux formation*. Spontaneous contrast is a contraindication for transesophageal, echo-guided electrical cardioversion.[65] The presence of significant mitral regurgitation reduces the incidence of left atrial thrombus formation and spontaneous contrast but may not reduce the risk of embolization.[50,53,110] Because of the recent clinical information concerning anticoagulation in patients with atrial fibrillation or atrial flutter, the diagnosis of left atrial thrombus has be-

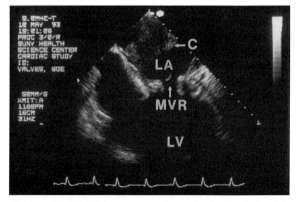

Figure 26-22. *This transesophageal view of the left atrium (LA) demonstrates thrombi (C). A prosthetic mitral valve (MVR) is present. LV, left ventricle.*

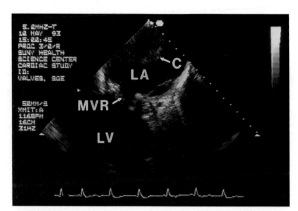

Figure 26-23. This is a second view of the thrombi (C) in the left atrium (LA) in the same patient shown in Figure 26-22. Channels have been created in the atrium by blood flow. MVR, mitral valve prosthesis; LV, left ventricle.

come crucial to the management of these patients.[5] It is not yet clear whether a negative echocardiographic study allows the immediate cardioversion of the patient without long-term anticoagulation.[65] Several reports have cautioned that embolic phenomema have occurred after electrical cardioversion despite a negative transesophageal study.[9,68] Until a larger multicenter study is available, the decision to perform electrical cardioversion based on transesophageal echocardiography must be made on an individual basis.[59] However, if electrical cardioversion is to follow transesophageal echocardiography, the patient should be on heparin and, if possible, the transesophageal probe should be left in place

during the cardioversion.[37] A follow-up transesophageal examination after cardioversion is indicated because of possible atrial stunning from the electrical shock, leading to thrombus formation.[36,42]

Recently, it has become clear that nonfibrillatory atrial tachycardias in congenital heart disease are associated with a high incidence of left atrial thrombus formation.[38] Patients with amyloidosis can form left atrial thrombi even though they remain in normal sinus rhythm.[30] Rarely, a free-floating or "ball" thrombus can be identified. Often these thrombi are seen in patients with mitral stenosis or prosthetic valves.[41] Ball thrombi can result in sudden cardiac death by the so-called hole-in-one phenomenon.[2] This occurs when the left atrial clot becomes lodged in the mitral valve inflow (Figs. 26-25 and 26-26). Recently, long linear strands have been identified on mitral valves, usually prosthetic mitral valves, that either embolize or are markers for a high risk of future embolization.[51] Spontaneous microbubbles, distinct from spontaneous contrast, have been noted with prosthetic mitral valve replacement and also may be a marker for the development of small thrombi.[75] If a left atrial thrombus is found prior to planned mitral commissurotomy, care must be taken not to disturb it during the procedure.[104] The differential diagnosis of left atrial thrombi includes mitral annular calcification with subsequent sterile abscess of the mitral ring, artifact, atrial myxoma, other tumors, and lipomatous hypertrophy. If there is any doubt about the diagnosis of left atrial thrombus, a transesophageal

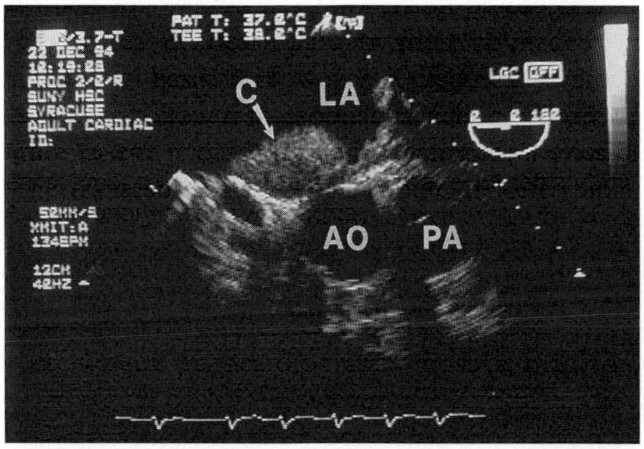

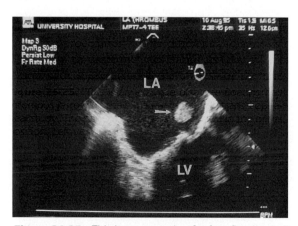

Figure 26-24. In this illustration, a thrombus (C) is noted near the mouth of the left atrial appendage. LA, left atrium; PA, pulmonary artery; AO, aorta.

Figure 26-25. This is an example of a free floating ball thrombus (arrow) in the left atrium (LA) on a transesophageal study. The patient has a prosthetic valve in the mitral position. Left ventricle (LV).

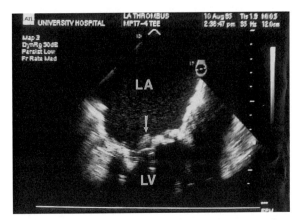

Figure 26-26. This example is from the same patient shown in Figure 26-25. The ball thrombus in this diastolic frame has lodged temporarily in the orifice of the mitral prosthesis. LA, left atrium; LV, left ventricle.

echocardiographic examination significantly improves the sensitivity. With a multiplane transesophageal echocardiographic study, even small thrombi can be identified. If a cardiac source of embolus is sought, the examination of choice is a transesophageal study.[21,56] Prosthetic valve thrombosis has been identified with transthoracic Doppler examination. Two-dimensional echocardiographic visualization of the thrombus is nearly impossible, but if the diagnosis is still in doubt after the transthoracic Doppler exam, a transesophageal study can provide indirect evidence of a thrombosed prosthetic valve.[43]

Right atrial thrombi are more difficult to visualize, as the right atrial appendage is blunter and less well defined echocardiographically. However, the right atrium may act as a reservoir for systemic thrombi that embolized to the heart and can be easily identified with transesophageal echocardiography.[3,24] These thrombi can then either cross through a probe patent foramen ovale into the arterial circulation or proceed to the pulmonary vascular bed, resulting in pulmonary thromboembolism.[28] In situ right atrial thrombi can also occur. They are often found in patients with pulmonary hypertension that results in right atrial enlargement and subsequent low-flow states. Such situations can occur in patients with chronic atrial arrhythmias, pulmonary hypertension, or cardiomyopathies. In addition, the number of patients receiving transvenous pacing catheters, Swan-Ganz catheters, and central venous catheters for parenteral nutrition has increased. Right atrial thrombi must be separated

from other causes of right atrial masses, including myxoma, secondary and primary tumors, and foreign bodies. In addition, normal right atrial structures such as the eustachian valve, chiari network, and thebesian vein of the coronary sinus must be distinguished. If the study is being done intraoperatively, an inverted right atrial appendage during the procedure can also mimic a right atrial thrombus. There is some concern that normal structures, such as the chiari network, may increase the likelihood of arterial embolization and stroke by directing the venous return flow directly at the foramen ovale.[92]

MISCELLANEOUS THROMBI

Thrombus formation can occur in areas easily seen on echocardiographic examination but not within the heart. A common example is the thrombus formation that occurs with sudden cardiac rupture. This situation can be due to blunt chest trauma, an iatrogenic device, or myocardial infarction. A characteristic thrombus forms that encases the heart and is associated with a small pericardial effusion (Fig. 26-27). Another area frequently involved with thrombus is the thoracic aorta. Usually associated with significant atherosclerotic plaque, aortic thrombi pose a significant risk (Fig. 26-28).

ENDOCARDITIS

Infective endocarditis is a destructive disease process that becomes potentially more fatal or disabling the longer it goes undiagnosed. It can destroy the heart

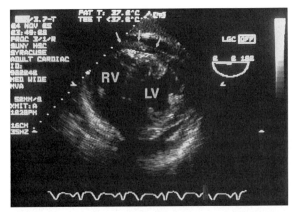

Figure 26-27. This transesophageal short axis view demonstrates the right ventricle (RV) and left ventricle (LV). There is a pericardial effusion with thrombus laminating along the posterior surface of the heart (arrows).

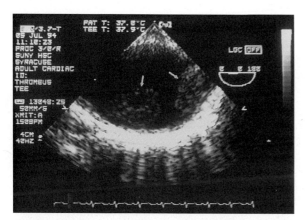

Figure 26-28. This is a transesophageal view of the descending aorta in short axis. Two prominent thrombi are seen (arrows).

valves, lead to congestive heart failure or embolization to other organs, and cause death if left untreated. Mortality over the last 25–30 years has remained relatively high at 25–40%.[35] Patients who are elderly, have congenital heart disease, or have prosthetic valves are at higher risk of developing significant complications and dying. The mortality rate is higher among specific subgroups and can reach nearly 100%.[35]

Endocarditis is caused by bacterial, yeast, or fungal infections that seed and grow on the valves of the heart, the papillary muscles, or, in some cases, the endocardial surface of the ventricles. The two main bacterial groups that cause endocarditis are staphylococci and streptococci. These account for more than 80% of the organisms isolated from blood cultures in patients with native valve infective endocarditis.[105] Staphylococcal infective endocarditis is reported to be more fatal than streptococcal varieties.[35] Infective endocarditis is classified as acute or subacute, depending on the nature of the responsible organism.

Vegetations form as a result of complex interactions between the immune system, the coagulation system, hemodynamic forces, and the invading microorganism. These interactions cause some vegetations to have certain general characteristics. For example, staphylococci and streptococci promote platelet adhesion and aggregation, and thus growth of the vegetations. These vegetations are often large and can have a stringy appearance on echocardiographic images. Organisms that are encapsulated,

such as *Escherichia coli* and other gram-negative microbes, usually form flat, more gelatinous vegetations that are by nature less adherent to damaged valves, perhaps explaining the low incidence of gram-negative endocarditis. The importance of the immune system in vegetation formation is illustrated by cases of nonbacterial thrombotic endocarditis (NBTE). NBTE includes all cases of endocarditis not due to an infectious process. Entities identified by older terms such as *murantic endocarditis* and *Libman-Sachs endocarditis* should be considered types of NBTE. Three events must occur to lead to NBTE: (1) endothelial damage, (2) development of a hypercoagulable state, and (3) a high-velocity jet flow.[12] If bacterial organisms are then injected into the area of NBTE by a high-velocity jet, infective endocarditis may result. The exact proportion of lesions that start as NBTE and become infective endocarditis is not yet known. As applied to clinical echocardiography, the hemodynamic forces tend to cause the vegetation to form on the low-pressure side of the involved heart valve. Thus, mitral and tricuspid vegetations are usually seen on the atrial surface of the valve, while aortic and pulmonic vegetations are found on the ventricular side of the valve, where diastolic pressure is quite low.

Patients with infective endocarditis can present with many signs and symptoms that are often nonspecific. Fever is the predominant clinical sign. In acute infective endocarditis the patient may present with a high fever and a rapid onset of a severe infection. The patient may have no heart murmurs in the early stages of the disease but in as little as a week can begin to develop murmurs as the infection destroys valve function, leading to congestive heart failure and embolization. With left-sided heart lesions, embolization can demonstrate petechiae and purpuric skin lesions, transient ischemic events, and stroke. With right-sided lesions, pneumonia-like symptoms can occur.

In subacute infective endocarditis, the onset of signs and symptoms may not lead the physician to suspect the heart as the site of infection. Common complaints include low-grade fever, fatigue, weight loss, cough, and weakness.[12] The infection can go on for weeks or months before the patient seeks medical help or the correct diagnosis is made and therapy started.

Blood cultures are drawn to make the diagnosis of infective endocarditis. In most cases, the cultures will demonstrate the offending organism. Once this is established, a cardiac source for the infection may be suspected. Blood cultures may not always demonstrate the presence of the infection. They can be accurate approximately 95% of the time when multiple blood samples are taken and analyzed.[111] Some organisms are difficult to detect. Fungal infections frequently have negative blood cultures. If antibiotic therapy is started for as little as 2 days, the ability to obtain an accurate diagnosis by blood cultures is lost.

When infective endocarditis is suspected, echocardiography is the diagnostic tool of choice to demonstrate the presence and extent of these lesions and their impact on the heart. Echocardiography can demonstrate the mass lesions that are formed by the organism. These lesions consist of microorganisms, leukocytes, fibrin, and thrombus and are called *vegetations*. Figure 26-29 is an apical four-chamber view demonstrating a mitral valve vegetation. This vegetation is associated with the anterior leaflet and prolapses into the left atrium. Ultrasound is limited in the size of the lesion that can be imaged. The frequency of the transducer, the depth of the lesion, and the method of focusing the sound beam all impact the size of the lesion that can be demonstrated. Under ideal circumstances, a vegetation as small as 2–3 mm can be diagnosed. Vegetations are irregularly shaped masses that can be laminated along the surface of the valve or valve apparatus. They can also be pedunculated masses attached to the surface of the valve and can be highly mobile.

A vegetation can grow large enough to create mechanical impedance to blood flow.

To demonstrate a vegetation adequately, the lesion must be defined in multiple planes with the highest resolution available. Consequently, transesophageal echocardiography is often the technique of choice to demonstrate the presence of a vegetation and its effect on valve function. The ability of this method to detect vegetations transthoracically (58%) is much lower than that of the transesophageal approach (90%).[69] While the vegetation in Figures 26-30 and 26-31 are only several millimeters thick, transesophageal echocardiography demonstrates the lesions well. In Figure 26-30 the vegetation is seen along the edges of the anterior leaflet. In Figure 26-31, the destruction of the valve leaflet is demonstrated by the flail segment of the anterior leaflet. Vegetations can also create tears in the leaflets and, in advanced cases, flail leaflets (Fig. 26-32). It can be difficult to determine how much of a mass is from vegetative debris and how much is disrupted valve leaflet. One must document the structure, extent, and mobility of each vegetation since these lesions are followed serially to demonstrate changes in cardiac function and to assess the timing of and need for surgical intervention.

Valvular vegetations are more likely to form on previously diseased valves. Valve thickening, prolapse, calcium deposits, and congenital defects, as well as atheromatous changes, can increase the likelihood of lesion formation. As valvular vegetations develop, they tend to disrupt the integrity of the

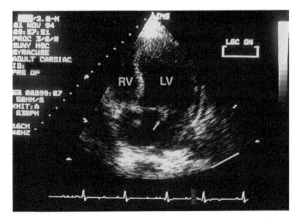

Figure 26-29. This is an apical four-chamber view demonstrating a mitral valve vegetation. LV, left ventricle; RV, right ventricle.

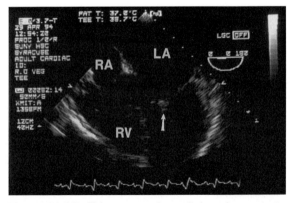

Figure 26-30. This transesophageal view demonstrates a mitral valve vegetation on the anterior leaflet (arrow). LA, left atrium; RV, right ventricle; RA, right atrium.

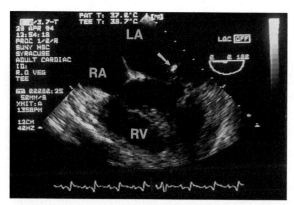

Figure 26-31. *This is the same patient shown in Figure 26-30 in a systolic frame. Note that part of the anterior leaflet is flail (arrow). LA, left atrium; RV, right ventricle; RA, right atrium.*

valve. Valvular regurgitation is a common complication of infective endocarditis and is often severe.[22] As the disease progresses, the severity of the regurgitation increases. It can cause heart failure and seed the adjacent valve with the offending organism. This is well demonstrated with aortic vegetations leading to acute severe aortic regurgitation and predisposing the adjacent anterior leaflet and chordal apparatus to infection. If the left ventricle has not had time to adjust to the increased load from the aortic regurgitation, the patient can rapidly develop congestive heart failure. Doppler echocardiography

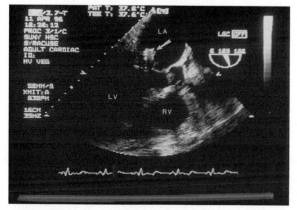

Figure 26-32. *A mitral valve vegetation is visualized on this transesophageal view. The vegetation (arrow) is seen in the left atrium (LA). Note the tear in the midportion of the anterior leaflet. This valve was determined to be partially flail and torn at surgery. RV, right ventricle; LV, left ventricle.*

is very helpful in demonstrating the presence of and changes over time in these regurgitant lesions. Even small, eccentric jets can be documented. This information can be helpful even if vegetations are small and poorly defined. Changes on subsequent studies can detail the course and progress of the disease.

Infective endocarditis can form vegetations on any of the cardiac valves. Echocardiographically, they appear as single or multiple masses along the surface of the leaflet. They can be pedunculated and mobile or more diffuse focal thickening of the leaflet. They tend to be fuzzy and echodense. Since vegetations are predisposed to occur on already deformed valves, they can be particularly difficult to detect on these valves when they are small. As the vegetations become larger over time, their presence becomes easier to detect and their destruction of valve function may make them obvious.

Vegetations occur more often on the left side of the heart and affect the mitral valve more often than the aortic valve.[76] Infection of both valves is also common in this disease. With the increase in intravenous drug use and infected indwelling venous catheters, right heart vegetations have become more common. Fungal vegetations create the largest masses and tend to be less destructive of the underlying valve leaflet. Some of these lesions can become large enough to create partial obstruction of the valve orifice or outflow tract.[113]

Perivalvular abscesses can develop as infective endocarditis advances. These abscesses can occur along the mitral and aortic rings and are typically extensions of active disease of the associated valve.[6,15,32] Antibiotic therapy may fail to penetrate and sterilize them. Early surgical intervention has been suggested by some authors to improve the outcome and avoid widespread tissue destruction.[23] Abscesses appear as sonolucent areas adjacent to the valve apparatus. They can be elongated and follow the contour of the surrounding anatomy. Figure 26-33 demonstrates a perivalvular aortic abscess in diastole that has been clearly separated from the aortic wall by multiplane scanning in Figure 26-34. Complications of fistulous communications with the left or right atrium or from the aortic valve to the left ventricle have been reported.[106] Great care should be taken to study all suspected perivalvular abscesses with Doppler for communication with adjacent structures. In patients who are not responding to antibiotic therapy, transesophageal imaging

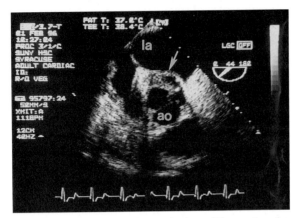

Figure 26-33. This is a short axis view of the aortic valve (ao) from a transesophageal exam. An abscess is noted (arrow) in the periaortic area adjacent to the left atrium (la).

may be indicated to search for possible perivalvular abscess.

Vegetations that occur on prosthetic valves are among the most difficult to diagnose. The ability to image a prosthetic valve is limited to the side that is closest to the transducer since the prosthesis will reflect all sound waves off the metal valve components and the dense sewing ring. Vegetations within the apparatus of both mechanical and bioprosthetic valves can easily be missed by shadows from the sewing ring or the valve itself. Prosthetic valves are predisposed to thrombus formation on the metallic surfaces and to pannus ingrowth from the sewing ring,

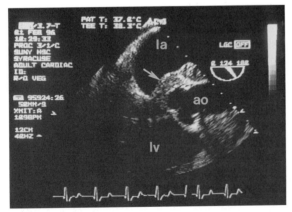

Figure 26-34. This is a transesophageal long axis view, in the same patient shown in Figure 26-33, of the aortic valve (ao) demonstrating the abscess (arrow) between the aorta and the left atrium (la). lv, left ventricle.

both of which further complicate the detection of vegetations. Transesophageal imaging performed carefully from multiple views can often detect these lesions. Perivalvular leaks are associated with prosthetic valve vegetations. In extreme cases, the valve itself may rock and become dehiscent.

Embolization of vegetations is a common complication of infective endocarditis.[45] Emboli can affect the coronary arteries, creating myocardial wall motion abnormalities, and the brain, causing stroke, as well as traveling to any other organ in the body. Embolization can occur early or late in the course of the disease, depending on the organism involved.[35] Staphylococcus infections tend to produce large vegetations that are friable and embolize readily.[70] These vegetations often produce multiple complications in remote organs. The prognosis for these patients is worse than with other organisms. In contrast, streptococcal infections tend to embolize less often and, when they do, they are usually single.[35,70]

Another complication of infective endocarditis, particularly with *Staphylococcus aureus,* is pericarditis. The mortality rate can be as high as 70%.[70] Pericarditis is more common with aortic or mitral ring abscess, but a pericardial effusion can be present even in its absence.[6]

Once the infection has been controlled and sterilized, changes in the appearance of the vegetations can be noted. Vegetations have been reported to be smaller and brighter in appearance.[98] This may be due to the fibrosis and calcium deposits as the healed vegetations begin to age. These changes can be noted from serial studies performed over the course of the disease. It is important to note the characteristics and locations of these lesions to avoid misdiagnosing old healed vegetations as new episodes of infective endocarditis.

False-Positive Cardiac Masses

There are several structures or normal variations within the heart that are not present in every patient. Some of these are congenital structures that persist and remain prominent, such as chiari networks, the eustachian valve, and the thebesian valve. Others are normal variants, such as atrial septal aneurysm, prominent moderator band, and false tendons. Lastly, manufactured objects such as pacemaker and internal cardiac defibrillator lead wires or infusion catheters need to be properly identified to avoid false interpretations.

The eustachian thebesian valves are remnants of the right venous valve. These valves are used in fetal life to help direct blood across the fossa ovalis to the left atrium. The eustachian valve, or valve of the inferior vena cava, is a band of tissue that extends from the inferior lateral wall of the right atrium to the posterior portion of the fossa ovalis[1] (Fig. 26-35). The thebesian valve is a band of tissue noted in the region of the coronary sinus as it enters the right atrium. Chiari remnants, or networks, have been described as a fenestrated right venous valve.[112] These networks can have a wider array of attachment points and swing widely throughout the atrium, even into the tricuspid valve orifice. Eustachian valves, being bands of tissue, tend to move in a more restricted manner. These structures can be seen in many infants, as well as in some adults. When they are present, care should be taken to image these structures from the apical four-chamber, right inflow tract, and subcostal views to distinguish them from tumor, thrombus, or vegetation in the right atrium. All of these structures appear as echodense, linear objects on echocardiography.

The right atrial walls themselves often have prominent trabeculations and folds, particularly on transesophageal studies. In off-axis views, the atrial appendage, along with the pectinate muscles, can be misinterpreted as a cardiac mass. In the right ventricle, the walls are heavily trabeculated and the moderator band is a prominent structure. The moderator band is a dense, muscular structure that carries a portion of the right bundle branch. The band is easily identified because its location is in the right ventricle, extending from the distal third of interventricular septum to the free wall of the right ventricle. The moderator band is well demonstrated in the apical four-chamber and subcostal views.

Another normal variant that is commonly found consists of false tendons of the ventricles. These fibrous bands transverse the ventricles in a variety of positions.[58] They can extend from the septum to the lateral, anterior, or inferior wall or parallel along the same wall. They can appear similar to the chordae tendineae of the atrioventricular valves or resemble more muscular bands. Echocardiographically, these bands need to be evaluated with two-dimensional imaging, as well as Doppler, to ensure that they do not obstruct flow, like subaortic membranes, or are confused with apical thrombus when noted near the apex. False tendons have not been associated with any specific pathology and are generally considered a coincidental finding.[58,69,109]

Manufactured objects within the heart are often easily identified, particularly when correlated with a brief clinical history. Prosthetic valves, Carpentier-Edwards valve rings, or pacemaker and internal cardiac defibrillator lead wires are all easily noted echocardiographically (Figs. 26-36 and 26-37). Their course through the heart needs to be documented, and detailed views from multiple planes will determine if any pathologic compromise has occurred, such as vegetations or thrombus formation. Most manufactured objects tend to create multiple reverberations or shadowing distal to the original struc-

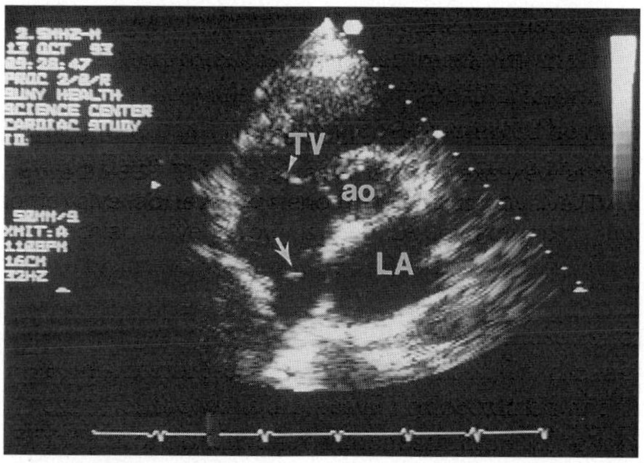

Figure 26-35. This is a parasternal short axis view at the aortic valve (ao) level. Posterior to the tricuspid valve (TV), a eustachian valve (arrow) is seen. LA, left atrium.

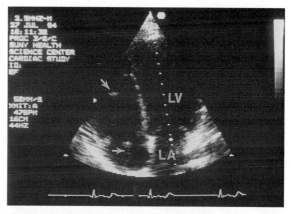

Figure 26-36. Two segments along a single pacemaker lead wire can be seen in this apical four-chamber view (arrows). The lead entering the right atrium is demonstrated and appears again in the right ventricle (arrow). LA, left atrium; LV, left ventricle.

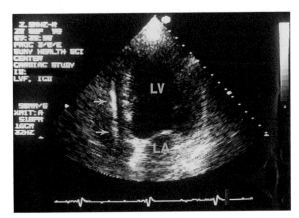

Figure 26-37. This apical four-chamber view demonstrates an internal cardiac defibrillator lead wire (arrows) traversing the right atrium and right ventricle. LA, left atrium; LV, left ventricle.

ture. Recognition of these artifacts will help eliminate false-positive reports. Figure 26-38 demonstrates a Greenfield filter that has migrated from the inferior vena cava through the right heart and has lodged in the right pulmonary artery. Each of the prongs that make up the filter can be noted in a circular pattern.

Summary

Cardiac masses have many different causes and varying impact on cardiac function. Echocardiography in its various forms can detail the location and extent of the dysfunction. Echocardiography, as a noninvasive tool, is uniquely suited to document the changes in these masses over the course of treatment. Serial studies are commonly requested to time surgical intervention and determine the effectiveness of medical therapy.

Echocardiography alone is usually not enough to allow the physician to determine the exact nature of the mass and plan a course of treatment. In nearly all cases, the diagnosis of a cardiac mass needs to be placed in the context of the patient's clinical history to form a complete diagnosis. The sonographer should always perform a detailed study, document a suspected cardiac mass from multiple views, and demonstrate its impact on function with Doppler and appropriate measurements.

REFERENCES

1. Aboliras E, Edwards W, Driscoll D. Cor Triatriatum Dexter: Two dimensional echocardiographic diagnosis. J Am Coll Cardiol. 1987;9:334.
2. Alam M, Jafri SM. Ball-valve thrombus obstructing a bioprosthetic mitral valve. Chest. 1993;103:1599–1600.
3. Alhaddad IA, Soubani AO, Brown EJ Jr, et al. Cardiogenic shock due to huge right atrial thrombus. Chest. 1993;104:1609–1610.
4. Ali S. Pleomorphic rhabdomyosarcoma of the heart metastatic to bone. Acta Cytol. 1995;39:555.
5. Archer SL, James KE, Kvernen LR, et al. Role of transesophageal echocardiography in the detection of left atrial thrombus in patients with chronic non-rheumatic atrial fibrillation. Am Heart J. 1995;130:287–295.
6. Arnett E, Roberts W. Valve ring abscess in infective endocarditis: Frequency, location and clues to clinical diagnosis from the study of 95 necropsy patients. Circulation. 1976;54:140.
7. Benator A. Prenatal pericardiocentesis: Its role in the management of intrapericardial teratoma. Obstet Gynecol. 1992;79:856.
8. Bikkina M, Alpert MA, Mulekar M, et al. Prevalence of intraatrial thrombus in patients with atrial flutter. Am J Cardiol. 1995;76:186–189.
9. Black IW, Fatkin D, Sagar KB, et al. Exclusion of atrial thrombus by transesophageal echocardiography does not preclude embolism after cardioversion of atrial fibrillation a multicenter study [see comments]. Circulation. 1994;89:2509–2513.
10. Bloor C. Cardiac tumors: Clinical presentation and pathologic correlations. Curr Probl Cardiol. 1984;9:7.

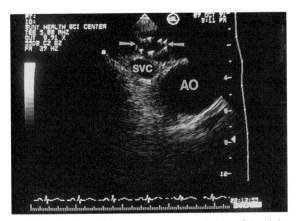

Figure 26-38. This is a transesophageal view of the right pulmonary artery. Six prongs from a Kimray Greenfield filter can be seen (arrows). AO, aorta; SVC, superior vena cava.

11. Bodenheimer MM, Sauer D, Shareef B, et al. Relation between myocardial infarct location and stroke [see comments]. J Am Coll Cardiol. 1994;24:61–66.

12. Braunwald E. Heart Disease. Philadelphia, WB Saunders; 1992:1077–1128.

13. Brickner ME, Friedman DB, Cigarroa CG, et al. Relation of thrombus in the left atrial appendage by transesophageal echocardiography to clinical risk factors for thrombus formation. Am J Cardiol. 1994;74:391–393.

14. Burke A. Cardiac myxoma—a clinicopathologic study. Am J Clin Pathol. 1993;100:671–680.

15. Byrd B, Shelton M, Wilson B. Infective perivalvular abscess of the aortic ring: Echocardiographic features and clinical course. Am J Cardiol. 1990;66:102.

16. Calchoo K. Mediastinal teratomas: Review of 15 pediatric cases. J Pediatr Surg. 1993;28:1161.

17. Cerel A, Burger AJ. The diagnosis of a pulmonary artery thrombus by transesophageal echocardiography. Chest. 1993;103:944–945.

18. Chen C, Koschyk D, Hamm C, et al. Usefulness of transesophageal echocardiography in identifying small left ventricular apical thrombus. J Am Coll Cardiol. 1993;21:208–215.

19. Clancy D. The heart in malignant melanoma: A study of 70 autopsies. Am J Cardiol. 1968;21:555.

20. Clancy D. Angiosarcoma of the heart. Am J Cardiol. 1968;21:413.

21. Comess KA, DeRook FA, Beach KW, et al. Transesophageal echocardiography and carotid ultrasound in patients with cerebral ischemia: Prevalence of findings and recurrent stroke risk. J Am Coll Cardiol. 1994;23:1598–1603.

22. Copeland S, Salomon N, Stinson E. Acute mitral obstruction from infective endocarditis. J Thorac Cardiovasc Surg. 1979;78:128.

23. Croft C, Woodward W, Elliot A. Analysis of surgical versus medical therapy in active complicated native valve infective endocarditis. Am J Cardiol. 1985;51:1650.

24. Crowley JJ, Kenny A, Dardas P, et al. Identification of right atrial thrombi using transesophageal echocardiography. Eur Heart J. 1995;16:708–710.

25. Davies M: Tumors of the heart and pericardium. *In* Pomerance A, Davies M (eds): The Pathology of the Heart. Philadelphia, JB Lippincott; 1975:413–439.

26. DePace N. Two-dimensional echocardiographic detection of intra-atrial masses. Am J Cardiol. 1981;48:954.

27. Derumeaux G, Mouton-Schleifer D, Soyer R, et al. High incidence of left atrial thrombus detected by transesophageal echocardiography in heart transplant recipients. Eur Heart J. 1995;16:120–125.

28. d'Ivernois C, Le Metayer P, Fischer B, et al. Life-threatening pulmonary embolism with right-sided heart thrombus. Rapid recovery with recombinant tissue plasminogen activator. Chest. 1994;105:1291–1292.

29. Dong C, Hurley E. Contralateral recurrent myxoma of the heart. Am Thorac Surg. 1976;21:59.

30. Dubrey S, Pollak A, Skinner M, et al. Atrial thrombi occurring during sinus rhythm in cardiac amyloidosis: Evidence for atrial electromechanical dissociation. Br Heart J. 1995;74:541–544.

31. Effert S. The diagnosis of the intra-atrial tumors and thrombi by the ultrasonic echo method. Gen Med Meth. 1959;4:1.

32. Ellis S, Goldstein J, Popp R. Detection of endocarditis—associated perivalvular abscesses by two-dimensional echocardiography. J Am Coll Cardiol. 1985;5:647.

33. Emami B. Heart and blood vessels. *In* Perez (ed): Principles and Practice of Radiation Oncology. Philadelphia, JB Lippincott; 1992;871–877.

34. Enberding R. Diagnosis of heart tumors by transesophageal echocardiography: Multicenter study in 154 patients. Eur Soc Cardiol. 1993;14:1223–1228.

35. Erbel R. Identification of high-risk subgroups in infective endocarditis and the role of echocardiography. Eur Soc Cardiol. 1995;16:588.

36. Fatkin D, Kuchar DL, Thorbum CW, et al. Transesophageal echocardiography before and during direct current cardioversion of atrial fibrillation: Evidence for "atrial stunning" as a mechanism of thromboembolic complications. J Am Coll Cardiol. 1994;23:307–316.

37. Fatkin D, Kelly RP, Feneley MP. Relations between left atrial appendage blood flow velocity; spontaneous echocardiographic contrast and thromboembolic risk in vivo. J Am Coll Cardiol. 1994;23:961–969.

38. Feltes TF, Friedman RA. Transesophageal echocardiographic detection of atrial thrombi in patients with nonfibrillation, atrial tachyarrhythmias and congenital heart disease. J Am Coll Cardiol. 1994;24:1365–1370.

39. Fenoglio J. Cardiac rhabdomyoma: A clinicopathologic and electron microscopic study. Am J Cardiol. 1976;38:241.

40. Glikson M, Agranat O, Ziskind Z, et al. From swirling to a mobile, pedunculated mass—the evolution of left ventricular thrombus despite full anticoagulation. Echocardiographic demonstration. Chest. 1993;103:281–283.

41. Gonzalez-Alujus T, Evangelista-Masip A, Garcia Del Castillo H, et al. Recurring free-floating thrombus in the left atrium in a patient with mitral prosthesis. Chest. 1994;106:303–304.

42. Grimm RA, Stewart WJ, Maloney JD, et al. Impact of electrical cardioversion for atrial fibrillation on left atrial appendage function and spontaneous echo contrast: Characterization by simultaneous transesophageal echocardiography. J Am Coll Cardiol. 1993;22:1359–1366.

43. Habib G, Cornen A, Mesana T, et al. Diagnosis of prosthetic heart valve thrombosis. The respective values of transthoracic and transesophageal Doppler echocardiography. Eur Heart J. 1993;14:447–455.

44. Herrmann M. Primary cardiac angiosarcoma: A clinicopathology study of SID cases. J Thorac Cardiovasc Surg 1992;103:655–664.

45. Herzog C, Houry T, Zimmer S. Bacterial endocarditis presenting as acute myocardial infarction: A cautionary note for the era of reperfusion. Am J Med. 1991;90:392–397.

46. Hoit BD, Shao Y, Gabel M. Influence of acutely altered loading conditions on left atrial appendage flow velocities. J Am Coll Cardiol. 1994;24:117–123.

47. Howamitz E. Pedunculated left ventricular rhabdomyoma. Ann of Thorac Surg. 1986;41:443–445.

48. Hwa J. Primary intravascular cardiac tumors in children: Contemporary diagnostic and management options. Pediatr Cardiol. 1994;15:233–237.

49. Hwang JJ, Kuan P, Chen JJ, et al. Significance of left atrial spontaneous echo contrast in rheumatic mitral valve disease as a predictor of systemic arterial embolization: A transesophageal echocardiographic study. Am Heart J. 1994;127:880–885.

50. Hwang JJ, Shyu KG, Hsu KL, et al. Significant mitral regurgitation is protective against left atrial spontaneous echo contrast formation, but not against systemic embolism. Chest. 1994;106:8–12.

51. Isada LR, Torelli JN, Stewart WJ, et al. Detection of fibrous strands on prosthetic mitral valves with transesophageal echocardiography: Another potential embolic source. J Am Soc Echocardiogr. 1994;7:641–645.

52. Kanemoto N. An adult case of cardiac fibroma. Intern Med. 1994;33:10–12.

53. Karatisakis GT, Gotisis AC, Cokkinos DV. Influence of mitral regurgitation on left atrial thrombus and spontaneous echocardiographic contrast in patients with rheumatic mitral valve disease. Am J Cardiol. 1995;76:279–281.

54. Kobayashi A. Bilocular pericardial cyst diagnosed by magnetic resonance imaging: A case report. Jpn Thorac Surg. 1992;45:1007–1009.

55. Kontny F, Dale J, Hegrenaes L, et al. Left ventricular thrombosis and arterial embolism after thrombolysis in acute anterior myocardial infarction: Predictors and effects of adjunctive antithrombotic therapy. Eur Heart J. 1993;14:1489–1492.

56. Labovitz AJ, Camp A, Castello R, et al. Usefulness of transesophageal echocardiography in unexplained cerebral ischemia. Am J Cardiol. 1993;72:1448–1452.

57. Li Mandri G. Detection of multiple papillary fibroelastomas of the tricuspid valve by transesophageal echocardiography. J Am Soc Echocardiogr. 1994;7:315–317.

58. Luetmer P. Incidence and distribution of left ventricular false tendons: An autopsy study of 483 normal human hearts. J Am Coll Cardiol. 1986;8:179–183.

59. Manning WJ, Silverman DI, Keighley CS, et al. Transesophageal echocardiographically facilitated early cardioversion from atrial fibrillation using short-term anticoagulation: Final results of a prospective 4.5-year study. J Am Coll Cardiol. 1995;25:1354–1361.

60. Manning WJ, Weintraub RM, Waksmonski CA, et al. Accuracy of transesophageal echocardiography for identifying left atrial thrombi. A prospective, intraoperative study. Ann Intern Med. 1995;123:817–822.

61. Markel ML, Armstrong WF, Waller BF. Left atrial myxoma with multicentric recurrence and evidence of metastasis. Am Heart J. 1986;111:409–413.

62. McAllister H. Tumors of the cardiovascular system. *In*: Atlas of Tumor Pathology. Washington, DC, Armed Forces Institute of Pathology; 1978.

63. Mendes LA, Magraw LL, Aldea GS, et al. Right ventricular thrombus: An unusual manifestation of Behcet's disease. J Am Soc Echocardiogr. 1994;7:438–440.

64. Minutello L. Usefulness of echocardiography in the differential diagnosis of a pericardial cyst simulating an aneurysm of the left ventricle. Minerva Cardioangiolo. 1994;42:313.

65. Missault L, Jordaens L, Gheeraert P, et al. Embolic stroke after unanticoagulated cardioversion despite prior exclusion of atrial thrombi by transesophageal echocardiography. Eur Heart J. 1994;15:1279–1280.

66. Mizushige K, DeMaria AN, Toyama Y, et al. Contrast echocardiography for evaluation of left ventricular flow dynamics using desitometric analysis. 1993;88(2):588–595.

67. Moggio R. Primary cardiac tumors. NY State Med J. 1992;49–52.

68. Moreyra E, Finkelhor RS, Cebul RD. Limitations of TEE in the risk assessment of patients before nonanticoagulated cardioversion from atrial fibrillation and flutter: An analysis of pooled trials. Am Heart J. 1995;129:71–75.

69. Mugge A. Echocardiographic detection of cardiac valve vegetations and prognostic implications. Infec Dis Clin of North Am. 1993;7:877–898.

70. Mugge A, Daniel W, Frank G. Echocardiography in infective endocarditis: Reassessment of prognostic implications of vegetation size determined by the transthoracic and transesophageal approach. J Am Coll Cardiol. 1989;14:631.

71. Mugge A, Kuhn H, Nikutta P, et al. Assessment of left atrial appendage function by biplane transesophageal echocardiography in patients with non-rheumatic atrial fibrillation: Identification of a subgroup of patients at increased embolic risk. J Am Coll Cardiol. 1994;23:599–607.

72. Munoz H. Prenatal sonographic findings of a large fetal cardiac fibroma. J Ultrasound Med. 1995;14:479.

73. Norifumi M. Angiosarcoma in Japan. Cancer. 1995;75:989.

74. Omori K. Treatment of pericardial cyst under thoracoscopy. Jpn J Thorac Surg. 1992;45:217.

75. Orsinelli DA, Pasierski TJ, Pearson AC. Spontaneously appearing microbubbles associate with prosthetic cardiac valves detected by transesophageal echocardiography. Am Heart J. 1994;128:990–996.

76. Pankey G. The prevention and treatment of bacterial endocarditis. Am. Heart J. 1979;98:102.

77. Pappo A. Biology and therapy of pediatric rhabdomyosarcoma J Clin Oncol. 1995;13:2123.

78. Parker M. Intracardiac teratoma 15 years after treatment of a non-serinomatous germ cell tumor. J Urol. 1993;150:478.

79. Prichard R. Tumors of the heart: Review of the subject and report of 150 cases. Arch Pathol. 1951;51:98.

80. Rashwan MA, Ayman M, Ashour S, et al. Endomyocardial fibrosis in Egypt: An illustrated review. Br Heart J. 1995;73:284–289.

81. Rechavia E, Imbar S, Bimbaum Y, et al. Protruding left ventricular thrombus formation following blunt chest trauma. Am Heart J. 1993;125:893–896.

82. Reimers C, Van Tosh A, Berger M, et al. Disappearance of a left ventricular aneurysm on radionuclide ventriculography due to formation of a mural thrombus. Chest. 1993;104:946–947.

83. Rettmar K. Primary angiosarcoma of the heart. Japanese Heart J. 1993;34:667–683.

84. Reyes L. Lipoma of the heart. Int Surg. 1976;61:179.

85. Reynen K. Cardiac myxomas. N Engl J Med. 1995;333:1610–1617.

86. Rittoo D, Sutherland GR. Acute pulmonary artery thromboembolism treated with thrombolysis: Diagnostic and monitoring uses of transesophageal echocardiography. Br Heart J. 1993;69:457–459.

87. Roberts W. The heart in acute leukemia: A study of 420 autopsy cases. Am J Cardiol. 1968;21:388.

88. Roberts W. Heart in malignant lymphoma (Hodgkin's disease, lymphosarcoma, reticulum cell sarcoma and mycosis fungoides): A study of 196 autopsy cases. Am J Cardiol. 1968;22:85.

89. Ryan P. Primary cardiac valve tumors. J Heart Valve Dis. 1995;4:222.

90. Sansoy V, Abbott RD, Jayaweera AR, et al. Low yield of transthoracic echocardiography for cardiac source of embolism. Am J Cardiol. 1995;75:166–169.

91. Santiago D, Warshofsky M, Li Mandri G, et al. Left atrial appendage function and thrombus formation in atrial fibrillation-flutter: A transesophageal echocardiographic study. J Am Coll Cardiol. 1994;24:159–164.

92. Schneider B, Hofmann T, Justen MH, et al. Chiari's network: Normal anatomic variant or factor for arterial embolic events? J Am Coll Cardiol. 1995;26:203–210.

93. Scully R. Weekly clinicopathological exercises. N Engl J Med. 1983;308:206.

94. Sethi K. Primary fibrosarcoma of the heart presenting as obstruction at the tricuspid valve: Diagnosis by cross-sectional echocardiography. Int J Cardiol. 1989;24:228–230.

95. Shih W. Diagnostic imaging for primary cardiac fibrosarcoma. Intern J of Cardiol. 1993;39:157–161.

96. Shrivastava S. Fibrosarcoma of the right ventricle—a case report. Int J Cardiol. 1985;9:234.

97. Simons M. Lipomatus hypertrophy of the arterial septum: Diagnosis by combined echocardiography and computerized tomography. Am J Cardiol. 1984;54:465–466.

98. Stafford A. Serial echocardiographic appearance of healing bacterial vegetations. Am J Cardiol. 1979;46:756.

99. Stoddard MF, Dawkins PR, Prince CR, et al. Left atrial appendage thrombus is not uncommon in patients with acute atrial fibrillation and a recent embolic event: A transesophageal echocardiographic study. J Am Coll Cardiol. 1995;25:452–459.

100. Steiner R. Radiologic aspects of cardiac tumors. Am J Cardiol. 1968;21:344.

101. Straus R, Merliss R. Primary tumor of the heart. Arch Pathol. 1945;39:74.

102. Sugita T. Pericardial cyst in the midline position. J Cardiovasc Surg. 1994;35:87.

103. Tarby I. Cavernous hemangioma of the heart: Case report and review of the literature. J Thorac Cardiovasc Surg. 1975;69:415.

104. Tessier P, Mercier LA, Burelle D, et al. Results of percutaneous mitral commissurotomy in patients with a left atrial appendage thrombus detected by transesophageal echocardiography. J Am Soc Echocardiogr. 1994;7:394–399.

105. Tunkel A, Mandell G. Infecting microorganisms. *In* Kay D (ed): Infective Endocarditis. New York, Raven Press; 1992:85–97.

106. Turnick P, Lefkow P, Kronzon I. Aorta to right atrium fistula caused by endocarditis: Diagnosis by color Doppler echocardiography. J Am Soc Echocardiogr. 1989;2:53.

107. Utley J, Mills J. Annular erosion and pericarditis. J Thorac Cardiovasc Surg. 1972;64:76.

108. Van Dantizig JM, Delemarre BJ, Bot H, et al. Doppler left ventricular flow pattern versus conventional predictors of left ventricular thrombus after acute myocardial infarction. J Am Coll Cardiol. 1995;25:1341–1346.

109. Vered Z. Prevalence and significance of false tendons in the left ventricle as determined by echocardiography. Am J Cardiol. 1989;53:330.

110. Wanishsawad C, Weathers LB, Puavilai W. Mitral regurgitation and left atrial thrombus in rheumatic mitral valve disease. A clinicopathologic study. Chest. 1995;108:677–681.

111. Werner A, Cobbs G, Kaye D. Studies on the bacteremia of bacterial endocarditis. JAMA. 1967;202:127.

112. Werner J, Cheitlin M, Gross B. Echocardiographic appearance of the chiari network: Differentiation from right-heart pathology. Circulation. 1981;63:1104.

113. Wyman AF. Principles and Practice of Echocardiography. Philadelphia, Lea & Febiger; 1994:1178.

114. Yansuoto S. Case report of pericardial diverticulum in the upper mediastinum: Surgical treatment in 2 cases. Jpn J Thorac Surg. 1994;48:242.

PART IX

Pericardial Disease

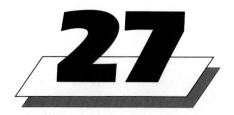

27

Echocardiographic Evaluation of Pericardial Disease

ALAN D. WAGGONER and CHRIS M. BAUMANN

Introduction

It has been 30 years since Feigenbaum et al. described the application of M-mode echocardiography in patients with pericardial effusion.[17] Our understanding of the utility of echocardiography in the diagnosis of pericardial effusion and tamponade has been expanded further with two-dimensional imaging.[4,11,12,14,16,22,26,35,46] Pulsed wave Doppler velocity recordings across the cardiac valves and hepatic and pulmonary veins are valuable in assessing alterations in ventricular filling that commonly occur in pericardial disease processes.[3,5,23,33,38,53] This chapter will review the applications of echocardiography in patients with pericardial disorders.

ANATOMY AND PHYSIOLOGY

The pericardium is a stiff, fibrous membrane with two layers, parietal (outer) and visceral (epicardial). The space between these layers normally contains a small amount (20 ml) of lymphatic fluid to decrease friction during cardiac contraction. The pericardium extends around the heart, encompassing the ventricular chambers, but terminates posteriorly at the atrial level and at the insertions of the pulmonary veins and vena cava. Superiorly, the pericardium is attached at the level of the great vessels just above the semilunar valve plane. When fluid accumulates in the pericardial space, it can be recognized initially in the posterior basal region. Further increases in the amount of fluid occur medially and laterally and involve the apex.

The mechanical function of the pericardium has been studied extensively.[60,61] One of its roles is to limit overdistention of the cardiac chambers with diastolic filling of the ventricles, more so in the right ventricle than in the left. The pericardium also acts to distribute diastolic pressures evenly in the chambers and may serve as a barrier to infection from an extracardiac source. Normal pressure in the pericardial space is subatmospheric, approximately the same as intrapleural pressure, and varies from -5 to $+5$ mm Hg. An important concept to understand is pericardial pressure. Although normally low, it is a determining factor in the transmural distending pressure (i.e., differences between intracardiac and intrapericardial pressure in millimeters of mercury). When changes occur in the diastolic ventricular size or pressure (of either chamber), there are resulting alterations in intrapericardial pressure. Abnormalities in the pericardial membrane (i.e., fibrosis or thickening) or increases in intrapericardial volume lead to increased intrapericardial pressure and a decrease in the transmural pressure gradient.

489

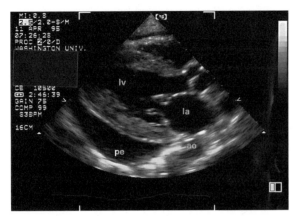

Figure 27-1. Parasternal long axis view with evidence of a moderate pericardial effusion (pe), primarily in the posterior portion of the heart. la, left atrium; ao, aorta; lv, left ventricle.

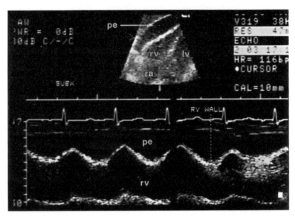

Figure 27-3. Subcostal four-chamber view with M-mode of a large pericardial effusion and RV diastolic collapse. pe, pericardial effusion; rv, right ventricle; ra, right atrium; lv, left ventricle.

THE ECHOCARDIOGRAPHIC EXAMINATION

A standard M-mode and two-dimensional study should include all possible views. Since pericardial fluid accumulates initially in the posterior portion of the heart, the parasternal long axis view is the most helpful one to identify pericardial effusion (Fig. 27-1). Most often, pericardial effusion is relatively echolucent, and a echo-free space is evident between the epicardium and parietal pericardium. When effusion is detected, the presence of intrapericardial densities or a pericardial mass should be sought, particularly when the patient has a malignancy. Serial short

axis views from apex to base should be obtained to determine the lateral and anterior extent of the effusion, its medial extension, and the possible presence of loculation (Fig. 27-2). M-mode in this view may be useful for timing right ventricular wall motion relative to mitral valve opening if diastolic collapse of the right ventricle is suspected (Fig. 27-3).

The apical views (four-chamber, two-chamber, long axis) are useful for determining the presence of effusion at the apex, evidence of chamber (left or right) collapse, and right ventricular size (Fig. 27-4). Our approach also entails the use of pulsed wave Doppler at the mitral and tricuspid leaflet tips

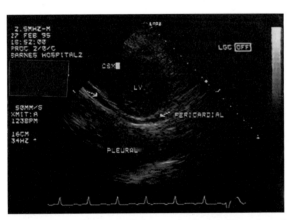

Figure 27-2. Parasternal short axis view (with reduced image gain) of a small pericardial effusion in the posterior aspect of the heart (arrows). LV, left ventricle; CSX, cross-section.

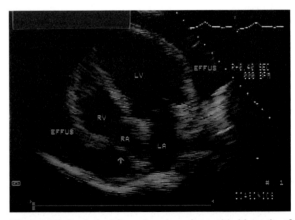

Figure 27-4. Apical four-chamber view with M-mode of a large pericardial effusion (EFFUS) and RA notching (arrow). RA, right atrium; RV, right ventricle; LA, left atrium; LV, left ventricle.

in the four-chamber view for flow velocities at early diastole (E) and atrial systole (A), as well as for measurement of deceleration time. Recording the Doppler signals at the slow speed of 25 mm/sec is helpful to detect evidence of respiratory variation. A nasal thermistor is very useful to record the respiratory cycle when a constrictive pericardial process is suspected. Pulmonary venous flow should be obtained in this situation as well.

The subcostal view provides information regarding the presence of pericardial fluid surrounding the right ventricle (RV). This view is important because the success of a subxiphoid approach in performing pericardiocentesis usually requires evidence of effusion over the right ventricular free wall and apex. The inferior vena should be examined for collapsibility, and pulsed Doppler in the left hepatic vein is required if constrictive pericarditis is suspected.

PERICARDITIS, PERICARDIAL EFFUSION, AND PLEURAL EFFUSION

Inflammation of the pericardium (pericarditis) can be caused by a variety of conditions, including viral syndromes, uremia, trauma, infection, metastatic invasion from malignancies, systemic diseases, congestive heart failure, acute myocardial infarction, chest radiation, or unknown causes (idiopathic). The clinical presentation of pericarditis usually consists of chest pain, fever, and diffuse ST-segment elevation recorded on a 12-lead electrocardiogram; a friction rub may be heard by auscultation. Pericardial effusion may occur as a consequence of pericarditis or in the absence of the typically clinical features (idiopathic). The normal fluid within the pericardium is serosanguineous (clear to straw-colored), originating from the subepicardial lymphatic system.[61] Increases in pericardial fluid result from interference with lymphatic drainage, such as in congestive heart failure, myxedema, or uremia. Hemopericardium may be a cause of effusion, as seen in trauma, acute myocardial infarction, neoplasm or malignancy, or aortic dissection. A "milky" effusion (chylopericardium) is a rare condition due to injury or obstruction of the thoracic duct.

CLINICAL SIGNS OF PERICARDIAL EFFUSION

Physical signs of pericardial effusion are related to the rapidity of accumulation and the resultant he-

modynamic consequences (Table 27-1). Jugular venous distention can occur as venous pressures become elevated due to increasing pericardial effusion and, with inspiration, may become more distended (Kussmaul's sign). There may also be "distant" heart sounds, the apical impulse may be difficult to palpate, and an inspiratory decrease in the systolic blood pressure below 10 mm Hg (pulsus paradoxus) can occur with a large pericardial effusion. The electrocardiogram may disclose low voltage or electrical alterans due to the swinging of the heart in larger effusions. The chest x-ray reveals an enlarged cardiac silhouette with a "water bottle" shape heart but clear lung fields. It is important to note that some physical signs may not be seen in all patients even when the pericardial effusion is large. Other conditions, such as cardiomyopathy with congestive heart failure, myxedema, or emphysema, can also result in physical signs of distant heart sounds, jugular venous distention, cardiomegaly, or pulsus paradoxus.

ECHOCARDIOGRAPHIC FINDINGS

M-mode, and particularly two-dimensional imaging, are the best techniques to detect pericardial effusion. The accumulation of fluid between the visceral and parietal pericardiums enlarges the pericardial space, providing recognition of the epicardial and pericardial echoes as distinctly separate and creating an echo-free space. Small effusions (<100 ml) are localized posteriorly or at the gravity-dependent regions of the heart. Moderate-sized effusions (100–500 ml) tend to extend the echo-free space laterally to the apical region and anteriorly between the RV wall and sternum, as viewed in the parasternal approach, or posterior to the diaphragm when viewed from a subcostal approach. Large effusions (>500 ml) extend posteriorly and lead to greater increases in the echo-free space in other areas. Swinging of the heart may be observed with distortion in the timing of ventricular wall motion and valvular motion. There is no accurate method to quantitate the volume of pericardial effusion, and generally its extent can be described in the terms outlined above.[64] Also, the type of pericardial fluid cannot be ascertained from the echocardiographic appearance of the echo-free space, although clotted blood from hemopericardium may be identified in some patients and fibrinous material may be evident in purulent pericarditis.

TABLE 27-1. CLINICAL AND ECHOCARDIOGRAPHIC SIGNS OF CONSTRICTIVE AND RESTRICTIVE CARDIOMYOPATHY

	Clinical Findings	Symptoms	M-Mode/2-D	Doppler
CONSTRICTIVE PERICARDITIS	Possible Kussmaul's sign Low-voltage ECG Atrial fibrillation Pleural effusion Pericardial knock Hepatomegaly Ascites Edema	Dypsnea on exertion Fatigue Orthopnea Cough Abdominal swelling	Normal LV/RV systolic function No LV hypertrophy Pericardial effusion Epicardial-pericardial tracking Thickened pericardium Flat LV posterior wall motion in mid to late diastole Abnormal septal motion Early pulmonary valve opening	Reciprocal changes in MV and TV flow velocities with inspiration, expiration Pulmonary and hepatic venous flow velocity respiratory variation Rapid early LV filling Normal TR jet velocity
RESTRICTIVE CARDIOMYOPATHY	Biventricular heart failure Low-voltage ECG Atrial fibrillation No pericardial knock Possible Kussmaul's sign Hepatosplenomegaly Ascites Edema	Dyspnea Palpitations Syncope Exercise intolerance Weakness Edema	LV and RV hypertrophy Low normal or impaired systolic function Decreased LV compliance Biatrial enlargement Normal pericardial thickness Atrial septal hypertrophy	Increased TR jet velocity Diastolic MR/TR Prolongued LV early diastolic filling Little or no respiratory variation in MVE or IVRT

Abbreviations: ECG, electrocardiogram; IVRT, isovolumic relaxation time; LV, left ventricle; MR, mitral regurgitation; MV, mitral valve; MVE, mitral wave E wave velocity; RV, right ventricle; TR, tricuspid regurgitation.

Careful attention to ultrasound system settings such as depth, gain, or transmit power levels is critical in identifying the echo-free space separating the parietal and visceral pericardiums. M-mode echocardiography may be useful to determine the timing of ventricular wall motion relative to the electrocardiogram or atrioventricular valve opening to diagnose diastolic chamber collapse. However, in cases of loculated effusion or when pericardial fluid extends behind the atrial wall, relying only on M-mode may be confusing or the effusion may be completely missed. Therefore, two-dimensional imaging is the preferred method to detect pericardial effusion, with its ability to use multiple imaging planes. When possible, it may be useful to have the patient assume an upright position to note the shift in fluid toward the apex in moderate or large effusions since loculated effusions may not show this change.

In a large study of patients who presented with primary acute pericardial disease, two-dimensional echocardiography revealed many cases of pericardial effusion. Clinically, nearly all of these patients had idiopathic pericarditis.[54] Less commonly observed were pericardial processes of a tuberculous etiology, neoplastic pericarditis, or bacterial (purulent) or viral pericarditis. An important finding in this study was the prevalence of large pericardial effusions and cardiac tamponade in the patients with neoplastic, tuberculous, or infectious etiologies. Nearly all of these patients had pericardial effusion, and a majority had cardiac tamponade. In contrast, only half of the patients with idiopathic or viral pericarditis had pericardial effusion and infrequently developed tamponade. Although hemopericardium is usually a sign of neoplastic involvement, this was observed in some patients with idiopathic pericarditis during pericardiocentesis.

Two-dimensional echocardiographic studies in patients with pericardiotomy syndrome after cardiac surgery found that a majority develop pericardial effusion. In many of these patients, small pericardial effusions develop in the early days following surgery, but they resolve over several weeks. Cardiac tamponade may develop but is rare,[67,77] and frequently these patients are noted to have excessive bloody chest tube drainage. There is often no correlation between the presence of effusion and a friction rub or chest pain.

Rarely, infectious or purulent pericarditis may

be suspected when two-dimensional evidence of pericardial effusion and fibrinous exudate exists within the pericardial space or attached to epicardial surface (Fig. 27-5). This may be seen in a patient with fever, bacteremia, and chest pain, particularly if chest trauma exists or surgery was performed.

It is not uncommon to encounter patients referred for echocardiography to rule out pericardial effusion who also have evidence of left pleural effusion. This often occurs in cases of metastatic carcinoma of the breast or lung. Careful attention to the position of the thoracic aorta in the parasternal long axis view should provide clear recognition of the echo-free space as pericardial or pleural (Fig. 27-6). Left pleural effusions are posterior or inferior to the thoracic aorta; pericardial effusion is anterior to the thoracic aorta and often tapers toward the left atrial wall. Within the pleural effusion there can be fibrinous strands or atelectasis of the left lower lobe of the lung. In some instances, these echo densities can be attached to the pericardium and mistaken for a tumor. In most patients with left pleural effusion, the sonographer can use a left subscapular approach (from the back) to view the heart in two different imaging planes. This can be useful for visualization of the posterior parietal pericardium and the pericardial space (Fig. 27-7). In our experience, these retrocardiac images are extremely useful to detect intrapericardial echo densities (i.e., clot, fibrin strands) and to measure the parietal pericardial

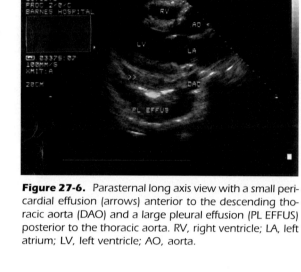

Figure 27-6. Parasternal long axis view with a small pericardial effusion (arrows) anterior to the descending thoracic aorta (DAO) and a large pleural effusion (PL EFFUS) posterior to the thoracic aorta. RV, right ventricle; LA, left atrium; LV, left ventricle; AO, aorta.

thickness. They can often be best employed when the patient is sitting upright.

INTRAPERICARDIAL ECHO DENSITIES AND PERICARDIAL THICKENING/CALCIFICATION

The presence of intrapericardial echoes that appear as thin strands attached to the epicardial surface and extending to the parietal pericardium is not unusual in patients with pericardial effusion (Fig. 27-8). They are composed of fibrin and can be seen in

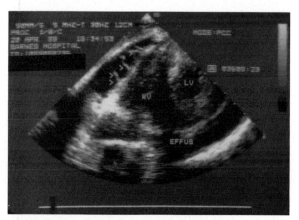

Figure 27-5. Transesophageal echocardiographic transgastric short axis view of pericardial effusion (EFFUS) with fibrinous exudate within the effusion (arrows). RV, right ventricle; LV, left ventricle.

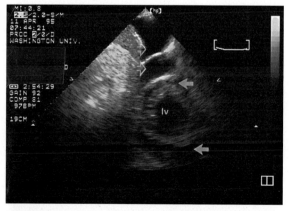

Figure 27-7. Left subscapular approach (from the back) through a moderate-sized left pleural effusion (open arrows) in a cross-sectional plane to visualize a small pericardial effusion (closed arrows). lv, left ventricle.

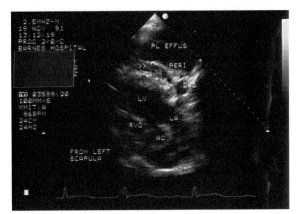

Figure 27-8. Left subscapular approach employing a long axis view with fibrinous strands within the pericardial effusion (arrows), clearly seen between the visceral and parietal layers of the pericardium. RVO, right ventricular outflow; LA, left atrium; LV, left ventricle; AO, aorta; DAO, descending thoracic aorta; PERI, pericardium; PL EFFUS, pleural effusion.

a variety of conditions, usually in association with hemopericardium. Initially, they were thought to be a precursor of a constrictive process and the development of pericardial thickening or calcification.[66] This has not been evident in the authors' experience; more often, these intrapericardial echoes are seen in patients with chronic effusions. They may also be seen as early as 48 hr after cardiac surgery.

Other uncommon causes of intrapericardial echo densities are pericardial cysts or tumors (primary or secondary). Pericardial cysts are rare and can be due to venous remnants of a left superior vena cava that does not regress during fetal growth. Pericardial tumors more often are metastatic (breast or lung) or lymphomas involving the pericardium in a diffuse manner. Primary tumors appear as a solid mass of echoes and can be due to mesothelioma, sarcoma, teratoma, fibroma, lipoma, or angioma.

Calcification or thickening of the pericardium is difficult to detect with echocardiography either anteriorly, due to the chest wall artifact, or posteriorly, due to attenuation and far-field resolution. Most cases are better diagnosed with computed tomography or magnetic resonance imaging.[75] Real-time visualization of "tracking" of the epicardial–pericardial interface may suggest a constrictive process, particularly in association with pericardial thickening. However, this conclusion may be only inferential. Also, increased pericardial thickness may not always result in a constrictive process.[9] The difficulties of recognizing increased pericardial thickness are compounded by the presence of epicardial fat distributed on the surface of the heart. This feature is common in the older obese patient and is generally seen on the anterior surface of the heart. The subcostal four-chamber view probably best displays this finding. The differentiation of fat from fluid can usually be done by location and echo density.

CARDIAC TAMPONADE

The use of two dimensional-Doppler echocardiography for diagnosis of cardiac tamponade requires an understanding of the hemodynamics in patients with this condition. As noted previously, intrapericardial pressure is lower than intracardiac pressure. However, increases in intrapericardial volume (i.e., due to fluid or blood) will lead to increased pericardial pressure. It is not necessarily the amount of effusion but rather the acuity or rate at which fluid accumulates that is important since the parietal pericardium is not a compliant membrane.

The pattern of cardiac tamponade differs in medical patients compared to those with penetrating cardiac injury; in the latter patients, accumulation of blood in the pericardial space is rapid.[2,24] Medical patients often have increased jugular venous pressure and pulsus paradoxus, though not all are hypotensive. Nearly one-third of patients with cardiac tamponade have a malignancy. Patients with large pericardial effusions can have elevated right atrial pressures (average, 14 mm Hg) and right ventricular end-diastolic pressures (>7 mm Hg) that are equal to intrapericardial pressure.[61] Pulmonary capillary wedge pressures and left ventricular end-diastolic pressures are also increased, with large amounts of pericardial fluid. When left heart diastolic pressures equal RV diastolic pressures, pulsus paradoxus occurs. If intracardiac volumes are maintained, such as occurs with intravenous volume loading, then no reduction in stroke volume occurs. However, any additional increase in pericardial pressure ultimately results in diminished cardiac filling and hence reduced chamber volumes, with a resultant decrease in stroke volume. It is common to observe increases in heart rate to maintain forward cardiac output in this situation.

Patients with left ventricular (LV) dysfunction and elevated LV diastolic pressures in the presence of cardiac tamponade have elevated right heart diastolic pressures and impaired right heart filling. However, the left-sided diastolic pressures do not equilibrate with intrapericardial pressure (even if markedly increased), and thus no pulsus paradoxus occurs in these patients despite significant hemodynamic compromise. This phenomenon also can be seen in patients with high right-sided intracardiac pressures (i.e., severe pulmonary hypertension with RV systolic dysfunction) in whom intrapericardial pressures may be extremely high but still do not equalize to the elevated RV end-diastolic pressure.[35]

Regional cardiac tamponade can occur and most often is seen in the post–cardiac surgery patient.[18] Compression of the right atrial (RA) or left atrial (LA) chamber alone by pericardial effusion can lead to hemodynamic derangement[39] since the atrial contribution to ventricular filling can be as much as 20%. Thus, the resultant impairment in atrial filling can produce a reduction in cardiac output. Generally, compression of both ventricles has a greater effect than tamponade confined to either right or left ventricle alone.[19] Regional tamponade affecting the right heart, however, tends to have a greater effect on cardiac output than tamponade affecting the left heart. As expected, the maximal hemodynamic effect of cardiac tamponade is containment of the entire heart by effusion.[19] Figure 27-9 is an example of regional cardiac tamponade.

The increase in intrapericardial pressures due to accumulating effusion will ultimately exceed intracardiac pressures and lead to chamber collapse during diastole (Fig. 27-10). This can be seen more often in right-sided chambers due to the relative thinness of the wall of the LA. Two-dimensional echocardiographic signs of early diastolic collapse of the RV wall can be seen in patients with clinical evidence of tamponade.[4] However, there are cases of RV diastolic collapse without clinical signs of tamponade. The effects of tamponade on RV wall motion have been studied in the canine model.[39] Early diastolic collapse of the RV is always associated with clinical evidence of cardiac tamponade and decreased cardiac output. When RV diastolic and systolic pressures are increased by pulmonary arterial constriction, RV diastolic collapse does not occur. These studies[4,22] and others[62] suggest that RV diastolic collapse occurs when intrapericardial pressures exceed RV diastolic pressures and result in decreased cardiac output, although arterial pressure may not fall (i.e., hypotension).

Late diastolic inversion of the RA free wall can be seen in patients with large pericardial effusions.[22] These patients may or may not have tamponade by clinical parameters, but prolonged inversion of the RA during diastole is associated with increased specificity. Diastolic collapse of the LV can be seen in postoperative cardiac surgery patients with clinical evidence of tamponade.[11,12,36,66] However, this rarely occurs due to the fact the LV wall thickness

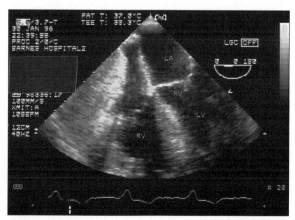

Figure 27-9. *Regional tamponade of the right atrium due to intrapericardial clot detected by transesophageal echocardiography. There is right atrial compression in the four-chamber view. RA, right atrium; RV, right ventricle; LA, left atrium; LV, left ventricle; MV, mitral valve.*

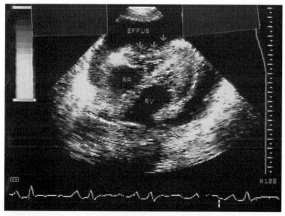

Figure 27-10. *Transthoracic subcostal four-chamber view demonstrating RV diastolic collapse (arrows). EFFUS, pericardial effusion; RA, right atrium; RV, right ventricle.*

is greater than RA or RV wall thickness. Thus, diastolic collapse can occur in any of the cardiac chambers, as it is related to equalization or increase in intrapericardial pressures relative to pressures within the chambers. RV or RA collapse in the presence of pericardial effusion may be influenced by changes in LV or RV preload or afterload[35] and may explain the false positives seen in some studies.[4,22] Also, RA compression may occur in patients with an intrapericardial hematoma[20] and may be mistaken for RA inversion.

Doppler echocardiography can be employed for assessment of cardiac tamponade. Pandian et al. first described exaggerated respiratory variation in the peak flow velocities across the cardiac valves in animals with experimental tamponade.[53] A marked inspiratory increase (>110%) in right-sided valvular velocities was noted, while corresponding left-sided valvular velocities decreased at least 40%. The use of Doppler-derived time-velocity integrals (TVI) obtained at each of the cardiac valves in patients with clinical tamponade revealed similar results.[38] Relief of cardiac tamponade produced near-normalization of the respiratory variation in the TVI. The mitral E/A velocity ratio decreases during inspiration, due mainly to the decrease in early diastolic filling. A small increase in atrial filling velocities is observed in this setting. These Doppler findings may be seen in patients with large effusions and is similar to patients with tamponade[3]; however, there is marked respiratory prolongation of the isovolumic relaxation time when clinical evidence of tamponade is present. Thus, pulsed Doppler combined with two-dimensional echocardiography may be more sensitive and specific than two-dimensional echocardiography alone in detecting tamponade. The patient's intravascular volume status may influence Doppler findings, just as it does two-dimensional echocardiographic findings. When performing pulsed Doppler to identify respiratory variation in flow velocities, it is useful to slow the monitor sweep rate to 25 mm/sec (Fig. 27-11). It should be recognized that respiratory variation in pulsed Doppler–determined flow velocities across the cardiac valves is not specific to cardiac tamponade; it can also be seen in patients with constrictive pericarditis. However, these patients generally do not have large pericardial effusions.

The presence of respiratory variation in Doppler flow velocities can be influenced by technical dif-

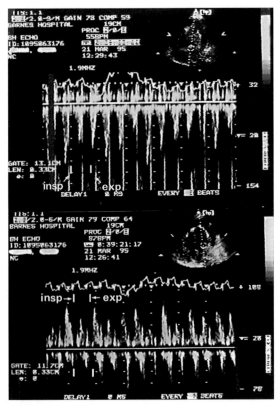

Figure 27-11. Pulsed wave Doppler of the left ventricular outflow tract (upper figure) and mitral valve inflows (lower figure) at a speed of 25 mm/sec obtained from the apical four-chamber view. Note that there is respiratory variation of flow velocities indicative of cardiac tamponade. insp, inspiration; exp, expiration.

ficulties when encountering a swinging heart in the setting of a large effusion. As one can appreciate, positioning a fixed pulsed Doppler sample volume site can be difficult in these patients. Another consideration when evaluating the patient is the pretest likelihood of tamponade based on clinical presentation and history. When the pretest probability is high, two-dimensional echocardiography nearly always shows tamponade. But when the pretest probability is low, two-dimensional echocardiography may also disclose signs of tamponade (i.e., RA inversion) suggesting a false-positive result.[14] These patients need to be carefully monitored, as they may have impending tamponade.[40] The sonographer needs to recognize that there is a continuum of hemodynamic changes that is usually related to the size of the effusion and the loading conditions.[58]

ECHOCARDIOGRAPHICALLY GUIDED PERICARDIOCENTESIS

Echocardiographic evidence of cardiac tamponade often necessitates pericardiocentesis or surgical creation of a pericardial window. Pericardiocentesis is often performed blindly or by an electrocardiographic monitoring lead attached to the pericardial needle. Blind pericardiocentesis can potentially lead to complications such as RV or RA laceration.[24] In acute tamponade secondary to trauma, this may be the method of choice if two-dimensional echocardiography is not immediately available. In stable patients, pericardiocentesis may be done in conjunction with right-sided cardiac catheterization and fluoroscopy.[56] This method allows measurement of intrapericardial and right-sided intracardiac pressures prior to and after the removal of the effusion to document relief of tamponade physiology. After successful needle placement, a catheter with multiple side holes is positioned in the effusion. Fluid is withdrawn with a large syringe connected to a three-way stopcock, with the other port connected to a closed drainage bag. The stopcock port can also be connected to a fluid-filled pressure transducer to measure intrapericardial pressure during pericardiocentesis.

An alternative method reported by some investigators,[7,10,51] and used in our institution, involves simultaneous two-dimensional echocardiography during pericardiocentesis. If a subxiphoid approach is used for needle placement, two-dimensional imaging is performed at another location (apical or parasternal). Two-dimensional visualization of pericardial needle placement may be possible, although it may not be seen in all patients. Agitated saline contrast injections through the pericardial needle can be used to verify needle position within the pericardial sac.[10] Continuous two-dimensional imaging from an apical four-chamber view and injection (5 ml) of agitated saline through the pericardial needle verifies the proper position of the needle in the pericardial space (Fig. 27-12).

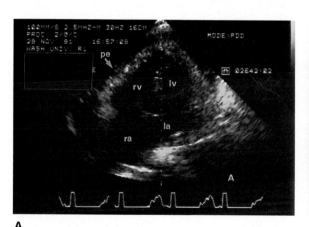

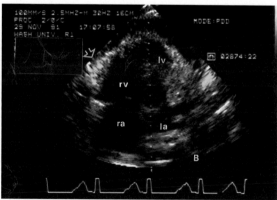

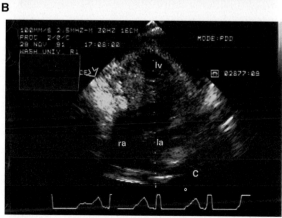

Figure 27-12. Series of apical four-chamber views before (**A**) and after injection of agitated saline contrast into the pericardial space (pe). The echodense area near the RV is a contrast effect (open arrows) moving in the pericardial effusion indicating the proper position of the pericardial needle (**B**), **C**). ra, right atrium; rv, right ventricle; la, left atrium; lv, left ventricle.

Two-dimensional echocardiographically guided pericardiocentesis (without saline contrast) has been used to determine the optimal pericardiocentesis puncture site based on the imaged effusion closest to the transducer position and may be either subcostal or in the chest.[7] There are rare complications, including pneumothorax, pneumopericardium, and ventricular puncture without sequelae. Thus, two-dimensional imaging, preferably with agitated saline contrast injections, should be done in conjunction with pericardiocentesis to decrease the complications associated with the procedure (particularly puncture of the atria or ventricles).

CONSTRICTIVE PERICARDITIS

In constrictive pericarditis, the patient may have exertional dyspnea and elevated jugular venous pressures but a normal heart size and clear lung fields.[43] A differential diagnosis of some form of restrictive cardiomyopathy must always be considered. Infections of the pericardium such as tuberculosis or viruses may be followed by an increase in pericardial thickness. Constriction may occur following cardiac surgery or cardiac trauma. Other possible etiologies are direct chest radiation therapy, collagen vascular disease, uremia, and neoplastic diseases (particular of the breast and lung).[44] Physical signs of cardiac constriction include distended neck veins with Kussmaul's sign and hepatomegaly, often with ascites and lower extremity edema. Often, no cardiac murmurs can be heard, although a pericardial "knock" may sometimes be present. However, these signs may not be present, and thus may make it difficult to distinguish a myocardial process from a primary pericardial process.[49] The 12-lead electrocardiogram will often show low voltage and atrial fibrillation. The chest x-ray may reveal a normal heart size or mild cardiomegaly due to the presence of pericardial fluid. In 40–50% of these patients, calcification of the pericardium can be demonstrated.[49] Cardiac catheterization is usually definitive and discloses equalization of diastolic pressures in the right heart and pulmonary capillary wedge position,[61] with an early diastolic dip and a plateau of the RV pressure tracings. Cardiac output is often within normal limits.

M-mode echocardiographic studies have demonstrated several key features of constrictive pericarditis,[76] including a thickened pericardium appearing as dense, parallel moving echoes; flat motion of the LV posterior wall during early diastole and through end diastole; abnormalities in septal motion; and premature pulmonary valve opening (Fig. 27-13). Though these signs are not specific,[9] they are important initial findings as possible indications of pericardial constriction.

Two-dimensional echocardiography may reveal pericardial effusion that often accompanies constrictive pericarditis.[41] Pericardial thickness, however, cannot be measured reliably, and overestimation is common with two-dimensional echocardiography.[52] Another acoustic window for measurement of posterior parietal thickness and visualization of pericardial tracking can be accomplished by imaging from the back, using a left subscapular plane in patients with left pleural effusion.[74] Several two-dimensional echocardiographic signs of constriction include early diastolic septal motion abnormalities and inferior vena cava plethora (lack of respiratory collapse and pericardial adhesions). These abnormalities have sensitivity of 62% and 79%, respectively, with a specificity of 93% and 80%, respectively, in patients with pericardial constriction.[27] Also, bright pericardial echoes have been described, with the parietal pericardium tracking LV epicardial motion during cardiac systole. Computed tomography or magnetic resonance imaging may be of value to visualize increased pericardial thickness, which is often >5 mm.[27,29,47,59,65,68]

Since constrictive pericarditis results in abnormalities of ventricular filling, Doppler echocardiography should be used to measure diastolic filling

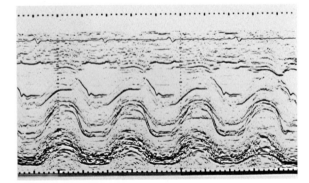

Figure 27-13. M-mode of the LV in a patient with constrictive pericarditis. The relaxation of the posterior wall in early diastole is abrupt (open arrow), with flat motion during mid and late diastole (closed arrow).

velocities across the mitral and tricuspid valves and in the pulmonary veins. The Doppler study will reveal distinctive variations in flow velocities, particularly during the respiratory cycle.[1,6,24,30,32,33,48,50,73] Hemodynamic findings of constriction alter the early mitral inflow characteristics, revealing increases in E velocities and shortened early diastolic deceleration times compared to controls (1.1 vs. 0.6 m/sec and 143 vs. 196 m/sec, respectively).[1] Marked changes in LV isovolumic relaxation times with respiration are also evident in constriction. Isovolumic relaxation times, along with early mitral and tricuspid flow velocities, vary between inspiration and expiration >25% from baseline.[25] The greatest changes are observed on the first beats of respiratory inspiration and expiration. These inspiratory changes in diastolic flow are manifested by a decrease in mitral E velocity, while tricuspid E velocity increases during inspiration. Since most ventricular filling occurs abruptly, mitral and tricuspid flow velocity deceleration times are usually shortened, and both mitral and tricuspid A wave velocities are decreased (Fig. 27-14). Venous flow velocity patterns are often abnormal in constrictive pericarditis. Left hepatic vein flow velocity patterns have been described as a W-shaped configuration, and abrupt reversal of flow late in systole and diastole.[73] Superior vena cava flow velocities are also abnormal in patients with constriction.[6] Pulmonary venous flow decreases in systolic and diastolic flow on inspiration and increases in diastolic flow during expiration.[33]

TRANSESOPHAGEAL ECHOCARDIOGRAPHY

Transesophageal echocardiography (TEE) has a potential role in patients with pericardial diseases. Studies comparing transthoracic echocardiography and TEE in the detection of pericardial thickening, pericardial metastases, or intrapericardial clot revealed that in each instance TEE was better, particularly in detecting intrapericardial clot.[62] TEE defines patients with increased pericardial thickness and constrictive processes more clearly than standard two-dimensional echocardiography. Comparisons of TEE-measured pericardial thickness to computer tomography or magnetic resonance imaging have been recently evaluated. These studies show that TEE had better sensitivity and specificity than computed tomography in distinguishing pericardial thickening.[42] The four-chamber and basal short axis planes are the best views to use, with measurements made at two different sites.[42] Pericardial thickness measures by TEE and magnetic resonance imaging agree closely in most patients with constrictive or effusive-constrictive pericarditis.[34]

ROLE OF DOPPLER AFTER PERICARDIECTOMY

Recent reports have described the use of two-dimensional Doppler echocardiography before and after pericardiectomy for constrictive pericarditis.[50,70] They have shown that the sensitivity of

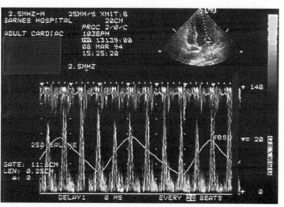

A   **B**

Figure 27-14. **(A)** Pulsed wave Doppler of mitral inflow velocity from the apical four-chamber view. The reduced deceleration time (dt) of 145 msec (0.145 sec) with increased early diastolic velocity and reduced atrial filling velocity (open arrow) are consistent with constrictive pericarditis. **(B)** Respiratory variation of the mitral inflow velocities on inspiration—upstroke of the respirometer tracing (resp).

Doppler is 88% in identifying patients with constrictive pericarditis. After pericardiectomy there is normalization of echocardiographic findings in most patients; some may continue to have restrictive mitral inflow patterns by Doppler (increased E wave, shortened deceleration time) but without respiratory variation.[50] These patients may continue to have symptoms of congestive heart failure. However, no preoperative Doppler parameters could be identified that predicted the postoperative response.[70]

CONSTRICTIVE PERICARDITIS AND RESTRICTIVE CARDIOMYOPATHY

Two-dimensional Doppler echocardiography can distinguish between constrictive pericarditis and restrictive cardiomyopathy. These conditions have similar clinical features and hemodynamic criteria but may not always be specific to a certain patient.[71] However, each condition can be best characterized by detection of abnormalities in ventricular filling. In constrictive pericarditis, nearly all diastolic filling is achieved in the first 50% of diastole and the atrial contribution is small. Ventricular filling in restrictive cardiomyopathy is prolonged throughout diastole, and the atrial contribution is greater unless there is significant LV systolic dysfunction. Also, the time to peak filling is usually shorter in constrictive pericarditis than in restrictive cardiomyopathy. Table 27-1 summarizes the clinical and echocardiographic findings.

Digitized M-mode[31] and, more recently, pulsed Doppler[25] echocardiography[57] or transesophageal have been used to help distinguish between the two conditions. Respiratory variation in isovolumic relaxation time greater than 30% between inspiration and expiration and >20% change in mitral E velocity[25] are more often seen in constriction. Increases in isovolumic relaxation time and decreases in mitral E velocity can also be observed at the beginning of inspiration, with the opposite response occurring at the beginning of expiration. Conversely, diastolic mitral or tricuspid regurgitation may be seen in restrictive cardiomyopathy but not in constrictive pericarditis. Patients with constriction and evidence of tricuspid regurgitation also generally have lower systolic jet velocities than those with restrictive cardiomyopathy since pulmonary hypertension is not common in these patients. The key finding is evidence of respiratory variation in pulmonary venous flow in patients with constriction, which is not present in restrictive cardiomyopathy.[57] Generally, patients with constrictive pericarditis have normal biventricular systolic function and ventricular wall thickness, while those with restrictive cardiomyopathy may have low normal or impaired systolic function with combined LV and RV hypertrophy.

CONGENITAL ABSENCE OF THE PERICARDIUM

This is a rare abnormality in which the left pericardium is absent, either partially or, less often, totally. Patients may have symptoms of chest pain and an abnormal chest x-ray that shows a prominent pulmonary artery and a unusual left heart border. Two-dimensional echocardiography reveals RV enlargement with paradoxical septal motion.[78] Enlargement of the LA appendage may also be observed. Computed tomography of the chest is the diagnostic technique for confirmation.

Conclusions

The diagnosis of constrictive pericarditis can be elusive and may require multiple modalities, both noninvasive (echocardiography, computed tomography) and invasive (catheterization). The patient's history must be carefully scrutinized for any predisposing clinical condition associated with constriction. M-mode findings of flat motion in early diastole of the LV posterior wall, abnormal septal motion, or thickened pericardium manifested as dense, parallel moving echoes should be cause for concern. Furthermore, two-dimensional findings of pericardial adhesion or inferior vena cava plethora with Doppler evidence of increased mitral/tricuspid early filling (E) velocities and decreased atrial (A) filling velocities with rapid deceleration times that vary with respiration are highly suspicious. Surgical resection of the pericardium may relieve the symptoms of heart failure in most, but not all, patients.

REFERENCES

1. Agatson AS, Rao A, Price RJ, et al. Diagnosis of constrictive pericarditis by pulsed Doppler echocardiography. Am J Cardiol. 1984;54:929–930.

2. Allen MN, Nanna M, Lichtenberg GS, et al. Blunt trauma causing delayed cardiac tamponade: Echocardiographic diagnosis. J Diagn Med Sonogr. 1988;4: 269–273.

3. Appleton CP, Hatle LK, Popp RL. Cardiac tamponade and pericardial effusion: Respiratory variation in transvalvular flow velocities studied by Doppler echocardiography. J Am Coll Cardiol 1988;11: 1020–1030.

4. Armstrong WF, Schilt BF, Helper DJ, et al. Diastolic collapse of the right ventricle with cardiac tamponade: An echocardiographic study. Circulation. 1982; 65:1491–1496.

5. Burstow DJ, Oh JK, Barley KR, et al. Cardiac tamponade: Characteristic Doppler observations. Mayo Clin Proc. 1989;64:312–324.

6. Byrd BF, Linden RW. Superior vena cava Doppler flow velocity patterns in pericardial disease. Am J Cardiol. 1990;65:1464–1470.

7. Callahan JA, Seward JB, Nishumara RA. Two-dimensional echocardiographically guided pericardiocentesis: Experience in 117 consecutive patients. Am J Cardiol. 1985;55:476–479.

8. Candel-Riera J, Del Castillo HG, Permanyer-Miraldo G, et al. Echocardiographic features of the interventricular septum in chronic constrictive pericarditis. Circulation. 1978;57:1154–1158.

9. Chandraratna PAN. Uses and limitations of echocardiography in the evaluation of pericardial disease. Echocardiography. 1984;1:55–74.

10. Chandraratna PAN, Reid CL, Nimalasuriya A, et al. Application of two dimensional contrast studies during pericardiocentesis. Am J Cardiol. 1983;52: 1120–1122.

11. Chuttani K, Pandian NG, Mohanty PK, et al. Left ventricular diastolic collapse: An echocardiographic sign of regional cardiac tamponade. Circulation. 1991;83:1999–2006.

12. D'Cruz IA, Kensey K, Campbell C, et al. Two dimensional echocardiography in cardiac tamponade occurring after cardiac surgery. J Am Coll Cardiol. 1985;5:1250–1252.

13. Eisenberg MJ, Oken K, Guerrero S, et al. Prognostic value of echocardiography in hospitalized patients with pericardial effusion. Am J Cardiol. 1992;70: 934–939.

14. Eisenberg MJ, Schiller NB. Bayes theorem and the echocardiographic diagnosis of cardiac tamponade. Am J Cardiol. 1991;68:1242–1244.

15. Engel PJ, Fowler NO, Tei C, et al. M-mode echocardiography in constrictive pericarditis. J Am Coll Cardiol. 1985;6:471–474.

16. Engel PJ, Hon H, Fowler NO, et al. Echocardiographic study of right ventricular wall motion in

cardiac tamponade. Am J Cardiol. 1982;50: 1018–1021.

17. Feigenbaum H, Waldhausen JA, Hyde LP. Ultrasound diagnosis of pericardial effusion. JAMA. 1965; 191:711–714.

18. Fowler NO. Regional cardiac tamponade: A hemodynamic study. J Am Coll Cardiol. 1987;10: 164–169.

19. Fowler NO, Gabel M. The hemodynamic effects of cardiac tamponade: Mainly the result of atrial, not ventricular compression. Circulation. 1985;71: 154–157.

20. Fyke FE, Tancredi RG, Shub C, et al. Detection of intrapericardial hematoma after open heart surgery: The roles of echocardiography and computed tomography. J Am Coll Cardiol. 1985;5:1496–1499.

21. Gibson TC, Grossman W, McLaurin LP, et al. An echocardiographic study of the interventricular septum in constrictive pericarditis. Br Heart J. 1976;38: 738–743.

22. Gillam LD, Guyer DE, Gibson TC, et al. Hydrodynamic compression of the right atrium: A new echocardiographic sign of cardiac tamponade. Circulation. 1983;68:294–301.

23. Gonzalez MS, Basnight MA, Appleton CP, et al. Experimental pericardial effusion: Relation of abnormal respiratory variation in mitral flow velocity to hemodynamics and diastolic right heart collapse. J Am Coll Cardiol. 1991;17:239–248.

24. Guberman BA, Fowler NO, Engel PJ, et al. Cardiac tamponade in medical patients. Circulation. 1981; 64:633–640.

25. Hatle LK, Appleton CP, Popp RL. Differentiation of constrictive pericarditis and restrictive cardiomyopathy by Doppler echocardiography. Circulation. 1989;79:357–370.

26. Himelman RB, Kircher B, Rockey DC, et al. Inferior vena cava plethora with blunted respiratory response: A sensitive echocardiographic sign of cardiac tamponade. J Am Coll Cardiol. 1988;12:1470–1477.

27. Himelman RB, Lee E, Schiller NB. Septal bounce, vena cava plethora and pericardial adhesion: Informative two dimensional echocardiographic signs in the diagnosis of pericardial constriction. J Am Soc Echocardiogr. 1988;1:333–340.

28. Hutchinson SJ, Smalling RG, Colletti P, et al. Comparison of transthoracic and transesophageal echocardiography in clinically overt or suspected pericardial heart disease. Am J Cardiol. 1994;74:962–965.

29. Isner JM, Carter BL, Bankoff MS, et al. Computed tomography in the diagnosis of pericardial heart disease. Ann Intern Med. 1982;97:473–479.

30. Isobe M, Yamaoki K, Tsuchimochi H, et al. Transmitral reversed blood flow during mid and end dias-

tole in constrictive pericarditis. Am Heart J. 1986; 112:855–888.

31. Janos GG, Arjunan K, Meyer RA, et al. Differentiation of constrictive pericarditis and restrictive cardiomyopathy using digitized echocardiography. J Am Coll Cardiol. 1983;1(2):541–549.

32. King SW, Pandian NG, Gardin JM. Doppler echocardiographic findings in pericardial tamponade and constriction. Echocardiography. 1988;5:361–372.

33. Klein AL, Cohen GI, Petro Lungo JF, et al. Respiratory changes in pulmonary venous flow distinguish constrictive pericarditis from restrictive cardiomyopathy (abstract). Circulation. 1991;84(suppl II):5.

34. Klein AL, Canale MP, Al-Assaad AN, et al. Transesophageal echocardiography is a useful technique in localizing pericardial thickening in patients with diastolic dysfunction compared to magnetic resonance imaging (abstract). J Am Coll Cardiol. 1995; 25:358A.

35. Klopfenstein HS, Cogswell TA, Bernath GA. Alterations in intravascular volume affect the relation between right ventricular diastolic collapse and the hemodynamic severity of cardiac tamponade. J Am Coll Cardiol. 1985;6:1057–1063.

36. Kronzon I, Cohen ML, Winer HE. Cardiac tamponade by loculated pericardial hematoma: Limitations of M-mode echocardiography. J Am Coll Cardiol. 1983;3:913–915.

37. Kronzon I, Cohen ML, Winer HE. Diastolic atrial compression: A sensitive echocardiographic sign of cardiac tamponade. J Am Coll Cardiol. 1983;2: 770–775.

38. Leeman DE, Levine MJ, Come PC. Doppler echocardiography in cardiac tamponade: Exaggerated respiratory variation in transvalvular blood flow velocity integrals. J Am Coll Cardiol. 1988;11:572–578.

39. Leimgruber PP, Klopefenstein HS, Wann LS, et al. The hemodynamic derangement associated with right ventricular diastolic collapse in cardiac tamponade: An experimental echocardiographic study. Circulation. 1983;68:612–620.

40. Levine MJ, Lorell BH, Diver DJ, et al. Implications of echocardiographically assisted diagnosis of pericardial tamponade in contemporary medical patients: Detection before hemodynamic embarrassment. J Am Coll Cardiol. 1991;17:59–65.

41. Lewis BS. Real time two-dimensional echocardiography in constrictive pericarditis. Am J Cardiol. 1982; 49:1789–1793.

42. Ling LH, Oh JK, Tei C, et al. Pericardial thickness measured by transesophageal echocardiography: Feasibility and potential clinical utility (abstract). J Am Coll Cardiol. 1995;25:103A.

43. Lorell BH, Braunwald E. Pericardial disease in heart disease. *In* Braunwald E (ed): A Textbook of Cardio-

vascular Medicine, 3rd ed. Philadelphia, WB Saunders; 1988:1501–1507.

44. Lorell BH, Grossman W. Profiles in constrictive pericarditis, restrictive cardiomyopathy and cardiac tamponade. *In* Grossman W (ed): Cardiac Catheterization and Angiography, 3rd ed. Philadelphia, Lea & Febiger; 1986:434–440.

45. Martin RP, Bowden RF, Filly K, et al. Intrapericardial abnormalities in patients with pericardial effusion. Findings by two dimensional echocardiography. Circulation. 1980;61:568–576.

46. Martin RP, Rakowski H, French J, et al. Localization of pericardial effusion with wide angle phased array echocardiography. Am J Cardiol. 1978;42: 904–912.

47. Moncada R, Baker M, Salinas M, et al. Diagnostic role of computed tomography in pericardial heart disease: Congenital defects, thickening, neoplasms and effusions. Am Heart J. 1982;103:262–282.

48. Nishimura RA, Abel MD, Hatle LK, et al. Assessment of diastolic function of the heart: Background and current applications of Doppler echocardiography. Mayo Clin Proc. 1989;64:181–204.

49. Nishimura RA, Connolly DC, Parkin TW, et al. Constrictive pericarditis: Assessment of current diagnostic procedures. Mayo Clin Proc. 1985;60:397–401.

50. Oh JK, Hatle LK, Seward JB, et al. Diagnostic role of Doppler echocardiography in constrictive pericarditis. J Am Coll Cardiol. 1994;23:154–162.

51. Pandian NG, Brockway B, Simonetti J, et al. Pericardiocentesis under two-dimensional echocardiographic guidance in loculated pericardial effusion. Ann Thorac Surg. 1988;45:99–100.

52. Pandian NG, Skorton DJ, Kieso RA, et al. Diagnosis of constrictive pericarditis by two-dimensional echocardiography: Studies in a new experimental model and in patients. J Am Coll Cardiol. 1984;4: 1164–1173.

53. Pandian NG, Wang SS, McInerney K, et al. Doppler echocardiography in cardiac tamponade: Abnormalities in tricuspid and mitral flow response to respiration in experimental and clinical tamponade (abstract). J Am Coll Cardiol. 1985;5:485.

54. Permanyer-Miralda G, Sagrista-Sauleda J, Soler-Soler J. Primary acute pericardial disease: A prospective series of 231 consecutive patients. Am J Cardiol. 1985;56:623–630.

55. Pool PE, Seagren SC, Abbasi AS, et al. Echocardiographic manifestations of constrictive pericarditis. Chest. 1975;68:684–688.

56. Reddy PS, Curtiss EI, O'Toole JD, et al. Cardiac tamponade: Hemodynamic observations in man. Circulation. 1978;58:265–272.

57. Schiavone WA, Calafiore PA, Salcedo EE. Transesophageal Doppler echocardiographic demonstra-

tion of pulmonary venous flow velocity in restrictive cardiomyopathy and constrictive pericarditis. Am J Cardiol. 1989;63:1286–1288.

58. Schutzman JJ, Obarski TP, Pearce GL, et al. Comparison of Doppler and two dimensional echocardiography for assessment of pericardial effusion. Am J Cardiol. 1992;70:1353–1357.

59. Sectern U, Tscholakoff D, Higgins CB. MRI of the abnormal pericardium. Am J Radiol. 1986;147:245–253.

60. Shabetai R. The pericardium: An essay on some recent developments. Am J Cardiol. 1978;42:1036–1043.

61. Shabetai R, Mangiardi L, Ross J, et al. The pericardium and cardiac function. Progr Cardiovasc Dis. 1979;22:107–134.

62. Singh S, Wann LS, Klopfenstein HS, et al. Usefulness of right ventricular diastolic collapse in diagnosing cardiac tamponade and comparison of pulsus paradoxus. Am J Cardiol. 1986;57:652–656.

63. Singh S, Wann LS, Schuchard GH, et al. Right ventricular and right atrial collapse in patients with cardiac tamponade—a combined echocardiographic and hemodynamic study. Circulation. 1984;70:966–971.

64. Smith MD, Waters JS, Kwan OL, et al. Evaluation of pericardial compressive disorders by echocardiography. Echocardiography. 1985;2:67–86.

65. Soulen RL, Stark DD, Higgins CB. Magnetic resonance imaging of constrictive pericardial disease. Am J Cardiol. 1985;55:480–484.

66. Steele RL, Perez JE. Left ventricular diastolic collapse provoking cardiac tamponade. Echocardiography. 1986;3:149–150.

67. Stevenson LW, Child JS, Laks H, et al. Incidence and significance of early pericardial effusions after cardiac surgery. Am J Cardiol. 1984;54:848–851.

68. Sutton FJ, Whitley NO, Applefield MM. The role of echocardiography and computed tomography in the evaluation of pericardial disease. Am Heart J. 1984;109:350–354.

69. Tei C, Child JS, Hiromitsu T, et al. Atrial systolic notch on the interventricular septal echogram: An echocardiographic sign of constrictive pericarditis. J Am Coll Cardiol. 1983;1:907–912.

70. Tokgozoglu SL, Kes S, Oram A, et al. Echocardiography in patients with constrictive pericarditis before and after pericardiectomy. Are there predictors of surgical outcome? Echocardiography. 1995;12:29–34.

71. Vaitkus PT, Kussmaul WG. Constrictive pericarditis versus restrictive cardiomyopathy: A reappraisal and update of diagnostic criteria. Am Heart J. 1991;122:1431–1441.

72. Voelkel AG, Pierto DA, Folland ED, et al. Echocardiographic features of constrictive pericarditis. Circulation. 1978;58:971–975.

73. Von Bibra H, Schober K, Jenni R, et al. Diagnosis of constrictive pericarditis by pulsed Doppler echocardiography of the hepatic vein. Am J Cardiol. 1989;63:483–488.

74. Waggoner AD, Stark PA, Gutierrez F, et al. Measurements of pericardial thickness by retrocardiac two dimensional echocardiography and computed tomography (abstract). J Am Soc Echocardiogr. 1995;8:374.

75. Wann LS. Echocardiography in pericardial disease (editorial). Echocardiography. 1984;1:111–113.

76. Wann LS, Weyman AE, Dillon JC, et al. Premature pulmonary valve opening. Circulation. 1977;55:128–135.

77. Weitzman LB, Tinker WP, Kronzon I, et al. The incidence and natural history of pericardial effusion after cardiac surgery—an echocardiographic study. Circulation. 1984;69:506–511.

78. Weyman AE. Principles and Practices of Echocardiography, 2nd ed., Philadelphia, Lea & Febiger; 1994:1132.

PART X

Congenital Heart Disease

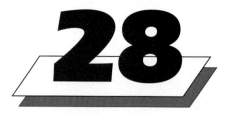

28

Cardiac Embryology

JAMES P. EICHELBERGER

Introduction

Formation of the cardiac system in the human embryo begins early in the course of development. Its onset in the third week after fertilization is necessary since diffusion of nutrients alone at this stage is not sufficient to maintain adequate nutrition for continued embryonic growth. In just a few weeks, a complex, functioning cardiovascular system is formed from the mesodermal germ layer that is capable of providing needed nutrients throughout the remainder of fetal development. Near the time of birth, this system normally undergoes modifications that are consequences of entry into a new environment. Abnormalities of development at any of these stages can lead to various congenital cardiac abnormalities. Therefore, a general comprehension of normal cardiovascular formation and modification is fundamental to understanding congenital heart disease. Knowledge of cardiovascular development not only provides a framework in which to explain various common congenital cardiac defects but also is helpful in understanding more complex cardiac abnormalities.

The objective of this chapter is to provide an introduction to basic cardiovascular formation so that the reader can more fully appreciate the origin and pathophysiology of common congenital cardiac anomalies. The chapter is not intended to provide a comprehensive or detailed discussion of cardiac development, but rather to highlight certain phases

in which linkages to common congenital cardiac anomalies are observed. In keeping with this goal, any common cardiac defect accompanying a particular phase of cardiac development will be included in the discussion of that phase. Although many different aspects of cardiovascular development occur simultaneously, or at least overlap, they will be discussed separately in this chapter to help illustrate their associations with various cardiac defects (Table 28-1).

Formation of the Heart Tube

As the superiorly located cardiogenic area in the embryo migrates ventrally in the fetus due to rapid cephalad expansion of the central nervous system, two lateral endothelial heart tubes migrate toward each other and eventually fuse to form a single straight cardiac tube (Fig. 28-1). This cardiac tube consists of a myocardial mantle lined with a core of cardiac jelly surrounding an inner single layer of endocardium. While the endocardium and cardiac jelly participate in the formation of endocardial cushions, among other functions, the outer myocardial mantle becomes the muscular wall of the heart enriched with contractile myocytes. The singular heart tube also segments longitudinally in a predictable and organized fashion, forming five primitive areas (Fig. 28-2): the sinus venosus (eventually forming the proximal vena cava), common atrium, common ventricle, conus cordis (future right and

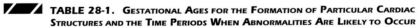 **TABLE 28-1.** Gestational Ages for the Formation of Particular Cardiac Structures and the Time Periods When Abnormalities Are Likely to Occur

Approximate Gestational Age (days)	Normal Development	Cardiac Defect
20	Blood vessels begin to form.	
21	Formation of right and left endocardial tubes.	
	Aortic arches begin to form.	
22	Further development of endocardial tubes and aortic arches. Primitive left and right atrium begin to form, as well as the sinus venosus.	
23–24	Myocardial mantle develops.	
	Single cardiac tube (bulbus cordis) begins to loop.	Corrected transposition
	Primitive atria begin a posterior ascent.	Double-outlet right ventricle
	Primitive ventricle begin to form.	Juxtaposition of atrial appendages
	AV canal formation.	
	Heart begins to beat.	
25–26	Bulbus cordis continues to loop, forming right ventricle, truncus arteriosus, and conus cordis.	Ventricular inversion
	Left ventricle forms.	Single ventricle
	Heart fills entire pericardial sac.	
	Septum primum begins.	
27–30	Development of muscular IVS.	Ventricular septal defect
	Formation of papillary muscles, moderator band, AV valve chordae tendineae, and trabeculations.	
	Endocardial cushions form.	Endocardial cushion defects
	Truncus begins to divide into aorta and pulmonary trunk.	Transposition of great vessels, truncus
	Single pulmonary vein forms. IVC and SVC start to develop.	
	Anterior cusp of TV forms.	Ebstein's anamoly
31–33	Enlargement of the AV canal.	
	Aortic pulmonary septum complete.	
	Primitive semilunar valve tissue starts to develop.	PV or AV stenosis
33–36	Mitral and tricuspid orfices form.	
	Conus swellings lead to development of RV.	Tetralogy of Fallot
37–42	Mitral valve is formed.	AV valve abnormalities
	Remainder of TV is formed.	Mitral or tricuspid atresia
	Further development of semilunar valves.	ASDs
	Septum secundum forms and migrates inferiorly toward septum primum (postnatally, these overlap to form the foramen ovale).	
	Membranous septum forms.	Perimembranous VSDs
55	Near-completion of fetal heart.	

Abbreviations: ASD, atrial septal defect; AV, atrioventricular; IVC, inferior vena cava; RV, right ventricle; SVC, superior vena cava; TV, tricuspid valve; VSD, ventricular septal defect.

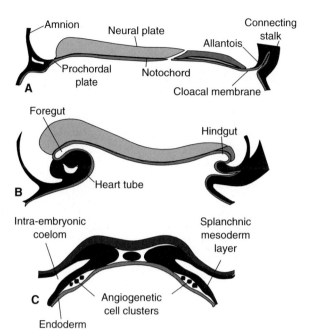

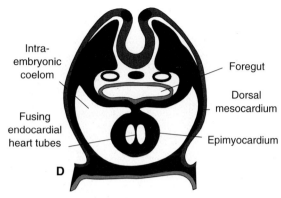

Figure 28-1. (**A,B**) The result of rapid brain growth shifting the cardiac position ventrally in the embryo. (**C,D**) Fusion of the two lateral heart tubes as they also migrate ventrally. (Used with permission. Sadler TW. Langman's Medical Embryology, fifth edition. Baltimore, Williams & Wilkins; 1985:170–171.)

left ventricular outflow tracts), and truncus arteriosus (which eventually divides to form both roots of the aorta and pulmonary arteries). At this stage, the heart functions as a tubular pump.

Since the heart tube grows much more rapidly than the surrounding pericardial cavity, elongation

of the tube is constrained in the longitudinal direction. Consequently, as the tube continues to grow, a bend or "loop" forms that is dictated by this constrained growth, active cell deformation, and a preexisting dorsal mesocardium acting as a tether. A simple analogy occurs when retrieving

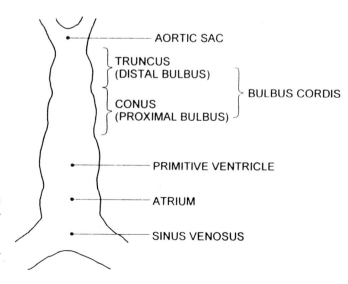

Figure 28-2. Traditional segmental organization of the heart tube. (From Van Mierop LHS. Morphological development of the heart. *In* Berne RM, (ed.): Handbook of Physiology, Section 2, Vol. I. Bethesda, Maryland, American Physiological Society; 1979:1–28.)

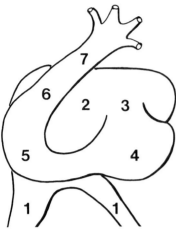

Figure 28-3. Rightward or dextro (d) looping of the heart tube. Right and left sinus venosum (1); common atrium (2); atrioventricular canal (3); primitive left ventricle (4); primitive right ventricle (5); conus cordis (6); truncus arteriosus (7).

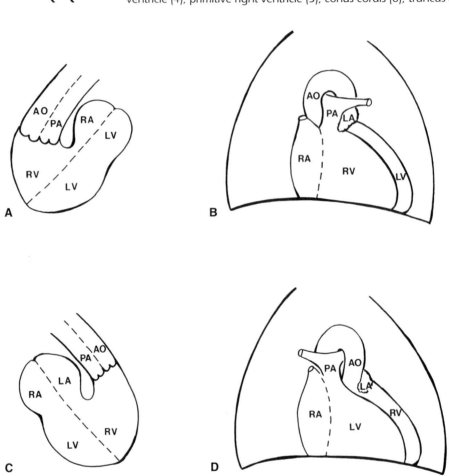

Figure 28-4. (**A**) Rightward or dextro (d) looping of the heart tube. Future normal septation is indicated by the broken line. (**B**) Normal or dextro (d) bulboventricular looping. Normal heart in the left chest. (**C**) Normally positioned atria with levo (l) looping of the remainder of the heart tube. (**D**) Congenitally corrected transposition. Normally positioned atria, levo (l) bulboventricular looping and transposed great arteries. The right-sided atrium empties into the right-sided, anatomic left ventricle, which empties into the pulmonary artery. The hemodynamic connections are correct; the anatomic connections are not. Ao, aorta; PA, pulmonary artery; RV, right ventricle; LV, left ventricle; RA, right atrium; LA, left atrium.

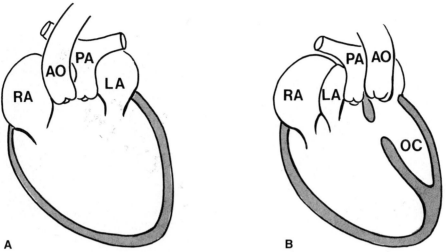

Figure 28-5. Double-inlet or single ventricle. (**A**) Single ventricle with dextro (d) transposed great arteries. (**B**) Single ventricle with levo (l) transposed great arteries and a primitive outflow chamber (OC). AO, aorta; RA, right atrium; PA, pulmonary artery; LA, left atrium.

a garden hose; as extra hose is brought in, it naturally tends to loop, as it has nowhere else to go. Cardiac looping occurs simultaneously with longitudinal segmentation and normally results in a posterior atrium, anterior and rightward conus cordis regions, and a truncus arteriosus region. This usual rightward direction of looping is termed *dextro* or *d-looping* (Fig. 28-3). If the heart loops abnormally to the left (*levo* or *l-looping*), then malposition of the ventricles and/or great vessels will result. This may take a variety of forms, most notably congenitally corrected transposition in which the right-sided atrium empties into the right-sided anatomic left ventricle, which then empties into the pulmonary artery. Likewise, the left-sided atrium empties into the left-sided anatomic right ventricle, which then empties into the aorta (Fig. 28-4).

If further differentiation of the heart tube is interrupted such that septation into right and left portions does not occur, then a single chamber may result. An example of this is a single ventricular chamber which gives rise to both great arteries and into which both atrioventricular valves empty. The resulting single ventricle, more commonly called the *double-inlet left ventricle,* can occur with l-looping or d-looping and is often associated with transposed great arteries. Occasionally, a primitive out-

flow tract chamber may accompany this abnormality (Fig. 28-5).

Development of the Sinus Venosus

The sinus venosus remains in its paired state longer than any other portion of the heart tube. As the left sinus horn is finally obliterated, all that remains is the oblique vein of the left atrium and the coronary sinus (Fig. 28-6). Rarely, cephalad drainage into the left sinus horn remains and forms a persistent left superior vena cava that drains into the coronary sinus. This can be easily discerned echocardiographically by the appearance of various contrast agents in an often prominent coronary sinus prior to its appearance in the right atrium after left arm intravenous injection.

With obliteration of the left sinus venosus, left-to-right venous shunts develop, contributing to right sinus venosus enlargement and the eventual formation of right superior and inferior vena cavae. The right-sided sinus venosus becomes incorporated into the right atrium as it grows, resulting in an atrial fold that helps to direct oxygenated inferior vena caval blood across the interatrial septum to the fetal systemic circulation. This fold, often called the *eustachian valve,* can persist to a variable degree in adulthood.

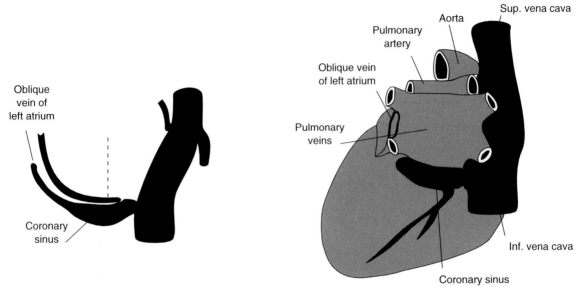

Atrial Septal Formation

As the primitive heart tube and cardiac looping grow, the common atrium expands and moves to a posterior and superior position. By the end of the fourth gestational week, a sickle-shaped crest begins to grow off the roof of the common atrium to eventually form the septum primum, which begins to divide the atrium into right and left halves. The remaining opening at the floor of the common atrium is called the *ostium primum* (Fig. 28-7A–D). Before closure of the ostium primum is complete, perforations appear more superiorly within the septum primum, which then coalesce to form the ostium secundum. Thus, at no time during fetal development are the right and left atria ever completely divided, again ensuring passage of maternally oxygenated blood across the atria to the fetal systemic circulation.

A second septum, or septum secundum, soon begins to form in the superior portion of the right atrium adjacent to the septum primum as a result of a fold created by enlargement of the superior portion of the right sinus venosus draining into the atrium. An oval-shaped opening that remains in the septum secundum as it develops more fully is called the *foramen ovale*. The portion of the septum pri-

mum adjacent to and covering the foramen ovale then acts as a flap valve, so that passage of blood from the right to the left atrium occurs as long as right atrial pressure exceeds left atrial pressure (Fig. 28-7D–G). At birth, when right atrial pressure decreases relative to left atrial pressure, the septum primum is pressed over the foramen ovale and eventually fuses. Fusion is not always complete, resulting in probe patency of the foramen ovale in about 25% of cases. Although usually benign, a persistently patent foramen ovale in adulthood has been associated with paradoxical embolization from the venous system across the interatrial septum to the systemic circulation.

A variety of congenital atrial septal defects can arise as a consequence of altered or arrested atrial septation. If atrial septation is arrested at the beginning of septum primum formation, then an inferior atrial septal defect, or ostium primum atrial septal defect, will result. This defect lies just above the atrioventricular valves and is often accompanied by some type of atrioventricular valve anomaly, most commonly a cleft anterior mitral leaflet. If development is arrested after closure of the ostium primum and formation of the ostium secundum, a more mid-level atrial septal ostium secundum defect will result. This can also be caused by excessive resorp-

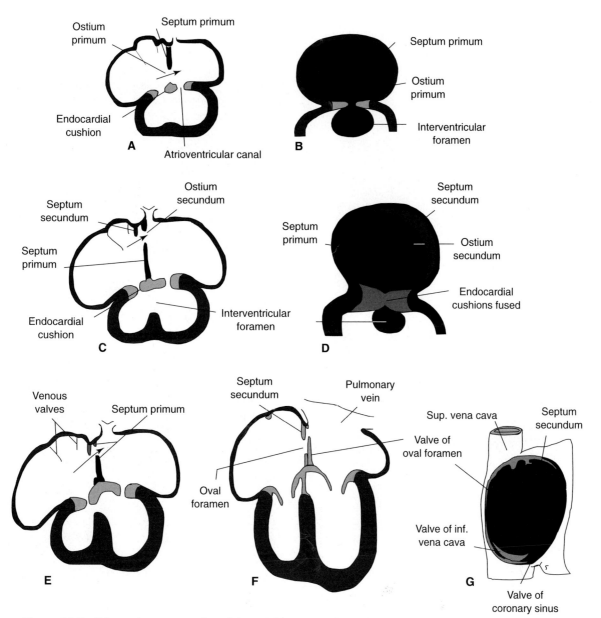

Figure 28-7. Schematic representation of the atrial septa at various stages of development. (**A**) At 6 mm (approximately 30 days); (**B**) same stage as in *A*, but seen from the right; (**C**) 9 mm (approximately 33 days); (**D**) same stage as in *C*, but seen from the right; (**E**) 14 mm (approximately 37 days); (**F**) newborn; and (**G**) view of the atrial septum seen from the right, same stage as in *F*. (Used with permission. Sadler TW. *Langman's Medical Embryology*, fifth edition. Baltimore, Williams & Wilkins; 1985:178.)

tion of the septum primum. Atrial secundum defects can be distinguished from atrial primum defects by a recognizable spur of atrial tissue inferiorly and the usual lack of associated atrioventricular valve anom-

alies. Abnormal positioning of the right sinus venosus in relation to the atrial septation may result in superior (in the case of the superior vena cava) or inferior (in the case of inferior vena cava) atrial septal defects involving these structures posteriorly, the so-called sinus venosus atrial septal defect. This type of atrial septal defect is frequently associated with partial anomalous pulmonary venous drainage into the right atrium.

Ventricular Septal Formation

At a time similar to atrial septation, the ventricle begins to expand more rapidly in its lateral aspects and more slowly in its medial portion, giving rise to a medial invagination that gradually fuses to form a portion of the interventricular septum (Fig. 28-8). A small opening near the level of the atrioventricular valves permits continued communication between the two ventricles until it is later closed by the membranous interventricular septum. Formation of the membranous and perimembranous portions of the interventricular septum arises by complex contributions from atrioventricular endocardial cushions (see "Formation of the Atrioventricular Canal") that divide the inflow into the ventricles and conus swellings (see "Outflow Tract and Aortic and Pulmonary Root Formation") that divide the outflow regions of the ventricles. Since proper development of this area of the interventricular septum is dependent on multiple factors, it is easy to understand that not only is a perimembranous interventricular

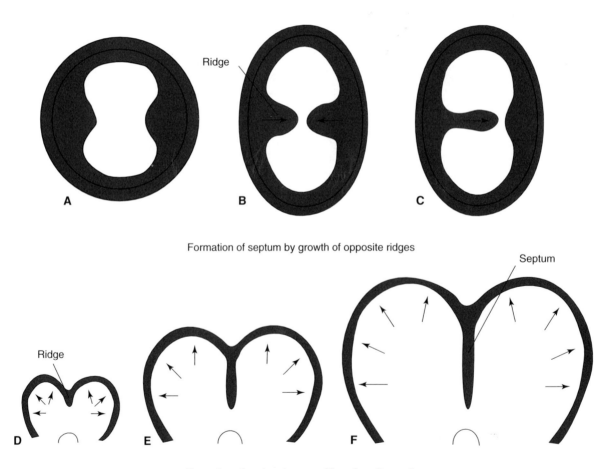

Formation of septum by growth of opposite ridges

Formation of septum by apposition of cardiac walls

Figure 28-8. Septum formation by two actively growing ridges which approach each other until they fuse (**A** and **B**). Sometimes the septum is formed by an actively growing single cell mass (**C**). (**D–F**) Septum formation by fusion of two expanding portions of the wall of the heart. Such a septum will never completely separate two cavities. (Used with permission. Sadler TW. *Langman's Medical Embryology,* fifth edition. Baltimore, Williams & Wilkins; 1985:177.)

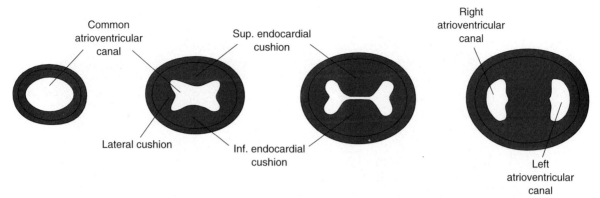

Figure 28-9. Formation of the septum in the atrioventricular canal. From left to right, 4-, 6-, 9-, and 12-mm stages, respectively. The initial circular opening becomes gradually widened in the transverse direction. (Used with permission. Sadler TW. Langman's Medical Embryology, fifth edition. Baltimore, Williams & Wilkins; 1985:177.)

defect a relatively common cardiac anomaly, but also that this defect is a common anomaly that accompanies other cardiac malformations. An example of the latter occurs in the case of tetralogy of Fallot, in which abnormal septation of the conus cordis results not only in an overriding aorta and a diminutive pulmonary infundibular area, but also in a perimembranous ventricular septal defect. Less often, single or multiple defects in the nonmembranous or muscular portion of the interventricular septum occur, probably as a result of inappropriate cell growth and cell death.

Formation of the Atrioventricular Canal

Around the perimeter between the common atrium and common ventricle, at the same time that each of these two chambers is being divided into left and right portions, four mesenchymal swellings begin to appear. These include two endocardial cushions and two lateral cushions, which begin to project into the lumen and ultimately fuse to divide the canal into right and left atrioventricular orifices (Fig. 28-9). The two endocardial cushions also are precursors to the septal leaflet of the tricuspid valve, as well as the anterior leaflet of the mitral valve and a portion of the inflow perimembranous interventricular septum, as noted above. The lateral cushions are responsible for forming the remaining anterior and posterior tricuspid leaflets, as well as the posterior leaflet of

the mitral valve. Valve formation is accomplished through a complex process of differential cell growth and cell death.

In addition to perimembranous ventricular septal defects, as discussed above, abnormal development of the atrioventricular canal can result in a variety of cardiac anomalies involving the tricuspid and/or mitral valves. When the cushions fail to fuse, a persistent atrioventricular canal defect results, with atrial and ventricular septal defect components separated by abnormal valve leaflets (Fig. 28-10A). Occasionally, partial fusion of the cushions occurs such that the interventricular septum closes but a low atrial septal defect and a cleft anterior mitral leaflet remain. This is known as the *ostium primum atrial septal defect* (Fig. 28-10D,E). Since the cushions also form the atrioventricular valves, various forms of mitral and/or tricuspid abnormalities may result from abnormal development at this stage. One important example of this is obliteration of the right atrioventricular orifice, leading to tricuspid atresia, which is always associated with both atrial and ventricular septal defects, underdevelopment of the right ventricle, and left ventricular hypertrophy. Various other forms of mitral and tricuspid stenosis can also occur, including Ebstein's anomaly, in which varying degrees of septal leaflet adhesion of the tricuspid valve to the interventricular septum lead to apparent atrialization of the right ventricle and some degree of tricuspid stenosis (Fig. 28-11).

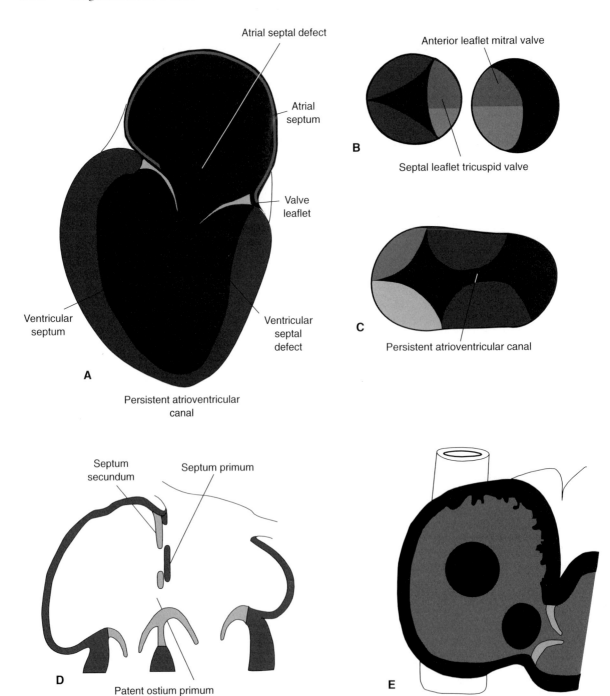

Figure 28-10. (**A**) Persistent common atrioventricular canal. This abnormality is always accompanied by a septum defect in the atrial as well as in the ventricular portion of the cardiac partition. (**B**) Valves in the atrioventricular orifices under normal conditions. (**C**) Split valves in the case of a persistent atrioventricular canal. (**D** and **E**) Ostium primum defect caused by incomplete fusion of the atrioventricular endocardial cushions. (Used with permission. Sadler TW. Langman's Medical Embryology, fifth edition. Baltimore, Williams & Wilkins; 1985:184.)

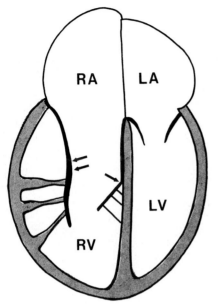

Figure 28-11. Ebstein's anomaly of the tricuspid valve. Note the lack of freeing of the septal leaflet (single arrow) and the long anterior leaflet (double arrow).

Outflow Tract and Aortic and Pulmonary Root Formation

Just as the endocardial cushions divide the inflow into the two ventricles, separate cushions in the conus cordis (conus cushions) divide the outflow tract into left and right portions. The conus cushions also contribute to the development of the outflow portion of the perimembranous interventricular septum. At about the same time, two swellings in the truncus arteriosus begin to grow to form a septum dividing the truncus into an aortic and a pulmonary channel. Division starts at the distal end of the truncus arteriosus and progresses toward the conus cordis. These two swellings twist around each other as they expand, creating the spiral relationship that exists between the aorta and pulmonary artery (Fig. 28-12). Tubercles on the main truncus swellings are responsible for formation of the aortic and pulmonic valves.

The most frequent abnormality seen in this region occurs when unequal division of the conus results in a narrowed right ventricular outflow tract, subsequent right ventricular pressure overload, and an interventricular septal defect (see "Ventricular Septal Formation"). The aorta arises directly above

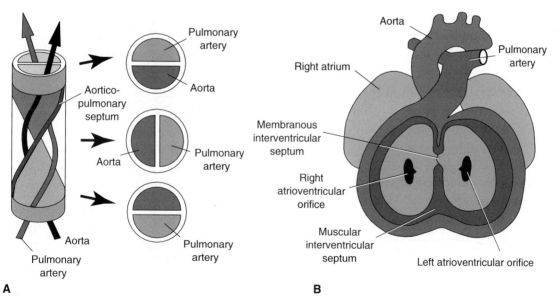

Figure 28-12. (**A**) Diagram to show the spiral shape of the aorticopulmonary septum. (**B**) Position of aorta and pulmonary artery at 25-mm stage (eighth week). Note how the aorta and pulmonary artery twist around each other. (Used with permission. Sadler TW. Langman's Medical Embryology, fifth edition. Baltimore, Williams & Wilkins; 1985:186.)

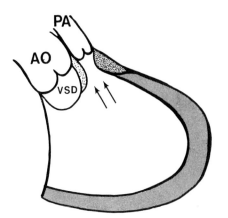

Figure 28-13. Tetralogy of Fallot viewed from the right ventricle. The main pulmonary artery and right ventricular outflow tract are narrow (arrows). There is a large ventricular septal defect below the large aortic root.

the interventricular septal defect, creating a tetrad of abnormalities known as *tetralogy of Fallot* (Fig. 28-13). If the truncoconal ridges fail to fuse, the pulmonary artery then arises some distance above the undivided portion of the truncus. This condition is known as a *persistent truncus arteriosus* and is always accompanied by a ventricular septal defect

for reasons previously explained (Fig. 28-14). Outflow valve cusps continue to form in the case of persistent truncus arteriosus, but can be variable in number and are usually regurgitant to some degree. In another anomaly, if the conotruncal septum fails to follow its normal spiral course and instead descends straight down, the aorta and pulmonary arteries become transposed with respect to their ventricular attachments. That is to say, transposition of the great arteries results in the aorta's originating from the right ventricle and the pulmonary artery originating from the left ventricle. Finally, interference with development at the time of aortic or pulmonary valve formation may result in various semilunar valve abnormalities, including bicuspid aortic valve and pulmonary valve atresia.

Formation of the Aortic and Pulmonary Arches

Beginning in the fourth week of development, six sets of symmetrically paired aortic arches form. Subsequently, the arch system loses its symmetric appearance as it changes into the adult arterial system. The third set of aortic arches becomes the common

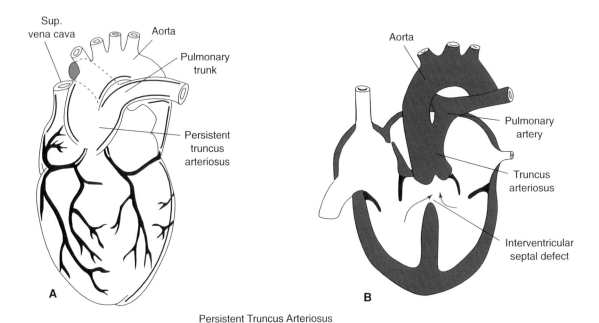

Persistent Truncus Arteriosus

Figure 28-14. (**A**) Persistent truncus arteriosus. The pulmonary artery originates from the common truncus. The septum in the conus and truncus has failed to form. (**B**) The abnormality is always combined with an interventricular septal defect. (Used with permission. Sadler TW. *Langman's Medical Embryology*, fifth edition. Baltimore, Williams & Wilkins; 1985:191.)

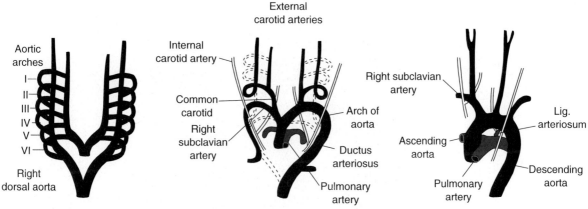

Figure 28-15. *Abnormal development of aortic arches. (Used with permission. Sadler TW. Langman's Medical Embryology, fifth edition. Baltimore, Williams & Wilkins; 1985:378.)*

and internal carotid artery bilaterally, the left fourth aortic arch develops into the aorta, and the sixth aortic arch becomes the right and left pulmonary arteries (Fig. 28-15). Most of the other arches obliterate with time. A distal portion of the left sixth aortic arch (to become the pulmonary artery) retains its connection to the arterial system during the rest of development and is known as the *ductus arteriosus*. This pulmonary-to-systemic shunt in the developing fetus helps divert unoxygenated blood from the right ventricle back to the placenta.

The ductus arteriosus may persist after birth and can exist as an isolated abnormality or in combination with other heart defects, particularly ones in which large differences between aortic and pulmonary pressures create a large volume of blood flow through the ductus. An example of this occurs with preductal aortic coarctation. In this anomaly, the descending aorta is significantly narrowed (due to intimal proliferation) above the entrance of the ductus arteriosus. Since the lower part of the body is thus supplied with blood by the ductus arteriosus to a larger degree, its normal closure is prevented. In the postductal type of aortic coarctation, the ductus arteriosus obliterates normally. Other abnormalities of the aorta can also occur, such as a double aortic arch, right aortic arch, interrupted aortic arch, or abnormal origin of the right subclavian artery.

Circulatory Changes at Birth

In the normal fetal circulation, blood from the placenta, which is about 80% saturated with oxygen,

travels to the fetus via the umbilical vein. The majority of this flow shunts past the liver through the ductus venosus directly into the inferior vena cava near its junction with the right atrium. This blood is preferentially shunted across the foramen ovale by the action of the eustachian valve and then proceeds out of the ascending aorta to supply the heart and brain with oxygen-rich blood. The least saturated blood returns from the upper body via the superior vena cava and is preferentially directed into the right ventricle, then across the ductus arteriosus to the lower body. Two umbilical arteries off the descending aorta direct flow toward the placenta for reoxygenation. Thus, preferential shunting patterns on the venous side direct most of the less oxygenated blood to reach the right ventricle for subsequent reoxygenation via the ductus arteriosus and umbilical arteries, and most of the more highly oxygenated blood to reach the left ventricle via the foramen ovale for subsequent myocardial and brain perfusion (Fig. 28-16).

Two main events at birth prompt abrupt changes in the fetal circulation. The first is a rapid, large decrease in pulmonary vascular resistance from various mechanisms that is triggered by oxygenation of the lung through the baby's first breath. This dramatically increases pulmonary blood flow, leading to increased left atrial pressure, which promotes coaptation of the two interatrial septa and eventual fusion. The second major event, disruption of the umbilical-placental circulation, leads to reduced flow through the ductus venosus and decreased right atrial pressure, thereby also

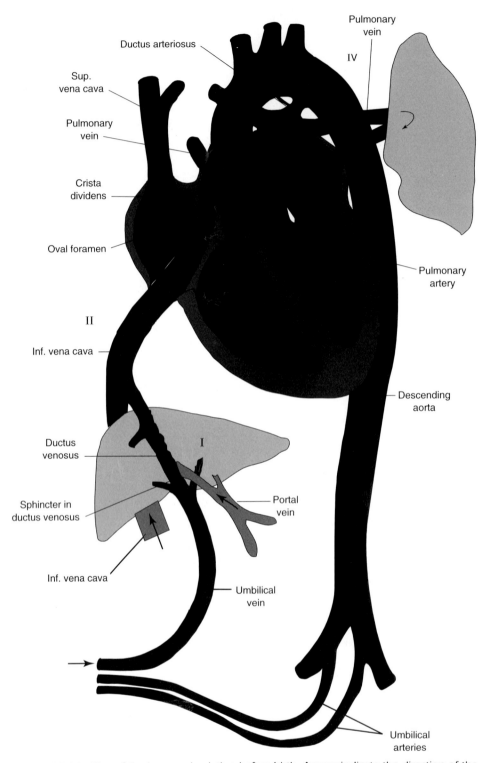

Figure 28-16. Plan of the human circulation before birth. Arrows indicate the direction of the blood flow. Note where the oxygenated blood mixes with deoxygenated blood: (I) in the liver, (II) in the inferior vena cava, (III) in the right atrium, and (IV) at the entrance of the ductus arteriosus into the descending aorta. (Used with permission. Sadler TW. Langman's Medical Embryology, fifth edition. Baltimore, Williams & Wilkins; 1985:210.)

aiding interatrial septal fusion. Other mechanisms, in addition to a change in pressure gradients, also contribute to abolishment of fetal shunting. In the case of the ductus arteriosus, active contraction of its muscular wall occurs soon after birth, probably mediated by bradykinin. This helps to promote its closure in the first hours or days of life. Until that time, flow through the ductus is reversed from a right-to-left conduit of blood to the aorta to a left-to-right conduit of blood to the lungs.

REFERENCES

1. Moss, Adams. Heart Disease in Infants, Children, and Adolescents Including the Fetus and Young Adult, 5th ed. Baltimore, Williams & Wilkins; 1995.
2. Langman J. Medical Embyrology, 4th ed. Baltimore, Williams & Wilkins; 1982.
3. Berman MC, Craig MC, Kawamura DM, eds. Diagnostic Medical Sonography: A Guide to Clinical Practice, Vol. 2. Philadelphia, JB Lippincott; 1991.
4. Moore KL. The Developing Human. Philadelphia, WB Saunders; 1988:4.

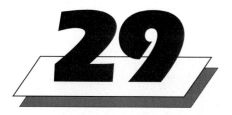

Congenital Heart Disease

SUSIE TRUESDELL

Introduction

Pediatric echocardiography is an exciting and challenging field. There is an infinite number of combinations of defects that can present in children's hearts. Abnormalities in situs place the heart in the right or left chest or at midline. There may be one or two right atria, one or two left atria, one or two ventricles, atrioventricular valves, and semilunar valves, or any combination of numbers and morphologies. Either atrium may communicate with a right ventricle, left ventricle, single ventricle, or no ventricle. Either ventricle may communicate with a pulmonary artery, an aorta, a single great vessel, or no great vessel. Due to the intricacies of these combinations of multiple defects, a pediatric echocardiogram must be meticulously performed, evaluating each connection and defining the morphology of each chamber and valve. The *segmental approach* to congenital heart disease will be described later in this chapter and should be used in every child in whom there is a question of complex congenital heart disease.

Children's attitudes and responses to a healthcare environment also vary widely. The frightened 5-year-old who lies rigid but still, quivering and silently crying; the 20-month-old who screams, kicks, bites, spits, and arches his back; the 10-year-old who discovers that when she takes a deep breath and holds it the entire two-dimensional (2D) image disappears—these are our patients, on whom we are supposed to make a detailed evaluation of every chamber and connection.

For these reasons, there is very little similarity between an adult echocardiogram and a pediatric echocardiogram. The equipment may be similar, but the behavior of the patient and the complexity of the anatomic relationships require additional expertise, patience, and concentration.

Although the segmental approach to congenital heart disease offers the most thorough assessment of anatomy and hemodynamics, it requires a fair amount of time to complete. Most children will not cooperate for the required period. For this reason, many infants and small children may require sedation to complete this study. It is often inappropriate to sedate a child in an outpatient clinic, however. Under these circumstances, pediatric sonographers discuss the priorities of the exam with the physician prior to taking the child to the echocardiographic lab. Then, based on those priorities, the echocardiographer starts at the top of the list and tries to answer as many questions as possible before the child becomes uncooperative. If the child is uncooperative, the report should state that the study was abbreviated due to the patient's behavior and should specify the portions of the study which were completed. A study under sedation at a future date may need to be scheduled to complete the evaluation.

Sedation, usually by oral chloral hydrate or intranasal midazolam (Versed), removes some of the child's apprehension and fear.[12] If an adequate level of sedation is achieved, the child will be quiet and cooperative for the study; he or she is usually awake and will still respond to outside stimuli. If sedation is heavy enough to induce sleep, the child must be watched closely until he or she awakens, for respiratory depression may accompany sedation. Thus, sedation of outpatients is used conservatively. For these reasons, we use other methods to quiet a child for the study rather than sedation.

There are a few tricks which may allow the completion of a study. Toys, especially musical toys, with the help of a parent may entertain a baby and allow the sonographer another 5–10 minutes for a study. If a baby is hungry, bottle feeding will often quiet him or her during the study; we have had little luck in performing an echocardiographic exam, however, while a child is breastfeeding. Another trick to use with infants and babies is a "sugar nipple"—fill a bottle nipple halfway with granular sugar and plug the hole with a 2 × 2 gauze square; add several drops of water to the gauze until the sugar dissolves. The pleasurable effects of the sugar nipple may last for 5 minutes.

In the older child, a strategically placed TV monitor with videos featuring well-known children's characters (particularly the Sesame Street characters) may allow the sonographer 10–15 minutes of quiet time. For the older child, short cartoons may help.

The primary rule is that the sonographer cannot become involved in distracting the child and still perform a satisfactory exam. If parents are unavailable or unhelpful, try to elicit the help of one of the nursing staff or another sonographer. The principal sonographer, however, must devote her or his full attention to the sonographic exam.

Nomenclature/Standard Views

In the discussions that follow, certain types of standard views are referenced. Since many views are not standard in the pediatric patient, the following illustrations and descriptions will aid the reader in obtaining the necessary views.

PARASTERNAL VIEWS

- *Long axis* (Fig. 29-1): The standard long-axis view, which allows visualization of left ventricular inflow and outflow with the interventricular septum perpendicular to the ultrasound plane, is the best view for M-mode measurements. From this orientation, the transducer is angled toward the

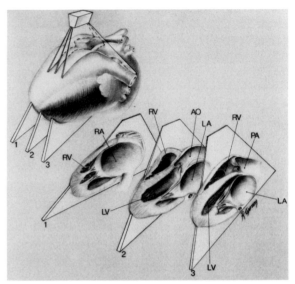

Figure 29-1. Parasternal long-axis views. These views are obtained by holding the transducer at the third to fourth left intercostal space, angled from the right shoulder to the left hip, and tilting from right to left. Plane 1 shows the right atrium (RA), tricuspid valve, and part of the right ventricular inflow tract. Plane 2 shows the left atrium (LA), mitral valve (MV), left ventricle (LV), aortic valve, and ascending aorta. In this plane, a portion of the right ventricle (RV) is also seen. In Plane 3, the right ventricular outflow tract, including the right ventricle, pulmonary valve, and main pulmonary artery (PA), is seen. (From Snider AR, Serwer GA. *Echocardiography in Pediatric Heart Disease.* Chicago, YearBook Medical Publishers; 1990:25. Reprinted with permission.)

head and tilted anteriorly; this view provides another view of the right ventricular outflow tract.
- *Short axis* (Fig. 29-2): With the transducer in the same position as for a long-axis view, the transducer is rotated 90 degrees clockwise. This view also allows good visualization of the left ventricle in cross section when angled toward the apex. When the transducer is angled toward the right shoulder, the aortic valve is seen in cross section and finally the right ventricular outflow tract (RVOT), pulmonary valve, main pulmonary artery, and left and right pulmonary arteries.

APICAL VIEWS (Fig. 29-3)

Although the standard orientation described in earlier chapters is accepted, most institutions performing pediatric echocardiograms prefer to have these views in the anatomically correct orientation—that is, with the image inverted so that the position of the transducer is at the bottom of the screen rather than at the top.

- *Four-chamber:* With the patient in the left lateral decubitus position, the transducer is held in a short-axis orientation, placed beyond the apex of the heart and angled toward the right shoulder. This view demonstrates pulmonary veins, both atria, atrioventricular (AV) valves, and ventricles.
- *Five-chamber:* In the same position as for the four-chamber view, the transducer is angled ante-

riorly. This view demonstrates the left atrium, mitral valve inflow, left ventricular outflow, aortic valve, and a short portion of the ascending aorta.

- *Long axis:* The transducer is held in the same position as for the four-chamber view and rotated 90 degrees counterclockwise. This view shows the left ventricular outflow tract (LVOT), especially the subaortic area. This view is best for color Doppler evaluation of left ventricular inflow and outflow.

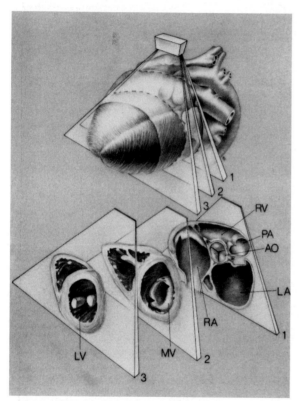

Figure 29-2. Parasternal short-axis views. These views are obtained by holding the transducer in the same position as the parasternal long-axis views but rotating it 90 degrees clockwise, then tilting from left hip to right shoulder. Starting with plane 3, the apices of the right ventricle (RV) and left ventricle (LV) and the mitral valve papillary muscles are seen. Sweeping toward the right shoulder, plane 2 demonstrates the mitral valve apparatus. In plane 1, the right atrium (RA), tricuspid valve, right ventricle, pulmonary valve, and a portion of the main pulmonary artery (PA) are seen. In addition, the three leaflets of the aortic valve (AO) are seen centrally. (From Snider AR, Serwer GA. *Echocardiography in Pediatric Heart Disease.* Chicago, YearBook Medical Publishers; 1990:29. Reprinted with permission.)

SUPRASTERNAL VIEWS (Figs. 29-4 and 29-5)

- *Aortic arch:* In this view, the reference point of the transducer is toward the left shoulder, allowing visualization of the aortic root and transverse arch. Rotating toward the left hip and keeping the transverse arch in view will allow visualization of the continuation to the descending aorta. This is a good view for color Doppler interrogation of the descending aorta. Unfortunately, this is not an easy view to obtain in newborn infants. In newborns, the arch can be seen more easily from the right supraclavicular area. If the infant is intubated or if the airway can be monitored, place a small pillow or rolled-up blanket under the shoulders and hyperextend the neck.

SUBCOSTAL VIEWS (Figs. 29-6 and 29-7)

- *Four-chamber:* This view is obtained by holding the transducer in a short-axis orientation in the subxiphoid area and angling anteriorly. This allows the best view of pulmonary veins and the best color Doppler interrogation of their flow characteristics. This is also the best view for evaluating all aspects of the interatrial septum with 2D and color Doppler. For patients with poor apical windows, this is also a good view for evaluating the relative sizes of atria and ventricles and AV valve flows.
- *Long axis:* In this view, the transducer is held in a plane parallel to the child's spine. The inferior vena cava (IVC), hepatic veins, descending aorta, liver, and part of the heart can be seen. Of particular interest in this view is the insertion of the IVC and superior vena cava (SVC) into the right atrium. Angling to the patient's left will demon-

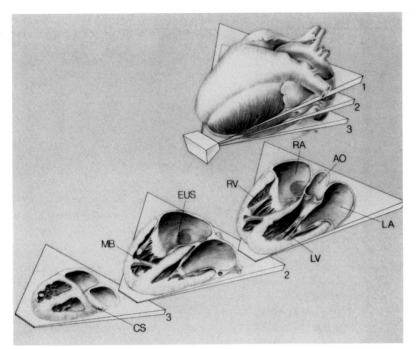

Figure 29-3. Apical four-chamber views. These views are obtained by holding the transducer at the apex, angled from the left axilla to the right hip, rotating posteriorly to anteriorly. Plane 3 is the most inferior view and shows the four chambers and the coronary sinus (CS). Plane 2 shows the four chambers, the tricuspid and mitral valve leaflets, the moderator band (MB) of the RV, and the eustachian valve (EUS). AO, ascending aorta; RA, right atrium; RV, right ventricle; LA, left atrium; LV, left ventricle. (From Snider AR, Serwer GA. *Echocardiography in Pediatric Heart Disease*. Chicago, Year-Book Medical Publishers; 1990:33. Reprinted with permission.)

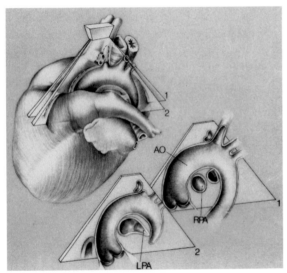

Figure 29-4. Suprasternal long-axis views. These views are obtained by holding the transducer in the suprasternal notch, angling from head to feet and rotating from right to left. In plane 1, the ascending aorta (AO), transverse aortic arch, and descending aorta are seen, as are the vessels coming off the top of the arch. Inside the arch is the right pulmonary artery (RPA) in cross section. In plane 2, the ascending aorta and transverse arch are seen, and the left pulmonary artery (LPA) is seen in a tangential view as it courses away from the right ventricle. (From Snider AR, Serwer GA. *Echocardiography in Pediatric Heart Disease*. Chicago, YearBook Medical Publishers; 1990:48. Reprinted with permission.)

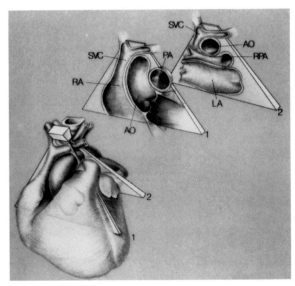

Figure 29-5. Suprasternal short-axis views. These views are obtained by holding the transducer in the suprasternal notch, rotating the transducer 90 degrees clockwise from the previous planes, and angling inferiorly and then superiorly. Plane 1 demonstrates the ascending aorta (AO), pulmonary artery (PA), superior vena cava (SVC), and right atrium (RA). Plane 2 demonstrates the SVC superiorly, the aorta (AO) in cross section, the right pulmonary artery (RPA), and the left atrium (LA). (From Snider RA, Serwer GA. *Echocardiography in Pediatric Heart Disease*. Chicago, YearBook Medical Publishers; 1990:51. Reprinted with permission.)

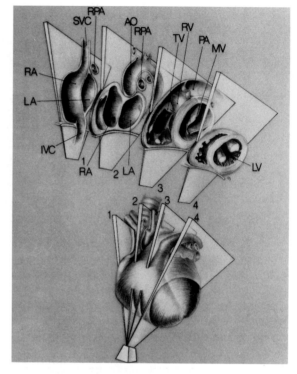

Figure 29-6. Subcostal short-axis views. These views are obtained by holding the transducer below the xiphoid process in the upper abdomen, angled from right to left and tilting from right to left. In plane 1, the superior vena cava (SVC), right atrium (RA), and inferior vena cava (IVC) are seen. In plane 2, the aortic arch (AO) is visualized, as are the right atrium (RA) and left atrium (LA). In plane 3, the right ventricular outflow tract is visualized with the tricuspid valve (TV), right ventricle (RV), and pulmonary artery (PV). In plane 4, the apices of both ventricles are seen, as are the mitral valve papillary muscles in the left ventricle (LV). RPA, right pulmonary artery. (From Snider AR, Serwer GA. *Echocardiography in Pediatric Heart Disease.* Chicago, YearBook Medical Publishers; 1990:44. Reprinted with permission.)

strate the right ventricular inflow and outflow tracts. To the left of the pulmonary valve is the aortic valve. Rotate the transducer toward the right shoulder to visualize the aortic root, ascending aorta, and transverse arch.

Segmental Approach

Identification of the visceral and intracardiac structures in complex heart disease requires knowledge of the characteristics of each structure.[16]

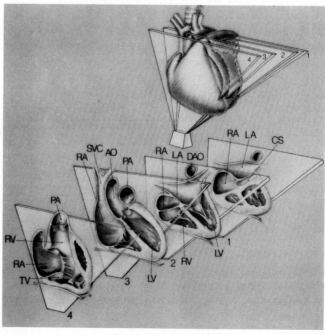

Figure 29-7. Subcostal four-chamber views. These views are obtained by holding the transducer below the xiphoid process in the upper abdomen, angled from right shoulder to left hip, and tilting from left to right. In plane 1, the right atrium (RA) with the entrance of the coronary sinus (CS) is seen. In plane 2, a small portion of the right atrium (RA) and right ventricle (RV) are seen. In addition, the left atrium (LA) in a transverse cut, the mitral valve, and the left ventricle (LV) are seen. In plane 3, the superior vena cava (SVC) and right atrium (RA) are well visualized. Also well seen in this plane are the left ventricle (LV), aortic valve, and aorta (AO). In plane 4, the right atrium, tricuspid valve (TV), right ventricular outflow tract (RV), and pulmonary artery (PA) are well seen. DAO, descending aortic arch. (From Snider AR, Serwer GA. *Echocardiography in Pediatric Heart Disease.* Chicago, YearBook Medical Publishers; 1990:40. Reprinted with permission.)

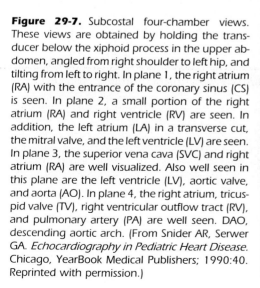

With the transducer at the midline of the abdomen and in a transverse plane, scan the abdomen, caudad to cephalad, to assess the configuration of the liver. In normal visceral situs, the majority of the liver is in the right portion of the abdomen, with a small "tail" extending across the midline to the left. On the opposite side of the abdomen is the stomach. With the transducer in a longitudinal plane, find the spine. The transducer is tilted to the left and right of the spine to define the IVC and aorta. A pulsed wave Doppler sample is placed in each of these vessels to confirm the configurations of arterial or venous flow. Follow the IVC cephalad, making sure that it communicates directly with the right atrium. If the IVC-to-right atrium connection cannot be found, hepatic veins may be the only venous structures emptying into the right atrium. If the IVC does not connect to the right atrium, locate the coronary sinus or SVC to help define the right atrium; each may anomalously return elsewhere, however.

If the major portion of the liver is to the right, the stomach is to the left, the IVC is on the right of the spine and enters the right atrium, the aorta is to the left of the spine, the visceral situs is assumed to be normal—*visceral situs solitus.* If all findings are the opposite of normal, then *visceral situs inversus* exists. If there are findings which do not fit either category, the term *visceral situs ambiguous* is used; it implies only that the classic configurations of situs solitus and situs inversus do not exist in this patient.

The initial evaluation of the heart should define the position of its long axis. If the long axis shows the apex to the left with the base at the midline, *levocardia* exists. If the long axis is opposite to this, so that the apex is to the right with the base at the midline, *dextrocardia* exists. *Mesocardia* exists if the apex is toward the midline, as is the base.

Finally, the intracardiac connections must be defined. In the longitudinal plane, the IVC should be seen running through the diaphragm into the heart. The entry of the *suprahepatic IVC* into the atrium defines this as a right atrium. Confusion can result from large hepatic veins entering the right atrium, as is seen with azygous continuation of the IVC to the SVC. Normally, the abdominal IVC courses cephalad into the right atrium, with hepatic veins entering the IVC defining this chamber as the right atrium. If the IVC does not enter the atrium, locate the coronary sinus, which will also define a right atrium if it is not unroofed.

With the transducer in a transverse plane, note the relationship between the right and left atria. If the morphologic right atrium is on the right and the morphologic left atrium is on the left, this is *atrial situs solitus.* If the reverse is seen, *atrial situs inversus* exists.

In the apical four-chamber view, the *morphologic right ventricle* is identified by the moderator band, by the more heavily trabeculated endocardium, and by the AV valve hinge points, which are deeper (further from the atrium) in the ventricle than are the left AV valve hinge points (Fig. 29-8). In addition, in a short-axis or long-axis view of the right ventricle, there is tissue between the tricuspid valve and the semilunar valve; there is essentially none in a left ventricle. Rotating and angling the transducer will locate the right ventricular outflow tract. There should be an identifiable outflow or infundibular portion, bordered on all sides by ventricular muscle.

In a parasternal short-axis view, visualize the great vessel coming off the right ventricle. If there is a bifurcation of this vessel, it is probably the *pulmonary artery.* Differentiate this vessel from the aortic arch, which will be identified later. Color Doppler may identify a ductus arteriosus entering near the left pulmonary artery, which will further assist in identifying this artery. In complex congenital heart

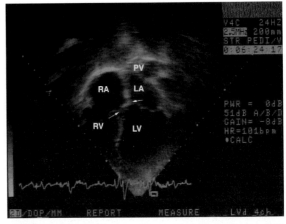

Figure 29-8. Relative positions of atrioventricular (AV) valves in the left and right ventricles. Note that the medial hinge point of the tricuspid valve (arrow between the right atrium [RA] and right ventricle [RV]) is more apical than the hinge point of the mitral valve (arrow between the left atrium [LA] and left ventricle [LV]). PV, pulmonary valve.

disease, some creative scanning is needed to define the plane of the bifurcation of the pulmonary artery. In a predominantly short-axis orientation, the transducer is moved in a cephalad and leftward position if the cardiac apex is to the left, caudad and rightward if the cardiac apex is to the right. On occasion, the only view of the bifurcation will be a subcostal view. This view is often difficult to obtain in infants, however. The short-axis subcostal view requires placement of the largest axis of the transducer in the smallest angle of the subcostal triangle and angling as far anterior as possible, which is difficult in small infants.

Once the great vessel associated with the right ventricle is identified, the anatomic evaluation of the right heart is complete. Attention should then be turned to the pulmonary veins; if they all enter one atrium, they will assist in identifying that atrium as a *morphologic left atrium* (Fig. 29-9). Next, evaluate the AV valve from the left atrium in the short axis; a *mitral valve* will have two leaflets and should have two distinct papillary muscles at the 4 o'clock and 8 o'clock positions. The mitral valve hinge points are higher (closer to the atrium) in the ventricle than all those of the tricuspid valve (Fig. 29-8).

A *morphologic left ventricle* is usually smooth-walled, with a slipper shape in the long axis and a circular shape in the short axis. There should be no infundibular chamber or tissue between the AV and semilunar valves on the echocardiogram. The out-flow tract is defined by IVS on one side and the mitral valve on the other.

The great vessel arising from the leftward ventricle is the last major structure to be identified. In the short-axis view, coronary ostia arising from this vessel help define this great vessel as an *aorta*. In the subcostal view, define the left ventricle, left ventricular outflow tract, ascending aorta, transverse arch, and a small portion of the descending aorta.

At this point in the study, identification of the connections between major veins and atria, atria and ventricles, and ventricles and great vessels should be complete. If any of the major structures cannot be located, more creative positioning and angling of the transducer and/or patient may be helpful.

MEASUREMENTS

Since pediatric patients range in weight from 0.5 to 100 kg and in height from 20 to 200 cm, normal values must be based on body size. Although there are normal values based on height, normalization by body surface area (BSA) is used since it takes into account both height and weight. All measurements listed below are based on BSA unless otherwise specified. To calculate BSA, the child's recent height and weight are necessary. Many ultrasound machine software packages or computer echo report software packages will calculate BSA when height and weight are input. The following formula can be used to calculate it manually:

$$BSA = 0.0001 \times 71.84 \times (weight)\, 0.425$$
$$\times (height)^{0.725}$$

Alternatively, Figure 29-10 can be used.

For M-mode measurements, see Figure 29-11.

For normal value diameters in millimeters, see Figure 29-12.

Qp:Qs

The magnitude of a left-to-right shunt is often important in clinical disease. From catheterization data, cardiologists evaluate shunts by comparing the volume of blood going to the lungs (Qp) with the volume of blood going to the aorta (Qs). Measurements made in the catheterization lab allow an estimation of the ratio of those flows (Qp:Qs). Measurements made in the echocardiography lab can also estimate that ratio. Since estimates of volume

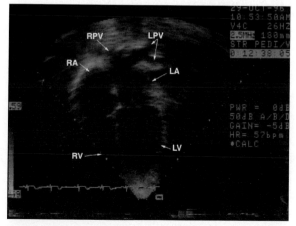

Figure 29-9. Pulmonary veins. In the apical four-chamber view, the right (RPV) and left (LPV) pulmonary veins can be seen entering the left atrium. LA, left atrium; LV, left ventricle; RA, right atrium; RV, right ventricle.

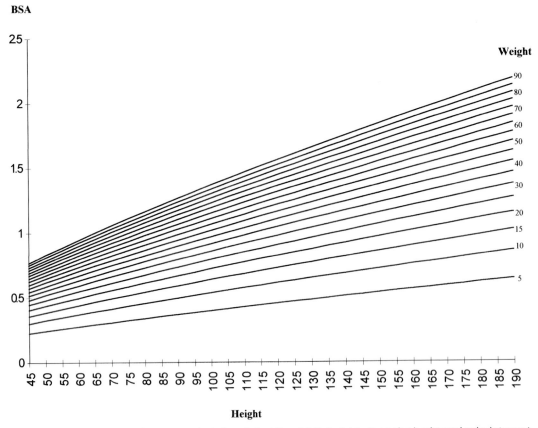

Figure 29-10. Body surface area calculation. Select the child's height along the horizontal axis; intersect it with the child's weight (on the right vertical axis); read across to the body surface area (BSA) on the left vertical axis.

in echocardiography are based on the area of the orifice through which the blood flows and the integral of the velocity profile, the use of the annulus size and flow characteristics across the annulus provides the measurements. In most cases, the pulmonary annulus and aortic annulus are the most appropriate structures for these measurements.

In certain circumstances, further changes in relative volumes occur after blood crosses these two valves, necessitating other measurements. For example, if there is a patent ductus arteriosus, such that increased pulmonary blood flow enters the pulmonary artery beyond the pulmonary valve, the valve used to estimate the pulmonary flow is the mitral valve (unless there is a coexistent atrial septal defect); systemic blood flow is estimated by flow returning to the right atrium across the tricuspid valve.

PULMONARY ARTERY PRESSURE ESTIMATES

To estimate pulmonary artery pressure, there must be communication between the pulmonary artery and a chamber or vessel whose pressure can be measured or inferred accurately. Thus, pulmonary artery pressure can be measured in any of the following circumstances:

- Patent ductus arteriosus (PDA) or systemic-to-pulmonary artery shunts
- Ventricular septal defect (VSD)
- Tricuspid insufficiency (TI)

All pulmonary artery pressure estimations are based on the modified Bernoulli equation[5]:

Pressure

$$= 4 \times velocity^2 \text{ (where velocity is in m/sec)}$$

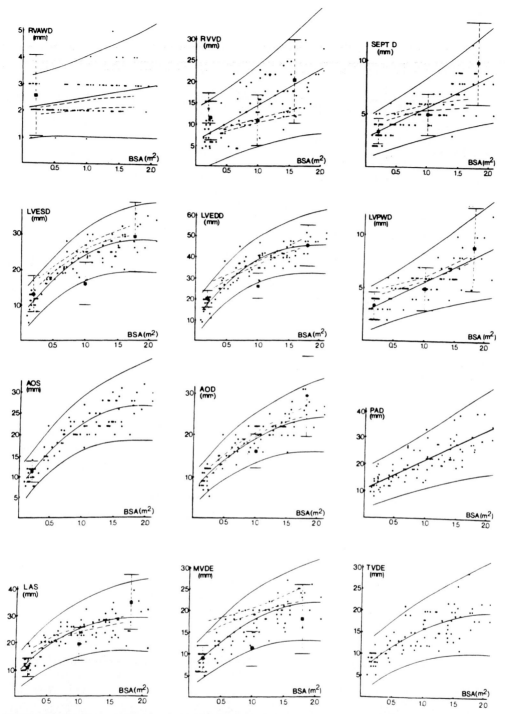

Figure 29-11. M-mode measurements by body surface area (BSA). For each measurement, select the correct BSA for the patient. Follow the graph vertically to see the 10%ile, 50%ile, and 90%ile for BSA. RVAWD, right ventricular anterior wall thickness in diastole; RVDD, right ventricular end-diastolic dimension; SEPT D, septal thickness at end diastole; LVESD, left ventricular end-diastolic dimension; LVEDD, left ventricular end-diastolic dimension, LVPWD, left ventricular posterior wall thickness at end diastole; AOS, aortic diameter in systole; AOD, aortic diameter in diastole; PDA, pulmonary artery diameter; LAS, left atrial dimension in systole; MVDS, anterior mitral valve leaflet excursion; TVDE, anterior tricuspid valve leaflet excursion. (From Roge CLL, Silverman NH, Hart PA. *Circulation*. 1978;57:288. Reprinted with permission.)

Measures of LV Function	Normals
Measurements of LV systolic function	
%FS = (LVDD − LVDS) / LVDD	>0.28
Ejection fraction = (LVEDv2 − LVESv^2) / LVEDv^2	50–70%
Vcf = (LVDD − LVDS) / (LVDD × LVET)	1.5 ± .04 (infants)
	1.3 ± .03 (2–10 years)
LV end-systolic wall stress (4) =	
$[(1.35)(P_{es})(D_{es})] / (4)(h_{es})[1 + (h_{es} / D_{es})]$ =	47.5 ± 7.0 g/cm^2
where P_{es} = end-systolic pressure,	
D_{es} = LVDs	
h_{es} = LVPWd	
Measurements of LV diastolic function (14):	
Mitral inflow velocity measures:	
E =	80 ± 20 cm/sec (adolescent)
	53.2 ± 9.3 cm/sec (day 1)
	50.2 ± 7.9 cm/sec (day 2)
	91 ± .11 cm/sec (>10 years)
A =	50 ± 20 cm/sec (adolescent)
	47.6 ± 5.8 cm/sec (day 1)
	48.7 ± 8.3 cm/sec (day 2)
	50 ± .08 cm/sec (>10 years)
E/A =	1.15 ± .17 cm/sec (1 day)
	1.00 ± .25 cm/sec (2 days)
	1.87 ± .39 cm/sec (>10 years)

Measures of LV Function	Normals
LV mass = $1.05 × \pi\{(b + t)2 × [2/3(a + t) + d − (d^3 / 3(a + t)^2)]$	66 ± 11 g/M2 (female)
$− b2 × [2/3(a) + d − (d^3 / 3a^2)]\}$	73 ± 13 g/M2 (male)
where b = (LVd Area SAX / π)1/2 SAX = short-axis endocardial	
t = (Lvd area SAXepi / π)1/2 − b SAXepi = short-axis epicardial	
a = left ventricle long-axis major length calculated from LVd length 4ch	
d = left ventricle long-axis minor length calculated from LVd length 4ch	

Since a *PDA* or *shunt* is a direct communication between the aorta and the pulmonary artery, and since aortic pressure can be measured accurately by a blood pressure cuff, the velocity of flow across the shunt will allow estimation of pulmonary artery pressure by subtracting the gradient across the shunt from the systolic cuff pressure:

Pulmonary artery (PA) pressure = aortic (Ao) pressure

− pressure gradient from Ao to PA

(So, if PDA maximum velocity = 4 m/sec and aortic pressure = 90 mm Hg, then PA pressure = (90 mm Hg − (4 × 42)) = (90 − 64) = 26 mm Hg).

If a *VSD* is present, left ventricular pressure can be estimated using Doppler evaluation if the left ventricular outflow tract (LVOT) is not obstructed.

If flow across the LVOT is laminar and of normal velocity, then assume that the left ventricular systolic pressure is the same as the cuff blood pressure. The gradient across the VSD can be subtracted from the systolic cuff pressure to estimate right ventricular pressure. To estimate pulmonary artery pressure accurately, the right ventricular outflow tract (RVOT) must also be without obstruction. If there is no gradient across the RVOT, then pulmonary artery pressure is assumed to be equal to right ventricular pressure.

If PA pressure = RV pressure (no gradient across RVOT) and LV pressure = Ao pressure (no gradient across LVOT), then

PA pressure = RV pressure = LV pressure

− VSD gradient

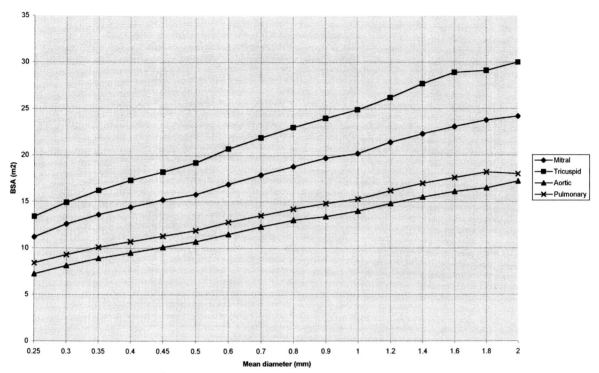

Figure 29-12. Valve diameters by body surface area (BSA). Mean diameter for each valve is indicated in millimeters. (Adapted from Rowlatt, *Surg Clin North Am.* 1963; and Stark J, deLeval M (eds). *Surgery for Congenital Heart disease.* London, Grune & Stratton; 1983.

For example, if aortic pressure = 90 mm Hg and VSD gradient = 350 cm/sec, then PA pressure = 90 mm Hg − (4 × 3.5²) = (90 − 50) = 40 mm Hg.

There are several pitfalls to this method of estimating pressures. Nonparallel Doppler tends to underestimate the velocity and therefore overestimate the right ventricular pressure. Also, it is difficult to interrogate a VSD or shunt/PDA from a position which is exactly parallel to flow. Therefore, a second estimate of right ventricular pressure via a tricuspid insufficiency jet can be used to confirm the pressure estimation. In the presence of *tricuspid insufficiency*, the maximum velocity can be measured by continuous wave Doppler from the apical four-chamber view. By TI gradient, the predicted right ventricular pressure is:

RV pressure = (4 × velocity2)

+ RA pressure (usually estimated as 10 mm Hg)

For example, if TI velocity = 300 cm/sec, then RV pressure = ([3² × 4] + 10) = (36 + 10) = 46 mm Hg. This gives two independent estimates of right ventricular pressure. In our institution, the TI estimate is usually more reliable.

Surgical Procedures in Pediatric Heart Disease and Postoperative Echocardiographic Exams

This section briefly describes surgical procedures used in the treatment of congenital heart disease in children. Each procedure is further described in the section on the specific form of heart disease for which it is utilized.

- *Atrial septal defect closure.* Some ASDs are closed with a suture, others with a pericardial patch. Postoperatively, the patch will appear brighter

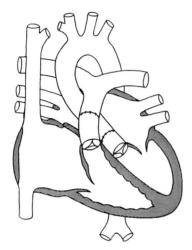

Figure 29-13. Arterial switch. The aorta and pulmonary artery are transected above the valve and coronary artery ostia. The appropriate vessel is attached to the existing stump from the transposed great vessel. (From Mullins CE, Mayer DC. *Congenital Heart Disease: A Diagrammatic Atlas.* Diagram 150. Chicago, YearBook Medical Publishers; 1990. Reprinted by permission of Wiley-Liss, Inc., a division of John Wiley & Sons, Inc.)

and thicker than the surrounding tissue but will move as a normal, intact atrial septum. Currently under investigation are devices inserted in the catheterization lab which permanently close the ASD.

- *Aortic/pulmonary valvulotomy.* Many children have sufficient relief of aortic or pulmonary valve obstruction with a valvulotomy; the commissures of the native valve are incised such that function of the valve is much more normal. This procedure is almost always associated with some degree of valvular regurgitation postoperatively.

- *Arterial switch* (Fig. 29-13). The aorta and pulmonary artery are transected above the valves and reanastomosed, establishing normal patterns of blood flow. Coronary arteries, which had arisen from the aorta on the right, are removed and reattached to the new aorta on the left.

- *Bidirectional Glenn procedure.* Like the Glenn shunt, which attaches the SVC to the pulmonary artery, this procedure divides the SVC near the point where the right pulmonary artery crosses it. The top part of the SVC is attached to the top of the right pulmonary artery; the bottom of the SVC is attached to the bottom of the right pulmonary artery. Thus blood flow from the SVC

goes into the right pulmonary artery; IVC blood goes into the right atrium. Any runoff from either vena cava can go either into the right atrium or pulmonary artery.

- *Coarctation of aorta repair.* There are two types of repair of coarctation of the aorta. In older children, the area of narrowing is simply excised and the two ends of the aorta are reattached (*end-to-end anastomosis*). In younger children, since this area of the aorta can be quite narrow, the subclavian artery is ligated and divided. This tissue is pulled down over the area of the coarctation and sewn into a longitudinal incision in the aorta, acting as a living tissue graft (*subclavian flap procedure*). Coarctation repairs which become stenotic are often addressed in the catheterization lab with balloon dilatation angioplasty.

- *Endocardial cushion defect (ECD) repair* (Fig. 29-14). Repair of ECD involves placement of patches which close both ventricular and atrial defects. The common AV valve is divided, and each side is reattached to the patch at the appropriate level.

- *Fontan procedure* (Fig. 29-15). The classic Fontan procedure separates the right atrium from the rest of the heart via a Gore-Tex baffle. The SVC and IVC blood flow into the right atrium. The right atrial appendage is attached to the pulmonary artery and the pulmonary valve is oversewn;

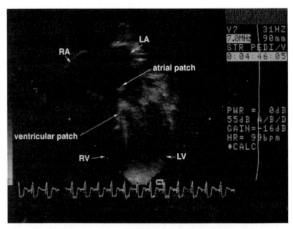

Figure 29-14. Repair of endocardial cushion defect. A patch is placed over the atrial septum to cover the atrial defect; a second patch is placed on the right ventricular (RV) side of the ventricular defect. RA, right atrium; RV, right ventricle; LA, left atrium; LV, left ventricle.

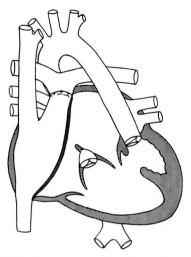

Figure 29-15. Fontan procedure. The pulmonary artery is transected and the proximal stump oversewn. Thus there is no exit of blood from the heart to the pulmonary artery. The right atrial appendage is sewn to the distal portion of the pulmonary artery, providing desaturated venous blood to the pulmonary artery. (From Mullins CE, Mayer DC. *Congenital Heart Disease: A Diagrammatic Atlas.* Diagram 157. Chicago, YearBook Medical Publishers; 1990. Reprinted with permission.)

thus right atrial systemic venous blood flows via the right atrial appendage into the pulmonary artery. Lately, the bidirectional Glenn procedure has been performed first; at a later date, the Gore-Tex baffle is inserted and the pulmonary valve oversewn.

- *Infundibular resection.* In children with dynamic RVOT obstruction, especially those with tetralogy of Fallot, resection of muscle tissue in the subvalvular area of the RVOT provides sufficient relief of obstruction.

- *Staged reconstruction of HLHS.* The staged reconstruction of HLHS is performed primarily in infants with hypoplastic left heart syndrome and has three stages. In the first stage, the Norwood procedure, the small aorta and the dilated pulmonary artery are combined to form one large great vessel. Since the coronary arteries come off the aorta, they are now part of the single great vessel. The branch pulmonary arteries are disconnected from the main pulmonary artery and a shunt is created between the descending aorta and the pulmonary arteries. The second stage is a Hemi-Fontan procedure in which the SVC is transected

and each end sewn into the right pulmonary artery (bidirectional Glenn shunt). At the third stage, the IVC and SVC are baffled away from the right atrium, such that systemic venous return does not enter the right atrium but goes directly to the pulmonary arteries. Pulmonary venous return thus enters the left atrium, crosses the atrial septum to the right atrium, passes through the tricuspid valve into the right ventricle and is pumped out the new aorta. Although morbidity and mortality are relatively high, many children survive these stages and live comfortably. Others require cardiac transplantation before the second or third stage.

- *Patent ductus arteriosus (PDA) ligation.* The PDA is usually ligated with two or three separate sutures through the ductus.

- *Pulmonary valvulectomy.* In some children with a very abnormal pulmonary valve, removal of the valve provides relief of obstruction and the degree of regurgitation is usually handled well. Some children, however, cannot tolerate the degree of pulmonary regurgitation and require insertion of a prosthetic valve at a later date.

- *Rastelli procedure* (Fig. 29-16). In children with double outlet right ventricle or pulmonary atresia

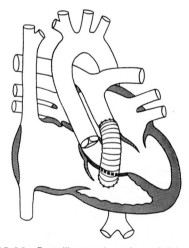

Figure 29-16. Rastelli procedure. A conduit is placed between the body of the right ventricle and the pulmonary artery, creating unobstructed from flow to the lungs. The ventricular septal defect is closed with a patch that commits the aorta solely to the left ventricle. (From Mullins CE, Mayer DC. *Congenital Heart Disease: A Diagrammatic Atlas.* Diagram 155. Chicago, YearBook Medical Publishers; 1990. Reprinted by permission of Wiley-Liss, Inc., a division of John Wiley & Sons, Inc.)

and VSD, the VSD is usually closed in such a way that the LV outflow exits only via the aorta. A tube graft with or without a valve is attached from the body of the right ventricle to the pulmonary artery. On echocardiography, the tube graft is often difficult to visualize. The VSD patch is clearly seen, as is the discontinuity between the aorta and the ventricular septum.

- *RVOT patch.* In children with narrow subpulmonary outflow tracts, especially those with Tetralogy of Fallot, an incision beginning near the bifurcation of the pulmonary artery and extending across the outflow tract into the body of the right ventricle is made. A diamond-shaped patch of Gore-Tex is sewn to the edges of this incision, forming a wider outflow tract than before. On 2D echocardiography this area will appear echogenic and will not contract with the rest of the ventricle. If the patch rests under the sternum, there may be a noticeable compression of the patch anteriorly.

- *Shunts.* In infants with obstruction to right ventricular outflow (Tetralogy of Fallot, pulmonary atresia, and many forms of complex congenital heart disease), a shunt can be placed which provides increased blood flow to the lungs. The most common anastomosis is the *Blalock-Taussig shunt*, a connection between the subclavian artery on the side opposite the aortic arch (usually the right subclavian artery) and the pulmonary artery on that side. The *Glenn shunt* (SVC to right pulmonary artery), *Potts anastomosis* (descending aorta to left pulmonary artery, and *Waterston shunt* (ascending aorta to pulmonary artery) may be seen in older children and young adults operated on in earlier years.

- *Unifocalization.* In children without a main pulmonary artery, the unifocalization procedure attempts to combine all separate pulmonary arteries into one central vessel which can eventually be connected to the RVOT.

- *VSD closure.* Most VSDs are closed from the right ventricular side with a patch of Gore-Tex. Immediately postoperatively, color Doppler flow can be seen as very narrow, high-velocity jets, crossing the ventricular septum, which probably represents small leaks between the sutures. These jets usually disappear by the end of the first postoperative week. The area of the patch remains echogenic and does not move with the rest of the ventricular septum since it has no contractile properties of its own.

- *Postoperative echocardiography.* The purpose of postoperative studies should be to evaluate the status of the surgical procedure and thus are specific to the type of defect. There are some issues, however, which are general to all postoperative cases and are common to all postoperative studies. There is always some bleeding from the incision for the first few days after surgery. Since the heart is contained within the pericardial sac, that blood may collect in the pericardium. Although there are tubes which should drain this fluid, they do not always work efficiently. Thus, one of the major areas to evaluate on a postoperative study is the pericardium. If anything more than a scant amount of fluid is visualized, evidence of tamponade should be sought. In the apical four-chamber view, you may see right atrial wall collapse into the atrium late in diastole; this is one sign of tamponade.[11] Another way to evaluate tamponade is to place a pulsed wave Doppler cursor in the aorta or pulmonary artery. With the paper speed slowed to minimum, record the Doppler outflow signal for a full minute. Measure the maximal and minimal peak velocities recorded during this time. If the difference is greater than 10%, tamponade is suggested.[2]

Patient Ductus Arteriosus

Isolated PDA (Table 29-1) is seen commonly in premature infants and less frequently in full-term infants. The left-to-right shunt across the PDA creates symptoms of congestive heart failure or respiratory problems in the premature infant and thus represents an acute medical problem affecting cardiovascular and respiratory stability.

ANATOMY

The ductus arteriosus is a vessel present in fetal life which connects the proximal left pulmonary artery with the descending aorta just below the left subclavian artery takeoff (Figure 29-17). In fetal life it provides a bypass route for blood entering the right heart to go directly to the descending aorta. Its cellular structure is different from that of either the pulmonary artery or the aorta. It's elastic properties are much greater than either of the great vessels and its diameter is affected by the oxygen saturation of blood flowing through it and by circulating Prostaglandins.

◢◢◢ TABLE 29-1. PATENT DUCTUS ARTERIOSUS

Question to Be Answered	Views	Comments
Antegrade flow across pulmonary valve	Short axis Long axis—RVOT Suprasternal	*Must* see antegrade flow from right ventricle to pulmonary artery to rule out ductal-dependent pulmonary blood flow.
Direction of ductal flow	Short axis Long axis—RVOT Aortic Arch	Is flow from aorta to pulmonary artery or from pulmonary artery to aorta?
Size of left atrium, left ventricle	Four-chamber Long axis—LVOT	If left-to-right flow is moderate to large in volume, left atrium will be dilated. M-mode for left atrium/aorta ratio will help define size of left atrium.
Pulmonary artery pressure	Suprasternal Short axis—second right intercostal space (2RICS)	Use continuous wave Doppler in PDA to estimate gradient from aorta to pulmonary artery.
Other associated defects	Four-chamber	*Must* evaluate entire heart and aortic arch for structural abnormalities.

PHYSIOLOGY

In fetal life, the ductus arteriosus allows oxygenated blood delivered by the placenta to bypass the lungs and enter the systemic circulation. While some blood flows from the RV into the main pulmonary artery (MPA) and to the lungs, most goes through the MPA and ductus to the descending aorta, providing oxygenated blood for the lower body. At the time of delivery, as a full-term infant begins to breathe, pulmonary vascular resistance drops rapidly. At the same time, the oxygen saturation in blood flowing through the ductus arteriosus rises. Prostaglandins which were provided by the placenta are now absent. Those prostaglandins, which are formed in the walls of the ductus arteriosus, are quickly catabolized in the lung once breathing is initiated. The combination of increased oxygen saturation in the blood flowing through the ductus and a decrease in circulating prostaglandins causes the ductus arteriosus in most newborns to constrict over the first few days of life and then to undergo cellular changes which involve eventual necrosis and scarring of the intima, preventing future patency of the vessel.

In some *full-term newborns*, the ductus arteriosus fails to constrict after delivery. Such newborn infants also seem to require a longer period of time for their pulmonary vascular resistance to drop. Since the degree of left-to-right shunting across the ductus arteriosus is related to the internal diameter of the ductus and the pressure across the ductus, and since the pressure gradient from aorta to pulmonary artery is still low, these infants have relatively low ductal flow in the perinatal period. With growth of the other vessels, even after the pulmonary resistance drops to near-adult levels, the relative size of

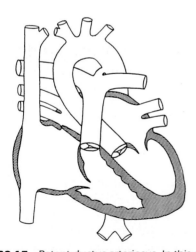

Figure 29-17. Patent ductus arteriosus. In this defect, all structures and connections are normal. The ductus arteriosus, between the descending aorta and left pulmonary artery, does not close spontaneously after birth. Thus there is excess blood flow into the lungs from the aorta via the ductus arteriosus. (From Mullins CE, Mayer DC. *Congenital Heart Disease: A Diagrammatic Atlas.* Diagram 53. Chicago, YearBook Medical Publishers; 1990. Reprinted by permission of Wiley-Liss, Inc., a division of John Wiley & Sons, Inc.)

the ductus is diminished and thus the left-to-right flow remains small. Thus, these infants rarely develop congestive heart failure from their PDAs.

In *premature infants*, the PDA plays a much different role. Pulmonary resistance may drop only slightly after delivery; a further decrease in resistance may take months, and resistance may never drop to normal levels. During fetal life, the diameter of the ductus arteriosus is the same as that of the aortic diameter. While pulmonary resistance is greater than systemic resistance, there is right-to-left shunting across the PDA. Unless there is a large pressure gradient however, the total volume of flow across the PDA will be small. As the pulmonary resistance begins to drop, however, the left-to-right flow across the ductus may be quite large. This increased flow into lungs which are immature can make these preterm infants very ill.

If flow through a PDA is from right to left, there will be no noticeable changes in chamber dimensions or contractility. Color Doppler will show no evidence of a PDA within the MPA or branch PAs. Doppler in the ductus itself will show low-velocity right-to-left flow with some left-to-right flow. Doppler in the aortic arch, however, will show flow coming from the ductus into the aorta, and pulsed wave Doppler will confirm it.

If flow through a PDA is from left to right, there is an increased volume of blood to the pulmonary arteries, and the pulmonary veins, left atrium, and left ventricle may be dilated. If the volume of flow is large enough, left ventricular contractility may be increased. Because of the increased flow to the left atrium, left ventricular volume will be increased and the atrial septum will bow to the right.

CLINICAL PROBLEMS

If flow through a PDA is from right to left, desaturated blood enters the systemic circulation below the left subclavian artery. Therefore, oxygen saturations measured in the upper extremities will be higher than those measured in the lower extremities. If pulmonary resistance is very high, there may be noticeable cyanosis in the infant's lower body.

The size of the shunt across the PDA is determined by the internal diameter of the ductus relative to that of the great vessels and the pressure gradient between the aorta and the pulmonary artery. If flow

through the ductus arteriosus is from left to right and the relative size of the ductus is small, the volume of left-to-right flow is usually not enough to cause clinical congestive heart failure. If the ductus is large, however, and the pressure gradient is also large, there may be a large enough volume of blood entering the lungs to cause congestive heart failure. In premature infants, prostaglandin synthetase inhibitors (indomethacin) are used to cause constriction of the ductus. This is successful in most but not all preterm infants and may cause only temporary constriction of the ductus. Some preterm infants require surgical closure of their PDA if indomethacin fails.

In a full-term infant with a PDA, congestive heart failure is rare. The volume of left-to-right flow is usually smaller than that of preterm infants, probably because the pulmonary resistance is slower to fall and the pulmonary arteries and lungs are more mature and therefore able to deal with the increased volume more easily. In these children indomethacin is not effective in closing the ductus arteriosus. In such children there is probably a cellular abnormality in the ductus arteriosus which makes it unable to constrict. Although most PDAs in full-term infants are closed by 2 weeks of age, those that persist require closure by either surgical ligation or occlusion in the catheterization laboratory.

ECHOCARDIOGRAPHIC EVALUATION

In most children, the PDA can be seen by both 2D and Doppler scanning. A small PDA, however, will not be visualized by a 2D scan because of the small size and the planes in which we are able to see the ductus.

In the full-term infant, from the short-axis orientation the transducer is moved cephalad and to the left. The ductus arteriosus is seen entering the LPA/MPA junction (Fig. 29-18). Color Doppler in this plane will usually show retrograde diastolic flow. Pulsed wave Doppler sampling in the ductus arteriosus demonstrates the direction of flow in all phases of the cardiac cycle and is used to quantify the predominant signal to estimate pulmonary artery pressure.

In the preterm infant, a subcostal long-axis view of the RVOT or a short-axis parasternal view is ideal. However, these views are often obscured by lung. Color Doppler may identify the left-to-right

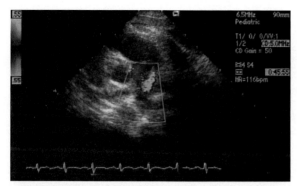

Figure 29-18. Patent ductus arteriosus. Color Doppler demonstrates retrograde diastolic flow in the pulmonary artery originating from the left pulmonary artery. This represents the source of increased pulmonary blood flow seen in these children. (See also Color Plate 70.)

shunting, despite poor 2D images. Likewise, a suprasternal view of the aortic arch with posterior angulation will demonstrate the pulmonary artery and ductus.

A ductus arteriosus should be evaluated from both sides of the ductus (pulmonary artery and aorta) and intraluminally if possible. Color and pulsed wave Doppler will provide documentation of the direction of flow. Continuous wave Doppler will allow estimation of pulmonary artery pressure using the following equation:

$$PA\ pres = systemic\ BP - (4 \times velocity^2).$$

One of the primary goals of echocardiographic evaluation of children with suspected PDA, especially in preterm infants, is to rule out ductal-dependent forms of congenital heart disease. *Ductal dependent* implies that the only source of pulmonary blood flow is from the aorta through the ductus arteriosus or vice versa. Thus, it is extremely important that a thorough anatomic scan be performed. In preterm infants with poor acoustic windows, it is especially important to document antegrade flow across the RVOT and into the pulmonary artery.

Once otherwise normal anatomy is established, evaluation of the degree of shunting is important. The size of the left atrium and left ventricle should be measured. Left ventricular contractility should be quantified. If requested, a Qp:Qs can be estimated. Since the shunting is occurring at the great vessel level, the aortic valve area and flow should be used for Qp and the pulmonary valve area and flow for Qs.

POSTOPERATIVE ECHOCARDIOGRAPHY

Premature infants with PDA will undergo a trial of indomethacin infusion. Indomethacin is a prostaglandin synthetase inhibitor and often causes closure of the PDA. If the indomethacin has no effect or if the child is older, the PDA is closed surgically. This repair usually involves ligation at each end of the ductus and may also include transection of the medial portion. In the cardiac catheterization laboratory, occlusion devices can be introduced into the ductus via a catheter.

On echocardiography, close attention should be paid to flow characteristics at each end of the PDA. On the aortic side some turbulence may be indicated by color Doppler; however, there should be only antegrade flow by pulsed wave Doppler. Left atrial and left ventricular sizes should normalize quickly after closure of the PDA, and contractility should return to normal. As in all postoperative evaluations, biventricular contractility, AV regurgitation, and the presence or absence of a pericardial effusion should be evaluated.

Atrial Septal Defects

ANATOMY

ASDs (Table 29-2) are described by their location: secundum, primum, or sinus venosus defects (Fig. 29-19). Secundum defects occur in the region of the fossa ovalis, and small secundum defects may be indistinguishable from a patent foramen ovale in newborn infants. The secundum ASD is the most common ASD and is usually an isolated defect. Primum defects represent failure of the endocardial cushions to merge and are part of the spectrum of endocardial cushion defects. The primum ASD can be associated with abnormalities of the AV valves or the inlet interventricular septum. Sinus venosus defects occur near the SVC/RA junction and are usually associated with anomalous drainage of the right upper pulmonary veins to the SVC.

PHYSIOLOGY

In most children with ASDs, intracardiac pressures are close to normal. With a communication between the atria, flow across the defect is from the higher-pressure left atrium to the lower-pressure right atrium. This causes an increased volume of blood in

TABLE 29-2. ATRIAL SEPTAL DEFECT

Question to Be Answered	Views	Comments
Position of ASD	Left atrium-right ventricle inflow Four-chamber Subcostal right atrium	Carefully evaluate each portion of septum. Remember that there may be multiple defects. Check SVC/right atrium junction for sinus venosus ASD. Color Doppler flow is seen crossing the defect.
Pulmonary venous return	Four-chamber Subcostal	Identify all four veins. Pay close attention to right pulmonary veins; may enter right atrium at SVC/right atrium junction.
Direction of flow across ASD	Subcostal	If flow is right to left, this means right-sided pressure is higher than left-sided pressure; look for reasons for high right heart pressure (right ventricular or pulmonary artery hypertension, obstruction to tricuspid inflow, increased right artery volume, total anomalous pulmonary venous return).
Size of right ventricle, right atrium	Left atrium—parasternal Four-chamber	M-mode for measurement of RVDD. Right ventricle size relative to left ventricle size.
Septal motion	Left atrium—parasternal	M-mode with attention to motion of IVS; note if flattened or paradoxical.

the right atrium, right ventricle, and pulmonary artery. The left atrium is also dilated due to the increase in pulmonary blood flow returning to it. The echocardiographic exam will reveal some degree of dilatation of right atrium, right ventricle, and main pulmonary artery. As the volume in the right ventricle increases, the length of the ventricle increases and the ventricular septum becomes flattened. In severe right ventricular volume overload, the ventricular septum actually bows into the LV, so that the RV becomes the circular ventricle in the short-axis view and the left ventricle takes on a more crescent-like shape.

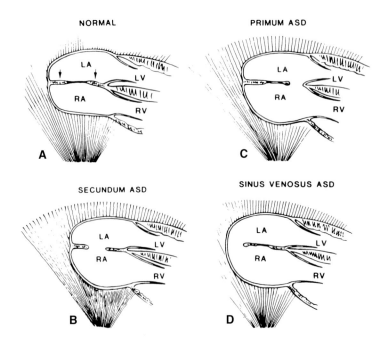

Figure 29-19. Atrial septal defects. Subcostal views of the atrial septum show a normal septum in (**A**), a secundum ASD in (**B**), a primum ASD in (**C**), and a sinus venosus ASD in (**D**). LA, left atrium; LV, left ventricle; RA, right atrium; RV, right ventricle. (From Shub O, et al. Sensitivity of two-dimensional echocardiography and the direct visualization of atrial septal defect utilizing the subcostal approach. *J Am Coll Cardiol.* 1983;2:127. Reprinted with permission.)

In some children with increased pulmonary vascular resistance, the right heart pressure is elevated enough to change the pressure gradient across the atrial septum such that flow is from right to left. Under these circumstances, the left atrium will be mildly dilated and the right atrium and right ventricle will be normal in volume. If right-to-left flow across an ASD is noted, it is critical to determine the cause of the increased right heart pressures or to rule out those defects which would cause them. Intracardiac defects which could cause these increased heart pressures can be divided into two groups. First are those defects which increase right atrial pressure primarily: tricuspid stenosis, tricuspid atresia, and total anomalous pulmonary venous return. Second are those defects which increase right ventricular pressure first and, as they become more severe, also increase right atrial pressure: RVOT obstruction (including severe branch pulmonary artery stenosis) or intrinsic lung disease. In cases of right-to-left shunting across an ASD, estimation of right ventricular pressure (see the section on "Pulmonary Artery Pressure Estimates") is of critical importance.

CLINICAL PROBLEMS

Clinically, few children with isolated ASDs develop congestive heart failure or cyanosis. If cyanosis is present, there are usually associated defects or a noncardiac reason for elevated pulmonary vascular resistance. Likewise, congestive heart failure rarely develops unless there are associated anomalies or abnormalities of ventricular function.

ECHOCARDIOGRAPHIC EVALUATION

The position of the defect must be evaluated from multiple views. The apical four-chamber will demonstrate a primum ASD and in younger children will also demonstrate a secundum ASD. Subcostal evaluation of the atrial septum will also demonstrate primum and secundum ASDs well. With anterior and superior angulation showing the SVC, a sinus venosus defect can be seen (Fig. 29-20).

Once the position of the defect is defined and the other areas of the septum have been evaluated, the direction of shunting should be determined. To evaluate shunt direction, the subcostal short-axis view of the atria is the most useful. In this view the direction of shunt flow is nearly parallel to the ultrasound beam in most types of ASD. In right-

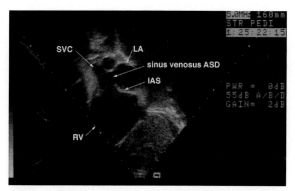

Figure 29-20. *Sinus venosus ASD. Angling superiorly to visualize the superior vena cava (SVC), the break in the atrial septum (IAS) is seen at the SVC/right atrial (RA) junction. LA, left atrium; RV, right ventricle.*

to-left shunting, quantification of right ventricular pressure is very important.

Proper anatomic definition of all pulmonary veins should be determined since anomalous pulmonary venous return (APVR) is always associated with an atrial-level communication (ASD or patent foramen ovale). APVR will cause an increase in blood volume returning to the right atrium, causing predominantly right-to-left shunting. The presence of a VSD or PDA may be used to quantify right ventricular pressure. Close evaluation of the tricuspid valve (to rule out an Ebstein's anomaly) and the RVOT (to rule out RVOT obstruction) is important.

If the flow across the ASD is predominantly from left to right, the right side of the heart may be dilated. The apical four-chamber view is best for evaluating right atrial and right ventricular size. In the parasternal long-axis view, a precise M-mode exam should be performed, carefully measuring the RV free wall and the RV diastolic dimension. The ventricular septal motion may be normal, flattened, or paradoxical. The more abnormal the septal motion, the larger the left-to-right shunt is likely to be.

Although the position of the defect and the degree of right ventricular dilatation are usually sufficient descriptive information, there are times when a quantitative measure of the degree of left-to-right shunting becomes important. Under these circumstances, Qp:Qs can be calculated. If there are no VSDs, the pulmonary valve should be used as the measure of pulmonary flow and the aorta as the measure of systemic flow.

PREOPERATIVE ECHOCARDIOGRAPHY

Since congestive heart failure develops only rarely in children with ASDs, follow-up is aimed at identifying any associated defects and watching for spontaneous closure (10–40% occurrence).[18] Repeat echocardiograms should evaluate the size of the right atrium and right ventricle, as well as IVS motion and, if significantly different, a Qp:Qs for further quantification of the change in the size of the shunt.

POSTOPERATIVE ECHOCARDIOGRAPHY

Most children with large ASDs have surgical repair within the first 5 years of life. Small ASDs may be closed with a single suture; larger ASDs are usually closed with a patch of either pericardium or prosthetic material. Some children will undergo device closure of their ASDs in the catheterization laboratory. The immediate postoperative echocardiographic exam should evaluate the site of repair, evidence of residual shunting, ventricular function, and the presence of a pericardial effusion. If the ASD is closed in the catheterization lab by the implantation of a device, 'postoperative' follow-up requires understanding of the structure of the devices and their expected 2D appearance when effectively positioned.

Ventricular Septal Defects

ANATOMY

VSDs (Table 29-3) are divided into four basic types based on their location in the ventricular septum: perimembranous, outlet, inlet, and muscular. Figures 29-21 and 29-22 graphically define the position of each of these defects.

The *perimembranous* defect is the most common and is seen in approximately 80% of all children with VSDs. Often there is an associated abnormality of the tricuspid valve. As time progresses, portions

◢◢◢ **TABLE 29-3.** Ventricular Septal Defect

Question to Be Answered	View	Comments
Position and number of defects	Long axis	See Figures 29-21, 29-22.
Size of defect	Short axis Apical four-chamber Apical five-chamber	Measure in multiple views; compare to diameter of aortic root.
Septal/aortic malalignment	Long axis Apical five-chamber	Anterior aorta and IVS should be seen in same plane. If the aorta is posterior to the IVS, the subaortic and aortic annulus diameters are measured.
Direction of flow	Long axis Short axis Apical four-chamber Apical five-chamber	Evaluation with color Doppler during systole.
Estimated right ventricular pressure	Apical four-chamber Long axis	Get TI gradient and VSD gradient, if possible.
Estimated pulmonary artery pressure	Short axis	Get gradient across RVOT.
Evidence of closure	Long axis Apical four-chamber	Is either TV or AoV tethered to IVS?
Aortic valve prolapse	Long axis Short axis	Is the AI? Try to visualize prolapse with color Doppler, try to identify which cusp prolapses.
Evidence of left ventricular hypertrophy	Long axis	Careful M-mode for contractility, size of IVS, left ventricle, LVPW, LA; contractility of left ventricle.
Tricuspid valve structure and function	Short axis Four-chamber	Is the tricuspid valve tissue redundant? Is there evidence of partial closure of VSD? Is there color Doppler evidence of a left ventricle to right atrium shunt?

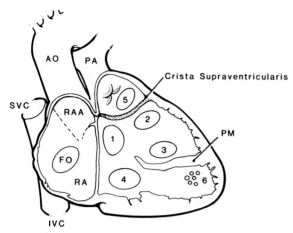

Figure 29-21. Position of ventricular septal defects. This figure demonstrates the following types of defects: 1, perimembranous. 2, outflow. 3, trabecular (muscular). 4, inflow. 5, supracristal. AO, aorta; RA, right atrium; SVC, superior vena cava; IVC, inferior vena cava; PA, pulmonary artery; RAA, right atrial appendage; PM, papillary muscle; FO, foramen ovale. (From Harvey Feigenbaum M. *Echocardiography*, 5th ed. Fig. 7-63. Philadelphia, Lea & Febiger; 1994:384. Reprinted with permission.)

ciated with aortic regurgitation, as the usual septal support for the right coronary cusp of the aortic valve is absent. This aortic leaflet tissue may prolapse through the VSD with sufficient tissue to create RVOT obstruction. For this reason, it is always important to measure the Doppler velocity in the RVOT. Spontaneous closure of these defects is extremely uncommon.

Muscular defects are responsible for 5–15% of defects and are further classified by the portion of the muscular septum in which they are found. Central or midmuscular defects and apical defects may have multiple channels on the right ventricular side which coalesce to form a single defect on the left ventricular side. Marginal defects are very difficult to visualize by 2D or color Doppler because they are positioned at the far lateral edge of the IVS where it

of the septal leaflet of the tricuspid valve may become adherent to the IVS just below the defect. This creates an "aneurysm" of the IVS and eventually closes the defect. The tricuspid valve septal leaflet may be deficient, causing a left ventricle-to-right atrial shunt.

Perimembranous defects may be associated with *malalignment* of the IVS and aorta. Usually, in the long-axis parasternal view, the IVS and the anterior aorta are continuous and in the same plane. Even in most perimembranous defects, the two structures appear to be in the same plane. If the IVS is malaligned posteriorly, the aorta appears to "override" the ventricular septum, as in tetralogy of Fallot. If the IVS is malaligned anteriorly, subaortic stenosis is usually present and complicates the surgical closure of the VSD.

Aortic regurgitation seen with perimembranous defects usually involves prolapse of either the right coronary cusp or the noncoronary cusp and is frequently associated with infundibular stenosis. Spontaneous closure of these defects is effected via tricuspid tissue tethering around the defect.

Outlet defects are seen in 5–7% of VSDs. These defects are also known as *supracristal, conal, infundibular, subpulmonary, subarterial,* or *doubly committed subarterial* defects. They are frequently asso-

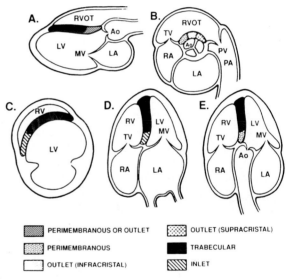

Figure 29-22. Color Doppler definition of the position of ventricular septal defects. In the parasternal long-axis view (**A**), the trabecular or muscular defects are seen, as are the perimembranous ones. In the parasternal short-axis view (**B**), perimembranous, outlet, and supracristal defects are visualized. In the parasternal short-axis view, angled toward the apex (**C**), both perimembranous and trabecular (muscular) defects are seen. In the apical four-chamber view, both trabecular (muscular) and inlet defects are seen. In the apical five-chamber view when the aorta is visualized, trabecular (muscular) and perimembranous defects are seen. RVOT, right ventricular outflow tract; Ao, aorta; LV, left ventricle; LA, left atrium; RV, right ventricle; RA, right atrium; TV, tricuspid valve; MV, mitral valve. (From Feigenbaum M. *Echocardiography*, 5th ed. Fig. 7-64. Philadelphia, Lea & Febiger; 1994:384. Reprinted with permission.)

meets the right ventricular free wall. These defects are usually numerous and may have multiple small, serpiginous tracts. Finally, there is the *Swiss cheese septum*, which defines the presence of multiple muscular defects which may be of several different subclassifications. Spontaneous closure of muscular defects is common and occurs via further tissue growth in the muscular septum.

Inlet defects are seen in 5–8% of patients with VSD and are often associated with endocardial cushion defects (see the section on "Endocardial Cushion Defects").

PHYSIOLOGY

In *fetal* life, pulmonary vascular resistance is high. Flow through a VSD during this time is bidirectional, with minimal flow volume. In *small to moderate-sized VSDs*, pulmonary resistance usually drops within the first 1–2 weeks of life and flow becomes predominantly left to right. Blood flow volume, velocity, and turbulence increase as the pressure difference between the left and right ventricles increases. As long as pulmonary vascular resistance and right ventricular pressure remain low, flow will remain left to right. If spontaneous closure occurs, turbulence will increase as the defect becomes smaller.

In *large VSDs*, pulmonary vascular resistance is slower to decrease, usually taking 1–2 months. During this time, the volume of blood flowing from left to right across the defect is moderate, and the velocity and turbulence of the flow are lower than in the small defect. The gradient between left and right ventricular pressures is less, and color Doppler flow is more laminar. When the pulmonary vascular resistance decreases to near-normal levels, there is a large increase in the volume of left-to-right shunting. With this increased volume to the pulmonary arteries, the arterioles dilate, which in turn causes the pulmonary veins to dilate, causing the left atrium to dilate and its pressure to increase. Eventually, this leads to left ventricular dilatation and later, left ventricular hypertrophy.

If there is no intervention in a child with a large VSD, the increased flow through maximally dilated pulmonary arterioles will cause increasing structural damage to the vessels; the walls of the vessels hypertrophy and impinge on the internal circumference of the vessels. This increases pulmonary vascular resistance and right ventricular pressure. These events reduce the volume of left-to-right shunting. In turn,

the size of the left atrium decreases, as does the size of the left ventricle. With continued work against an increased vascular resistance, right ventricular hypertrophy is seen. Once this kind of damage to the pulmonary arterioles becomes irreversible, the child is said to have *Eisenmenger's complex*. This implies a permanent increase in pulmonary vascular resistance, with further increases expected over time. Once pulmonary vascular resistance increases over systemic resistance, the shunting across the VSD becomes right to left. With decreased pulmonary blood flow, the child becomes cyanotic and has lowered exercise tolerance. Death due to right ventricular failure or pulmonary hemorrhage usually occurs in the third to fourth decade of life. To prevent this predictable demise, the identification and surgical closure of large VSDs within the first several months of life is important.

CLINICAL PROBLEMS

Children with isolated small VSDs rarely require surgery. If the VSD is perimembranous or muscular, there is a strong chance (>50%) of spontaneous closure. For children with moderate-sized perimembranous or muscular defects, close clinical follow-up is required. If they develop signs of congestive heart failure, failure to thrive, or pulmonary hypertension, surgical closure will be considered. Because of the high incidence of development of aortic regurgitation with outlet VSDs, these children will also require close clinical follow-up. In some institutions, surgical closure will be performed as soon as the defect is discovered to protect the aortic valve and its supporting structures; in other institutions, surgery will be considered if aortic regurgitation develops.

ECHOCARDIOGRAPHIC EVALUATION

The position of the defect must be evaluated in several different views: parasternal or apical four-chamber, long axis, and short axis. In each view, close evaluation of the 2D image should be followed by superimposition of the color Doppler image. If any area of turbulence is seen, the transducer should be "torqued" slowly in all directions in an attempt to visualize the entire VSD tract. Once the tract of the VSD is defined, the next step is to find a transducer position which puts the flow parallel to the beam. This will rarely be in one of the standard views; however, it is imperative that the flow across the VSD be parallel to the ultrasound beam before initiating a Doppler evaluation. Once the flow is parallel, pulsed wave Doppler is used to evaluate the direction of flow during the cardiac cycle. Steerable continuous wave Doppler will allow an evaluation of the maximum velocity. Assuming that there are no other areas of high-velocity flow within the heart, a Pedoff evaluation of the VSD jet is important; often the highest, most parallel approach to the VSD jet is from an area with suboptimal 2D images.

The size of the defect can be estimated from 2D images. It must never be assumed that a VSD is a circular structure. Measurements must be made in several different planes and reported as diameters in each plane.

Since there may be multiple defects in a septum (Swiss cheese septum), close evaluation in all planes for other defects is important. These may vary in size, shape, and placement. Careful evaluation, however, should elucidate the number and placement of defects with better detail than catheterization.

In a parasternal long-axis view with the IVS perpendicular to the beam, the septum and the anterior aorta should be contiguous or, if a perimembranous VSD is present, should appear to be in the same plane. If this is not the case,[24] the position of the anterior portion of the aorta relative to the IVS should be determined. If the aorta is anterior to the IVS, it is said to override the IVS and conotruncal defects should be considered. If the aorta is posterior to the IVS, evaluate the LVOT closely by 2D and color Doppler. Measuring the diameter of the subaortic area versus the aortic annulus is helpful; in posterior malalignment there often will be subaortic stenosis with a long, narrow subaortic area. Once a parallel Doppler evaluation of the VSD flow is accomplished, estimations of right ventricular pulmonary artery pressure can be made.

Since VSDs can be associated with infundibular or valvular pulmonary stenosis, it is always important to evaluate the RVOT by 2D, color Doppler, and pulsed wave or continuous Doppler. If the velocity in the MPA is <200 cm/sec, the increase in flow is probably (though not always) related to the increased volume of blood passing through the valve; this does not indicate RVOT obstruction. If the velocity is >200 cm/sec, some of the increase in velocity is probably due to structural abnormalities. Under these circumstances, it is necessary to mea-

sure RVOT velocity by continuous wave Doppler. This can be done in the parasternal short-axis view or the subcostal long-axis view of the right ventricle. Once a peak velocity is obtained, the gradient is estimated via the modified Bernoulli equation: RVOT gradient = $4 \times \text{velocity}^2$. Using the previously made estimate of RV pressure, the pulmonary artery pressure can be estimated as follows:

Pulmonary artery pressure

= (estimated RV pressure − RVOT gradient)

If the defect is perimembranous, a close evaluation in the apical four-chamber and the parasternal short axis of the septal leaflet of the tricuspid valve may show evidence of its being tethered over the defect. This finding predicts eventual spontaneous closure. Serial scans of a patient with muscular VSD demonstrating a decrease in the size of the defect or the width of the color Doppler band also predict eventual closure of the defect.

Finally, in all but lower muscular VSDs, the aortic valve should be evaluated closely for evidence of prolapse into the defect. In the parasternal long-axis view, the cusps of the aortic valve should be seen in the same plane when closed. If the anterior leaflet seems to "sag" or buckle into the LVOT, prolapse is present. Likewise, the discovery of aortic regurgitation in the absence of a bicuspid aortic valve suggests that the aortic valve is not sufficiently supported and may be prolapsing. If aortic regurgitation is found, the aortic valve should be evaluated in the short-axis view with color Doppler to define the origin of the aortic regurgitation. With outlet VSDs it is usually the left coronary cusp that prolapses; with perimembranous VSDs, it may be the right or noncoronary cusps.

In some cases, an estimate of the amount of right-to-left shunting may be necessary. In these cases, Qp:Qs can be estimated by echocardiography. In the absence of RVOT obstruction or other shunt defects, the pulmonary valve and velocity can be used to estimate Qp, and the aortic valve and velocity can be used to estimate Qs.

PREOPERATIVE ECHOCARDIOGRAPHY

After a thorough anatomic scan to define the position, size, and number of defects and to estimate right ventricular and pulmonary artery pressures, follow-up exams are usually done to evaluate any changes in the patient's clinical status, physical findings, or noninvasive tests. Although any further testing should be tailored to the specific questions asked, the following information should always be obtained: direction of flow across the defect, size of left atrium and left degree of right and left ventricular hypertrophy, estimated gradient across the VSD, estimated RV pressure, estimated PA pressure, and presence or absence of aortic regurgitation.

POSTOPERATIVE ECHOCARDIOGRAPHY

Surgery for VSDs involves placement of a patch, either pericardial or prosthetic, over the defect. If the defect is in the outlet septum or associated with aortic regurgitation, an attempt to resupport the aortic annulus is made by the surgeon. In the immediate postoperative period, there may be multiple small "leaks" between sutures around the patch. However, within the first few days to weeks, most leaks disappear. The long-term prognosis after surgical closure of isolated VSDs is excellent. A few children will have a residual small shunt; in all, however, the size of the shunt will be diminished. The immediate postoperative echocardiographic exam should evaluate biventricular function, the site of the repair, evidence of residual shunting, aortic valve function, and the presence of a pericardial effusion. Within the first few weeks after surgery, left atrial and left ventricular size should normalize. Ventricular hypertrophy will regress, but over a much longer period of time. The area of the IVS now covered with a patch will remain echodense. If the defect was in the perimembranous portion of the IVS, septal motion on M-mode will appear flat, since the area of the septum involved in the M-mode measurements is now a prosthetic material which will move only in relation to pressure differences between the two ventricles.

Endocardial Cushion Defects

ANATOMY

The spectrum of endocardial cushion defects (ECDs) (Table 29-4), also referred to as *atrioventricular canal defects (AVCDs)*, involves failure of complete growth of the endocardial cushions. Since the endocardial cushions make up the interventricular septum, interatrial septum, and AV valve annuli,

▰▰▰ **TABLE 29-4.** Diagnosis of Endocardial Cushion Defect

Question to Be Answered	Views	Comments
VSD size and direction of flow	Four-chamber Subcostal	VSD should be seen best in four-chamber view, just below AV valves; may be very small or may encompass most of septum.
ASD size and direction of flow	Four-chamber Subcostal	ASD is in primum portion of atrial septum, just above AV valves; may be small or encompass most of septum; may see multiple defects.
AV valves	Four-chamber Subcostal	If there is a cleft mitral valve and complete ECD, no medial hinge point of the AV valves is seen; there will be a "common" bridging leaflet extending across the medial portions of the right and left atria. Identify chordal attachments in four-chamber view and left atrium.
Other VSDs	Four-chamber Long axis Subcostal	Evaluate septum for muscular VSDs.
Aorta/IVS continuity	Long axis Subcostal	Is aorta committed entirely to left ventricle? If not, is there coexisting tetralogy of Fallot?
Pulmonary artery	Short axis Long axis	Pulmonary artery flow should be laminar and normal in velocity. If child is >2 months old, pulmonary artery should be dilated, suggesting increased pulmonary blood flow.
AV regurgitation	Four-chamber Subcostal	AV valves usually are insufficient, ranging from mild and unilateral to severe and bilateral. Quantification of ventricular pressure from AV regurgitation is usually impossible, since jets overlap. To evaluate right ventricular pressure, use flow across VSD.

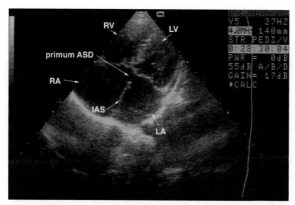

Figure 29-23. Partial endocardial cushion defect. There is a break in the primum portion of the atrial septum (IAS). In addition, the medial hinge points of the tricuspid and mitral valves are at the same level. ASD, atrial septal defect; RA, right atrium; RV, right ventricle; LV, left ventricle; LA, left atrium.

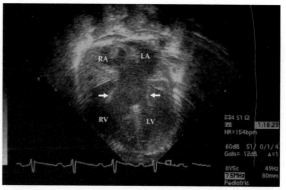

Figure 29-24. Complete endocardial cushion defect. In addition to the break in the primum portion of the atrial septum, there is a break in the inflow portion of the ventricular septum and a lack of tissue centrally for attachment of the atrioventricular valves. RA, right atrium; RV, right ventricle; LA, left atrium; LV, left ventricle.

a wide variety of defects is seen in this category. ECDs can be partial or complete. A complete ECD includes all the components; a partial ECD may include one or several components. The main distinction between a partial and a complete ECD is the presence of two distinct AV valve annuli in a partial defect.

A *partial ECD* (Fig. 29-23) involves one or more of the following defects:

- Primum ASD
- Inlet VSD
- Cleft anterior mitral valve leaflet
- Cleft tricuspid valve

A partial ECD may be associated with any of the following: secundum ASD, persistent left SVC to the coronary sinus, pulmonary stenosis, subaortic stenosis, tricuspid stenosis or atresia, coarctation of the aorta, patent ductus arteriosus, membranous VSD, or hypoplastic left ventricle.

A *complete ECD* (Fig. 29-24) is defined as having the following:

- Common AV valve
- Deficient membranous portion of the IVS
- Foreshortened LV length
- Increased length of the apex to the aortic valve, forming the "gooseneck" deformity of the outflow tract
- AV valve with usually five leaflets, three attached to the ventricular free walls and, two bridging the medial portions of the ventricles

- Left papillary muscles closer together than usual
- Possible attachment of chordae from the papillary muscles of the anterior ridging leaflet to the crest of the IVS

ECD is seen most frequently in children with trisomy 21. Intracardiac defects associated with ECD include Tetralogy of Fallot, double outlet right ventricle (DORV), D-transposition of the great vessels, asplenia, and polysplenia. The combination of ECD and tetralogy of Fallot is most often seen in trisomy 21. DORV with ECD is most often seen in the asplenia syndrome. Often the left ventricular cavity is smaller than the right ventricular cavity or is even hypoplastic. Subaortic stenosis is seen with ECD, as is Ebstein's anomaly.

The common atrium associated with two ventricles is thought to be a manifestation of a severe partial ECD. This combination is usually associated with complex congenital heart disease, including the polysplenia syndrome, asplenia syndrome, D-transposition of the great vessels, DORV, anomalous pulmonary venous return, or univentricle with a single AV valve.

PHYSIOLOGY

A complete or partial ECD with a large atrial component and abnormal AV valves will usually present in infancy with a left-to-right shunt at the atrial level and AV valve regurgitation, especially mitral regurgitation. With the increase in pulmonary blood flow, these infants usually develop congestive heart failure. Even if their congestive heart failure is compensated, they may experience failure to thrive. A small primum ASD with normal AV valves may present few if any problems during infancy.

If left unrepaired, the increase in pulmonary blood flow will cause progressive obliteration of the pulmonary arterioles. These changes cause an irreversible increase in vascular resistance in the pulmonary vascular bed. As pulmonary artery pressure increases, there is a decrease in left-to-right shunting as pulmonary blood flow decreases. This change allows resolution of the child's congestive heart failure symptoms. When pulmonary artery pressure surpasses systemic pressure, however, there is an increase in right-to-left shunting, with increased cyanosis and dyspnea. This leads to a prolonged downward course with early death. This process is even more accelerated in children with trisomy 21. For these reasons, it is important to repair complete ECDs and large partial ECDs within the first year of life.

PREOPERATIVE ECHOCARDIOGRAPHY

Because of the association of complex congenital heart disease with ECDs, a segmental assessment must be made.[13] Orientation of the great vessels should be defined, as well as the entrance of pulmonary and systemic veins. Careful evaluation of the relationship between the IVS and the anterior aorta may demonstrate malalignment, which suggests a coexisting tetralogy of Fallot or DORV. An apical four-chamber view will usually demonstrate the break in the primum interatrial septum (IAS) (Fig. 29-23). The size of the defect should be estimated and color Doppler used to define the direction of flow across the defect, as well as the degree of AV valve regurgitation. In most ECDs, both partial and complete, there is an anterior leaflet common to the mitral and tricuspid valves which nearly spans the base of the heart, as seen on the four-chamber view. When the leaflet opens and moves out of the 2D plane, the large defects in the IAS and IVS are clearly seen. Pulmonary venous drainage must be defined in this setting. In this and other views, the secundum portion of the IAS should be evaluated since there is often an additional secundum defect. Careful evaluation of ventricular volumes is necessary

since unequal volumes may make surgical repair more complex, if not impossible. In the long-axis parasternal view and then the short-axis view, the ventricular septum should be scanned, first for an inlet defect and then for muscular or membranous defects. The short-axis parasternal view is also good for evaluating the relationship between the two AV valves. Subcostal views are usually best for defining the size and position of atrial defects.

After the perinatal period, left-to-right shunting may cause dilatation of the RVOT, pulmonary arteries, and left atrium. There is usually mild to moderate RV hypertrophy on 2D. The aorta may be dextroposed. The subaortic area may be elongated, with a tunnel-like obstruction. Using multiple views, it is important to assess the relative volumes of the ventricles, which should be nearly equal. Finally, the aortic arch must be evaluated, as coarctation of the aorta is sometimes seen with ECD.

Preoperative evaluation should monitor atrial sizes, ventricular volumes, degree of AV regurgitation, size of the subaortic area and the degree of obstruction. If the ventricular defect is small, each study should attempt to estimate right ventricular pressure.

POSTOPERATIVE ECHOCARDIOGRAPHY

The immediate postoperative echocardiogram should include the usual evaluation of ventricular function and pericardial fluid status. Residual leaks around the ASD or VSD patches should be described precisely so that they can be followed. The degree of AV regurgitation may vary considerably from day to day as the child's fluid status and ventricular function change. During all evaluations, close attention should be paid to the subaortic area. In addition, repair of the mitral valve may lead to the development of mitral stenosis, often several years after repair. Therefore, careful attention should be given to the 2D, color, and pulsed wave Doppler evaluations of mitral inflow.

Conotruncal Defects

Failure of conotruncal septation results in an array of defects including: Tetralogy of Fallot, pulmonary atresia with VSD, DORV, and truncus arteriosus (Table 29-5). In all defects, the relationship of the IVS and the great vessels is abnormal, with one great

▰▰◢ TABLE 29-5. CONOTRUNCAL DEFECTS

Question to Be Answered	Views	Comments
Orientation of great vessels	Short axis	Define anterior-posterior and left-right relationships.
Size of VSD	Long axis Four-chamber	Should have laminar flow into by color Doppler.
Degree of aortic override	Long axis Subcostal	If aorta is not at least partly associated with LVOT, consider DORV.
Presence/degree of semilunar regurgitation	Long axis Apical left atrium	Define width and length of regurgitation jet.
Level and degree of right ventricular outflow tract obstruction	Left atrium-right ventricle Subcostal	Check infundibulum, supravalve area, branch pulmonary arteries: Use pulsed wave and continuous wave Doppler to interrogate pulmonary arteries.
Size of MPA and branches	Long axis-right ventricle Short axis Subcostal	Measure diameter of MPA and each branch; measure ratio of MPA to aorta.
Coronary arteries	Short axis	Need to know origin and course of left anterior descending artery.
Other defects: VSDs	Four-chamber Left atrium	Look closely at muscular septum.
ASD	Four-chamber Subcostal	?Associated secundum ASD.
Coarctation of aorta	Suprasternal	
Absent pulmonary valve	Long axis-right ventricle Short axis	Will see more PI than with intact valve.
Right ventricle-pulmonary artery continuity	Left atrium-right ventricle	Make sure there is color Doppler flow from right ventricle to pulmonary artery; otherwise this is probably pulmonary atresia.

vessel overriding the IVS, allowing blood from both ventricles to exit partially or completely via that great vessel. This combination of defects accounts for 10–15% of the cases of congenital heart disease in infants.

TETRALOGY OF FALLOT/PULMONARY ATRESIA WITH VSD

Anatomy

Tetralogy of Fallot comprises four defects (Fig. 29-25): aorta overriding IVS, VSD, infundibular stenosis, and right ventricular hypertrophy. Since the aorta overrides the septum, flow from either ventricle may exit via the aorta; this decrease in blood flow to the pulmonary artery reduces the size of the pulmonary artery and causes an incremental increase in the size of the aorta. The size of the pulmonary arteries is important in defining the surgical repair and in anticipating the child's prognosis. Flow through the RVOT may be so diminished that the pulmonary

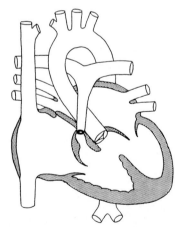

Figure 29-25. Tetralogy of Fallot. This defect consists of four associated defects: ventricular septal defect, overriding aorta (due to posterior malalignment of the ventricular septum), infundibular stenosis (thickening of the muscle below the pulmonary valve), and right ventricular hypertrophy (due to obstruction of pulmonary blood flow). (From Mullins CE, Mayer DC. *Congenital Heart Disease: A Diagrammatic Atlas.* Diagram 55. Chicago, YearBook Medical Publishers; 1990. Reprinted by permission of Wiley-Liss, Inc., a division of John Wiley & Sons, Inc.)

valve is atretic; likewise when there is a larger volume of flow across the RVOT, the pulmonary valve may be close to normal in size, with larger pulmonary arteries. A less common manifestation of tetralogy of Fallot includes an absent pulmonary valve. In this case, there is moderate to severe pulmonary regurgitation and large pulmonary arteries. In all cases of Tetralogy of Fallot, there is a high incidence of coronary artery anomalies, particularly an anomalous left anterior descending artery from the right coronary artery which crosses the RVOT or a single coronary artery where a major branch crosses the RVOT.

In pulmonary atresia with VSD (Fig. 29-26), only the aorta takes blood away from the heart. The main pulmonary artery may be in its proper place, but without communication with the right ventricle; it may also be nonexistent. There may or may not be communication between the right and left pulmonary arteries; in fact, there may be no discernible pulmonary arteries. In severe cases, pulmonary blood flow is provided exclusively from bronchiolar collaterals off the descending aorta.

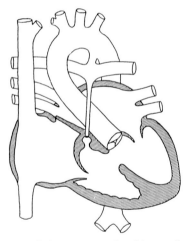

Figure 29-26. Pulmonary atresia with ventricular septal defect. This defect is similar to tetralogy of Fallot and is also called *tetralogy of Fallot with pulmonary atresia.* In this anomaly, the pulmonary valve is atretic; thus, no blood flow reaches the pulmonary artery across the pulmonary valve. There is a very small pulmonary artery, usually some infundibular stenosis, and a large ventricular septal defect. Pulmonary blood flow comes solely from left-to-right flow across the ductus arteriosus. (From Mullins CE, Mayer DC. *Congenital Heart Disease: A Diagrammatic Atlas.* Diagram 70. Chicago, YearBook Medical Publishers; 1990. Reprinted by permission of Wiley-Liss, Inc., a division of John Wiley & Sons, Inc.)

Physiology

Blood flow in tetralogy of Fallot is as follows: IVC/SVC to right atrium to right ventricle; at this point, blood can go out the aorta or the pulmonary artery. The amount of blood flow to each great vessel depends on the resistance met in each great vessel. If the pulmonary artery is normal in size and the pulmonary vascular resistance has started to drop, there will be more blood flow to the pulmonary artery than to the aorta. If there is severe narrowing of the pulmonary arteries, pulmonary atresia, or severe infundibular narrowing, most or all of the blood entering the right ventricle will cross the VSD and go to the aorta. Pulmonary venous return enters the left atrium, goes to the left ventricle and then out the aorta. Since desaturated blood from the right ventricle is entering the aorta, the child will be cyanotic.

In pulmonary atresia with VSD, all blood from both circuits can leave the heart via the aorta. Pulmonary blood flow is provided through the ductus arteriosus. For this reason, once this diagnosis is confirmed, these children are started on prostaglandin E1 (PGE1) to maintain patency of the ductus until surgical repair or until a surgical shunt can be placed to provide for pulmonary blood flow.

Echocardiographic Evaluation

Since there are several manifestations of this defect, echocardiographic evaluation should be via the segmental approach. The parasternal long-axis view will best demonstrate the aorta overriding the IVS. The short-axis parasternal view, with slow angulation cephalad, will demonstrate the RVOT and may show the infundibular hypertrophy below the pulmonary valve. The apical four-chamber and subxiphoid views will further demonstrate the size and configuration of the VSD.

Especially difficult is the definition of the communication between right ventricle and pulmonary arteries. Normally, the parasternal short-axis view is used to define this anatomy. In these children, however, the pulmonary arteries are often difficult to see in this plane. Instead, a subcostal evaluation of the RVOT, or a high parasternal view in the short-axis orientation, angling down toward the heart, will better define this anatomy.

The definition of pulmonary artery anatomy is particularly difficult in pulmonary atresia with VSD.

A high right parasternal or subcostal view is used to define the aortic arch. Color Doppler is used to trace the ductus back from the aorta to the pulmonary artery. Not uncommonly, however, the pulmonary artery anatomy is not seen well on echocardiography in pulmonary atresia with VSD.

The definition of coronary artery anatomy is likewise difficult. Identification of a single coronary artery ostia guarantees that the anatomy is abnormal; definition of two ostia in the appropriate places, however, does not guarantee that the anatomy is normal. Cardiac catheterization with an ascending aortic injection is often necessary to define the coronary artery anatomy prior to definitive repair.

Since the VSD is large in both tetralogy of Fallot and pulmonary atresia with VSD, right ventricular pressure will be close to or equal to systemic pressure. In tetralogy of Fallot, the gradient across the RVOT is important; continuous wave Doppler should be used to estimate the total gradient across the RVOT.

Postoperative Echocardiography

Surgical repair of tetralogy of Fallot involves closure of the VSD, resection of the infundibulum, and/or placement of a patch across the RVOT. Postoperative echocardiography is used to evaluate the RVOT for the degree of pulmonary regurgitation, diameter of the RVOT, and gradient across the RVOT. In addition, the IVS should be evaluated by color Doppler for a residual VSD, and the LVOT should be evaluated by color Doppler for the development of aortic regurgitation (this may be a short- or long-term complication and is related to the repair of the VSD where it impinges on the aortic annulus). As always, ventricular function and the presence of pericardial fluid should be evaluated in the immediate postoperative period.

Surgical repair of pulmonary atresia with VSD depends on the anatomy of the pulmonary arteries. If only collaterals are coming from the aorta to the pulmonary arteries, a unifocalization procedure to bring all the pulmonary artery segments together and place a graft from them to the RVOT may be done. If an MPA exists, a patch or conduit from the right ventricle to the MPA may be placed. The VSD is also closed. The postoperative echocardiographic exam should look at the same features as the postoperative tetralogy exam.

TRUNCUS ARTERIOSUS

Anatomy/Physiology

In truncus arteriosus, one large great vessel carries both right and left ventricular outflow. Unlike pulmonary atresia and aortic atresia, in which one great vessel exits the heart and the other is atretic, the great vessel in truncus arteriosus serves as both aorta and pulmonary arteries. In fact, the pulmonary arteries arise from the truncal vessel in one of three major areas (Fig. 29-27): (1) the MPA arises from the truncus (type I) and then branches to the right and left pulmonary arteries; (2) left and right pulmonary arteries arise from the truncus adjacent to one another (type II); (3) left and right pulmonary arteries arise from the truncus on opposite sides of the great vessel from one another (type III). In all cases, the truncus carries output from both ventricles, with the pulmonary arteries exiting the truncus. Depending on the relative size of the pulmonary arteries and the size of the opening into them, there may be too little or too much pulmonary blood flow. Thus, these children may be profoundly cyanotic, in congestive heart failure, or somewhere between the two.

The truncal valve is always abnormal, usually having more than three cusps. It is often mildly insufficient and may be severely insufficient.

Associated defects include interrupted aortic arch (usually associated with DiGeorge syndrome), right aortic arch, unilateral absence of a pulmonary artery, and coronary artery abnormalities.

Clinical Problems

As discussed earlier, if there is stenosis at the pulmonary artery takeoff, the child will be cyanotic due to decreased pulmonary blood flow. More common, however, is the development of congestive heart failure as the pulmonary vascular resistance drops and pulmonary blood flow increases. The child may be further compromised by a moderate to severe degree of truncal valve regurgitation.

Echocardiographic Evaluation

A large overriding great vessel seen in the long-axis parasternal view can represent either tetralogy of Fallot, truncus arteriosus, or DORV (Fig. 29-28). The differentiation is in the placement of the pulmonary arteries. For this reason, identification of

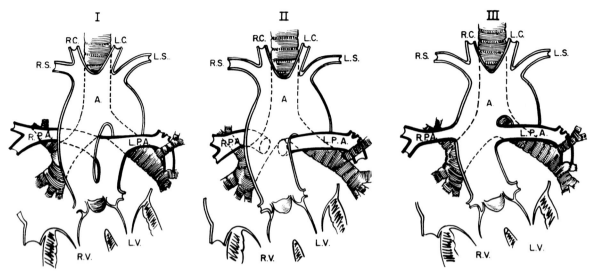

Figure 29-27. Truncus arteriosus. In this defect, there are usually normal-sized atria and ventricles; mitral and tricuspid valves are usually normal, and blood flow into the ventricles is normal. There is one large great vessel coming off the top of the heart; both ventricles eject blood to this vessel via a large ventricular septal defect. There are three main types of pulmonary artery attachments in truncus arteriosus. In type I, the pulmonary trunk arises from the truncus and shares the common valve annulus. In type II, the pulmonary artery branches arise separately but in close proximity. In type III, the pulmonary arteries arise separately and more laterally from the truncus. (From Emmanouilides GC, Riemenschneider TA, Allen HD, et al. *Heart Disease in Infants, Children, and Adolescents.* Baltimore, Williams & Wilkins; 1995:1028. Reprinted with permission.)

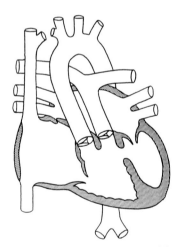

Figure 29-28. Double outlet right ventricle. In this defect, there is posterior malalignment of the ventricular septum such that the aorta is committed to the right ventricle, as is the pulmonary artery. There is a large ventricular septal defect which allows blood from the left ventricle to exit one or both great vessels. (From Mullins CE, Mayer DC. *Congenital Heart Disease: A Diagrammatic Atlas.* Diagram 64. Chicago, YearBook Medical Publishers; 1990. Reprinted by permission of Wiley-Liss, Inc., a division of John Wiley & Sons, Inc.)

pulmonary arteries and their origins is absolutely essential. In a high right parasternal short-axis orientation, with the transducer angled toward the apex, color Doppler is used to identify the origin of both pulmonary arteries off the truncus (Fig. 29-29). Steerable continuous wave Doppler interrogation of both pulmonary arteries is performed to determine the degree of obstruction on either side. In the parasternal long-axis view, evaluation of the truncal valve for regurgitation is important. This evaluation should be repeated in the apical long-axis view. Close evaluation of the coronary arteries in the parasternal short-axis view and identification of both ostia and the takeoff and course of the left anterior descending artery are essential.

Postoperative Echocardiography

Surgical repair usually involves closure of the VSD, excision of the pulmonary arteries from the truncus, and placement of a valved conduit from the RV to the pulmonary arteries. Postoperative evaluation should include color Doppler evaluation of the degree of truncal valve regurgitation, ventricular func-

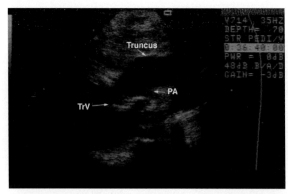

Figure 29-29. Truncus arteriosus. In a suprasternal long-axis view of the aortic arch, the dilated truncus is visualized. One of the pulmonary arteries (PA) is seen coming off the truncus posteriorly. The truncal valve (TrV) is seen inferiorly.

tion, color Doppler flow characteristics through the conduit and into the pulmonary arteries, and continuous wave Doppler estimation of the total gradient across the new RVOT.

DOUBLE OUTLET RIGHT VENTRICLE

Anatomy

There are three major components to the diagnosis of DORV: (1) there are two great vessels, both of which arise from the morphologic right ventricle; (2) there is a VSD through which blood in the left ventricle must pass to reach the aorta; (3) there is no fibrous continuity between either AV valve and either semilunar valve. There is often pulmonary or subpulmonary stenosis. With DORV there may be one of four great vessel orientations: (1) aorta posterior to the PA (normal); (2) aorta to the right of the pulmonary artery with the valves at same level (side by side); (3) aorta to the right and anterior to the pulmonary artery (transposed); (4) aorta to the left and anterior to the pulmonary artery. There are four types of VSDs associated with DORV: (1) subaortic, where the VSD lies directly below the aortic valve; (2) subpulmonary, where the VSD lies directly below the pulmonary valve; (3) doubly committed, where the VSD is very large and equally committed to each great vessel; and (4) remote, where the VSD

is at a distance from either great vessel. There is a variant of DORV, called the *Taussig-Bing anomaly*, which includes a supracristal, subpulmonary VSD. In this case the aorta is to the right of the pulmonary artery with a side-by-side orientation and a dilated pulmonary artery.

Associated defects include pulmonary stenosis, secundum ASD, subaortic stenosis, interrupted aortic arch, coarctation of the aorta, mitral valve abnormalities (parachute mitral valve, cleft mitral valve, straddling mitral valve, supramitral ring), and coronary artery anomalies.

Physiology

Physiologic characteristics of DORV depend on the orientation of the great vessels, the presence or absence of a VSD and its position, and the condition of the pulmonary vascular bed. In all cases, blood flow from the left and right ventricles mixes at the ventricular level and exits via both great vessels. The degree of mixing and the relative volumes going to each great vessel depend on the positions of the VSD and the great vessels.

Clinical Problems

Children without pulmonary or subpulmonary stenosis and a normal pulmonary vascular bed will have increased pulmonary blood flow and therefore suffer congestive heart failure. Those with RVOT obstruction will have diminished pulmonary blood flow and therefore will be cyanotic.

Preoperative Echocardiography

Because of the complex combinations of defects in DORV, a segmental approach should be used. Important features of this evaluation include placement and size of the VSD, great vessel relationships, color Doppler evaluation of flow across the pulmonary outflow tract, and definition of the proximal coronary artery course. To evaluate for fibrous continuity of the AV valves and semilunar valves, each ventricular outflow tract should be identified from a long-axis view. With both the AV and semilunar valves visualized, evaluate the hinge points of each. If there is fibrous continuity, the distance between the hinge points will be very short (Fig. 29-30). If there is no continuity the distance between the

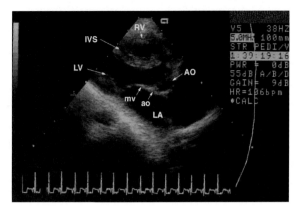

Figure 29-30. Double outlet right ventricle. In the normal parasternal long-axis view, the hinge point of the posterior aortic valve leaflet is within a few millimeters of the hinge point of the anterior mitral valve leaflet. In the double outlet right ventricle, there is "fibrous discontinuity" between these two hinge points, creating a tunnel-like left ventricular outflow tract. LA, left atrium; LV, left ventricle; RV, right ventricle; IVS, interventricular septum; MV, mitral valve hinge point; AO, aorta; ao, aortic valve hinge point.

two will be greater, defining a separate outflow chamber.

Postoperative Echocardiography

Surgery for DORV has three goals: (1) establish left ventricle-to-aorta continuity, (2) establish right ventricle-to-pulmonary artery continuity, and (3) repair associated defects. In most cases, the left ventricle-to-aorta continuity is established by closing the VSD with a patch which extends anteriorly and superiorly to enclose the aortic annulus. The right ventricle-to-pulmonary continuity is established in several ways, ranging from a small patch in the RVOT to a valved conduit between the RV and pulmonary artery. In the Taussig-Bing anomaly, closure of the VSD results in D-transposition of great vessel physiology and is therefore performed in association with a Mustard or Senning procedure or an arterial switch procedure.

Postoperative evaluation should define the VSD patch, any residual shunting across the VSD, and the color and pulsed wave Doppler characteristics of flow between left ventricle and aorta. It should also include the color and pulsed wave Doppler characteristics of flow between the right ventricle and pulmonary artery.

Transposition of the Great Vessels

Although D-transposition of the great vessels (DTGV) and L-transposition of the great vessels (LTGV) may be very different in a morphologic, morphogenetic, and clinical sense, they are very similar to a sonographer and their differences are often very confusing (Table 29-6). From a short-axis view, if the aorta is anterior to the pulmonary artery, the diagnosis is transposition of the great vessels (TGV). In the diagnosis of TGV, the biggest challenge is determining whether it is L- or D-transposition.

The parasternal short-axis view (Fig. 29-31) is best to define the aorta's anterior position relative to the pulmonary artery. It is important to define the right-left orientation of the aorta relative to the pulmonary artery. If the apex of the heart is to the left and the aorta is anterior and to the right of the pulmonary artery, the diagnosis is DTGV (D = *dextro*, Latin for "right"). If the aorta is to the left, the diagnosis is LTGV (L = *levo*, Latin for "left"). If the great vessels are essentially on top of each other or side by side, the examination must be done following the guidelines discussed earlier for the segmental approach to complex congenital heart disease.

In DTGV, there is one "wrong" connection or mismatch. Although the correct atrium is connected to the correct ventricle, the wrong great vessel is attached to each ventricle. This is illustrated in Figure 29-32.

In LTGV (also called *corrected transposition*) there are two "wrongs" or mismatches: the atria are connected to the wrong ventricles, which are connected to the wrong great vessels. And, although our mothers always told us that "Two wrongs don't make a right," in congenital heart disease they do. When there are two wrong connections, the overall connection is "right" or correct. Thus, in LTGV, despite the mismatches, blood flows through the heart appropriately, with desaturated blood coming into the right atrium and going out the pulmonary artery to the lungs; saturated blood comes back to the left

▰▰▰ **TABLE 29-6.** TRANSPOSITION OF GREAT VESSELS

Question to Be Answered	Views	Comments
Is aorta anterior to pulmonary valve?	Short axis	This defines it as transposed great vessels (TGV).
Is aorta to right or left of pulmonary valve?	Short axis	If aorta is to the right, D(dextro)-TGV; if the aorta is to the left, L(levo)-TGV; if side by side or one on top of another: if aorta (Ao) comes off right ventricle and pulmonary artery comes off left ventricle, then it is DTGV. If Ao comes off left ventricle and pulmonary artery comes off right ventricle, then it is LTGV.
Is there a VSD? • Placement • Size	Long axis Four-chamber Subcostal	If muscular, look for multiple defects. If inlet VSD, look at AV valves.
Are ventricles normal in size and shape?	Four-chamber	If ventricles are not equal in volume, look closely at AV valves and semilunar valves.
Is the subpulmonary area narrow?	Short axis Long axis RVOT Subcostal	Color Doppler examination in MPA.
Is there malalignment of the IVS and anterior pulmonary artery?	Long axis Subcostal	If the VSD is large, closely examine the plane of the IVS as it relates to the anterior pulmonary artery. If IVS is posterior to anterior pulmonary artery, consider DORV.
Is aortic arch clear?	Suprasternal Subcostal	Must rule out coarctation of aorta, interrupted aortic arch.
Size of ASD; direction of flow	Four-chamber Subcostal	Size of ASD; what direction is flow across ASD and is it laminar?
Size of PDA; direction of flow	Short axis Suprasternal Subcostal	Size of PDA, width of color Doppler flow and direction.
AV valves	Four-chamber	Is there evidence of Ebstein's anomaly of the left AV valve?

atrium and goes out the aorta to the body. The child is not cyanotic or acidotic and, unless there is a large VSD, is not in heart failure. Figure 29-33 demonstrates the two "wrongs."

At this point in the examination, you should know whether you are dealing with DTGV or LTGV. It is also important to have more specific information about each of the defects.

D-Transposition of the Great Vessels

ANATOMY/PHYSIOLOGY

DTGV is a common cardiac cause of cyanosis in a newborn infant. These infants suffer severe cyanosis, acidosis, and death within a short period of time unless there is a large atrial-level shunt or a PDA. Even with a large VSD, there is not enough mixing

to keep the infant well oxygenated. Thus, a large ASD is an absolute necessity for these infants. Without any intervention, most of them die within the first year of life. Thus, the diagnosis of DTGV represents a medical emergency necessitating immediate intervention. Currently, the most common intervention involves the use of PGE1 infusion, which inhibits the natural closure of the ductus arteriosus and may actually cause its dilatation. The infusion of PGE1 establishes a source of shunting which is usually sufficient to stabilize the infant for several days to weeks.

The most common defect associated with DTGV is VSD. The VSD may be in any position and may be single or multiple. The most common location is in the perimembranous septum. If an inlet VSD is noted, the AV valves should be closely evaluated for associated abnormalities. Alignment

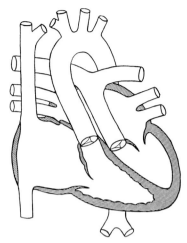

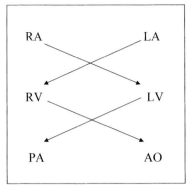

Figure 29-33. L-transposition of the great vessels. Blood flow in this case is rerouted twice, once at the ventricular level and once at the great vessel level. Although the rerouting is more complicated than in D-transposition of the great vessels, the outcome is relatively normal. Desaturated blood returns to the right atrium (RA) and exits via the pulmonary artery (PA) to become saturated with oxygen in the lungs; saturated blood returns to the left atrium (LA) and exits via the aorta (AO) to the body to supply the cells with oxygen. RV, right ventricle; LV, left ventricle.

Figure 29-31. D-transposition of the great vessels. The right ventricle gives rise to an aorta, the left ventricle to a pulmonary artery. Desaturated blood returns to the right atrium, passes through the tricuspid valve to the right ventricle, and exits via the aorta to the body; thus the child is cyanotic. Saturated blood returns to the left atrium, passes through the mitral valve to the left ventricle, and exits via the pulmonary artery to the lungs. Unless there is an atrial or ventricular septal defect or ductus arteriosus, this represents two parallel circulatory patterns; oxygenated blood cannot get to the body to provide oxygen and remove metabolic byproducts. (From Mullins CE, Mayer DC. *Congenital Heart Disease: A Diagrammatic Atlas.* Diagram 82. Chicago, YearBook Medical Publishers; 1990. Reprinted by permission of Wiley-Liss, Inc., a division of John Wiley & Sons, Inc.)

of the IVS and PA must be evaluated closely in DTGV since malalignment of these structures represents a problem for surgical repair. If the

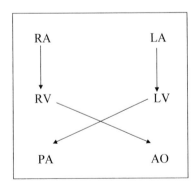

Figure 29-32. D-transposition of the great vessels. Blood flow, which is usually from the right atrium (RA) to the right ventricle (RV) to the pulmonary artery (PA) and left atrium (LA) to the left ventricle (LV) to the aorta (AO), is rerouted. The only rerouting, however, occurs at the level of the great vessels.

pulmonary artery is malaligned anteriorly and overrides the IVS, there is essentially a DORV with a subpulmonary VSD, the Taussig-Bing anomaly. The subaortic area in this defect may be narrow and may be associated with hypoplasia of the aortic arch or interrupted aortic arch. If the pulmonary artery is malaligned posteriorly, there may be varying degrees of subpulmonary outflow obstruction with annular hypoplasia or even pulmonary valve atresia.

In DTGV there is a 25% incidence of LVOT (subpulmonary) obstruction.[10] If the ventricular septum is intact, there may be mild dynamic subpulmonary obstruction due to bulging of the septum into the pulmonary outflow tract. There may also be fixed subvalvular obstruction with a fibrous ridge or a discrete membrane. If there is a VSD, there is a higher likelihood of more severe subpulmonary outflow obstruction. There may be a subvalvular ring, a long tunnel-like narrowing, or muscular obstruction in this region. There may be abnormal AV valve chordae that attach to the muscular outlet septum, obstructing outflow.

Other, less frequently seen defects associated with DTGV include abnormal chordal attachments of the tricuspid valve, coarctation of the aorta, and interrupted aortic arch.

CLINICAL PROBLEMS

Children with DTGV and intact ventricular septum (IIVS) have two parallel circulation patterns with little or no mixing. Desaturated blood enters the right atrium, flows to the right ventricle, and is pumped to the aorta. Desaturated blood is circulated through the body and returns to the right atrium. Saturated blood from the lungs enters the left atrium, flows to the left ventricle, and is pumped to the pulmonary artery where it flows through the lungs back to the left atrium. Thus, oxygenated blood is unable to reach the systemic circulation and desaturated blood is unable to reach the lungs. During fetal life, the ductus arteriosus provides a source of shunting between the two circulations. After delivery, while the ductus is open, there is bidirectional shunting, which allows some desaturated blood to be delivered to the lungs. The infant appears cyanotic, however, because desaturated blood is mixed with the saturated blood from the left heart via the ductus arteriosus. If the desaturation is severe, the infant becomes increasingly acidotic and dies. If the flow through the ductus and/or the ASD is high (either naturally or after infusion of PGE1), the infant is less cyanotic and less acidotic and may be clinically stable for days to weeks.

PREOPERATIVE ECHOCARDIOGRAPHY

As with all other complex congenital heart defects, the segmental approach should be used in the ultrasound evaluation of children with DTGV. Using either the short-axis view at the base or the short-axis subcostal view, the great vessel should be followed out of each ventricle until it is defined as the aorta or pulmonary artery. In DTGV, the vessel coming off the right ventricle will be an aorta. It is important to confirm ductal flow off the aortic arch (Fig. 29-34).

Once the systemic circuit has been defined, identification of the pulmonary venous atrium in the subcostal or parasternal long-axis view and its ventricle is important. With the high incidence of LVOT obstruction, close attention must be paid to the alignment of the IVS and PA, the subpulmonary area, and the pulmonary valve. Color Doppler evaluation of the LVOT will provide assistance in determining the site of obstruction. Finally, the aorta and arch must be evaluated for the possibility of coarctation or interruption.

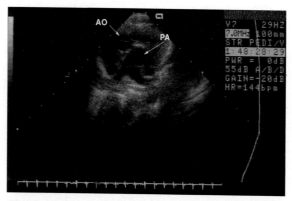

Figure 29-34. D-transposition of the great vessels. In the parasternal short-axis view, the aorta (AO) is seen to be anterior and to the right of the pulmonary artery (PA). The pulmonary artery is defined by the bifurcation to the right and left pulmonary arteries.

POSTOPERATIVE ECHOCARDIOGRAPHY (Table 29-7)

In the infant with DTGV, if early primary surgical repair is not to be considered, a Rashkind procedure (balloon atrial septostomy) performed in the catheterization laboratory within the first few days of life increases atrial-level mixing and therefore improves systemic oxygenation. Echocardiographic evaluation of these patients is directed at the degree of shunting across the atrial septum and the size of the defect created.

At least three different surgical procedures are available for repair of the child with DTGV. The *Mustard* and *Senning* procedures (Fig. 29-35) involve "transposing" the atrial functions and therefore rerouting blood to the appropriate great vessel. After the procedure, systemic venous blood returns via the IVC and SVC into the interatrial baffle and is directed across the mitral valve, into the left ventricle, and out the pulmonary artery. Oxygenated blood returning via the pulmonary veins passes around the atrial baffle, across the old atrial septum to the tricuspid valve, into the right ventricle, and out the aorta. Thus oxygenated and desaturated circulations are separate, and each arrives at its appropriate great vessel.

The *arterial switch* procedure (see Fig. 29-13) involves surgically transposing the aorta and pulmonary artery trunks and reimplantation of coronary arteries. After this procedure, systemic venous blood returns to the right atrium, crosses the tricus-

◢◣ TABLE 29-7. POSTOPERATIVE ECHOCARDIOGRAPHY: D-TRANSPOSITION OF GREAT VESSELS

Question to Be Answered	Views	Comments
MUSTARD/SENNING		
Biventricular function	Short axis Four-chamber Subcostal	Compare contractility of two ventricles in 2D in multiple planes.
SVC/IVC return	Short axis Subcostal	Color Doppler in SVC and IVC as they enter right atrium may demonstrate turbulence at site of anastomosis and may indicate obstruction; use pulsed wave Doppler to confirm.
Pulmonary venous return	Short axis Four-chamber Subcostal	Color Doppler in pulmonary veins will show increased velocity and turbulence if there is posterior obstruction in the left atrium.
Subpulmonary flow	Subcostal	Color Doppler in pulmonary outflow in a long axis view of the LVOT may show turbulence below the valve; define by 2D.
ARTERIAL SWITCH		
Biventricular function	Subcostal Short axis	Segmental left ventricular wall motion and comparative contractility of two ventricles; coronary stenosis can occur.
Suprapulmonary area	Subcostal Short axis	At the anastomosis line, obstruction above the pulmonary valve is more common than obstruction above the aorta. Look with color Doppler and pulsed wave or continuous wave for confirmation of velocity; also look for narrowing and acceleration in the distal pulmonary arteries.
RASTELLI		
Biventricular function	Short axis Apical four-chamber	Carefully evaluate segmental left ventricular wall motion since coronary stenosis may develop.
Conduit valve function	Short axis Subcostal	Color Doppler in the RVOT may demonstrate turbulence at the site of anastomosis above the pulmonary valve.
Flow characteristics in conduit	Short axis Subcostal	RV function may deteriorate over time. Conduit valve may become stenotic or insufficient. Color Doppler in subcostal views may be best window for conduit; MPA may dilate at site of insertion of conduit.
MPA size	Short axis Subcostal	Conduit may become narrow along entire length. Color Doppler with turbulence should be evaluated closely. Follow with pulsed wave Doppler to try to identify specific sites of obstruction.
Predicted right ventricular pressure	Four-chamber	As conduit and/or valve becomes stenotic, right ventricular pressure will increase; look for TI to estimate right ventricular pressure.

pid valve into the right ventricle, and exits the pulmonary artery. Pulmonary venous blood returns to the left atrium, crosses the mitral valve into the left ventricle, and exits the aorta. This procedure is the primary repair for children with intact ventricular septum. In children with a large VSD, many institutions will place a pulmonary artery band first, allow the left ventricle to hypertrophy for several days to weeks, and then perform the arterial switch procedure.

The *Rastelli* procedure (see Fig. 29-16) is performed on children with DTGV, large VSD, and

severe LVOT (subpulmonary) obstruction. This procedure involves removing the pulmonary artery from the pulmonary annulus, oversewing the pulmonary annulus, closing the VSD with a patch that connects the LV to the aorta, and placing an external valved conduit from the body of the right ventricle to the transected pulmonary artery. After this repair, systemic venous blood enters the right atrium, goes across the tricuspid valve to the right ventricle and out the valved conduit to the pulmonary arteries. Pulmonary venous blood returns to the left atrium, crosses the mitral valve into the left

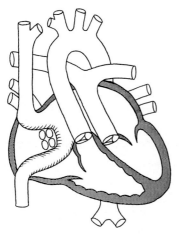

Figure 29-35. Mustard procedure for D-transposition of the great vessels. In this operation, blood flow is rerouted at the atrial level. A "pair of pants" is constructed from an artificial substance. The "legs" are sewn at the entrance of the superior vena cava and inferior vena cava into the right atrium. The "waist" of the pants is sewn over the mitral valve annulus. Thus, desaturated blood returns from the superior and inferior venal cava into the "legs," through the body of the pants, out the "waist," and across the mitral valve annulus. From there it enters the left ventricle and is pumped to the lungs via the pulmonary artery. Saturated blood returns from the pulmonary veins to the left atrium. It cannot cross the mitral annulus because the pants "waist" is sewn over the annulus, so it crosses the atrial septal defect to the right atrium. Here it flows across the tricuspid valve to the right ventricle and out the aorta to the body. (From Mullins CE, Mayer DC. *Congenital Heart Disease: A Diagrammatic Atlas*. Diagram 148. Chicago, YearBook Medical Publishers; 1990. Reprinted by permission of Wiley-Liss, Inc., a division of John Wiley & Sons, Inc.)

ventricle and is directed through the VSD to the aorta.

Each surgical procedure has its own short- and long-term complications. Children undergoing the *Mustard* or *Senning* procedures are at risk of developing systemic venous and pulmonary venous obstruction.[27] The systemic obstruction is at the site of the surgical anastomosis of the interatrial baffle, i.e., at the SVC/RA junction or the IVC/right atrium junction. Obstruction at the SVC/right atrium junction usually results in SVC obstruction and SVC syndrome, with increased SVC pressure and edema of the upper body and head. Obstruction at the IVC/right atrium junction usually leads to increased IVC pressure with hepatomegaly and eventual ascites. A color Doppler study in an apical four-chamber or a subcostal short-axis view will show aliasing in

the vessel with obstruction; pulsed wave Doppler will show turbulent high-velocity flow.

Pulmonary venous obstruction is usually related to the interatrial baffle impeding the laminar return of pulmonary venous blood to the left atrium. It may also be a structural stenosis within the individual pulmonary veins. Pulmonary venous obstruction causes increasing exercise intolerance, dyspnea, tachypnea, and coughing in these children. A color Doppler study in an apical four-chamber or a subcostal short-axis view will show turbulence in the pulmonary veins in question or in the back of the left atrium. If pulmonary venous pressure is elevated, there may be dilated pulmonary arteries, pulmonary regurgitation, dilated right ventricle, tricuspid regurgitation, and dilated right atrium.

Complications of the *arterial switch* procedure are related to the surgical anastomoses.[7] Suprapulmonary stenosis is a common complication and may be severe enough to require intervention. Supra-aortic stenosis is much less common. The "new" aortic root is usually somewhat dilated, and there may be aortic regurgitation. Finally, obstruction at the site of coronary artery anastomoses may lead to coronary artery stenosis and decreasing ventricular function. Echocardiographic studies of children after the arterial switch procedure should involve close attention to the suprapulmonary and supra-aortic areas, in their respective long-axis views, with color Doppler to evaluate the site of obstruction and continuous wave Doppler to evaluate the degree of obstruction. Both ventricles should be evaluated systematically in several views for global contractility and both AV valves interrogated for the determination of diastolic ventricular function.

With the *Rastelli* procedure there is a risk of external conduit stenosis, necessitating reoperation and replacement of the conduit. This obstruction may occur at the site of the conduit insertion into the right ventricle, at the conduit valve, or at the site of the conduit insertion into the pulmonary artery, or it may be a tunnel-like narrowing along the length of the conduit. The conduit valve may become stenotic or insufficient. Evaluation of the external conduit by echocardiography is often difficult since the conduit is directly below the xiphoid and runs parallel to the chest wall. Subcostal or apical views are best for evaluating the external conduit by color Doppler and continuous wave Doppler.

L-Transposition of the Great Vessels

ANATOMY/PHYSIOLOGY

LTGV is an uncommon defect characterized by discordance or mismatch of atrial-to-ventricular connections and discordance of ventricular-to-great vessel connections (Fig. 29-36). As discussed earlier, this combination of two mismatches ultimately leads to acyanotic and usually asymptomatic heart disease in young children. Often these children are not recognized as having congenital heart disease until later in life unless they also have other coexisting defects such as VSD, pulmonary stenosis, or abnormalities of the left AV valve. In 5% of children with LTGV there will be situs inversus (both abdominal and thoracic organs on the opposite site), and in 25% there will be dextrocardia (heart in the right chest, apex to the right) or mesocardia (heart in the midline, apex to the left or midline). Many children with LTGV will have abnormalities of the left-sided, morphologic tricuspid valve structure,

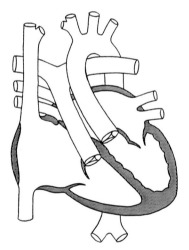

Figure 29-36. L-transposition of the great vessels. In this defect, although blood flows in a relatively normal pattern, the ventricles have been transposed, creating a connection of the right atrium to the morphologic left ventricle and a connection of the left atrium to the morphologic right ventricle. Likewise, the morphologic left ventricle is attached to the pulmonary artery and the morphologic right ventricle to the aorta. Blood flow, however, is from systemic veins to pulmonary artery and from pulmonary veins to systemic artery. (From Mullins CE, Mayer DC. *Congenital Heart Disease: A Diagrammatic Atlas.* Diagram 91. Chicago, YearBook Medical Publishers; 1990. Reprinted by permission of Wiley-Liss, Inc., a division of John Wiley & Sons, Inc.)

ranging from subclinical abnormalities to chordae which straddle a VSD, to Ebsteinization of the valve leaflets. There is also a higher incidence of coarctation of the aorta. In addition to structural defects, the conduction system in LTGV is in an abnormal position, so often the only hint of the defect is an abnormal electrocardiogram (EKG).

PREOPERATIVE ECHOCARDIOGRAPHY

With the high incidence of situs abnormalities and heart position abnormalities in children with LTGV, it is important to evaluate these children with a segmental approach. Beginning in the abdomen, in a transverse plane, if the aorta is on the right and the IVC on the left, there is situs inversus; if the aorta is on the left and the IVC on the right, the situs is probably normal; if they are both on the same side of the spine, there is situs ambiguous. The IVC is followed to the systemic atrium in a longitudinal view to determine whether the systemic atrium is on the right or left relative to the other atrium. With the transducer angled 90 degrees to a transverse plane, this atrium is followed to its ventricle and evaluated for the morphology of that ventricle (a moderator band and deeper AV hinge points suggest morphologic right ventricle; a smooth-walled ventricle and higher AV hinge points suggest morphologic left ventricle) (see Fig. 29-8). This information is confirmed from an apical four-chamber view. Using this ventricle as a reference, the outflow tract is followed to a semilunar valve and then to a pulmonary artery. There should be no visible infundibulum; the AV valve hinge point and pulmonary hinge point should be in continuity. From an apical four-chamber view, the pulmonary venous atrium is identified by following blood across the pulmonary AV valve to the pulmonary ventricle; this ventricle should have the appearance of a morphologic right ventricle. In a subcostal transverse view, this ventricle should be seen to give rise to an aorta through an infundibular area (the subaortic conus); in this view and a long-axis view, the right-sided AV valve should *not* be in continuity with the aortic valve.

With a high incidence of VSDs, close attention is paid to the different areas of the ventricular septum with 2D and color Doppler. Close evaluation of the pulmonary outflow tract is carried out by 2D and color Doppler. The left AV valve may be structurally abnormal and may have some degree of regurgitation.

POSTOPERATIVE ECHOCARDIOGRAPHY

Surgical repair of the large VSD associated with LTGV is more complicated than that of a large VSD and normally related great vessels. First, the conduction system runs anterior to the VSD in LTGV, which makes the risk of postoperative complete heart block high. Second, the AV valve in many of these hearts is abnormal; repair of the VSD has no effect on the degree of AV valve regurgitation and may therefore have little effect on the overall clinical status of the child. Postoperative studies should evaluate the ventricular function, the status of the VSD patch, and the pericardial space. In addition, close attention should be paid to the amount of left AV valve regurgitation.

Right Ventricular Outflow Tract Obstruction

RVOT obstruction (Table 29-8) encompasses a variety of defects ranging from subclinical to often fatal prognoses. The level of obstruction may be below, at, or above the pulmonary valve. Subvalvular obstruction involves hypertrophy of the infundibulum and is not seen as an isolated entity; it is usually associated with tetralogy of Fallot, pulmonary valve stenosis, or DTGV. It will therefore be discussed with its associated defect. Valvular obstruction may be in the form of a bicuspid pulmonary valve, varying degrees of pulmonary valve stenosis, or pulmonary atresia. Obstruction above the valve is usually in the form of discrete stenoses of the branch pulmonary arteries. A nonobstructive lesion of the RVOT, absent pulmonary valve, is an uncommon but interesting anomaly which is usually associated with tetralogy of Fallot and is discussed in that section.

ANATOMY

Pulmonary valve stenosis is expressed in two major forms—fusion of the raphe, often with a *bicuspid pulmonary valve* which domes, or severely thickened valve tissue with a tricuspid valve (*dysplastic pulmonary valve*). The dysplastic pulmonary valve is most often associated with Noonan's syndrome, which includes dysmorphic features, and pulmonary stenosis. Isolated pulmonary valve stenosis with a nondysplastic pulmonary valve is not generally associated with other defects or syndromes. *Branch pulmonary artery stenosis* can be a single area of stenosis in one of the major branches or multiple narrowings of the more peripheral vessels. Although it can occur alone, branch pulmonary artery stenosis is often associated with congenital rubella syndrome, Noonan's syndrome, Williams syndrome (in association with supravalvular aortic stenosis), Alagile syndrome, and Ehlers-Danlos syndrome.

TABLE 29-8. RIGHT VENTRICULAR OUTFLOW TRACT OBSTRUCTION

Question to Be Answered	Views	Comments
Right ventricular size	Four-chamber Long axis—RVOT	Is right ventricular cavity size similar to that of left ventricle?
Infundibulum	Short axis Long axis—RVOT Subcostal	Is area under pulmonary valve narrow or is muscle thickened? Does color Doppler show turbulence below pulmonary valve?
Pulmonary valve	Short axis Long axis—RVOT Subcostal	Is valve thickened? Does it move well? If leaflets are not seen well, could this represent absent pulmonary valve? Does color Doppler turbulence begin at level of valve? Evaluate velocity with steerable continuous wave Doppler and Pedoff.
Supravalvular area	Short axis Long axis—RVOT	Is turbulence beginning above pulmonary valve?
Branch pulmonary arteries	Short axis Long axis—RVOT	Does turbulence begin after bifurcation of main pulmonary artery? Measure velocity with steerable continuous wave Doppler and Pedoff.
Tricuspid valve annulus—size	Apical four-chamber	Measure diameter of tricuspid valve annulus.

PHYSIOLOGY

The development of right ventricular hypertrophy due to pulmonary outflow obstruction is usually related to the degree of obstruction. Mild pulmonary valvular stenosis or branch pulmonary artery stenosis rarely causes right ventricular hypertrophy. As the degree of obstruction increases, the thickness of the right ventricular wall and IVS increases, and the right ventricular cavity size appears to become smaller. As the obstruction increases still further, the infundibular muscle hypertrophies, producing an accompanying subvalvular obstruction.

CLINICAL PROBLEMS

Most infants with RVOT obstruction are asymptomatic. As long as there is a reasonable pulmonary annulus, most infants will thrive. If the degree of stenosis is moderate to severe, they will have a loud systolic murmur which will be recognized within the first few days to months of life. Since the right ventricle is not built to withstand high pressure and resistance for long periods of time, early surgical repair is necessary to relieve the stress on the right heart. Mild to moderate stenoses are well tolerated, are unlikely to progress, and usually require no surgical intervention.

Pulmonary atresia (Fig. 29-37) presents a much more grave situation. Infants with pulmonary atresia have no pulmonary blood flow except that provided by the ductus arteriosus. These infants tend to be cyanotic, and they usually present emergently in the newborn period. There are two main manifestations of pulmonary atresia—those with intact interventricular septum (IIVS) and those with a large VSD. Pulmonary atresia with VSD is very similar in anatomy and physiology to severe tetralogy of Fallot and is discussed in that section. Pulmonary atresia with IIVS continues to carry a poor prognosis despite the use of new surgical techniques. The major problem precluding successful repair is the status of the right ventricle. Since there is no blood exiting the right ventricle during development, the tricuspid valve is either severely stenotic/atretic or insufficient. In either case, flow into the ventricle is compromised, and it does not grow appropriately during fetal development. Thus the right ventricle is usually very small and noncompliant and contracts minimally. If surgical pulmonary valvulotomy and shunting are performed, severe pulmonary insufficiency usually follows, with

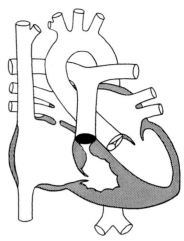

Figure 29-37. *Pulmonary atresia with intact ventricular septum. The pulmonary valve is atretic; thus, no blood can flow from the right ventricle across the pulmonary valve to the pulmonary artery. Since there is no ventricular septal defect, there is no way for blood to exit the right ventricle except back across the tricuspid valve annulus. These right ventricles tend to be very small, round, and muscle-bound. The pulmonary artery may be small or nonexistent. Blood flow to the pulmonary arteries comes from flow through the ductus arteriosus. (From Mullins CE, Mayer DC. Congenital Heart Disease: A Diagrammatic Atlas. Diagram 91. Chicago, YearBook Medical Publishers; 1990. Reprinted by permission of Wiley-Liss, Inc., a division of John Wiley & Sons, Inc.)*

progression in severity. The retrograde PI jet shows the course of blood flow through the right heart: aorta → PDA → pulmonary artery → right ventricle → right atrium. If the child recovers forward flow into the pulmonary artery through the pulmonary valve postoperatively, it is usually after a long and difficult course. Furthermore, these ventricles often have abnormal connections with the coronary arteries. It is hypothesized that these abnormal connections cause myocardial ischemia and further complicate the problem of poor right ventricular compliance. In general, these children do poorly; the few who survive have relatively normal right ventricular function in childhood (probably those with more normal tricuspid valves and no abnormal ventricle-to-coronary artery anomalies); many will die during the postoperative period. Those who survive, but with poor ventricular function, may be candidates for a Fontan procedure.

PREOPERATIVE ECHOCARDIOGRAPHY

Although the RVOT can be visualized in many views, the three most useful ones are the short-axis parasternal view, parasternal long-axis view of the right ventricle, and subcostal long-axis view of the right ventricle. In the *short-axis parasternal view*, the PV is seen with its leaflets perpendicular to the ultrasound beam. Since the transducer is closer to the pulmonary valve in this view than in any other, it is usually the best view for defining the pulmonary valve anatomy. In systole, the valve tissue may dome upward into the main pulmonary artery if there is moderate to severe pulmonary valve stenosis. Evaluation of the relative thickness of the pulmonary valve leaflets compared to the aortic valve leaflets aids in distinguishing stenosis from a thickened, dysplastic valve that is unlikely to be relieved by a balloon angioplasty. Color Doppler should be used to evaluate the degree of pulmonary regurgitation and to define the origin of the turbulent flow through the RVOT; this will define at least the first level of obstruction. If the flow velocity is within the transducer's Nyquist limits, place the pulsed wave Doppler transducer below the pulmonary valve and then above the pulmonary valve to determine how much of the total gradient is valvular versus subvalvular. From this view, the infundibulum is also visualized just anterior to the aortic valve. In defects such as tetralogy of Fallot, this area will show thickening and turbulence on color Doppler scanning.

The short-axis parasternal view is also very helpful in defining branch pulmonary artery stenosis. Once first-level of branching of the pulmonary artery is visualized, color Doppler in this area will indicate turbulence if there is proximal stenosis. If the stenoses are distal, echocardiography may or may not be helpful in defining the site. If this view is obscured, the *RVOT in the long axis* can be visualized by turning the transducer 90 degrees to the left and angling toward the left shoulder. This view can sometimes give a clear picture of the RVOT in its long axis, from the apex of the right ventricle to the pulmonary valve and proximal main pulmonary artery. Either of these views may be used to measure the pulmonary annulus. The *subcostal view of the RVOT* gives a combination of the parasternal short- and long-axis views and is excellent for evaluating both right ventricular inflow and outflow. If the child is small enough for these images to be well visualized, the infundibulum and pulmonary valve wall can be seen well. Color Doppler evaluation of these areas will be helpful in small children but less so in larger children because of the distance from the transducer.

POSTOPERATIVE ECHOCARDIOGRAPHY

Relief of RVOT obstruction comes in the form of surgery or balloon angioplasty. In either case, the goal is to open the pulmonary valve to provide a larger orifice for pulmonary outflow. In the case of branch pulmonary artery stenosis, the stenosis is not surgically correctible and is approached by balloon angioplasty or stent placement during cardiac catheterization.

Postoperative evaluation for RVOT reconstruction should focus on the color Doppler signal through the outflow tract and the degree of regurgitation. If the infundibulum is resected, there will continue to be turbulence in that area for a while, but the velocity of flow should be normal. After pulmonary valvulotomy, many children will show evidence of dynamic subvalvular obstruction immediately after surgery. This is a result of a hypertrophied, hypercontractile ventricle which has had acute relief of distal obstruction; in several weeks, the hypertrophy in the subvalvular area will begin to resolve, as will the hypercontractile state of the ventricle.

Left Ventricular Outflow Tract Obstruction

Although the four main forms of LVOT obstruction (Table 29-9) will be discussed separately, it is important to remember that they often occur in combination and may occur with abnormalities of the left ventricular inflow tract (LVIT) in *Shone's complex*. For this reason, the echocardiographic evaluation of all children with LVOT disease must include the methodical evaluation of all areas of the left ventricular inflow and outflow tracts. Likewise, the preoperative and postoperative echocardiographic evaluations are essentially the same and will be discussed at the end of this section.

BICUSPID AORTIC VALVE/AORTIC STENOSIS

Aortic valve disease in children ranges from the subclinical bicuspid aortic valve to severe aortic valve stenosis requiring emergency surgical intervention in the newborn period to aortic atresia, a lethal form of congenital heart disease. Although a child may begin life with a subclinical form of aortic valve disease, the condition will probably progress. Al-

▰▰▰ TABLE 29-9. LEFT VENTRICULAR OUTFLOW TRACT OBSTRUCTION

Question to Be Answered	Views	Comments
Size of left ventricular cavity	Long axis Four-chamber	M-mode for measurements; left ventricular size relative to that of right ventricular in four-chamber view. Evaluate septal motion and percent FS, size of left atrium, MR. Look at size of mitral and aortic annulus.
Structure of mitral valve	Short axis Long axis Four-chamber	Are there two papillary muscles at 4 and 8 o'clock? Does the anterior leaflet move well? Is there any cleft in the anterior leaflet? Do both leaflets move normally in the long axis? Is there systolic anterior motion of the mitral valve? Does the annulus diameter appear normal?
Function of mitral valve	Four-chamber	Color and pulsed wave Doppler evaluation of mitral inflow. Evaluate maximum velocity, E/A slope, E/A ratio, presence of turbulence. Identify mitral regurgitation.
Adequacy of the subaortic area	Apical and parasternal Long axis	Is subaortic area widely patent with laminar color Doppler flow? Look for subaortic ridge in subaortic area of IVS or anterior leaflet of mitral valve; evaluate in *multiple* views.
Structure of aortic valve	Short axis Long axis	Unicuspid, bicuspid, tricuspid valve? Any redundant or thickened valve tissue? Leaflets should move freely. Color Doppler to look for aortic regurgitation, turbulence above aortic valve. Pulsed and continuous wave Doppler in LVOT to evaluate total inflow tract gradient.
Supravalvular area	Long axis Subcostal	? Narrowing above aortic valve leaflets. Color Doppler to look for turbulence beginning above valve.
Aortic arch	Suprasternal Subcostal	Evaluate course of aorta; should be like candy cane. Look for area of narrowing in area of ductus arteriosus (coarctation of aorta). Evaluate diameter of aorta at ascending, transverse, and descending areas.

though the disease may present no life-threatening emergencies during the early years, very close clinical observation is required to prevent permanent damage to the LV and to provide for optimum timing of surgical repairs.

Anatomy

While the normal aortic valve has three leaflets of equal size, area, and function, there are many children with aortic valves which are mildly to severely abnormal. The mildest form of aortic valve disease is bicuspid aortic valve (Fig. 29-38). In most bicuspid aortic valves there is fusion at one of the raphes, transforming what should have been two normal leaflets into one large leaflet with variably limited excursion. A rarer form of aortic valve disease is the unicuspid or monocuspid valve, in which the valve leaflets have either one or no lateral attachments; there may be just a central orifice. In the congenitally abnormal aortic valve, thickening of the valve tissue and calcification may occur throughout life. Aortic valve stenosis may be associated with PDA,

coarctation of the aorta, VSD, or pulmonary valve stenosis. There is a rare combination of defects, Shone's complex, which may include supramitral ring, parachute mitral valve, subaortic stenosis, aortic valve stenosis, and coarctation of the aorta.

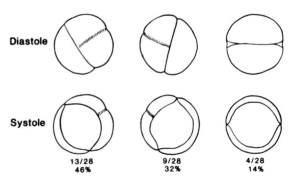

Figure 29-38. Bicuspid aortic valve. This diagram shows the three most common forms of bicuspid aortic valve in systole and diastole. The percentages refer to the prevalence of each type. (From Feigenbaum M. *Echocardiography*, 5th ed. Baltimore, Williams & Wilkins; 1994:368. Fig. 7-32. Reprinted with permission.)

Physiology

As the valve becomes more stenotic, the left ventricle must work harder to provide an adequate volume and pressure to the body. In response to this increased need, the left ventricular muscle hypertrophies and the pressure in the left ventricle increases. If the obstruction is severe and surgery is not performed to relieve it, the pressure in the left ventricle continues to rise and the ventricle continues to hypertrophy until no further hypertrophy is possible. With the increase in left ventricular mass, the resistance within the myocardium increases. Although coronary arteries supplying blood to the myocardium have the capacity to dilate to meet increased myocardial oxygen needs, there is a limit to this capacity. After maximum dilatation occurs and with increasing myocardial resistance, the cumulative coronary flow to the myocardium decreases. As the myocardial cells receive less than the needed oxygen, they become ischemic and may die. The result is a decrease in ventricular contractility. The heart compensates for this decrease in contractility by dilating, thus having more blood available for each contraction. Once the ventricle begins to dilate, the myocardial cells are assumed to have been damaged. Surgery performed at this point will improve the gradient across the outflow tract but may not improve the function of the ventricle since damage to the myocardial cells may be permanent. For these reasons, the timing of repair for children or young adults with congenital aortic stenosis is critical.

Clinical Problems

Most children with aortic valve stenosis are asymptomatic. On physical examination there will be a murmur and a click. On EKG there will be evidence of increased left ventricular pressure load if the stenosis is significant. Until the degree of left ventricular hypertrophy is such that coronary artery dilatation is unable to provide for the increased myocardial oxygen demands during exercise, there will be no chest pain or exercise intolerance. Children rarely present initially with myocardial ischemia-induced chest pain; instead, they are usually followed by pediatric cardiologists for years before they require surgery. Under these circumstances, surgery is scheduled at a time when the stenosis has reached a moderate level but has not yet led to irreversible changes in the ventricular myocardial cells. The criteria for surgery vary from institution to institution and may include a peak gradient exceeding 50 mm Hg, signs of LV dysfunction, abnormal exercise test, or resting EKG changes.

SUBVALVULAR AORTIC STENOSIS

Narrowing of the subvalvular area in the LVOT may take one of three major forms. The first is the *discrete subvalvular membrane* (Fig. 29-39); this membrane is seen in the subvalvular area of the IVS and extends into the outflow tract. The membrane usually extends around the IVS and involves the anterior leaflet of the mitral valve. Surgery for this defect involves removing the ridge and attempting to free the anterior mitral leaflet from the ridge. Postoperatively there may be residual obstruction, damage to the support of the aortic valve with resultant regurgitation, damage to the mitral valve involving the development of regurgitation or stenosis, and injury to the conduction system.

The second form of subvalvular stenosis is *dynamic muscular subaortic stenosis* (Fig. 29-40), often associated with global left ventricular hypertrophy and often related to a systemic illness such as muscular dystrophy or glycogen storage disease. Finally, there are several *other forms of congenital heart disease* which may be associated with an anatomically narrow outflow tract, such as complete ECD with abnormal insertion of the mitral papillary muscles at the crest of the ISD.

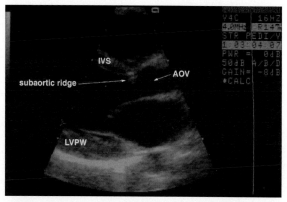

Figure 29-39. Subaortic ridge. In the parasternal long-axis view, there is an echobright ridge in the left ventricular outflow tract below the aortic valve (AOV). It may be isolated to this anterior surface or it may form a membrane which wraps around the entire outflow tract and adheres to the anterior mitral valve. LVPW, left ventricular posterior wall; IVS, interventricular septum.

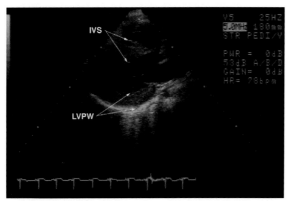

Figure 29-40. Dynamic muscular subaortic stenosis. In the parasternal long-axis view, both the ventricular septum (IVS) and the left ventricular posterior wall (LVPW) are thick (left ventricular hypertrophy). The ventricular septum, however, is much thicker than the posterior wall. As the underlying disease progresses, the end-diastolic and end-systolic volumes decrease as the muscle mass takes up more and more of the cavity. As this happens, there will be an increase in the velocity of blood exiting the left ventricle. In severe stenosis, there will be no appreciable cavity in end systole.

SUPRAVALVULAR AORTIC STENOSIS

Unlike other forms of LVOT obstruction, supravalvular aortic stenosis is usually associated with other defects. There are two major groups of associated defects: (1) familiar supravalvular aortic stenosis and branch pulmonary artery stenosis and (2) nonfamilial Williams syndrome. In the first group, there is usually a family history of supravalvular aortic stenosis and pulmonary artery branch stenosis; absent, however, are the facial anomalies or mental retardation associated with Williams syndrome. In the second group, Williams syndrome is associated with abnormal facial characteristics (*elfin facies*), mental retardation, and abnormalities of calcium metabolism. Most of these cases are nonfamilial and reflect a disease affecting multiple organ systems.

There are three major types of supravalvular aortic stenosis: isolated narrowing above the sinus of Valsalva, circumferential discrete membrane, or diffuse hypoplasia of the ascending aorta. In each of these cases, the coronary arteries arise proximal to the area of obstruction, so they are subject to the elevated left ventricular pressure. These coronary arteries may be tortuous in course and undergo accel-

erated atherosclerotic changes. The aortic valve may appear thickened.

AORTIC ATRESIA

Aortic atresia is very rarely seen in association with other defects. Its most common presentation is in conjunction with mitral atresia and hypoplastic left ventricle in what is termed *hypoplastic left heart syndrome* (Fig. 29-41).[8] In this syndrome, blood flow through the right heart is normal. Pulmonary venous return, however, enters the left atrium, meets a solid bar across the mitral annulus, and exits the left atrium across the IAS to the right atrium. There is no egress from the heart except via the pulmonary artery. In utero and in the immediate postnatal period, systemic blood flow is provided by pulmonary outflow crossing the ductus arteriosus into the aorta. As it enters the aorta, some blood flow goes superiorly to supply the upper body and around the arch to the coronary arteries; the remainder courses inferiorly to supply the trunk and lower

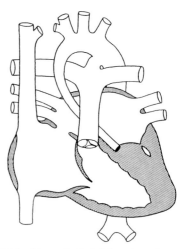

Figure 29-41. Hypoplastic left heart syndrome. This syndrome usually consists of mitral atresia and aortic atresia. Since there is no flow into the left ventricle (mitral atresia) and no flow out of the left ventricle (aortic atresia), the left ventricular cavity is very small and round, with bright endocardial walls and poor contractility. Color Doppler will demonstrate retrograde flow in the ascending aorta which fills the coronary arteries. (From Mullins CE, Mayer DC. *Congenital Heart Disease: A Diagrammatic Atlas.* Diagram 27. Chicago, YearBook Medical Publishers; 1990. Reprinted by permission of Wiley-Liss, Inc., a division of John Wiley & Sons, Inc.)

body. Without a PDA, this defect is obviously lethal. Treatment is surgical and involves a staged reconstruction (a series of three operations ending in the Fontan procedure) or neonatal heart transplant.

Preoperative Echocardiography

The initial echocardiographic evaluation of a child with left ventricular outflow obstruction should involve a complete, thorough study of the entire heart, but with special attention paid to all aspects of left ventricular inflow and outflow. The *mitral valve apparatus* can be evaluated in the short-axis parasternal view for placement of papillary muscles and for overall function (see Fig. 29-2). Apical four-chamber or subcostal transverse views allow evaluation for mitral regurgitation by color Doppler.

The parasternal short-axis view of the LV, starting at the apex and sweeping up to the level of the aortic valve, will give a good evaluation of the *LVOT* and left ventricular mass. Parasternal long-axis views allow M-mode measurement of left ventricular thickness and fractional shortening. In this view, the interventricular septum (IVS) *must* be perpendicular to the plane of the ultrasound beam; otherwise, the thickness of the IVS and left ventricular posterior wall (LVPW) will be overestimated. The M-mode trace should be placed at the tips of the mitral valve leaflet so that leaflet motion is seen but the entire excursion of the leaflet is not appreciated. The parasternal long-axis view also gives a good look at the subaortic area. If there is a thin membrane in the LVOT, it may not be seen in the parasternal long-axis view. Therefore, the LVOT should *also* be evaluated by 2D and color Doppler in the apical long-axis view or the subcostal long-axis view. With the same long-axis transducer orientation, the transducer is moved toward the right shoulder to evaluate the first 1–2 cm of the supravalvular area by 2D. The apical long-axis and subcostal views allow other planes of the ascending aorta to be evaluated.

The *aortic valve* is best evaluated in the short-axis view; the number of cusps and the orientation of the raphe are best defined in this view. The normal aortic valve leaflets are of equal size, with equal distances between the hinge points. In the closed position the valve leaflets resemble the "Mercedes Benz" insignia (upside down). Mild abnormalities of the aortic valve, represented in Figure 29-38, are variations of *bicuspid aortic valve*. If aortic regurgitation is present, a long-axis parasternal and apical view will give a good estimation of the width and length of the aortic insufficiency (AI) jet and its source. With the transducer in a parasternal long-axis orientation, move the transducer toward the right shoulder, following the course of the ascending aorta. In this view, look for evidence of *supravalvular narrowing*. It is also important to evaluate the *aortic arch* for evidence of coarctation of the aorta.

If there is only a bar of tissue in the mitral position, a thin slit-like left ventricle, and a thread-like aorta with a diameter of less than 4 mm, this indicates *hypoplastic left heart syndrome* (HLHS). From a parasternal short-axis view, identification of the coronary arteries as they come off the aortic root is important; often they are larger in diameter than the aortic root. Color Doppler in the ascending aorta should show retrograde flow from the aortic arch to the aortic root. Color Doppler in the four-chamber view will confirm no flow into the left ventricle from the left atrium and a large left-to-right shunt across the interatrial septum.

Once the anatomy is defined and understood, hemodynamic information should be obtained. A pulsed wave Doppler evaluation of mitral inflow and aortic outflow provides valuable information. Evaluation of aortic outflow should include pulsed wave Doppler evaluation in the subvalvular area, just above the aortic valve, in the supravalvular area, and in the descending aorta below the site of a coarctation. Color Doppler evaluation should assist in defining the site of obstruction. Continuous wave Doppler in one of the long-axis orientations will provide maximum instantaneous velocity, which, via the Bernoulli equation, can estimate the gradient across the LVOT. If there is aortic or mitral regurgitation, it should be graded according to the length of the flame, and comments made about the width of the flame and the site of the regurgitation.

Postoperative Echocardiography

Postoperative echocardiographic evaluation will depend upon the type of surgery performed. If an aortic valvulotomy is performed, look closely at the degree of aortic regurgitation and its source. If aortic valve replacement was performed, refer to the discussion in Chapter 16 on the configuration of flow across prosthetic aortic valves. If a subaortic ridge was resected, look closely at the function and motion of the anterior mitral valve leaflet, look for a new VSD in the position of the subaortic ridge, and carefully evaluate any residual gradient across the area.

Surgery for congenital aortic valve stenosis usually involves aortic valvulotomy; aortic valve replacement is uncommon in childhood. An excellent surgical result provides maximal relief of obstruction without the development of aortic regurgitation. Unfortunately, a suboptimal result may fail to relieve the gradient sufficiently or may cause moderate to severe aortic regurgitation. Postoperative echocardiography should therefore evaluate the degree of obstruction and regurgitation. Careful measurement of each, in addition to the M-mode measurement of LV dimensions, provides a baseline against which future measurements can be compared.

Surgery for HLHS involves either a heart transplant or the staged reconstruction. A description of the echocardiographic evaluation of each stage of the Norwood procedure is beyond the scope of this chapter. Evaluation of the posttransplant heart is similar to that in adult cardiology.

Aortic Arch Anomalies

Although many forms of aortic arch anomalies (Table 29-10) are seen in children, three types are most common: coarctation of the aorta, interrupted aortic arch, and right aortic arch. Although these represent different embryologic processes, they are discussed together in this section because they involve findings from the same portion of the echocardiographic study.

COARCTATION OF THE AORTA

Coarctation of the aorta usually consists of a discrete area of stenosis in the descending aorta just below the takeoff of the left subclavian artery and across from the insertion of the ductus arteriosus. Coarctation represents 6–8% of congenital heart defects. It may be associated with VSD, PDA, and aortic and mitral valve abnormalities. Occasionally, the combination of coarctation of the aorta and VSD in infants causes severe symptoms of congestive heart failure. More commonly, however, the presence of the coarctation is unknown for several months to years.

Anatomy and Physiology

Since coarctation of the aorta is found most often opposite the insertion of the ductus arteriosus, blood flow in utero is undisturbed since flow coming from the ascending aorta has the ductal insertion point as a "detour" around the coarctation. As the ductus arteriosus closes near the aorta, the detour

TABLE 29-10. AORTIC ARCH ANOMALIES

Question to Be Answered	Views	Comments
Intact aortic arch?	Suprasternal notch Subxiphoid	Does arch appear intact?
Flow characteristics in descending aorta	Suprasternal notch	Is color Doppler in arch continuous between ascending and descending aortas? Is pulsed wave Doppler velocity the same in descending and ascending aortas?
If other anomalies seen, what side is aorta on?	Suprasternal notch Longitudinal	Find tracheal rings. Tip transducer each way until you see descending aorta. Is it to the right or left of the trachea?
Adequacy of subaortic area	Parasternal Long axis	Measure diameter of subaortic area. Use color Doppler to look for turbulence in subvalvular area. Quantify with continuous wave Doppler.
Structure of aortic valve	Parasternal Short axis	How many leaflets are seen? Any redundant or thickened valve tissue? Leaflets should move freely. Color Doppler should look for AI, turbulence above aortic valve. Use pulsed and continuous wave Doppler in LVOT to evaluate total outflow tract gradient.
Structure of mitral valve	Long axis Short axis	Does the mitral valve open fully? Are papillary muscles in appropriate positions? Is color Doppler inflow normal and laminar? Use pulsed wave Doppler to quantify E and A wave inflow velocities. Use color Doppler to look for mitral regurgitation.

becomes narrower. When the ductus is completely closed, there little detour is left; blood flow is therefore turbulent, with high velocity around this narrow area. This high-velocity jet usually impacts the aortic wall distal to the coarctation in such a way as to create an area of dilatation (called *poststenotic dilatation*) and intimal disruption. In this area, there is the potential for the development of bacterial endocarditis.

Because of the obstruction to blood flow presented by the coarctation, the resistance in the systemic arterial circulation is increased distal to the coarctation. If there is a coexisting VSD, as the pulmonary vascular resistance drops after birth, blood flows preferentially to the pulmonary artery since the systemic resistance is increasing (as the ductus closes) while the pulmonary resistance is decreasing. This may lead to large volumes of excess blood flow to the pulmonary artery, leading to congestive heart failure.

Although a discrete narrowing is the usual form of coarctation, there may be a long area of narrowing instead; this is often associated with a narrow transverse arch. These coarctations are more difficult to approach surgically. Coarctation can also occur infrequently in other areas of the aorta, distal to the usual site, and may even occur in the abdominal aorta.

Coarctation of the aorta can be associated with many other intracardiac abnormalities.[29] The most common ones are bicuspid aortic valve, VSD, valvular aortic stenosis, subaortic stenosis, endocardial cushion defect, DTGA with VSD, and DORV. In fact, bicuspid aortic valve has been reported in up to 85% of children with coarctation of the aorta.

Clinical Problems

If the coarctation is isolated (i.e., there are no other associated defects), the child is asymptomatic. He or she is referred to the cardiologist if a new murmur (from the collateral vessels which form off the aorta) or high blood pressure develops. The high blood pressure exists only in the arteries proximal to the coarctation (head and arms); blood pressure distal to the coarctation is normal to slightly decreased (legs and torso). For this reason, pediatric cardiologists always recommend that blood pressure be checked in the arms and legs in all patients with high blood pressure.

Preoperative Echocardiography

The thoracic aorta is best viewed in the suprasternal and subxiphoid views. In the suprasternal view, the diameters of the ascending aorta, transverse arch, and descending aorta are compared. Careful evaluation of the descending aorta in the region of the ductus arteriosus and the takeoff of the left subclavian by color Doppler should be part of the study. Although the direction of blood flow is changing in that area, color Doppler should still suggest laminar flow. Using pulsed wave Doppler, the sample volume is placed in the ascending aorta and maximal flow velocity is measured. Sample volume in the descending aorta beyond the point where the coarctation would be seen allows measure maximal velocity here. There should be very little difference between the two velocities in the normal aorta. If color Doppler suggests turbulence in the descending aorta, the pulsed wave cursor and then the continuous wave cursor are placed in the area of turbulence and the maximal velocities are measured. Once both maximal velocities are obtained, the predicted gradient across the coarctation can be estimated by the following equation:[22]

Proximal pressure − distal pressure

$$= 4(\text{distal velocity}^2 - \text{proximal velocity}^2)$$

Thus, if velocity is 4 m/sec in the descending aorta and 1.5 m/sec in the ascending aorta, the estimated pressure gradient across the coarctation would be

$$4(4^2 - 1.5^2) = 4(16 - 2) = 56 \text{ mm Hg}$$

From the subxiphoid view, excellent images of the ascending aorta and aortic arch can be obtained. The same information should be obtained from this view. Doppler evaluation may be more difficult from this view, however, since aortic flow is close to perpendicular to the plane of the image in the descending aorta.

After the arch has been interrogated, a thorough evaluation of intracardiac anatomy should be performed. Close attention should be paid to the left heart. Coarctation of the aorta may be part of Shone's complex. Therefore, careful visualization of the mitral valve apparatus and attachments, aortic valve leaflets, and subaortic and supra-aortic areas should be performed. Since 85% of children with coarctation have bicuspid aortic valve, close attention should be paid to the structure and position of the aortic valve leaflets and commissures. Color and pulsed wave Doppler evaluation of inflow/outflow of each of these valves should be carried out.

Postoperative Echocardiography

Surgical repair of coarctation usually consists of an end-to-end anastomosis or a subclavian flap. Both of these procedures are discussed in the section on surgical descriptions. Postoperatively, flow should be laminar through the repaired area unless the repair contorts the shape of the descending aorta. Aside from the usual postoperative evaluation, a careful color and pulsed wave or continuous wave Doppler evaluation of the area of the surgical repair should be undertaken. It is very important to estimate the residual gradient across the area of coarctation.

INTERRUPTED AORTIC ARCH

Anatomy

Interrupted aortic arch (IAA) consists of the complete separation of the ascending and descending aortas. While there are nine described types of IAA,[23,30] there are three major types. In type A, the interruption is distal to the left subclavian artery; thus, all neck vessels come off the ascending aorta. In type B, the interruption is between the carotid and subclavian arteries; in this case, there is one neck vessel coming off the descending aorta and two from the ascending aorta. In type C, the interruption is between the carotid arteries. In this type, there is one neck vessel arising from the ascending aorta and two from the descending aorta. Type A IAA is associated with an aortopulmonary window, with an intact ventricular septum and DTGA. Type B IAA is more common and is usually associated with conotruncal abnormalities. This is the type seen in children with DiGeorge syndrome. Type C IAA is very rare, and there are no acknowledged associations specific to this type. All three types of IAA may also have some degree of subaortic obstruction.

Physiology

With IAA, blood flow from the left ventricle enters the ascending aorta and goes to the neck vessels. Since there is no communication between the ascending and descending aortas, no blood exiting the left ventricle enters the descending aorta. Thus, descending aorta flow (and perfusion of the kidneys, gut, liver, spleen, and lower extremities) depends on flow from the pulmonary artery across the ductus arteriosus into the descending aorta. If the ductus arteriosus closes, the child suffers profound cardiovascular collapse, and usually requires resuscitation and PGE1 infusion to reestablish descending aorta blood flow.

Preoperative Echocardiography

Since the best images of the aorta are obtained from the suprasternal and subxiphoid windows, these views should be attempted first. The classic view of an IAA shows the ascending aorta leaving the left ventricle and traveling in the direction of the head only; there is no reason for it to form an arch since there is no communication with the descending aorta. Thus, a classic IAA is easy to visualize. There are some, however, which resemble a severe coarctation of the aorta since the ascending and descending aortas overlie each other. Color Doppler may help define the source of blood flow for each of the neck vessels.

Since IAA is associated with complex congenital heart disease, close attention should be paid to the evaluation of intracardiac structures and hemodynamics.

Postoperative Echocardiography

Surgical repair of IAA depends on the degree of subaortic obstruction. If the subaortic area is 5–6 mm or more in diameter, a primary repair can be accomplished.[31] In addition to repair of the other intracardiac anomalies, the two ends of the aorta are reanastomosed. If the subaortic area measures less than 3 mm in diameter, a Norwood procedure is usually performed. The postoperative echocardiographic study should closely evaluate the other aspects of intracardiac repair. It should also examine the characteristics of flow through the new aortic arch. Using color Doppler, areas of turbulence are identified and carefully interrogated with pulsed and continuous wave Doppler. The 2D image should allow measurement of the diameters of the ascending and descending aortas. Finally, the subaortic area should be visualized and color Doppler used to evaluate the characteristics of flow in this area. Continuous wave Doppler will help to quantify the maximal velocity across the subaortic area.

RIGHT AORTIC ARCH

Anatomy/Physiology

Most aortic arches course to the left; the initial portion of the descending aorta is to the left of the spine.[15] In a right aortic arch, the aorta crosses over the right mainstem bronchus and descends, usually on the right side of the spine. This anomaly is seen most frequently in tetralogy of Fallot; it is reported to occur in 13–34% of children with this condition. It is also seen in children with DTGV and an intact ventricular septum. Unless there is an anomalous vessel which swings around the posterior side of the bronchus, causing a vascular ring, there are no symptoms associated with a right aortic arch; thus, no surgical repair is necessary.

Echocardiography

Echocardiographic determination of the side of the arch is often difficult since the exam is performed in small children, in whom a suprasternal notch view is very difficult. This author prefers a suprasternal notch or infraclavicular area in a longitudinal plane. The transducer is tipped toward the right shoulder and angled slowly toward the left shoulder. When tracheal rings (a series of parallel echolucent lines perpendicular to the ultrasound beam) are visualized, the transducer is tipped first to one side and then to the other to visualize the descending aorta. If the descending aorta is seen to the left of the tracheal rings, it is assumed to be a left aortic arch; if it is seen to the right, it is assumed to be a right aortic arch.

Atrioventricular Valve Abnormalities

AV valve abnormalities (Table 29-11) include tricuspid atresia (see the section on "Single Ventricle"), Ebstein's anomaly of the tricuspid valve, mitral atresia (see the section on "Single Ventricle"), mitral regurgitation, mitral valve prolapse, cleft mitral valve, mitral stenosis, supramitral stenosing ring, and cor triatriatum.

EBSTEIN'S ANOMALY OF THE TRICUSPID VALVE

Anatomy and Physiology

In Ebstein's anomaly of the tricuspid valve, the tricuspid valve leaflets are displaced toward the apex of the right ventricle (Fig. 29-42). In addition, they are adherent to the ventricular walls, thus forming an extension of the atrium into the ventricle (called *atrialization of the right ventricle*). The valve tissue is usually redundant, but if adherence to the right ventricular wall is significant, the movement of the unadhered valve leaflets may be limited. In mild Ebstein's anomaly, the displacement is minimal and the clinical picture is that of mild tricuspid regurgitation. In severe Ebstein's anomaly, the tricuspid valve closure point is close to the apex; thus, the right ventricular cavity is very small and the right atrial cavity is quite large. A severe abnormality is usually associated with moderate to severe regurgitation; there may be some degree of inflow and outflow obstruction. Associated defects include ASD, VSD, pulmonary stenosis, and pulmonary atresia.

Clinical Problems

In moderate to severe Ebstein's anomaly, there is poor closure of the valve and thus variable degrees of tricuspid regurgitation. If the right ventricular cavity is small, its contraction pattern may be inefficient in propelling blood through the pulmonary valve, and a functional pulmonary atresia may exist. Either of these two factors may cause an increase in right atrial pressure, leading to right-to-left shunting at the atrial level. For this reason, these children are usually cyanotic. They also have an increased incidence of dysrhythmias, especially supraventricular tachycardia.

Medical management of these children involves treatment of congestive heart failure and dysrhythmias. As the degree of tricuspid regurgitation decreases, however, the heart failure becomes more difficult to treat medically. Eventually, most children with a moderate to severe abnormality will require surgery. In those in whom antegrade pulmonary artery flow is limited, a Blalock-Taussig shunt may be indicated early in life. For those with predominantly tricuspid regurgitation, valve replacement is usually attempted, along with release of the excessive tricuspid tissue in the body of the right ventricle and closure of the ASD. For those with arrhythmias not amenable to medical therapy, ablation of accessory pathways may be attempted in the operating room at the time of surgery. Unfortunately, defect still has a poor overall prognosis.

◢◤◢◤ TABLE 29-11. ATRIOVENTRICULAR VALVE ABNORMALITIES

Question to Be Answered	Views	Comments
TRICUSPID VALVE		
Structure and function of tricuspid valve, right ventricle	Short axis	Are hinge points of tricuspid valve deeper in ventricle than those of mitral valve? Look at degree of valve regurgitation. How does size of right ventricular cavity compare to that of left ventricular cavity? How does size of right atrium compare to that of left atrium? With pulsed wave Doppler, look at inflow velocity and configuration. Measure valve annulus.
RVOT	Short axis Subcostal	Look at size of RVOT, color Doppler signal across RVOT, pulsed wave Doppler velocity, and degree of PI.
Right ventricle pressure		With continuous wave Doppler, interrogate TI jet; estimate right ventricular pressure (RVP).
IAS	Four-chamber Subcostal	Look closely at IAS for breaks in the septum and bowing of septum.
IVS	Long axis	Look with 2D and color Doppler for associated VSDs.
Other defects: VSDs, ASD, C/A, absent pulm, valve, right ventricle-pulmonary artery continuity	Four-chamber Subcostal Suprasternal Left atrium Short axis	Look closely at muscular septum. Will see more PI than with intact valve. Make sure there is color Doppler flow from right ventricle to pulmonary artery; otherwise, this is probably pulmonary atresia.
MITRAL VALVE		
Mitral valve structure	Short axis Long axis Apical four-chamber	Where are papillary muscles and how many are there? How many leaflets do you see? Is there a defect in either of the leaflets? In long axis, how well do leaflets move? Does valve prolapse? Measure valve annulus.
LV function, size	Long axis Apical four-chamber	M-mode for measurement of %fs, LVDD, VCF, left atrium. With pulsed wave Doppler, interrogate mitral inflow for evaluation of diastolic function. How much mitral regurgitation is there?
Pulmonary veins	Apical four-chamber Subcostal	Do all four pulmonary veins return to left atrium? Measure flow velocity in each vein. Is flow through the left atrium laminar by color Doppler?
Left atrium	Long axis Apical four-chamber Subcostal	Size of left atrium relative to right atrium. Are there any anomalous structures in the posterior left atrium or behind the mitral valve leaflets?
LV, Aorta	Long axis Short axis Suprasternal	Because of associated defects of mitral valve and LVOT, look closely at subaortic area, aortic valve, supravalvular area, aortic arch.

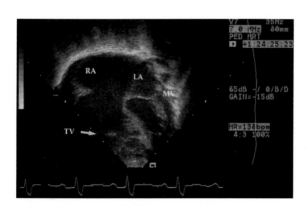

Figure 29-42. Ebstein's anomaly of the tricuspid valve. The hinge points of the tricuspid valve appear displaced toward the apex of the right ventricle. The portion of the heart functioning as an atrium is increased, while the portion functioning as a ventricle is decreased. These valves are usually incompetent, and valve regurgitation increases with time. RA, right atrium; LA, left atrium; MV, mitral valve; TV, tricuspid valve.

Preoperative Echocardiography

Because of the variety of associated defects, the segmental approach should be used when Ebstein's anomaly of the tricuspid valve is suspected. In the apical four-chamber view, the closure point of the tricuspid valve should be seen displaced toward the apex.[25] A careful color Doppler examination of the tricuspid valve should be carried out to determine the number of tricuspid regurgitation jets, and continuous wave Doppler should be employed to estimate the right ventricular pressure. In the parasternal short-axis and subcostal short-axis views, close evaluation of the RVOT, especially by color Doppler, is important. The degree of pulmonary regurgitation and the outflow velocity should be noted. In the subcostal short-axis plane, the atrial septum is evaluated for ASD. In the apical four-chamber and parasternal long-axis views, the ventricular septum is examined for VSD.

Postoperative Echocardiography

Close evaluation of the tricuspid valve in the postoperative study is essential; multiple "creative" views may be necessary to obtain good images of the valve and its function. Evaluation of the valve in each view with color Doppler is necessary to evaluate regurgitation and the inflow pattern. Quantification of the inflow velocity with pulsed wave Doppler should be performed. In the apical four-chamber and parasternal short-axis views, the contractile qualities of the right ventricle can be examined. Evidence of removal of tricuspid valve tissue from the body of the right ventricle may be visualized. Evaluation of the RVOT with color and pulsed wave Doppler will help define the degree of regurgitation and obstruction. Finally, an attempt should be made to estimate right ventricular pressure via tricuspid regurgitation.

MITRAL REGURGITATION, MITRAL VALVE PROLAPSE, AND CLEFT MITRAL VALVE

Anatomy/Physiology

The most common isolated structural causes of mitral regurgitation in children are cleft mitral valve and mitral valve prolapse. In addition, systemic diseases and ventricular function may also affect the mitral valve. Secondary causes of mitral regurgitation are acute inflammatory processes (rheumatic heart disease, viral myocarditis, Kawasaki's disease), dilated and hypertrophic cardiomyopathy, connective tissue diseases (Marfan's syndrome, Ehlers-Danlos syndrome), and metabolic diseases (mucopolysaccharidoses).

Despite the cause, anything more than a mild degree of regurgitation will cause dilatation of the left atrium. As the regurgitation increases, left atrial pressure increases; this pressure will be transmitted into the pulmonary vascular bed. Thus, pulmonary artery pressure rises, right ventricular pressure rises, and the tricuspid valve may become incompetent, allowing echocardiographic estimation of right ventricular pressure.

Cleft mitral valve is most commonly associated with complete or partial AV canal defects. It is rarely seen as an isolated defect. The cleft may occur in the anterior or posterior leaflet and can cause moderate to severe mitral regurgitation.

Mitral valve prolapse, which is discussed at length in Chapter 13, is also a cause of regurgitation, though it is usually mild in childhood. The definition of mitral valve prolapse in children follows the guidelines for adults. The diagnosis of mitral valve prolapse in children is usually not made before the age of 5 years.

Clinical Problems

In most children, mild to moderate mitral regurgitation is not associated with noticeable symptoms. Moderate to severe mitral regurgitation causes dyspnea, decreased exercise tolerance, and signs of congestive heart failure. Medical management of congestive heart failure may improve the clinical symptoms for months to years. There is also an increased risk of atrial thrombus when the left atrium becomes dilated.

Preoperative Echocardiography

The study is started with the transducer in the parasternal long-axis view, allowing evaluation of left ventricular function, mitral valve motion, and left ventricular outflow by 2D and color Doppler. In the parasternal long-axis view, the valve is evaluated for normal motion; the leaflets should close in a straight line between their hinge points. If the closed leaflets "sags" back into the left atrium, it prolapses. The presence of mitral regurgitation can be documented with color Doppler. In the parasternal short-axis view, the mitral valve is seen in cross section. Both leaflets should be carefully interrogated for evidence of a cleft. The transducer should be swept from apex to base to identify the area of dropout in one of the leaflets.

Postoperative Echocardiography

Surgery for mitral regurgitation usually involves prosthetic valve replacement. Flow characteristics of the prosthetic valves are discussed in Chapter 16 and are comparable for children. Look for residual mitral regurgitation, the size of the left atrium, and left ventricular function, and, if possible, estimate right ventricular pressure by continuous wave Doppler velocity of tricuspid regurgitation.

MITRAL STENOSIS, SUPRAMITRAL STENOSING RING, AND COR TRIATRIATUM

Although supramitral stenosis and cor triatriatum are not technically abnormalities of the mitral valve, they cause an effective mitral stenosis and, as such, are discussed in this section.

Anatomy/Physiology

Congenital mitral stenosis is rare and is seen most often as a result of a double orifice mitral valve, fused commissures, or parachute mitral valve. *Double orifice mitral valve* is the result of anomalous tissue which divides the mitral orifice into two smaller openings. *Parachute mitral valve*[6,26] involves attachment of all chordae to a single papillary muscle; the chordae are usually shortened, and motion of the mitral valve is restricted. Parachute mitral valve is associated with other levels of left ventricular inflow and outflow obstruction.

Cor triatriatum (Fig. 29-43) is due to late stenosis of the common pulmonary vein as it enters the left atrium; the result is a "chamber" posterior to the left atrium which has an orifice through which pulmonary venous return must pass to enter the left atrium. Since this chamber presents obstruction to flow into the left ventricle, its consequences are similar to those of valvular mitral stenosis.

Supramitral stenosing ring involves connective tissue in the left atrium, just above the mitral valve, which encroaches on the mitral valve leaflets and may obstruct mitral inflow.

In all cases of mitral stenosis, left atrial pressure is increased, pulmonary artery pressure is increased relative to left atrial pressure, and congestive heart

failure may be present. Medical management involves treatment of congestive heart failure. Surgery will be required in almost all of these children.

Preoperative Echocardiography

Since there is an association with congenital mitral stenosis and other defects, a careful evaluation via the segmental approach should be performed, with special attention to left ventricular inflow and outflow. If the mitral valve appears structurally normal, the left atrium and pulmonary veins should be evaluated closely. If there appears to be a membrane in the left atrium, the diagnosis is either cor triatriatum or supramitral stenosing ring. This distinction is made by the position of the foramen ovale and left atrial appendage: they are located between the membrane and mitral valve in cor triatriatum and behind the mitral valve and ring in supramitral stenosing ring.

Postoperative Echocardiography

In children with valvular mitral stenosis, surgery to replace the mitral valve may provide some improvement if the valve annulus is large enough to allow a valve which will accommodate the child's growth over several years. In smaller children, mitral valvuloplasty may be attempted, though it is considered as a palliative procedure only; valve replacement will probably be required in time.

In supramitral stenosing ring and cor triatriatum, surgery is aimed at removing the membrane between pulmonary venous return and the mitral valve. In supramitral stenosing ring, the membrane may be so adherent to the mitral valve tissue that it cannot be removed without replacing the mitral valve.

The postoperative echocardiogram should carefully evaluate the pulmonary venous return by color and pulsed wave Doppler, mitral inflow configuration, and evidence of mitral regurgitation. In addition, close attention should be paid to left ventricular function.

Situs Abnormalities

The echocardiographic evaluation of a child with a known cardiac malposition or suspicion of abnormal situs (Table 29-12) is perhaps the most challenging of all studies. Under these circumstances, the *only* way to assess the intracardiac anatomy and hemody-

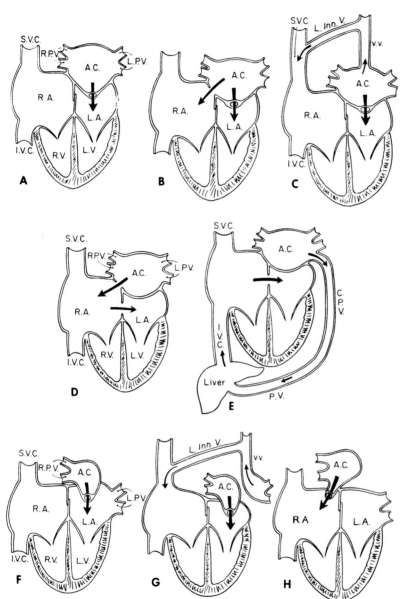

Figure 29-43. Cor triatriatum. These diagrams represent the many variants of cor triatriatum. In all forms, some or all of the pulmonary veins enter an accessory chamber which is posterior to the left atrium. Flow from this chamber usually goes into the left atrium through an opening between the two chambers; it can go anomalously to the superior or inferior vena cava. (From Emmanouilides GC, Riemenschneider TA, Allen HD, et al. *Heart Disease in Infants, Children, and Adolescents.* Baltimore, Williams & Wilkins; 1995: 864. Reprinted with permission.)

TABLE 29-12. DIAGNOSIS OF SITUS ABNORMALITIES

Question to Be Answered	Views	Comments
Visceral situs	Transverse Abdomen	If the bulk of the liver is to the right, the stomach to the left, and the IVC goes directly into the right atrium, *visceral situs solitus*.
Atrial situs	Subcostal Apical four-chamber	If rightward atrium receives systemic veins and coronary sinus and leftward atrium receives pulmonary veins, *atrial situs solitus*.
Dextrocardia Levocardia Mesocardia	Parasternal	If apex to left, base midline, *levocardia;* if apex to right, base midline, *dextrocardia;* if apex midline, base midline, *mesocardia.*
IVC-right atrium	Subcostal	Follow suprahepatic IVC to right atrium, SVC to right atrium. Is this atrium on right or left of heart?
Right atrium-right ventricle	Subcostal Apical four-chamber	Are hinge points of this AV valve deeper in ventricle than those of other valve? Are there several papillary muscles? Does AV valve have three leaflets? Does ventricle have moderator band at apex? Does ventricle have infundibular or outflow chamber? If all these apply, this is *tricuspid valve* and *morphologic right ventricle.*
Right ventricle-pulmonary artery	Short axis Long-axis—RVOT	From this ventricle, which great vessel arises? Must see pulmonary artery branch. Look for PDA by color Doppler. Look at size of this great vessel relative to that of other vessel.
Pulmonary veins-left atrium	Apical four-chamber Subcostal	Find leftward atrium. If pulmonary veins enter this atrium, this is *left atrium.* Perform color Doppler evaluation of pulmonary valve.
Left atrium-left ventricle	Apical four-chamber Subcostal	Does this AV valve have two papillary muscles and two leaflets? Are its hinge points higher in the ventricle than those of the other valve? If so, this is a *mitral valve.* A *morphologic left ventricle* should be smooth-walled, circular in cross section, and slipper-shaped in long axis; the LVOT should be defined by the IVS and anterior mitral leaflet. Evaluate relative ventricular volumes. Look for a VSD.
Left ventricle-aorta	Long axis Subcostal	Does this ventricle give rise to an aorta? Is the aorta committed only to this ventricle? Look at the relative size of the great vessels above the semilunar valves. Evaluate ventricular outflow tract with color Doppler.
Pulmonary artery/aorta orientation	Short axis	Is pulmonary artery anterior or posterior to aorta?

namics correctly is to use the segmental approach. Careful delineation of systemic venous return, with precise definition of the morphology of each chamber and valve and its relationship to its associated chambers and vessels, *must* be performed. Any other attempt will certainly end in both an erroneous diagnosis and a frustrated sonographer.

Although there are some anomalies which are more commonly associated with certain forms of situs abnormalities, a sonographer should assume that any intracardiac abnormality may be present in every one of these patients. Efforts to rule in or rule out each of those abnormalities should be made before proceeding to the next stage of the evaluation. In addition, although the visceral (abdominal) situs and thoracic situs are almost always the same, the sonographer should assume that the association of abdominal structures to thoracic ones is a random event and set out to prove the situs in both areas.

The anatomy, physiology, and clinical aspects of each of the defects associated with situs abnormalities is described in detail in the chapter related to each defect. This section focuses on the echocardiographic challenges involved in initially determining the diagnosis.

ECHOCARDIOGRAPHIC EVALUATION

Identification of the visceral and intracardiac structures in complex heart disease requires knowledge of the identifying characteristics of each structure.

In a transverse plane, scan the abdomen from caudad to cephalad to assess the configuration of the liver. In the normal visceral situs, the major bulk of the liver is located in the left portion of the abdomen, with a small "tail" extending across the midline to the left. The stomach is seen on the opposite side of the abdomen. With the transducer in a longitudinal plane, find the spine. Rotating the transducer to the left and right of the spine, define the IVC and aorta. Place a pulsed wave Doppler sample in each of these vessels to confirm the configurations of arterial or venous flow. Follow the IVC cephalad, making sure that it communicates directly with the right atrium. If the IVC is not seen entering the RA, hepatic veins may be the only venous structures emptying into the right atrium. If the IVC does not connect to the right atrium, locating the coronary sinus or SVC will help define the right atrium, although each may return anomalously elsewhere. As discussed earlier, the SVC and IVC are best visualized in the subxiphoid planes, with the plane of the transducer parallel to the spine and to the left of the midline. Both the SVC and IVC are large venous structures; color Doppler will demonstrate laminar low-velocity flow coming toward the right atrium. Pulsed wave Doppler will demonstrate flow velocity which is low, variable, and continuous. The coronary sinus is best visualized in the short-axis orientation in the subxiphoid position and is seen as a large, echo-free structure posterior to the atrium; color Doppler flow will also be low velocity, continuous, and laminar.

If the major portion of the liver is to the right, the stomach is to the left, the IVC is on the right of the spine and enters right atrium, and the aorta is to the left of the spine, then the visceral situs is assumed to be normal—*visceral situs solitus*. If all findings are the opposite of normal, then *visceral situs inversus* exists. If there are findings which do not fit either category, the term *visceral situs ambiguous* is used; it implies only that the classic configuration of situs solitus and situs inversus do not exist in this patient.

The initial evaluation of the heart should be done to define the orientation of the long axis of the heart. In *levocardia*, the long axis shows the apex to the left, with the base at the midline. In *dextrocardia*, the long axis is opposite to this, so that the apex is to the right, with the base at the midline. *Mesocardia* indicates that the apex is toward the midline, as is the base.

Finally, the intracardiac connections must be defined. In a longitudinal plane, the IVC is followed through the diaphragm into the heart. The entry of the *suprahepatic IVC* into the atrium defines this as right atrium. Large hepatic veins entering the right atrium, as can happen with azygous continuation of the IVC to the SVC, may be confused with the IVC. The abdominal IVC courses cephalad into the right atrium, with hepatic veins entering the IVC; this defines the atrium as the right atrium. If the IVC does not enter the atrium, locate the coronary sinus, which will also define a right atrium if it is not unroofed.

Turning the transducer in a transverse plane, note the relationship between the right and left atria. If the morphologic right atrium is on the right and the morphologic left atrium is on the left, this is *atrial situs solitus*. If the reverse is seen, then *atrial situs inversus* exists.

In the apical four-chamber view, the *morphologic right ventricle* is identified by the moderator band and by the AV valve hinge points, which are deeper in the ventricle than are the left AV valves' hinge points. In addition, in a short-axis or long-axis view of the right ventricle, there is tissue between the tricuspid valve and the semilunar valve; there is none in a left ventricle. The *morphologic tricuspid valve* has three leaflets and is seen in the short axis. Rotating and angling the transducer, find the RVOT. There should be an identifiable outflow or infundibular portion, bordered on all sides by ventricular muscle.

In a parasternal short-axis view, the great vessel can be seen coming off the right ventricle. If this vessel bifurcates, it is probably a *pulmonary artery*. Make sure that this vessel is different from the aortic arch, which will be identified later. Color Doppler may identify a ductus arteriosus entering near the left pulmonary artery, which will further assist in identifying this as pulmonary artery. In complex congenital heart disease, nonstandard "creative" views may be necessary to document the bifurcation of the pulmonary artery. In a predominantly short-axis orientation, the transducer is moved in a cephalad and leftward position if the cardiac apex is to the left, caudad and rightward if the cardiac apex is to the right. On occasion, the only view of the bifurcation will be a subcostal view; this is often difficult to obtain in infants, however, because the pulmonary artery is the most anterior structure. A short-axis subcostal view requires placement of the largest axis of the transducer in the smallest angle of the subcostal triangle and angling as far anterior as possible.

Once the great vessel associated with the right ventricle is identified, the anatomic evaluation of the right heart is complete. Attention should then be turned to the pulmonary veins; if they all enter one atrium, they will assist in identifying that atrium as a *morphologic left atrium*. Next, evaluation of the AV valve from the left atrium is made in the short-axis view; a *mitral valve* should have two distinct papillary muscles at 4 o'clock and 8 o'clock and two leaflets, one anterior and one posterior (the tricuspid valve will have three leaflets and several smaller papillary muscles). The mitral valve hinge points are higher in the ventricle than are those of the tricuspid valve.

A *morphologic left ventricle* is usually smooth-walled, with a slipper shape in the long axis and a circular shape in the short axis. There should be no infundibular chamber or tissue between the AV and semilunar valves by echocardiography. The outflow tract is defined by the IVS on one side and the mitral valve on the other.

The great vessel arising from the leftward ventricle is the last major structure to be identified. In a short-axis orientation, the presence of coronary ostia and the finding of two distinct vessels exiting the heart define this great vessel as an *aorta*. The subcostal views will usually demonstrate the left ventricle, LVOT, ascending aorta, transverse arch, and a small portion of the descending aorta. The pulmonary artery must be positively identified in order to define the other great vessel as the aorta.

Once each connection is defined, abnormal connections are sited to define the abnormality. In the case of situs inversus or ambiguous, abdominal scans to determine the presence or absence of spleens, and the number of spleens (polysplenia vs. asplenia) if present, are performed. The results of these scans will add further information to the explanation of the defects.

Surgery and prognosis are based on the specific defects seen. They vary from isolated VSD, with an excellent outcome, to very complex disease with a high mortality.

Criss-Cross Heart

There is an unusual entity, called *criss-cross heart*, in which pulmonary and systemic venous inflows cross at the crux of the heart.[19] Pulmonary venous return enters a right-sided atrium and crosses a VSD into a left-sided ventricle. Systemic venous return enters the left-sided atrium and crosses the VSD into a right-sided ventricle. The ventricles may or may not be inverted; the ventricle-arterial connection may be concordant or discordant. The ventricles are usually in a superior-inferior orientation, and the streaming from AV valves into ventricles is such that there is little mixing across the VSD.

The clue to the existence of such an anomaly is a four-chamber view with two atria and AV valves, one normal-appearing ventricle, and one small, round ventricle with no color Doppler inflow. The evaluation of this anomaly is very difficult and, again, should be performed only with the segmental approach. Particularly helpful are the subxiphoid views, which allow easier transitions between ventricles, atria, and great vessels.

Single Ventricle

Single ventricle (*common ventricle, univentricular heart*) (Table 29-13) describes a group of defects in which there is mixing of pulmonary venous and systemic venous flow in one ventricle, which then directs blood flow to both great vessels. This is usually the case with atresia of an AV valve (tricuspid atresia, mitral atresia), but it can also occur with double inlet ventricle.

In single ventricle, since pulmonary venous and systemic venous blood mix in a common chamber before egress to the great vessels, the oxygen saturation in pulmonary artery and aorta are equal; thus, these children are at least mildly cyanotic. Pressure in the great vessels will be equal unless there is obstruction either at or below the semilunar valve.

The volume of blood flow to each great vessel is determined by the resistance in each arterial circuit. Resistance in the pulmonary circuit is determined by the presence of structural obstruction (subvalvular,

TABLE 29-13. SINGLE VENTRICLE

Question to Be Answered	Views	Comments
AV valves/ventricles	Subcostal Apical four-chamber	Is either valve atretic? If so, what is the relative size of the associated ventricle? Try to define morphology of ventricle.
Right ventricle-pulmonary artery	Short axis Long-axis—RVOT	From the rightward ventricle, which great vessel arises? To define *pulmonary artery*, must see it branch. Look for PDA by color Doppler. Look at size of this great vessel relative to that of other vessel.
Pulmonary veins-left atrium	Apical four-chamber Subcostal	Define the leftward atrium. If pulmonary veins enter this atrium, this is *left atrium*. Perform color Doppler evaluation of pulmonary veins.
Left ventricle-aorta	Long-axis—LVOT Subcostal	Does this ventricle give rise to an *aorta*? Is the aorta committed only to this ventricle? Look at relative size of great vessels above semilunar valves. Evaluate ventricular outflow tract with color Doppler.
Pulmonary artery/ aorta orientation	Short axis	Is pulmonary artery anterior or posterior to aorta in short axis?
VSD	Four-chamber Left atrium	How large is VSD? What is its position? Direction of flow?

valvular, supravalvular, or branch pulmonary artery stenoses), pulmonary arteriolar resistance, and left atrial pressure (determined by the ease with which blood finds its way out of the left atrium, either across the mitral valve or across the atrial septum; if either causes obstruction to blood flow, left atrial pressure will be elevated). Unless pulmonary resistance is greater than systemic resistance, there will be an increase in the volume of flow to the pulmonary artery compared to the aortic flow. This will cause symptoms of congestive heart failure in these children. In many of these defects, however, there will be subpulmonic obstruction, which limits flow to the lungs and therefore provides some protection to the pulmonary vasculature.

TRICUSPID ATRESIA

Anatomy

Since transposition of the great vessels and ventricular inversion can occur with tricuspid atresia, the term *systemic venous ventricle* is used to define the ventricle associated with systemic venous return and the term *pulmonary venous ventricle* is used to define the ventricle which receives pulmonary venous return. Tricuspid atresia (Fig. 29-44) defines the absence of tricuspid valve tissue with no communication between the right atrium and the systemic venous ventricle. There will always be an ASD, al-

lowing blood to leave the right atrium and travel via the left atrium and pulmonary venous ventricle to the systemic circulation. There must also be a communication between the systemic and pulmo-

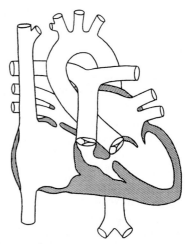

Figure 29-44. Tricuspid atresia. In this defect the tricuspid valve is atretic and does not allow blood to flow from the right atrium to the right ventricle. Blood therefore leaves the right atrium via an atrial septal defect, enters the left atrium via the mitral valve, and exits the left ventricle either across the aortic valve to the aorta or across the ventricular septal defect to the pulmonary artery. (From Mullins CE, Mayer DC. *Congenital Heart Disease: A Diagrammatic Atlas.* Diagram 6. Chicago, YearBook Medical Publishers; 1990. Reprinted by permission of Wiley-Liss, Inc., a division of John Wiley & Sons, Inc.)

▰▰▰ **TABLE 29-14. MAJOR MANIFESTATIONS OF TRICUSPID ATRESIA**

Anatomy	Clinical Status
NORMALLY RELATED GREAT VESSELS (74%)	
Intact ventricular septum, pulmonary atresia	Cyanosis
Small VSD, pulmonary stenosis, small pulmonary artery	Cyanosis
Large VSD, normal-sized pulmonary artery	Normal, occasional congestive heart failure
DTGV (23%)	
VSD, pulmonary atresia	Cyanosis
VSD, pulmonary stenosis	Normal to increased cyanosis
VSD, no pulmonary outflow obstruction	Congestive heart failure
LTGV (3%)	
Subpulmonary stenosis	Normal to increased cyanosis
Subaortic stenosis	

Source: Adapted from Rosenthal A, Dick M. Tricuspid atresia. *In* Moss, Adams Heart Disease in Emmanouilides GC, Riemenschneider TA, Allen HD, Gutgesell HP (eds.): *Infants, Children and Adolescents Including the Fetus and Young Adult,* 5th ed., Vol. 1, Baltimore, Williams & Wilkins; 1995:903.

nary circulations for pulmonary blood flow to exist. Since there is no flow into the systemic venous ventricle via the tricuspid valve, it is hypoplastic and usually does not contract well. If there is a VSD, a portion of the blood entering the left ventricle will cross the VSD and enter the PA. If there is no VSD, then flow to the pulmonary artery must be through the PDA and the pulmonary valve will be atretic. Tricuspid atresia can be seen with normally related great vessels, as well with DTGV and LTGV. The major manifestations of tricuspid atresia are listed in Table 29-14.

The most common associated defects, other than those described above, are persistent left SVC, coarctation of the aorta, and patent ductus arteriosus.

Physiology

Blood flow in *tricuspid atresia with normally related great vessels* is from the SVC and IVC into the right atrium. Since there is no tricuspid valve, all systemic venous return flow crosses the atrial septum into the left atrium, joins the pulmonary venous return

via the pulmonary veins, and then crosses the mitral valve to the left ventricle. If there is no VSD, blood is ejected into the aorta, with some entering the pulmonary artery via the ductus arteriosus. If there is a small VSD, some blood crosses the ventricular septum and goes to the pulmonary artery, though the pulmonary artery is usually small if the VSD is small, so the total pulmonary blood flow is diminished. If the VSD is large, as the pulmonary resistance drops after birth, an increasing amount of blood flow goes across the VSD to the right ventricle and out a dilated pulmonary artery.

If there is *tricuspid atresia with DTGV*, blood flow is from the left ventricle to the pulmonary artery. A portion of the ventricular inflow will cross the VSD and enter the aorta. If there is *tricuspid atresia with LTGV*, the blood flow is from the right atrium across the morphologic mitral valve to the morphologic left ventricle to the pulmonary artery, pulmonary veins to the left atrium, and across the atrial septum to the mitral valve.

In both normally related great vessels and DTGV, there may be variable amounts of pulmonary outflow obstruction from subvalvular to valvular to supravalvular stenoses. The more significant the obstruction, the less flow to the pulmonary arteries.

Clinical Problems

Most children with tricuspid atresia experience one of two clinical problems: congestive heart failure or cyanosis. Those with congestive heart failure obviously have increased pulmonary blood flow. Those with cyanosis have diminished pulmonary blood flow. *Congestive heart failure* is likely to develop in children with a large VSD and a large pulmonary artery or in children with DTGV when there is no subpulmonary obstruction. If the child develops subpulmonary stenosis, this will decrease the amount of pulmonary blood flow and the child may be stable for a period of time. *Cyanosis* develops in children with an obstruction to pulmonary outflow: intact interventricular septum with pulmonary atresia, small VSD with small pulmonary artery, DTGV with pulmonary atresia, or any combination of these conditions with subpulmonic obstruction. In the newborn period, the infusion of PGE1 in such a cyanotic child will allow the ductus arteriosus to remain patent, thus stabilizing pulmonary blood flow for a few days to weeks. Cyanosis in a child who was previously acyanotic may signal closure of a ductus arteriosus, a decrease in the relative size of the VSD and thus the amount of flow across it, or an increase in the degree of pulmonary outflow obstruction.

Echocardiographic Evaluation

As with any form of complex congenital heart disease, a segmental approach to the echocardiographic evaluation should be undertaken. It is important to define the morphology of the ventricles, making sure that there is no ventricular inversion. The size of the atrial defect and the flow characteristics across it are extremely important since the ASD is the only outlet by which systemic venous blood is delivered to the ventricle. Color Doppler flow should be laminar, and pulsed wave Doppler should show low-velocity, biphasic flow. The size of the ventricular defect, if present, is important, as is the color Doppler flow across the defect. If color Doppler flow across the defect is turbulent, the defect may be restricting flow to the pulmonary artery. The relationships and relative sizes of the great vessels will help define the most appropriate surgical approach. The characteristics of the pulmonary outflow tract will help predict future problems; if there is infundibular narrowing or if the pulmonary artery is small, the amount of pulmonary blood flow will probably decrease over time.

The morphology of the single ventricle and, if present, of the outflow chamber, must be looked at carefully. A morphologic left ventricle has a smooth endocardium, and there is no infundibular chamber leading out of a left ventricle to its associated great vessel. A morphologic right ventricle has a trabecular, irregular-looking endocardium and should have an infundibular chamber associated with its connection to a great vessel.

Preoperative Follow-up

For those children who were cyanotic at birth, *increasing cyanosis* may be a problem. Increasing cyanosis may be due to closure of the PDA; relative diminution in the size of the VSD, and therefore a decrease in the flow across it to the pulmonary artery, or increasing pulmonary outflow tract obstruction. The echocardiographic examination should closely evaluate these areas and compare them to previous studies. Increasing *heart failure* is expected in children with unrestricted pulmonary artery flow as pulmonary vascular resistance drops after birth. Echocardiographic evaluation should document increased pulmonary blood flow relative to aortic flow. A Qp:Qs measured at the pulmonary and aortic valves would indicate the relative flow to each circuit. Ventricular function should be evaluated in the short-axis veiw by a slow sweep from apex to base. Although measurement of %FS is not appropriate in a single ventricle, if quantification is needed, an ejection fraction via biplane volumes might be helpful. Generally, however, a 2D evaluation of segmental contractility will suffice.

Prior to performing the Fontan procedure, several areas must be evaluated. Children with mitral regurgitation do not tolerate a Fontan procedure well, nor do those with elevated pulmonary artery pressure or ventricular dysfunction. Therefore, echocardiography should look closely at the mitral valve and ventricular function and should attempt to estimate the pulmonary artery pressure.

Postoperative Follow-up

The first operation on these children will be based on their clinical status. If the child is cyanotic, a systemic-to-pulmonary artery shunt (usually a *Blalock-Taussig shunt*) (Fig. 29-45) may be used to in-

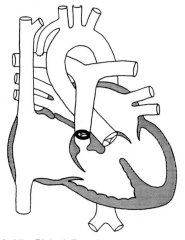

Figure 29-45. Blalock-Taussig shunt. In this operation, the right subclavian artery is transected; the proximal portion is attached to the right pulmonary artery and provides unobstructed flow to the pulmonary arteries. The side of the operation (right versus left) is determined by the position of the aortic arch. (From Mullins CE, Mayer DC. *Congenital Heart Disease: A Diagrammatic Atlas.* Diagram 138. Chicago, YearBook Medical Publishers; 1990. Reprinted by permission of Wiley-Liss, Inc., a division of John Wiley & Sons, Inc.)

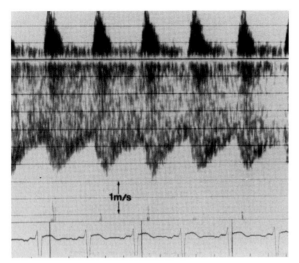

1m/s

Figure 29-46. Doppler flow in a Blalock-Taussig shunt. Continuous wave Doppler sampling in a Blalock-Taussig shunt shows flow throughout the cycle with systolic pulsatility. The peak velocity of 350 cm/sec implies a gradient from the aorta to the pulmonary artery of (3.5, *3.5, *4) 49 mm Hg. (From Snider AR, Serwer GA. *Echocardiography in Pediatric Heart Disease.* Reprinted with permission.)

crease pulmonary blood flow. In these children, the echocardiogram can evaluate the shunt flow. From a short-axis orientation, starting at the base or slightly higher, the pulmonary arteries are identified. Turbulent flow will be seen entering the branch pulmonary artery in which the shunt is placed. Continuous wave Doppler evaluation in the shunt stream will demonstrate continuous flow into the pulmonary artery from the shunt (Fig. 29-46) and will allow estimation of pulmonary artery pressure. If the child is experiencing heart failure, a pulmonary artery band may be necessary to protect the pulmonary vascular bed. Using continuous wave Doppler, the gradient across the pulmonary artery band is obtained.

Most of these children will go on to have a Fontan procedure. Some may have this procedure staged, with a bidirectional Glenn shunt placed first and the Fontan procedure completed at a later time. The *bidirectional Glenn shunt* interposes the right pulmonary artery with the SVC such that the superior SVC brings blood into the upper portion of the right pulmonary artery. The SVC/right atrium junction is patched so that SVC blood cannot enter the right atrium. The lower end of the SVC is anastomosed to the underside of the right pulmonary artery in preparation for the Fontan procedure. The postoperative echocardiogram should evaluate the

site of the SVC/right atrium junction to document lack of communication between the two structures. The area of the SVC and right pulmonary artery (RPA) anastomosis should be evaluated by color Doppler for laminar, low-velocity, biphasic flow. Since SVC obstruction can occur with the Glenn shunt, this evaluation with pulsed wave Doppler is very important.

The *Fontan procedure* (see Fig. 29-15) essentially reroutes the systemic venous return directly to the pulmonary arteries, usually bypassing the heart. At the time of the Fontan procedure, one of two basic repairs is performed based on the underlying anatomy. If there is a right ventricle with an outflow tract, the anastomosis is from the right atrium to the RVOT with a valved conduit or a nonvalved graft. The VSD is closed, as is the ductus arteriosus and any systemic-to-pulmonary artery shunt. If there is no RVOT or if the right ventricle is deemed too small, the anastomosis is from the right atrium to the pulmonary artery. If there is a preexisting bidirectional Glenn shunt, the IVC flow is tunneled into the SVC where the SVC meets the underside of the pulmonary artery. Postoperatively, there may be swelling of the face and head, as in SVC syndrome. In the postoperative period, the velocity and waveform of SVC flow from the head into the pulmonary artery and flow characteristics from the IVC into the pulmonary artery should be evaluated.[9] Careful attention to ventricular contractility and AV valve regurgitation is important in these children.

MITRAL ATRESIA

Mitral atresia, the absence of mitral valve tissue and the absence of communication between the left atrium and left ventricle, is a rare and potentially lethal heart defect. In association with aortic valve atresia, it makes up hypoplastic left heart syndrome and is discussed in the section on "Left Ventricular Outflow Tract Obstruction." Other than in hypoplastic left heart syndrome, mitral atresia is most commonly associated with single ventricle and DTGA, though it may also be part of DORV and may be associated with VSD.

DOUBLE INLET VENTRICLE

Double inlet ventricle describes one ventricle which receives inflow from both AV valves. There are four types of double inlet ventricle based on the morphology of the predominant ventricle: double inlet left ventricle, double inlet right ventricle, double inlet ventricle of mixed morphology (absence of IVS), and double inlet ventricle of indeterminate morphology. Of these four, the most common form is double inlet left ventricle.

Double inlet left ventricle is usually associated with double outlet great vessel connections, usually from the morphologic right ventricle. AV valves may be abnormal with such anomalies, ranging from hypoplasia and stenosis to straddling or atresia and parachute deformity of the left AV valve. Pulmonary outflow tract obstruction is seen frequently, and subaortic obstruction may occur if the aorta is associated with the small outlet chamber; the bulbo-ventricular foramen may be obstructive. In addition, conduction abnormalities similar to those with LTGV are often seen.

Echocardiography

Because of the variety of associated defects and the various forms of double inlet ventricle, a thorough segmental evaluation should be performed, with close attention paid to ventricular morphology, great vessel orientation and relationship to the ventricle, great vessel outflow tracts, and color Doppler flow across the bulboventricular foramen.

Anomalies of Pulmonary Venous Return

Anomalous pulmonary venous return (Table 29-15) refers to a condition in which one, several, or all pulmonary veins do not return directly to the left atrium. It comprises three separate diagnostic entities: partial anomalous pulmonary venous return (PAPVR), total anomalous pulmonary venous return (TAPVR), and cor triatriatum. In PAPVR and TAPVR, some or all of the pulmonary veins return either directly to the right atrium or to vessels which drain directly into the right atrium. In cor triatriatum, pulmonary veins return to the left atrium, but through a posterior channel which usually obstructs flow into the left atrium. This entity is discussed in the section on "Atrioventricular Valve Abnormalities" since clinically and physiologically it resembles mitral stenosis.

PARTIAL ANOMALOUS PULMONARY VENOUS RETURN

Anatomy

In PAPVR, any number of pulmonary veins, in any combination, may drain to any of several venous structures (Fig. 29-47). The most common connections, in order of frequency of occurrence, are (1) right pulmonary veins to SVC, (2) right pulmonary veins to right atrium, (3) right pulmonary veins to IVC, and (4) left pulmonary veins to coronary sinus. Fifteen percent of children with PAPVR have an associated ASD.

Physiology

Any combination of PAPVR implies a decrease in the volume of pulmonary venous return to the left atrium and an increase to the right atrium. If there

---

TABLE 29-15. ANOMALOUS PULMONARY VENOUS RETURN

Question to Be Answered	Views	Comments
Status of atrial septum	Four-chamber Subcostal	Make sure sinus venosus portion of IAS is intact.
Relative size of IVC, SVC	Subcostal	Is one vessel larger than the other (implies more flow into that vessel)? Is flow velocity increased?
Size of coronary sinus	Long axis	Is coronary sinus dilated? If so, anomalous veins may return to the coronary sinus.
Confluence of pulmonary veins	Subcostal Supraclavicular	Is/are there vessels behind left atrium with venous flow configuration? Trace vessel into heart or circulation. If IVC is dilated, look for a large vessel entering IVC near liver; flow may be turbulent. If SVC dilated, look for vessel entering SVC above SVC/right atrium junction; flow may be turbulent. Once site of insertion is found, perform color and pulsed wave Doppler evaluation of venous inflow—turbulent, high velocity from right ventricle to pulmonary artery? Otherwise, this is probably pulmonary atresia.

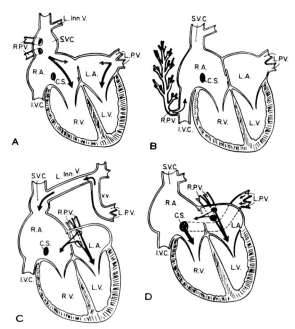

Figure 29-47. Partial anomalous pulmonary venous return—most common forms. In (**A**) right pulmonary veins (R.P.V) return to the superior vena cava (S.V.C). In plate (**B**) the right pulmonary veins are abnormal, multiple, and return to the inferior vena cava (I.V.C.). In (**C**) the left pulmonary veins return to a vertical vein (v.v.) and then to the innominate vein (L. Inn. V.). In (**D**) the left pulmonary veins return to the coronary sinus (C.S.). R.A., right atrium; L.A., left atrium; R.V., right ventricle; L.V., left ventricle; L.P.V., left pulmonary veins. (From Emmanouilides GC, Riemenschneider TA, Allen HD, et al. *Heart Disease in Infants, Children, and Adolescents.* Baltimore, Williams & Wilkins; 1995:841. Reprinted with permission.)

is no ASD, the assumption is that for each pulmonary vein which returns abnormally, there is a 20% increase in blood flow in the right atrium. A single pulmonary vein returning to the right atrium provides such a small volume change that it is probably not noticed clinically. Two or more anomalous veins may cause abnormal physical findings, an abnormal chest X-ray, and an abnormal EKG. The presence of an associated ASD increases the size of the left-to-right shunt, so that the Qp:Qs may be quite large if the ASD is large.

Defects associated with PAPVR include: polysplenia, asplenia, ASD (especially the sinus venosus type), Turner's syndrome, Noonan's syndrome, and tetralogy of Fallot.

Clinical Problems

Most children with PAPVR are asymptomatic and acyanotic. If there are several anomalous veins, they may be subject to frequent respiratory infections. Otherwise, the only findings will be changes in heart sounds, a murmur, increased pulmonary blood flow and cardiomegaly on chest X-ray, and an abnormal EKG.

Echocardiography

Since the defects associated with anomalous pulmonary venous return can be complex, the initial evaluation of a child with this suspected condition should be via a segmental approach. Anomalous veins may return to the IVC or SVC. Close attention to the diameter of these vessels and identification of their course away from the heart will aid in diagnosing anomalous vessels. In addition, there is a high incidence of ASD, especially sinus venosus ASD, associated with anomalous pulmonary veins. In the apical four-chamber and subxiphoid short-axis views, careful documentation of the insertion point of each of the pulmonary veins into the left atrium is important.

TOTAL ANOMALOUS PULMONARY VENOUS RETURN

In TAPVR, all veins return to the right atrium or to one of the systemic veins. Figure 29-48 shows the major types of TAPVR. There are three main classifications of TAPVR: venous connection to the right atrium, venous connection "above the heart" (SVC, azygous vein, left innominate vein, coronary sinus), and venous connection "below the diaphragm" (portal vein, ductus venosus). In TAPVR, since pulmonary venous flow does not return to the left atrium, there must be a large ASD to provide the left atrium and ventricle with blood flow.

In *TAPVR to the right atrium*, all four veins may enter the right atrium, or the veins from both lungs may coalesce with a common vein entering the right atrium. Stenosis of the pulmonary veins under these circumstances is rare.

In *TAPVR above the heart*, the common cardinal vein may enter either the coronary sinus or the left innominate vein. If the ascending vein passes between the MPA and the bronchus, there can be extrinsic compression of the vessel, causing obstruction to venous flow. If the veins return to the coro-

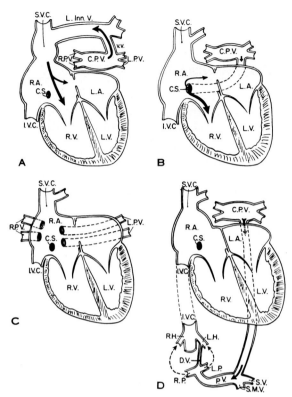

Figure 29-48. Total anomalous pulmonary venous return—most common forms. In (**A**) the veins return to a common pulmonary vein (C.P.V.), through a vertical vein (v.v.), to the left innominate vein (L. Inn. V.) to the superior vena cava (S.V.C.). In (**B**) the veins return to a common pulmonary vein and then to the coronary sinus (C.S.). In (**C**) the right pulmonary vein (R.P.V.) and left pulmonary vein (L.P.V.) both return to the right atrium (R.A.). In (**D**) the pulmonary veins return to a common pulmonary vein through an anomalous vertical channel to the portal vein (P.V); this is known as *total veins below the diaphragm.* R.V., right ventricle; R.A., right atrium; I.V.C., inferior vena cava; L.V., left ventricle; L.A., left atrium; R.H., right hepatic vein; L.H., left hepatic vein; D.V., duodenal vein; L.P., left pulmonary veins. (From Emmanouilides GC, Riemenschneider TA, Allen HD, et al. *Heart Disease in Infants, Children, and Adolescents.* Baltimore, Williams & Wilkins; 1995:848. Reprinted with permission.)

nary sinus, there may be obstruction at the site of the junction between the common vein and the coronary sinus or within the coronary sinus.

In *TAPVR below the diaphragm,* the pulmonary veins come together in the common cardinal vein, descending through the diaphragm and joining the portal vein or ductus venosus. In this situation, there is almost always pulmonary venous obstruction.

TAPVR without pulmonary venous obstruction results in decreasing right-to-left shunting as pulmonary vascular resistance drops after delivery. As pulmonary blood flow increases, there will be dilatation of the right atrium, right ventricle, and pulmonary artery with increasing right ventricular hypertrophy. Congestive heart failure is frequently seen.

Physiology/Clinical Problems

In TAPVR, systemic veins return blood to the right atrium, which delivers blood to the right ventricle and pulmonary artery. Pulmonary veins return either via the SVC, IVC, or coronary sinus to the right atrium. In order for blood to enter the left ventricle and aorta, there must be a large ASD with right-to-left flow. Because pulmonary and systemic veins enter the same chamber (right atrium), saturations in the atria, ventricles, and great vessels are equal. As pulmonary vascular resistance drops after delivery, there is less right-to-left flow across the ASD and increasing blood flow to the lungs. Left unchecked, this will lead to massive congestive heart failure.

In TAPVR with obstruction, the pattern of circulation is the same as that described above. The difference is that the pulmonary veins have difficulty emptying; there is engorgement of the pulmonary veins proximal to the obstruction, with changes in osmotic pressure such that pulmonary edema develops. These children will quickly develop right heart failure and tricuspid regurgitation if surgery is not performed.

TAPVR may be associated with asplenia and polysplenia syndromes.

Echocardiography

The echocardiographic examination[28] is the same as with PAPVR, except that the lack of pulmonary venous return to the left atrium will be obvious: the right atrium will be dilated, while the relative size of the left atrium is small. The common cardinal vein must be identified, usually in a suprasternal or high parasternal short-axis view, and traced to its insertion point. Using color and pulsed wave Doppler, flow along these channels is identified and interrogated for evidence of obstruction (high-velocity, turbulent flow). If direct visualization is difficult, the relative sizes of the IVC and SVC can be compared; if one is noticeably larger than the other, the chances are that the anomalous flow comes into that vein. Tracing that vein backward may reveal the source of the large volume of inflow. Careful attention to the size of the coronary sinus in the long-axis parasternal view may indicate the site of insertion, particularly if it is dilated. Finally, there will be right-to-left flow across the ASD.

Preoperative Evaluation

There should be little clinical change in a child with either PAPVR or TAPVR during the period prior to surgical repair. Those with two or more anomalous veins may develop congestive heart failure with dilated right heart, but this should become evident within the first few months of life. Any of the defects with pulmonary venous obstruction will cause increasingly severe symptoms, and these children will be sent for surgery quickly.

Postoperative Evaluation

Most children with TAPVR, PAPVR, or cor triatriatum will do well after surgical repair. Once the pulmonary venous obstruction is relieved, their pulmonary artery pressures return to normal, with no evidence of permanent damage to the lungs. Therefore, postoperative evaluation would likely be infrequent unless changes in physical exam or EKG/chest x-ray findings occur.

Cardiomyopathies

Diseases affecting the myocardium—cardiomyopathies (Table 29-16)—are a fascinating group of diseases which affect an otherwise structurally normal heart. These cardiomyopathies are usually not seen in association with other forms of heart disease. Some are acute infectious diseases affecting otherwise healthy, normal myocardium; others consist of inherently abnormal myocardium which may or may not be inherited.

HYPERTROPHIC CARDIOMYOPATHY

Anatomy/Physiology

There are many different manifestations of hypertrophic cardiomyopathy (HCM); they all have in common, however, hypertrophy of the myocardium without dilatation of the ventricular cavity. In most forms of HCM, certain areas of the myocardium are more hypertrophied than others. Although the most common site of hypertrophy is the IVS below

◢◢◢ TABLE 29-16. Cardiomyopathies

Question to Be Answered	Views	Comments
Left ventricle thickness	Long axis Short axis	Perform a careful M-mode exam for measures of LVDD, LVDS, EPSS, left atrium, %FS, Vcf. Compare each measurement with normals for BSA.
Left ventricle function	Short axis Apical four-chamber	Perform a slow sweep from apex to base, evaluating segmental contractility. With pulsed wave Doppler, interrogate mitral inflow for diastolic function.
LVOT	Long axis Apical left atrium	Is there SAM of the mitral valve? Look at LVOT with color Doppler. In apical left atrium, put pulsed wave and continuous wave Doppler in LVOT and measure outflow tract velocity. With color Doppler, define the site of obstruction.
Mitral valve	Apical left atrium Subxiphoid	Mitral regurgitation?
RVOT	Short axis	With color and pulsed wave Doppler, is there obstruction in the RVOT from the thick IVS?
Coronary arteries	Short axis	Make sure the left coronary artery communicates with the aorta; unless you see the ostium, assume there is an anomalous right coronary artery from the pulmonary artery; then evaluate pulmonary artery in short axis for the ostium of the left coronary artery.
Pericardium	Apical four-chamber Long axis Short axis	Is there a pericardial effusion? If there is, is there evidence of tamponade (compression of atrial wall by fluid under pressure)?

the aortic valve (see Fig. 29-40), the left ventricular posterior wall may be affected; the affected areas may be small and discrete, or there may be generalized hypertrophy. Although 20–25% of patients with HCM will also have obstruction to left ventricular outflow, most have no evidence of outflow obstruction.[20] Serial echocardiographic studies have shown that the increased hypertrophy and obstruction seen in childhood and adolescence plateaus in early adulthood, with little further progression.[21] In addition, many patients have structural abnormalities of the mitral valve which are assumed to be primary in origin, that is, they are part of the disease process. These abnormalities range from redundant valve tissue to anomalous insertion of papillary muscles. As the degree of hypertrophy progresses, the mitral valve becomes thickened, probably as a result of its contact with the thickened IVS and the endocardium in this area. The thickening of the IVS endocardium leads to the formation of a plaque, which is easily seen on 2D as an echogenic line along the endocardial surface of the IVS just below the aortic valve. At the microscopic level, the myocardial cells in HCM have abnormal shapes and are not aligned in the usual parallel fashion but rather in a disorganized fashion. At autopsy, 80% of patients with HCM demonstrate coronary arteries which are abnormally narrow, with thickened walls. In addition, patchy areas of scarring are seen within the myocardium. These findings imply that "small vessel disease" may contribute to areas of myocardial ischemia, necrosis, and scar formation. These areas may be responsible for the diastolic dysfunction and ventricular arrhythmias seen in this group of patients.

In a small number of patients, obstruction to left ventricular outflow will develop. Although the IVS may be quite thick, the obstruction is caused by systolic anterior motion of a redundant anterior mitral valve leaflet. In infants and young children, the septal hypertrophy can also cause obstruction to right ventricular outflow.

Clinical Problems

In most patients with HCM, symptoms develop in adulthood, usually in the second to fourth decade; however, such symptoms may develop at any age. Symptoms of HCM include exercise limitation, fatigue, chest pain, light-headedness, and fainting. Most children are initially diagnosed based on referral for a heart murmur. Severe HCM seen in infancy leads quickly to signs and symptoms of congestive heart failure and carries a poor prognosis despite medical and surgical intervention.

Sudden death occurs in some of these patients, usually in childhood and early adulthood (12–35 years of age). Most patients are asymptomatic prior to sudden death; most die while engaging in quiet activity. Approximately one-third of the patients with HCM who die suddenly, however, die during or immediately following vigorous physical activity.

In those patients who do not die suddenly from their HCM, some will develop congestive heart failure as their ventricle loses its systolic function; the ventricular walls thin, contractility decreases, the ventricle dilates, and congestive heart failure ensues.

Treatment initially includes beta blockers and verapamil. For those patients with severe symptoms who have outflow obstruction, surgery is recommended. This involves resection of the septal muscle mass. Most patients experience a decrease in outflow gradient and a reduction in systolic anterior motion of the mitral valve after surgery. Likewise, there is usually a decrease in symptoms.

Echocardiography

Echocardiography is important in defining the degree of hypertrophy, the areas of hypertrophy, left ventricular diastolic function, and the presence or absence of outflow tract obstruction. Beginning with a parasternal long-axis view, an M-mode scan through the left ventricle allows accurate measurements of left ventricular thickness. Careful attention to the 2D image prior to performing the M-mode scan will give a general estimate of the relative thicknesses of the IVS and LVPW. It may be difficult to distinguish the right ventricular free wall from the IVS on M-mode. Turning to a parasternal short-axis view may allow the M-mode cursor to be placed in the best position to make that distinction. Likewise, the LVPW may be difficult to define, especially the epicardial surface. Again, using both short-axis and long-axis views, a slow sweep from apex to base in the short-axis view should be used to evaluate segmental contractility. In the long-axis view, systolic anterior motion (SAM) of the mitral valve can be seen. If there is any question, place an M-mode cursor through the mitral valve leaflets. In a short-axis view, the RVOT should be evaluated with 2D and color Doppler. The RVOT velocity should be measured by pulsed wave Doppler.

From an apical long-axis or apical five-chamber view, the subaortic area is evaluated by color Doppler. Careful definition of the site of obstruction is made by 2D. With continuous wave Doppler, the maximum velocity across the LVOT should be measured and LV pressure estimated. Color Doppler is used to evaluate mitral inflow; with pulsed wave Doppler the mitral inflow velocity is evaluated; the ratio of the peaks will be used to quantify diastolic function.

Postoperative Echocardiography

The postoperative study should include all of the above. In addition, close evaluation of the aortic outflow tract for aortic regurgitation is made. The degree of SAM and the measurements of LV thickness should be compared to those noted in the preoperative study.

DILATED CARDIOMYOPATHY/MYOCARDITIS

Anatomy/Physiology

Dilated cardiomyopathy is a disease of the myocardium in which the ventricle contracts poorly and is dilated. Dilated cardiomyopathy may be related to a structural anomaly (anomalous origin of the left coronary artery from the pulmonary artery [ALCA]), toxins (cancer chemotherapy drugs, amphetamines), viral or bacterial infections, abnormal nutritional status (hypocalcemia, elevated copper level, iron deficiency, selenium deficiency, thiamine deficiency, carnitine), or long-standing tachyarrhythmias. Other than the nutritional deficiencies and ALCA, there are no reversible causes of dilated cardiomyopathy. Although the etiology may be any one of the aforementioned, the result is a poorly contractile left ventricle which is dilated, thin-walled, and unable to provide adequate cardiac output for all the patient's needs. As the left ventricle dilates, the mitral annulus dilates and mitral regurgitation is usually seen. With increasing mitral regurgitation and left atrial dilatation, left atrial pressure increases; this pressure increase is transferred to the pulmonary vascular bed, leading to increased pulmonary artery pressure and eventually right heart failure. The increase in pulmonary venous pressure causes pulmonary edema; the increased right heart pressure is transmitted to the liver, and the liver enlarges.

Clinical Problems

These children suffer from congestive heart failure; therefore, they may experience diminished ability to perform low-level activities, coughing, shortness of breath, and increased abdominal girth with abdominal pain. They usually present in acute distress, and appear anxious and unable to breathe effectively. If there is a nutritional deficiency, replacement may reverse the course of the disease. Otherwise, these children are treated with aggressive medical management. Many of those with an underlying infectious process will recover some or all of their ventricular function. For those who do not recover function, cardiac transplantation may be considered.

Echocardiography

The initial echocardiogram on these children is done to confirm the diagnosis of cardiomyopathy and look for structural, potentially reversible, etiologies. Close evaluation of the proximal coronary arteries in the parasternal short-axis and apical four-chamber views will demonstrate the origin of the left coronary artery from the aorta; anomalous origin of the left coronary artery will cause a dilated cardiomyopathy. A complete study should be performed to rule out any other coincident forms of structural heart disease.

In analyzing the left ventricle and its function, it is best to begin with a parasternal long-axis view; a good 2D image in real time will quickly convey the degree of severity of the dysfunction. The M-mode cursor placed through the left ventricle at the level of the chordae of the mitral valve will allow accurate M-mode measurements. Close attention must be paid to the plane of the IVS and the exact position, as subsequent measurements must be made at the same point; movement of the cursor in either direction may give very different measurement of % FS and will *certainly* give different absolute measurements of LVDD and LVDS. In addition to the above-mentioned measurements, the motion of the mitral valve and an EPSS should be part of the exam. The pericardium should also be evaluated to rule out an effusion. From a parasternal short-axis orientation, a slow sweep from apex to base should be made to evaluate the motion of all segments of the left ventricle. From an apical four-chamber view, the mitral valve is evaluated with color Doppler to define the degree of mitral regurgitation and the size of the left atrium; these are other parameters which can be followed over the course of therapy. Diastolic function of the ventricle is evaluated by placing the pulsed wave Doppler cursor in the mitral inflow area.

Acute Diseases Affecting the Heart

Pericarditis and endocarditis are seen in children infrequently; their presentation and echocardiographic evaluation are similar to those in adults, and they should be evaluated in the same manner. There are two acute diseases specific to children which will be discussed here: Kawasaki's disease and acute rheumatic fever. Both affect the heart, and both may have long-lasting complications (Table 29-17).

KAWASAKI'S DISEASE

Kawasaki's disease is an acute disease occurring in children <5 years of age which is characterized by fever of at least 5 days' duration, reddening and swelling of the hands and feet, a total body rash, bilateral conjunctival reddening, reddening and swelling of the lips and tongue, and enlarged cervical lymph nodes. Without treatment, the acute process lasts for 1–2 weeks, and over the next 2–4 weeks the skin of the hands and feet peels in long sheets, usually starting under the nails. Abnormal laboratory values include an elevated erythrocyte sedimentation rate, C-reactive protein, alpha-1 antitrypsin, white blood cell count, protein, and white cells in the urine.

During the first 10 days of the illness, there is a vasculitis which occurs throughout the body, causing the physical findings listed above; this vasculitis also affects the coronary arteries. This inflammatory process appears to occur in all layers of the coronary arteries and disrupts the elastic properties of the vessels. Acutely, the coronary arteries appear dilated (Fig. 29-49). If the vasculitis remains untreated, aneurysms of the coronary arteries may develop, with subsequent acute thrombosis, infarction, and sudden death.

Treatment is aimed at diminishing the inflammatory process before irreparable damage is done

TABLE 29-17. DIAGNOSIS OF ACUTE DISEASES AFFECTING THE HEART OR PERICARDIUM

Question to Be Answered	Views	Comments
Left ventricle size	Long axis Four-chamber	Need M-mode with BSA normals. Compare left ventricle volume to right ventricle volume.
Left ventricle function	Long axis Short axis	M-mode with BSA normals. Look at global, then segmental contractility. Is one area less contractile than others?
Pericardial effusion	Left atrium Four-chamber Subcostal	Look posteriorly and anteriorly. Look laterally. Look posteriorly to atria.
Tamponade	Subcostal Short axis	Does right atrial wall move independently of heart motion? Does it collapse into right atrium?
AV valve regurgitation	Four-chamber Long axis	Look at amount of regurgitation, width of jet, depth of jet into atrium, relative sizes of atria. Need M-mode through left atrium if MR is seen.
Semilunar valve regurgitation	Long axis	Look at parasternal and apical left atrium since jet direction should be nearly parallel to ultrasound beam. Look at width and depth of band.
Vegetations	Four-chamber Subcostal Long axis	Watch for restriction of movement of valve leaflets, valve regurgitation. Look carefully at areas of existing defects or surgical repair.
Coronary artery dilatation/aneurysm	Short axis	At level of aortic valve, look at first 1–2 cm of right and left main arteries; make sure you see bifurcation of LAD and circumflex arteries; measure diameters of left main and right main arteries (should be <3 mm). Look in AV groove at the right main and left main/LAD arteries. If dilation or aneurysm seen, look more closely at wall motion in region supplied by that coronary artery.

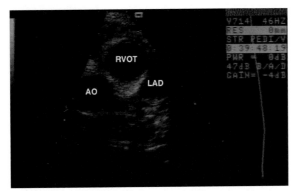

Figure 29-49. Aneurysm of left anterior descending coronary artery. The aortic root (Ao) is seen in cross section, with the right ventricular outflow tract (RVOT) anterior to it. The left main coronary artery is seen coming off the aortic root in the 4 o'clock position. It is mildly dilated (normal coronary artery diameter is 3–4 mm). At the bifurcation, the left anterior descending artery (LAD) becomes severely dilated as it angles anteriorly.

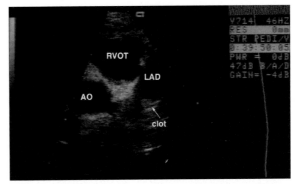

Figure 29-50. Aneurysm of the left anterior descending coronary artery with clot formation posteriorly. The aortic root (AO) is seen in cross section, with the right ventricular outflow tract (RVOT) anterior to it. The left main coronary artery is seen coming off the aortic root in the 4 o'clock position. It is mildly dilated (normal coronary artery diameter is 3–4 mm). At the bifurcation, the left anterior descending artery (LAD) becomes severely dilated as it angles anteriorly. In the posterior portion of the LAD just behind the bifurcation is an echodense structure with bright borders and an irregular shape. This represents a clot.

to the coronary arteries. Treatment usually consists of intravenous gamma globulin followed by high-dose aspirin until the inflammatory process appears to have subsided.

Anatomy/Physiology

Nearly half of all children with Kawasaki's disease show signs of coronary artery dilatation during the acute phase. These may progress to aneurysms which may be fusiform, saccular, cylindrical, or segmented (looking like a series of beads) (Fig. 29-50). These aneurysms are most likely to occur in the left main and left anterior descending coronary arteries but may occur anywhere in the coronary system, either proximally or distally.

Echocardiographic Evaluation

Echocardiography has been shown to be effective in defining proximal dilatation and aneurysm formation in the coronary arteries in these children.[3] The short-axis view at the level of the aortic valve shows the takeoff of both coronaries; moving the transducer 1–2 cm cephalad and angling down to the base of the heart demonstrates their proximal course for 1–3 cm in length. If the coronary arteries appear dilated, their diameter at reproducible points should be measured. In children <5 years of age,

if the coronary artery is >3 mm in diameter or if one segment of the coronary artery is >1.5 times the diameter of its adjoining segment, the coronary artery is assumed to be dilated. If the coronary artery measures >8 mm in diameter, the aneurysm is defined as "giant."

Echodense masses may be seen within the lumina of these vessels (see Fig. 29-50) which may represent thrombus. Since coronary artery inflammation may cause diminished myocardial function, the evaluation of LV function is imperative. In the short-axis parasternal view, a slow sweep from apex to base evaluates segmental motion of the left ventricle. In the long-axis parasternal view, an accurate M-mode assessment of LV contractility is performed. In the apical long-axis view, color Doppler is used to visualize mitral regurgitation (usually a sign of increased LV compliance associated with dysfunction).

Since the long-range outcome of these children with or without coronary aneurysms is still unknown, most institutions follow children without aneurysms with yearly cardiology evaluations and echocardiographic studies. Children with aneurysms are followed more frequently. If there are signs of obstruction, these children are treated as adults with coronary artery disease.

ACUTE RHEUMATIC FEVER

Acute rheumatic fever (ARF) is the leading cause of acquired heart disease in children and young adults. After a decline in its incidence in the last few decades, there has been an increase in the number of cases since 1985. ARF occurs within 3 weeks following an untreated strep throat infection (group A streptococcus). Although this discussion of ARF will involve only the cardiac manifestations, ARF can affect many other organ systems. The damage to the heart is assumed to result from the immune reaction to the strep infection rather than from the bacterium itself.

ARF is characterized by low-grade fever, arthritis or arthralgia of several joints, Sydenham's chorea (involuntary movements of large muscle groups like those of the face, neck, or arms), a characteristic rash, nodules on the extensor surfaces of joints, and certain laboratory abnormalities.

The carditis caused by ARF usually involves the AV valves (usually mitral), semilunar valves (usually aortic), myocardium, and/or pericardium. Acutely, damage to the valves results in regurgitation; this may become severe enough to warrant valve replacement or it may progress over several years to stenosis. Myocardial damage is seen as diminished LV contractility. Pericardial inflammation usually accompanies other forms of carditis and results in a pericardial effusion.

Clinical Problems

Acutely, children with ARF and carditis develop congestive heart failure, either from the acute mitral or aortic regurgitation or from the myocardial dysfunction. With medical management and bed rest, they are watched closely until the heart failure and inflammatory process resolve. Surgery to replace a valve during an acute episode of ARF is reserved for those children who cannot be managed medically.

Echocardiographic Evaluation

During the acute phase of ARF, echocardiography is used to define the extent and severity of carditis. Although ARF usually causes damage to mitral and aortic valves, all valves should be evaluated closely for evidence of regurgitation. Each valve should be evaluated in several different planes with color Doppler. If necessary, transesophageal echocardiography may be considered in children with poor acoustic windows. Myocardial function, including systolic function or contractility and diastolic function, should be studied carefully at each study and compared with previous measurements. Close attention should be paid to the pericardial space in multiple views; if a pericardial effusion is present, the anatomic landmarks and the depth of the effusion should be recorded.

Miscellaneous Anomalies

There are two defects which do not fit into the previous categories: anomalous origin of the coronary artery and aortopulmonary window. Anomalous origin of the left coronary artery is usually identified outside the neonatal period and may, in older children, cause chest pain and congestive heart failure. Aortopulmonary window is usually identified in the neonatal period and usually causes a loud murmur and congestive heart failure early in life (Table 29-18).

ANOMALOUS ORIGIN OF THE LEFT CORONARY ARTERY FROM THE PULMONARY ARTERY

Anatomy/Physiology

In this defect, the left main coronary artery comes off the pulmonary artery rather than the aorta (Fig. 29-51). The fetus is not affected by this since the pressures and saturations in both great vessels are nearly equal. After birth, however, as pulmonary artery pressure falls, the pressure and saturation of blood flow into the left coronary artery are less than those of the right coronary artery. The left coronary vessels dilate maximally to increase flow to the left ventricular myocardium but reach their maximal dilatation early. After this point myocardial ischemia occurs, initially with exertion (feeding, crying). As myocardial oxygen demands increase with growth and development of the child, the episodes of myocardial ischemia increase in frequency and portions of the left ventricular free wall become infarcted. Collateral circulation will develop between the normally placed right coronary artery and the left. Since pressure through the left coronary artery will reflect the lower pulmonary artery pressure, flow in the collateral vessels tends to be from the right coronary artery into the collaterals into the left main coronary artery and then into the pulmonary artery. The steal

◢◣◤◥ **TABLE 29-18. MISCELLANEOUS CONDITIONS**

Question to Be Answered	Views	Comments
ANOMALOUS ORIGIN OF LEFT CORONARY ARTERY		
Origin of left coronary artery	Short axis	Make sure LAD artery is from aorta; if not seen clearly, evaluate root of pulmonary artery. Color Doppler in that area may help identify the origin.
Left ventricle function	Long axis Short axis	Accurate M-mode measurement of left ventricle dimensions and %fs will give insight into the degree of myocardial dysfunction. Slow, careful sweep in short axis from apex to base may show areas of akinesis or dyskinesis, particularly in upper IVS.
Mitral valve function	Long axis Short axis	Is there mitral regurgitation? If so, quantify. Evaluate mitral motion in both planes. Sometimes papillary muscle is ischemic and thus mitral motion is diminished.
AP WINDOW		
Pulmonary artery	Short axis	Look at RVOT with color Doppler; are there any sites of turbulent or retrograde flow?
Left atrium	Long axis Apical four-chamber	Is the left atrium dilated?
Left ventricle	Long axis Short axis	Careful M-mode measurement of left ventricle dimensions and %fs. Is left ventricle dilated? Slow sweep in short axis will show any areas of diminished contractility.

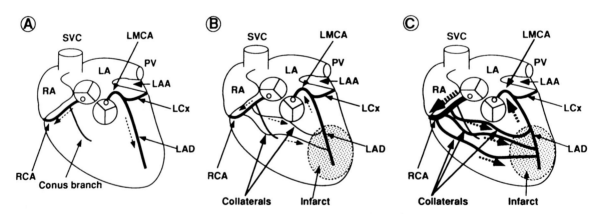

Figure 29-51. Anomalous origin of the left main coronary artery from the pulmonary artery. In fetal life (**A**), both coronaries receive forward flow, each from its respective great vessel. After birth (**B**), before collateral vessels have developed, there may be an infarct in the area supplied by the left anterior descending (LAD) coronary artery since it is perfused with desaturated blood. After collaterals develop (**C**), there is high flow in the right coronary artery, through the collaterals, and retrograde through the left coronary artery into the pulmonary artery. (From Emmanouilides GC, Riemenschneider TA, Allen HD, et al. *Heart Disease in Infants, Children, and Adolescents.* Baltimore, Williams & Wilkins; 1995. Reprinted with permission.)

of saturated blood from the left coronary artery causes further ischemia and infarction of the free wall of the left ventricle. Congestive heart failure with diminished ventricular function ensues. If the papillary muscles have been infarcted, mitral regurgitation develops, and symptoms of congestive heart failure may occur earlier and be more severe. Although some people will survive into adulthood with this anomaly, nearly half will die suddenly.

Clinical Problems

Infants may exhibit irritability, pallor, sweating, and dyspnea during episodes of myocardial ischemia. Unfortunately, these conditions may be attributed to colic and the symptoms ignored. If the condition remains undiagnosed, many of these children will develop signs and symptoms of congestive heart failure later in childhood. The age at presentation may vary from months to years.

Echocardiographic Evaluation

In many of these children, the degree of myocardial ischemia and infarction will cause left ventricular dilatation and diminished contractility. Therefore, careful M-mode evaluation of left ventricular dimensions and contractility is important. Since mitral regurgitation may develop either from infarction of the papillary muscles or from dilatation of the mitral ring accompanying left ventricular dilatation, an apical long-axis view with color Doppler evaluation of mitral inflow and regurgitation is necessary.

To evaluate the coronary arteries,[17] the transducer is placed in the short-axis orientation and positioned slightly higher on the chest than in the usual parasternal window. The transducer is angled down toward the base of the heart and rotated until the left coronary system is visualized. The left system may be followed back to the pulmonary artery. Although it may appear to exit from the aortic root, color Doppler will indicate that, in fact, flow in the left coronary artery is retrograde, that is, toward the pulmonary artery. It is extremely important to be able to identify the site of insertion into the pulmonary artery, as that will affect the surgical repair.

In the parasternal short-axis orientation, a slow, methodical sweep from the apex to the base of the left ventricle is done to evaluate for areas of dyskinesis or akinesis. Careful description of these areas will be helpful in the evaluation of postoperative recuperation.

Postoperative Evaluation

Surgery for this condition involves removing the left main coronary artery from the pulmonary trunk and reimplanting it into the aortic root. Postoperatively, echocardiography should be able to demonstrate antegrade color Doppler flow into the left main coronary artery. Hopefully, left ventricular function will improve as it is perfused with higher-pressure oxygenated blood. Areas of infarction, however, are less likely to improve. Close evaluation of segmental contractility in the short-axis view, by sweeping from apex to base, is important in the serial postoperative evaluation of these children. We have seen noticeable improvement in left ventricular contractility and decreased mitral regurgitation in children who were repaired in childhood, though complete resolution of function was not reached.

AORTOPULMONARY WINDOW

Anatomy/Physiology/Clinical Problems

The aortopulmonary (AP) window (Fig. 29-52) involves a connection between the aorta and the pulmonary artery, usually circular in shape and midway between the pulmonary valve and the bifurcation of the main pulmonary artery. Less commonly, the communication may occur between the aorta and the right pulmonary artery. Rarely, the communica-

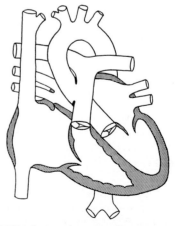

Figure 29-52. Aortopulmonary window. Atria and ventricles are normal in size and morphology; great vessels are normally oriented. There is a defect connecting the aorta and pulmonary artery above the valve annuli. (From Mullins CE, Mayer DC. *Congenital Heart Disease: A Diagrammatic Atlas.* Diagram 54. Chicago, YearBook Medical Publishers; 1990. Reprinted by permission of Wiley-Liss, Inc., a division of John Wiley & Sons, Inc.)

tion is large and involves the entire main pulmonary artery out to the right pulmonary artery. As pulmonary vascular resistance drops in the first few weeks of life, there is an increasing left-to-right shunt across this defect. Therefore, signs and symptoms of congestive heart failure develop within the first few weeks of life.

Associated defects include interrupted aortic arch, tetralogy of Fallot, anomalous origin of the right coronary artery from the pulmonary artery, right aortic arch, VSD, pulmonary or aortic atresia, DTGV, and tricuspid atresia.

Echocardiographic Evaluation

The defect may be visualized on 2D but not always. Color and pulsed wave Doppler will help distinguish this from a PDA; flow in an AP window is antegrade into the branch pulmonary arteries, and color Doppler turbulence may be seen at the insertion site in the main pulmonary artery. The left atrium and left ventricle will be dilated, and the degree of dilation is related to the size of the shunt.

Postoperative Evaluation

Surgery involves closure of the defect and attention to associated defects. The postoperative echocardiogram should demonstrate laminar color Doppler flow in the MPA and aorta, with a diminishing size of the left atrium and left ventricle.

REFERENCES

1. American Society of Echocardiography Committee on Standards. Recommendations for quantitation of left ventricle by two-dimensional echocardiography. *J Am Soc Echocardiogr.* 1989;2:5:358–367.
2. Appleton CP, Hatle LK, Popp RL. Cardiac tamponade and pericardial effusion: Respiratory variation in transvalvular flow velocities studied by Doppler echocardiography. *J Am Coll Cardiol.* 1988;11:5:1020–1030.
3. Arjunan K, Daniels SR, Meyer RA, et al. Coronary artery caliber in normal children and patients with Kawasaki disease but without aneurysms: An echocardiographic and angiographic study. *J Am Coll Cardiol.* 1986;8:5:1119–1124.
4. Colan SD, Borow KM, Neumann A. Left ventricular end-systolic wall stress-velocity of fiber shortening relation: A load-independent index of myocardial contractility. *J Am Coll Cardiol.* 1984;4:715–724.
5. Currie PJ, Seward JB, Chan KL, et al. Continuous wave Doppler determination of right ventricular pressure: A simultaneous Doppler-catheterization study in 127 patients. *J Am Coll Cardiol.* 1985;6:4:750–756.
6. Davachi R, Moller JH, Edwards JE. Diseases of the mitral valve in infancy: Anatomic analysis of 55 cases. *Circulation.* 1971;43:565–579.
7. Duncan WJ, Freedom RM, Rowe RD, et al. Echocardiographic features before and after the Jatene procedure (anatomical correction) for transposition of the great vessels. *Am Heart J.* 1981;102:227–232.
8. Farooki ZZ, Henry JG, Green EW. Echocardiographic spectrum of the hypoplastic left heart syndrome: A clinicopathologic correlation in 19 newborns. *Am J Cardiol.* 1976;38:337–343.
9. Fogel MA, Chin AJ. Imaging of pulmonary venous pathway obstruction in patients after the modified Fontan procedure. *J Am Coll Cardiol.* 1992;20:1:181–190.
10. Fyler DC, Buckley LP, Hellenbrand WE, et al. Report of the New England Regional Infant Cardiac Program. *Pediatrics.* 1980;65:432–436.
11. Gilliam LD, Guyer DE, Givson TC. Hydrodynamic compression of the right atrium: A new echocardiographic sign of cardiac tamponade. *Circulation.* 1983;68:294–301.
12. Guidelines for Monitoring and Management of Pediatric Patients during and After Sedation for Diagnostic and Therapeutic Procedures. *Pediatrics.* 1992;89:6:1110–1115.
13. Hagler DJ, Tajik AJ, Seward JB, et al. Real-time wide-angle sector echocardiography: Atrioventricular canal defects. *Circulation.* 1979;59:140–150.
14. Hard K, Shiota T, Takahashi Y, et al. Doppler echocardiographic evaluation of left ventricular output and left ventricular diastolic filling changes in the first day of life. *Pediatric Res.* 1994;35:4:506–509.
15. Hastreiter AR, Dcruz IA, Cantez T, et al. Right sided aorta I: Occurrence of right aortic arch in various types of congenital heart disease. II: Right aortic arch, right descending aorta and associated anomalies. *Br Heart J.* 1966;238:722–739.
16. Huhta JC, Hagler DJ, Seward JB, et al. Two dimensional echocardiographic assessment of dextrocardia: A segmental approach. *Am J Cardiol.* 1982;50:1351–1360.
17. King DH, Danforth DA, Huhta JC, et al. Noninvasive detection of anomalous origin of the left main coronary artery from the pulmonary trunk by pulsed Doppler echocardiography. *Am J Cardiol.* 1985;55:608–609.
18. Mahoney LT, Truesdell SC, Krzmarzick TR, et al. Atrial septal defects that present in infancy. *Am J Dis Child.* 1986;140:1115–1118.

19. Marino B, Sanders SP, Pasquini L, et al. Two-dimensional echocardiographic anatomy in crisscross heart. *Am J Cardiol.* 1986;58:325–333.

20. Maron BJ, Epstein SE. Clinical significance and therapeutic implications of the left ventricular outflow tract pressure gradient in hypertrophic cardiomyopathy. *Am J Cardiol.* 1986;58:1093–1096.

21. Maron BJ. Hypertrophic cardiomyopathy. *In* Emmanouilides GC, Riemenschneider TA, Allen HD, et al. (eds). *Heart Disease in Infants, Children, and Adolescents.* Baltimore, Williams & Wilkins; 1995: 1349.

22. Marx GR, Allen HD. Accuracy and pitfalls of Doppler evaluation of the pressure gradient in aortic coarctation. *J Am Coll Cardiol.* 1986;7:6:1379–1385.

23. Oppenheimer DA, Gittenberger de Groot AC, Roozendaal H. The ductus arteriosus and associated cardiac anomalies in interruption of the aortic arch. *Pediatr Cardiol.* 1982;2:185–193.

24. Roberson DA, Silverman NH. Malaligned outlet septum with subpulmonary ventricular septal defect and abnormal ventriculoarterial connection: A morphologic spectrum defined echocardiographically. *J Am Coll Cardiol.* 1990;16:2:459–468.

25. Shiina A, Seward JB, Edwards WD, et al. Two-dimensional echocardiographic spectrum of Ebstein's anomaly: Detailed anatomic assessment. *J Am Coll Cardiol.* 1983;3:356–370.

26. Shone JD, Sellers RD, Anderson RC, et al. The developmental complex of "parachute mitral valve," supravalvular ring of left atrium, subaortic stenosis and coarctation of the aorta. *Am J Cardiol.* 1963; 11:714–725.

27. Smallhorn JF, Gow R, Freedom RM, et al. Pulsed Doppler echocardiographic assessment of the pulmonary venous pathway after the Mustard or Senning procedure for transposition of the great arteries. *Circulation.* 1986;73:765–774.

28. Sreeram N, Walsh K. Diagnosis of total anomalous pulmonary venous drainage by Doppler color flow imaging. *J Am Coll Cardiol.* 1992;19:1577–1582.

29. Tawes RL, Berr CL, Averdeen E. Congenital bicuspid aortic valve associated with coarctation of the aorta in children. *Br Heart J.* 1969;31:127–128.

30. Weinberg PM. Aortic arch anomalies. *In* Emmanouilides GC, Riemenschneider TA, Allen HD, et al. (eds), *Heart Disease in Infants, Children, and Adolescents.* Baltimore, Williams & Wilkins; 1995: 810–837.

31. Weinberg PM. Aortic arch anomalies. *In* Emmanouilides GC, Riemenschneider TA, Allen HD, et al. (eds), *Heart Disease in Infants, Children, and Adolescents.* Baltimore, Williams & Wilkins; 1995: 828–837.

PART XI

Diseases of the Aorta

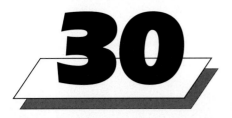

Echocardiographic Evaluation of the Aorta

PRISCILLA J. PETERS

The aorta has been described as the ultimate conductance vessel. It is the main trunk of the systemic arterial system and carries approximately 200 billion liters of blood to the body during the average lifetime.[1] It is composed of three layers: a thin inner tunica (a membrane or structure covering a body part or organ) intima; a thicker middle tunica media; and a thin outer layer, the tunica adventitia. The tunica media is the most important of these layers, comprising more than 80% of the aortic wall. It is composed of multiple interwoven elastic sheets arranged in a spiral fashion to provide maximal tensile strength.

The elasticity of the aortic wall allows for damping (or storing) of the force generated by the ventricle in systole and expulsion of the stored energy in diastole, enabling passage of blood through the peripheral vessels. Thus, wide surges in systemic arterial pressure are avoided and a relatively constant perfusion pressure is maintained.

Normal Anatomy

The aorta can be divided into three principal anatomic regions: the *ascending aorta*, the *aortic arch*, and the *descending aorta*, which is further divided into thoracic and abdominal segments[2] (Fig. 30-1). In the adult patient, each of these segments of the aorta is examined from separate echocardiographic windows, and the information is combined to provide total assessment of the aorta (Table 30-1).

The *ascending aorta* is approximately 5 cm in length, beginning at the aortic valve, coursing anterior and rightward, crossing the right pulmonary artery, and continuing to the second costal cartilage, where it joins the aortic arch. The proximal portion of the ascending aorta is contained within the pericardium. Posterior to the ascending aorta are the left atrium, the right pulmonary artery, and the right mainstem bronchus. The standard parasternal long axis view (PLAX) provides the best delineation of the key segments of the proximal ascending aorta, which are designated the *annulus* (valve insertion), the *sinuses of Valsalva*, the *sinotubular junction*, and the *ascending aorta* (Fig. 30-2). The aortic diameter is smallest at the level of the annulus, increases at the level of the sinuses, and decreases slightly from the sinus diameter at the beginning of the tubular portion. The diameter of the tubular portion of the aorta should be no less than that measured at the annulus. Dimensions should be taken at end-diastole. Values increase slightly with age[3] (Table 30-2).

The *aortic arch* begins at the second right costal cartilage and curves slightly leftward in front of the trachea, then passes inferior to the left of the trachea and esophagus. The arch gives rise to the innominate, left common carotid, and left subclavian arteries. The suprasternal notch views allow for relatively easy visualization of the arch; identifying all the branch vessels is somewhat more difficult, but (at

599

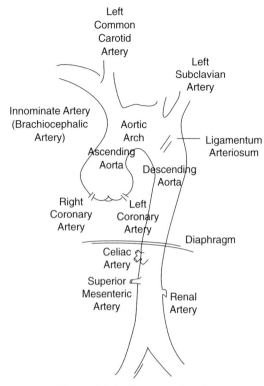

Figure 30-1. The normal aorta.

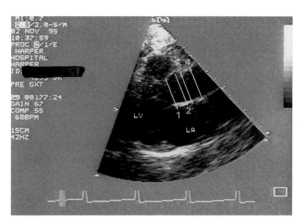

Figure 30-2. Normal transthoracic image of the aorta from the parasternal long axis view. The annulus (1), sinuses of Valsalva (2), sinotubular junction (3), and proximal ascending aorta (4) are seen. LV, left ventricle; LA, left atrium.

least in children) the common carotid and subclavian arteries can be seen in up to 92% of patients and the innominate artery in up to 60%.[4] *Imaging from the suprasternal notch should be considered routine in all adult patients.*

◤◢ TABLE 30-1. TRANSTHORACIC ECHOCARDIOGRAPHIC VIEWS REQUIRED TO IMAGE THE AORTA

View	Segment of Aorta Imaged
Left parasternal	Proximal ascending and descending thoracic aorta
Right parasternal	Ascending aorta; proximal aortic arch
Suprasternal notch	Entire aortic arch; proximal descending aorta
Modified apical	Descending thoracic aorta
Subcostal	Distal descending thoracic and abdominal aorta
	Proximal ascending aorta

Source: Goldstein SA, Mintz GS, Lindsay J. Aorta: Comprehensive evaluation by echocardiography and transesophageal echocardiography. J Am Soc Echocardiogr. 1993;6:634–639. Reprinted with permission.

The normal arch appears as an arcuate (or bow-shaped), echo-free structure and is approximately 4.5 cm long. Its normal diameter is 2.5–3 cm, increasing to 3.5 cm in patients more than 60 years old. Segments of the ascending aorta (left of the suprasternal view), descending aorta (right of the suprasternal view), and right pulmonary artery (center of the view below the arch) are also seen when the arch is imaged. The origins of the left common carotid and left subclavian arteries are noted to the right of the scan plane (Fig. 30-3).

The *descending thoracic aorta* continues beyond the arch, initially posteriorly and to the left of the vertebral column. It eventually courses in front of the vertebral column as it descends and assumes a position behind the esophagus. From a parasternal long axis view, the descending aorta is seen as a

◤◢ TABLE 30-2. NORMAL ADULT AORTIC DIMENSIONS FROM THORACIC IMAGE

Site Being Measured	Normal Range
Annulus	1.4–2.6 cm
Sinus of valsalva	2.1–3.5 cm
Sinotubular junction	1.7–3.4 cm
Ascending aorta	2.1–3.4 cm
Aortic arch	2.0–3.6 cm

Source: Adapted from Normal cross-sectional values. *In*: Weyman AE: Principles and Practice of Echocardiography, 2nd ed. Philadelphia, Lea & Febiger; 1994:1290. Used with permission.

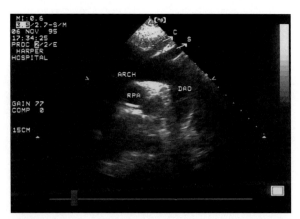

Figure 30-3. The aorta as viewed from the suprasternal notch. The arch, left common carotid (C), left subclavian (S), and descending aorta (DAO) are seen, as well as the right pulmonary artery (RPA).

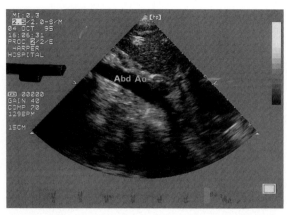

Figure 30-5. A subcostal view demonstrating the proximal abdominal aorta (Abd Ao).

pulsatile circular structure beneath the atrioventricular (AV) groove as it passes behind the left side of the heart (Fig. 30-4). The descending aorta can also be seen from the apical four-chamber and apical long axis views; transesophageal imaging provides the most extensive evaluation. The normal descending thoracic aorta is smaller than both the aortic root and the ascending aorta. The diameter narrows as the vessel descends from about 2.5 cm to 2.0 cm.[5] The *aortic isthmus* is an important segment of the aorta just distal to the left subclavian at which the arch and the descending aorta join. This is the site at which coarctation commonly occurs. It is also the point at which the mobile segments of the aorta (ascending and arch) become fixed to the thorax. At this site the aorta is particularly vulnerable to traumatic injury. The *abdominal aorta* begins at the diaphragm and has an average diameter of 2.0 cm. From a subxiphoid transducer position a good portion of the abdominal aorta can be seen, and can be evaluated for aneurysms and dissecting flaps (Fig. 30-5). In patients with severe aortic regurgitation, holodiastolic flow reversal can be recorded in the abdominal aorta.

Structural Abnormalities

OBSTRUCTIVE LESIONS

Supravalvular aortic stenosis is a congenital narrowing of the ascending aorta that begins just distal to the insertion of the coronary arteries. It is the least common type of left ventricular outflow tract obstruction and is rare.[6] The obstruction may be localized or diffuse. There are three principal anatomic types: an "hour glass"-shaped, discrete narrowing just above the aortic sinuses; a fibrous membrane with a narrow opening; and a diffuse narrowing (hypoplasia) of the ascending aorta.[7] The hour glass type is the most common. The cusps of the aortic valve may also be thickened with this lesion, and some degree of associated pulmonary artery steno-

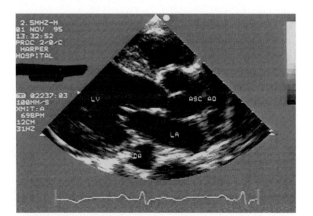

Figure 30-4. The descending aorta (DA) as viewed from the parasternal long axis plane. LV, left ventricle; LA, left atrium; ASC AO, proximal ascending aorta.

sis, either supravalvular or peripheral, is commonly seen. Williams' syndrome is the association of supravalvular aortic stenosis with an abnormal facial appearance ("elfin facies"), infantile hypercalcemia, and mental retardation.[8]

Supravalvular aortic stenosis is identified on the echocardiogram as a decrease in the aortic diameter just above the sinuses of Valsalva. In adults this narrowing may not be well seen from standard PLAX views, so high left or right parasternal views may be necessary. Interestingly, because the coronary arteries insert proximal to the site of obstruction, they are subject to the elevated left ventricular pressure; in the short axis views, the coronary arteries are usually quite prominent. An apical five-chamber view may identify the site of narrowing in the proximal aorta; the suprasternal views, especially in children, can confidently identify the area of obstruction. This lesion is not easily assessed by Doppler, but occasionally the site of obstruction can be pinpointed with pulsed wave or localized by turbulent color flow; continuous wave Doppler can record the maximum velocity, but this can be unreliable in hour glass lesions as the aorta reexpands distal to the obstruction and allows pressure recovery. Doppler gradients tend to exceed those at cardiac catheterization; catheterization is usually indicated in these patients because of anatomic variability and the associated peripheral pulmonary stenosis.

Coarctation ("to make tight") of the aorta is a localized deformity of the aortic media causing narrowing of the vessel lumen. It represents up to 8% of all congenital heart disease and is more common in males.[9] Coarctation is divided into preductal and postductal types. The preductal type typically presents in infancy and is most often associated with other abnormalities of the left heart, including congenital mitral stenosis, left ventricular outflow tract obstruction, and ventricular septal defects. The postductal (or adult) type occurs in the region of the ductus arteriosus and the left subclavian artery and is usually not associated with other left-sided abnormalities, with the notable exception of a bicuspid aortic valve, which is seen in more than 50% of all cases.[10,11] Coarctation is symptomatic at two stages of life: in early infancy and after the age of 20. In the older child or young adult, the diagnosis should be suspected by the discovery of systolic hypertension, with significant upper to lower extremity blood pressure or pulse differential. Even though survival to adulthood is not unusual with untreated coarctation, on average death occurs in the mid-30s.[12]

Echocardiography is invaluable in the diagnosis of coarctation. Special attention should be paid to the anatomy of the aortic valve in the basal short axis view, and to left ventricular size, thickness, and function (hypertension may predispose to premature coronary artery disease). The subcostal views may provide a useful clue to the diagnosis by establishing a *lack of pulsation* in the abdominal aorta. Suprasternal views of the arch and the descending thoracic aorta may provide direct visualization of the obstruction; however, reliable imaging of the anatomy depends on the size and age of the patient. Coarctation will appear as a localized decrease in aortic diameter, typically in the region just distal to the left subclavian (which may be dilated) (Fig. 30-6A). Color flow mapping will demonstrate turbulence in the region of the obstruction, but the width of the color jet does not represent the degree of narrowing accurately. Doppler interrogation should be directed to the descending aorta in the area of obstruction. The continuous wave exam should demonstrate a classic "sawtooth" pattern (diastolic flow through the obstruction is delayed) and can be used to derive the pressure drop across the lesion (Fig. 30-6B). The peak gradient alone often overestimates the true gradient because the precoarctation velocity may be significantly elevated if the aortic valve is abnormal. Hence the preobstruction (or proximal) velocity, as measured by pulsed Doppler, if greater than 1.5 m/sec, should be subtracted from the postobstruction (or distal) velocity, as determined by continuous wave Doppler ($\Delta P = V_2 CW - V_1 PW$). Also, peak velocities may underestimate the gradient in the adult patient with well-developed collateral vessels around the coarctation.

ANEURYSMS

Aneurysms are localized areas of abnormal dilation of a blood vessel wall, usually an artery. They may be saccular (limited to a portion of the vascular wall) or fusiform (involving the entire circumference of the vessel). Aneurysms of the aorta may be congenital or acquired. Common congenital aneurysms are those that arise from a sinus of Valsalva or those associated with Marfan's syndrome or other diseases of the connective tissue. Acquired aneurysms result

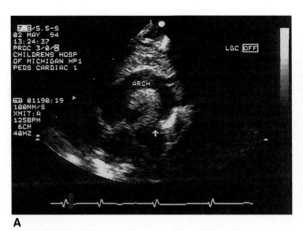

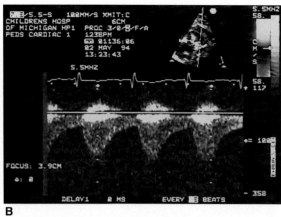

A   **B**

Figure 30-6. (**A**) Coarctation of the aorta (arrow). (Courtesy of Dr. Richard Humes, Children's Hospital of Michigan.) (**B**) Continuous wave Doppler across the coarctation demonstrating the typical "sawtooth" appearance. (See also Color Plate 71.)

from atherosclerosis, syphilis, or trauma; most acquired aneurysms are the result of atherosclerosis.[13]

SINUS OF VALSALVA ANEURYSMS

Congenital aneurysms of the sinuses of Valsalva are uncommon, and result from a weakness at the junction of the aortic media and the annulus fibrosa. The weakness in the aorta sets the stage for aneurysm formation; while the developmental anomaly is present at birth, with rare exceptions the aneurysm is not.[14,15]

Most sinus of Valsalva aneurysms originate in the right sinus or the right portion of the noncoronary sinus and protrude or rupture into the right ventricle or right atrium or into both right heart chambers.[16] They frequently occur in association with defects of the ventricular septum and the aortic valve.[17] Unruptured aneurysms can be asymptomatic and incidental findings or may protrude into the right ventricular outflow tract and cause obstruction.[18] With abrupt rupture, chest pain and dyspnea often initiate the onset of heart failure in association with a loud, continuous murmur, but the physiologic and hemodynamic consequences of rupture depend on the size of the shunt, the rapidity with which it develops, and the recipient chamber.[19] Thus, small perforations in otherwise normal hearts are likely to progress slowly, with initially good hemodynamic compensation.[20] These patients may be without cardiac symptoms. Volume overload of the left heart always occurs (rupture to the right heart > pulmonary bed > left atrium > left ventricle > aorta); when the right ventricle is the recipient chamber, it will dilate; with right atrial shunts, all four chambers will deal with the additional volume load.[19] Rupture of the left sinus into left-sided chambers is exceptional.[21]

Sinus of Valsalva aneurysms are best assessed with the echocardiogram from the basal short axis views (Fig. 30-7A–D). The affected sinus will demonstrate some outpouching and will be thinner than the adjacent sinuses. With rupture, color flow usually identifies the continuous flow into the recipient chamber. The flow is *continuous* with *high velocity* because the aortic pressure is higher than the pressure in the receiving chamber in both systole and diastole. The important echocardiographic differential diagnosis is between a ruptured sinus and a membranous ventricular septal defect (VSD) with an aneurysm. The distinction can usually be made from the parasternal long axis views, in which the membranous VSD arises *below* the annulus and the ruptured sinus originates *above* the aortic valve. Occasionally, even this anatomic distinction is difficult, and the timing of shunt flow (systolic for a VSD and continuous for a ruptured sinus) can make the diagnosis. Higher-resolution transesophageal imaging should resolve any anatomic uncertainty. Normal sinuses of Valsalva may become infected and perforate in patients with infective endocarditis of the aortic valve.

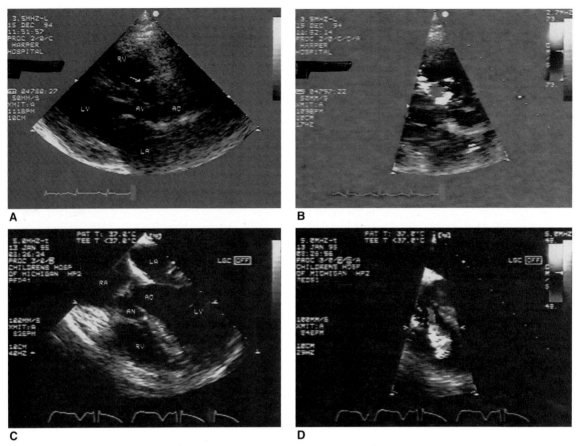

Figure 30-7. (**A**) Parasternal long axis view of a ruptured right sinus of Valsalva aneurysm (arrow). Note that the rupture is above the level of the valve. LV, left ventricle; LA, left atrium; AV, aortic valve; AO, aorta, RV, right ventricle. (**B**) Color flow through the ruptured sinus. (See also Color Plate 72.) (**C**) Four-chamber transesophageal view demonstrating the aneurysmal sinus. AN, aneurysm; RA, right atrium; RV, right ventricle; LA, left atrium; LV, left ventricle. (**D**) Color flow through the ruptured sinus into the right ventricle. The sinus had perforated into both the right ventricle and the right atrium. (See also Color Plate 73.)

MARFAN'S SYNDROME

Marfan's syndrome is a connective tissue disorder characterized by manifestations in primary organ systems, specifically eye (ectopia lentis); skeletal (excessive limb length, pectus excavatum); cardiovascular (dilatation of the aortic root, aortic dissection, mitral valve prolapse); and occasional pulmonary, skin, and central nervous system derangements.[22] Cardiovascular abnormalities are commonly seen in classic Marfan's syndrome, with aortic ectasia and mitral valve prolapse now being identified in up to 95% of these patients[23]; cardiovascular involvement, specifically aortic dissection, is the most important

cause of early death in this condition.[24] Children tend to be more affected by mitral valve problems; aortic dilatation, regurgitation, and dissection are progressive and tend to appear in adolescence and early adulthood.[25,26]

On the echocardiogram the aortic root is dilated, sometimes strikingly so (Fig. 30-8). Dilatation begins at the valve and involves the sinuses and the distal ascending aorta. Long axis views are straightforward and demonstrate a markedly ectatic vessel and stretched aortic leaflets. As the root continues to dilate, aortic regurgitation will result. In the short axis views, the sinuses of Valsalva are sym-

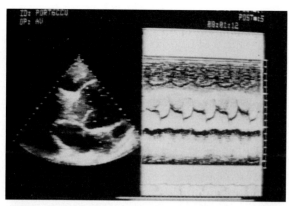

Figure 30-8. Parasternal long axis view of the aorta in a patient with Marfan's syndrome. The aorta measured approximately 7.2 cm just above the level of the valve.

metrically dilated; occasionally, the aortic root appears to compress the left atrium. The involvement of the sinuses is characteristic of Marfan's syndrome. In addition to evaluation of the aorta, careful inspection of the mitral valve is important to assess for the presence of prolapse or myxomatous changes of the valve and supporting apparatus. Color and spectral Doppler are important to the identification and quantification of both mitral and aortic regurgitation.

Serial echocardiograms on at least an annual basis are of great importance in patients with Marfan's syndrome to follow the size of the aorta and to establish the presence and severity of regurgitant lesions. Survival beyond the fourth decade is unusual in patients with significant root involvement.[27] Currently, elective surgical replacement of the aortic root and valve is recommended when the aorta reaches a diameter of 6 cm, as the risk of dissection increases significantly with the size of the aorta.[28] Occasionally, mitral regurgitation is the dominant lesion. Surgery for mitral regurgitation in Marfan's syndrome is somewhat problematic, as valve repair may be less feasible in these patients and dehiscence of a prosthesis is not uncommon in individuals with connective tissue disorders.[29] Also, cross-clamping an aneurysmal aorta creates the risk of dissection. Surgery for mitral regurgitation may sometimes be delayed until the patient requires concomitant root replacement.

The *Ehler's-Danlos syndrome* is another connective tissue disorder associated with abnormalities of the aorta (usually abdominal) and mitral valve pro-

lapse, especially Ehler's-Danlos syndrome type IV.[30] Spontaneous rupture of vessels originating from the aortic arch can occur. If the ascending aorta is involved, echocardiographic findings in this syndrome may be similar to those in Marfan's syndrome. Women with Ehler's-Danlos or Marfan's syndromes are particularly prone to aortic dissection or rupture during the third trimester of pregnancy and during labor and delivery.[31]

ATHEROSCLEROTIC ANEURYSMS

Aneurysms secondary to atherosclerosis are the most common type of aneurysm, and most are found in the abdominal aorta. However, approximately 25% of atherosclerotic aneurysms involve the thoracic aorta. The atherosclerotic process leads to weakening of the aortic wall, medial degeneration, and localized vessel dilatation. Hypertension is an important cause of diseases of the aorta, and contributes to undermining the strength of the aortic wall and to expansion of the aneurysm. The arch and the descending aorta are the most common sites of aneurysm formation in the thoracic aorta.[32]

Symptoms of thoracic aortic aneurysms are related to their size and location and occur when the aneurysms are large enough to impinge on adjacent structures. Thus, wheezing, cough, dyspnea, hemoptysis, hoarseness, or dysphagia may result from compression of the left mainstem bronchus, the recurrent laryngeal nerve, or the esophagus by the aneurysmal segment.[33] As these lesions are frequently associated with widespread atherosclerosis, symptoms of cerebral or coronary arterial disease may dominate the clinical picture.

Diagnosis of thoracic aneurysms is usually made by mediastinal widening on the chest X-ray, but this is not specific. Localized saccular aneurysms can be missed. Computed tomography (CT) with contrast is reliable for identification and sizing of thoracic aortic aneurysms. Angiography is still considered the gold standard for the diagnosis and provides comprehensive evaluation of the branch vessels. Angiography can, however, miss aneurysms that are layered with thrombus because the thrombosed sac may not opacify. Magnetic resonance imaging (MRI) is an excellent technique for the evaluation of aneurysms, particularly because it does not require contrast material. Atherosclerotic aneurysms of the aorta are seen with transthoracic echocardiographic imaging, using both the long and short axis parasternal windows (Fig. 30-9*A*,*B*); right parasternal views can be particularly useful in the evaluation of the ascending aorta, but imaging from the right parasternum can be difficult in many adult patients. Transesophageal imaging provides additional extensive evaluation of the arch and descending aorta, and can confidently detail thrombus and atherosclerotic plaque, as well as increased echogenicity ("smoke") of slow blood flow in aneurysmal segments. Survival in patients with atherosclerotic aneurysms appears to be dependent on size: aneurysms more than 7 cm in diameter are prone to rupture and to produce symptoms of compression of surrounding structures.[34]

AORTIC DISSECTION

Dissection of the aorta is a catastrophic event initiated by a sudden tear in the intima. Degeneration of the media is probably prerequisite for the development of dissection, typically manifested by deterioration of elastic tissue. This process is *cystic medial necrosis* and usually results from chronically increased wall stress, such as that from long-standing hypertension. Over half of all patients with dissection are hypertensive.[35] Most dissections arise in one of two locations: the ascending aorta just proximal to the aortic valve and the descending thoracic aorta just beyond the origin of the left subclavian artery.[36] Men are more frequently affected than women overall; half of all aortic dissections in

women under the age of 40 occur during the last trimester of pregnancy,[37] when isolated coronary artery dissection may also be seen. The most common presenting symptom is excruciating—*tearing, ripping, stabbing*—pain. It is typically most severe at onset, unlike the pain of myocardial infarction, which is usually progressive in intensity. The pain tends to radiate in the path of the dissection.

Patients with acute dissection appear clammy and as though they are in shock, but most patients with dissection are *hypertensive*. Patients with proximal dissections may have severe aortic regurgitation with resultant heart failure.

Individuals with suspected aortic dissection require immediate and accurate diagnosis to facilitate the appropriate therapeutic interventions. Issues to be determined include the (1) involvement of the ascending aorta; (2) site of entry; (3) presence of aortic regurgitation; (4) presence of pericardial effusion; (5) extent of the tear; (6) involvement of branch vessels, including coronary arteries; and (7) thrombus within the false lumen (Table 30-3). Ascending involvement usually mandates surgery, even if the entry site is in the arch, because dissection may progress retrograde as well as antegrade. The location of the entry site will determine the surgical approach, that is, median sternotomy or lateral thoracotomy. New aortic regurgitation requires urgent surgery; the presence of a pericardial effusion makes surgery emergent. Knowing the extent of the tear and associated major branch involvement helps to

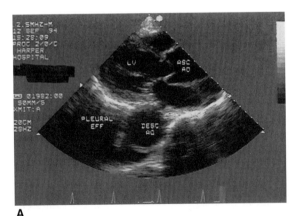
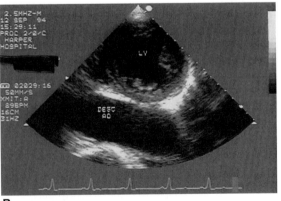

A   **B**

Figure 30-9. (**A**) Aneurysm of the descending thoracic aorta as seen in the parasternal long axis view. LV, left ventricle; Asc AO, proximal ascending aorta; PLEURAL EFF, pleural effusion; DESC AO, descending aorta. (**B**) The same aneurysm seen from the short axis plane. LV, left ventricle; DESC AO, descending aorta.

TABLE 30-3. AORTIC DISSECTION: THE QUESTIONS

- Is the ascending aorta involved?
- Where is the entry site?
- Is the aortic valve competent?
- Is there a pericardial effusion?
- What is the extent of the tear?
- Are major branch vessels involved?
- Is the false lumen thrombosed?

define the surgical risk and complications and may mandate vascular stenting. Thrombosis of the false lumen improves the prognosis but can be a diagnostic dilemma.

Current imaging modalities employed to diagnose dissection include aortography, CT, MRI, and transesophageal echocardiography (TEE). Each technique has strengths and weaknesses, and none is ideal for all patients. A reasonable understanding of the advantages and limitations of each technique is desirable.[38–44]

Both aortography (long the diagnostic gold standard) and CT have high sensitivity for the diagnosis of dissection but are less accurate than MRI. Both modalities require contrast agents, a disadvantage in a population that frequently has impaired renal or cardiac function. In addition, spiral CT scanning requires a fair amount of postprocessing time, a disadvantage in an emergency setting. Also, CT cannot evaluate branch vessels or assess aortic regurgitation. Aortography yields little information regarding the aortic wall and periaortic structures (it can easily miss a thrombosed false lumen), carries the risk of an invasive procedure, and is associated with a delay in assembling the personnel necessary to perform the procedure.[38–44]

MRI can address all the pertinent diagnostic questions (Fig. 30-10). The entire aorta and all its major branches can be assessed, with the following advantages: (1) MRI is noninvasive; (2) it provides a large field of view in any plane, unimpeded by air, bone, or increasing depth; and (3) it requires no contrast agent. MRI also has significant limitations, however, including the inability to image patients with any implanted metal or electronic devices and the logistical difficulty of placing of hemodynamically unstable and mechanically supported patients in the magnet, out of easy reach in an emergency. Some patients also have significant and prohibitive

claustrophobia and cannot tolerate the procedure. In addition, thoracic MRI currently requires electrocardiographic gating, and conduction abnormalities will compromise the data.

TEE shares with MRI the advantages of being noninvasive and requiring no contrast medium. In addition, TEE can be performed quickly *at the bedside. No other procedure offers this advantage.* For the thoracic aorta, it matches MRI in diagnostic sensitivity and specificity.[40] When combined with color Doppler, TEE can identify aortic regurgitation, flow through intimal tears, and motion of the intimal flap; the false lumen may be furthered characterized by "webs" that represent incompletely sheared ribbons of media[45] and by its slower flow.

TEE does have limitations. It cannot reliably assess the abdominal aorta, and it provides only limited evaluation of the arch vessels. Furthermore, TEE is semi-invasive, requires sedation and local anesthetic, and carries a small but definite risk. Complications range from transient changes in blood pressure or rhythm to esophageal perforation and death; they may be related to the ultrasound probe itself, the procedure, or the drugs used during the procedure.[46] In patients with suspected aortic dissection undergoing TEE, special attention should be paid to minimizing the hemodynamic and mechanical effects of the procedure,[47] especially pro-

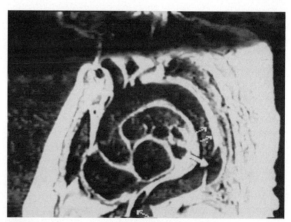

Figure 30-10. Parasagittal spin-echo MRI image showing the entry site in the distal descending aorta (solid arrow) and the reentry site in the proximal abdominal aorta (single arrow). There is retrograde progression of the dissection with thrombus in the false lumen (double arrow). (Courtesy of Dr. Renate Soulen, Harper Hospital, Detroit.)

viding adequate sedation to suppress the gag reflex and to minimize the hypertensive response. Serious complications overall occur in less than 1%. TEE is precluded in patients with conditions that make probe passage difficult or unsafe. Dysphagia, pathologic conditions of the esophagus, or recent esophageal surgery are absolute contraindications, while esophageal varices, active upper gastrointestinal pathology, and inability to flex the neck are relative contraindications. The risk:benefit ratio must be weighed in patients with these relative contraindications (Table 30-4).

CT scanning is less accurate than either MRI or TEE,[39,40] requires a large volume of contrast, and should be done as the first-line diagnostic procedure only if neither MRI nor TEE is available. Aortography is indicated only if other modalities are not available. MRI is ideal in the stable patient without contraindications because it is the most comprehensive and is highly accurate, with no overt risk. TEE, equally accurate in a somewhat more limited way, is preferable in the unstable patient or in one whose arrhythmia would degrade MRI. Both MRI and TEE are well suited to follow-up of patients with chronic dissections.

The hallmark of aortic dissection by two-dimensional echo cardiography is the demonstration of an intimal flap, an abnormal linear density within the aorta seen in more than one plane. Several observers have defined the criteria for diagnosing a flap to include (1) oscillation independent of the aorta

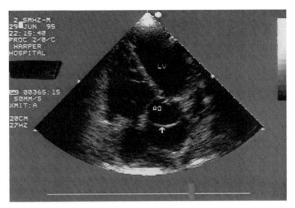

Figure 30-11. Apical five-chamber view demonstrating a proximal dissecting flap (arrow). LV, left ventricle; AO, aorta.

itself; (2) visualization in more than one view; and (3) distinction from other structures, such as aortic calcification, arteriosclerotic plaque, or intracardiac monitoring lines.[43] Transthoracic imaging can identify a flap in the proximal ascending aorta (Fig. 30-11) and can quickly determine the presence of pericardial fluid. Its usefulness is otherwise limited because of the inconsistent quality of the image of the ascending aorta, arch, and descending aorta. TEE is necessary to establish the diagnosis and the extent of dissection. TEE can distinguish the true and false lumina[43] (Fig. 30-12*A–C*). The false lumen is usually larger than the true lumen. The intimal flap moves toward the false lumen in systole

TABLE 30-4. COMPARISON OF TEE AND MRI IN EVALUATION OF AORTIC DISSECTION

	TEE	MRI
ADVANTAGES	• Bedside exam • Real time • No contrast medium required • Sensitivity/specificity 98% for thoracic aorta	• Noninvasive • Large field of view in any plane • No contrast medium • Most comprehensive exam • Sensitivity/specificity 98% each
LIMITATIONS	• No evaluation of abdominal aorta • Limited evaluation of arch and branches • Is semi-invasive, requires sedation and local anesthetic • Dysphagia, pathologic conditions of the esophagus, recent esophageal surgery are absolute contraindications • Esophageal varices, active upper gastrointestinal tract bleed, inability to flex the neck are relative contraindications	• Implanted electronic devices, ocular metal, thermodilution catheters, and most cerebral aneurysm chips are absolute contraindications • Requires special nonferromagnetic support equipment for critically ill patients • Gating required for thoracic imaging • Claustrophobia

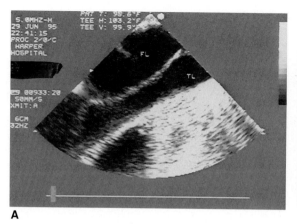

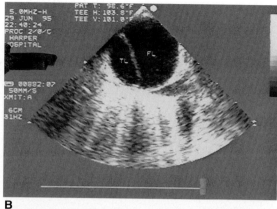

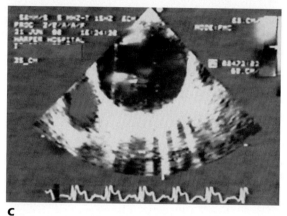

Figure 30-12. (**A**) Transesophageal longitudinal view of aortic dissection. The intimal flap divides the true (TL) and false (FL) lumen. (**B**) TEE short axis view of the dissection. TL, true lumen; FL, false lumen. (**C**) Color Doppler demonstrating flow from the true to the false lumen in this short axis view. (See also Color Plate 74.)

and toward the true lumen in diastole. Spontaneous contrast is often present in the false lumen. Color flow Doppler can also assist in distinguishing the true from the false lumen. Flow in the true lumen tends to be more rapid and flow in the false lumen is usually slower; hence, the color in the false lumen will be a duller shade of red/blue, indicating the absence of turbulence. If an entry site is identified (sometimes only by color), flow will be from the true to the false lumen. Color flow is also used to assess for the presence and severity of aortic regurgitation (Fig. 30-13*A,B*).

ATHEROMATOUS DEBRIS

Until recently, little attention was paid to the embolic potential of atheromatous debris within the aortic arch and proximal descending aorta.[48,49] Transesophageal imaging now makes possible reliable assessment of arteriosclerotic plaque within

the arch. The esophagus is adjacent to the thoracic aorta, and the higher-frequency transducers provide superior imaging of all segments of the aorta. In a recent important study, Karalis et al. prospectively identified intra-aortic debris in 38 of 556 consecutive patients studied by TEE.[50] An embolic event occurred in 11 (31%) of the 36 patients with debris. The authors characterized debris as *simple* (or simple plaque) if it was focal thickening extending less than 5 mm from the aortic wall into the lumen, without overlying shaggy, mobile material and no evidence of disruption of the intimal surface. *Complex* plaque (atheromatous debris) was defined as disruption and irregularity of the intimal surface, with overlying shaggy material extending > 5 mm into the aortic lumen. Complex debris could be either broad-based and immobile or pedunculated and highly mobile. This study and several others established aortic debris, especially of the complex, mobile type, as a likely source of systemic embo-

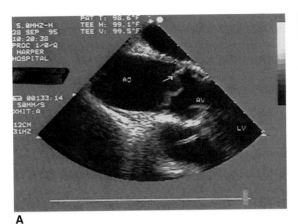

A

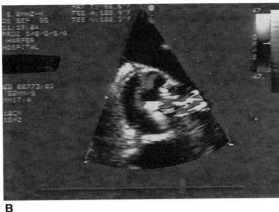

B

Figure 30-13. (**A**) Transesophageal view in the horizontal plane of a proximal dissection with a highly mobile flap (arrow). AO, aorta; AV, aortic valve; LV, left ventricle. (**B**) Aortic regurgitation in the same patient. There was intermittent prolapse of the flap through the aortic valve. (See also Color Plate 75.)

lus.[51,52] In addition, the identification of debris is extremely important in patients undergoing cardiac surgery, allowing the surgeon to make appropriate modifications to cannulation, perfusion, and operative techniques in order to reduce detachment of mobile atheroma and resultant stroke.[53] Echocardiography is a far more sensitive technique for the detection of aortic plaque than simple aortic palpation[53] (Figs. 30-14, 30-15). Pathologic evaluation of complex debris shows it most often to be a combination of fatty atheromatous material and thrombus (Fig. 30-16). Some early data suggest that anticoagulation may be appropriate in certain patients with complex debris.[54]

TRAUMA

Blunt trauma to the aorta most commonly occurs with high-speed deceleration injuries resulting from motor vehicle accidents.[55,56] In effect, when the steering wheel stops, the aorta keeps moving, and this creates enormous shear forces that act maximally on those areas where the mobile segments of the aorta join the fixed segments. The most frequent site of injury is the aortic isthmus, just distal to the origin of the left subclavian.[57] As previously noted, the isthmus is where the mobile ascending aorta and arch become fixed to the thorax, making this segment particularly vulnerable.

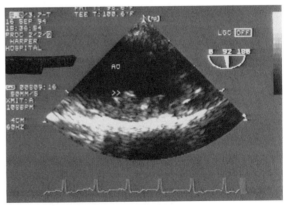

Figure 30-14. Transverse (short axis) transesophageal image demonstrating a simple aortic plaque (arrow). AO, aorta.

Figure 30-15. Longitudinal image demonstrating complex atheromatous debris (arrow). AO, aorta.

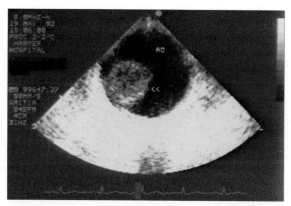

Figure 30-16. Short axis TEE view of a highly mobile mass lesion in the proximal descending aorta (arrow). The lesion was found to be thrombus at surgery. AO, aorta.

Most patients with traumatic injury to the aorta have numerous other injuries, and the diagnosis may often be overlooked, especially since one-third of all patients with aortic rupture have no evident chest wall injury.[58] Pursuit of this diagnosis should be undertaken on the basis of the mechanism of injury, as survival depends on early and correct diagnosis. Emergency aortography has long been the standard diagnostic imaging method. Smith and colleagues, of the University of Kentucky, attempted TEE in 101 patients admitted to their emergency room with suspected aortic trauma. Successfully performed in 93 patients, 11 studies demonstrated rupture of the aorta near the isthmus. There was one false-positive echocardiogram (the patient had a negative aortogram); in the remaining 10 patients, the findings were confirmed by aortography and surgery (9 patients), or autopsy (1 patient), yielding a sensitivity of 100% and a specificity of 98%. Importantly, even in critically ill patients, TEE was performed *at the bedside* without complications, within a mean period of 29 min from the time of arrival at the emergency room.[59] This timely evaluation of critically ill, unstable patients is a principal advantage of TEE over other diagnostic procedures for the evaluation of acute pathology of the aorta. One special additional advantage of TEE in the trauma patient is that it can be performed while other diagnostic procedures or stabilization measures are being undertaken. The need to move patients to the MRI or angiography suite, or to wait for appropriate personnel, is a serious drawback to these techniques.

The principal disadvantages to the use of TEE in the setting of serious trauma are two: (1) it cannot be undertaken in combative patients or those with unstable head or neck injuries, and (2) it cannot reliably evaluate the innominate, left carotid, or subclavian artery. While injuries to these vessels are rare (and usually clinically evident), they do occur, and aortography is indicated when such injuries are suspected. *TEE in thoracic trauma should be performed only by experienced operators.*

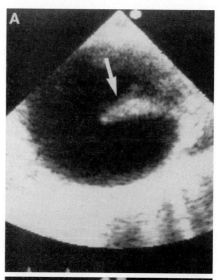

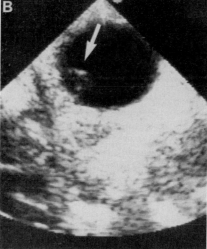

Figure 30-17. (**A,B**) TEE short axis images of a ruptured thoracic aorta. Intraluminal defects indicative of aortic wall disruption (arrows) are noted. (From Kearney PA, Smith DW, Johnson SB, et al. Use of TEE in the evaluation of traumatic aortic injury. J Trauma. 1993;34:696. Reprinted with permission.)

The typical appearance of aortic rupture (or transection) is that of a mobile, echogenic flap (2–3 cm, not typically traversing the aorta) located distal to the isthmus (Fig. 30-17). Occasionally, the injury does have an appearance similar to that of a dissection, with the flap traversing the lumen but found only in a localized region of the aorta.[59] The disruption of the aorta may also have the appearance of a protruding mass, which is usually thrombus overlying the aortic tear.

TEE is highly sensitive and specific for the evaluation of aortic injury. Early objections to single-plane technology related to its inability to image a small segment of the upper ascending aorta because of interposition of the air-filled trachea, although this region of the aorta is rarely involved by trauma. Biplane and multiplane techniques have eliminated this blind spot.[60] TEE is quick, is safe when performed by experienced operators, and is reliable in the evaluation of the critically ill trauma patient with multiple injuries.

REFERENCES

1. Eagle K, De Sanctis R. Diseases of the aorta. *In* Braunwald E (ed): Heart Disease. A Textbook of Cardiovascular Medicine, 4th ed. Philadelphia, WB Saunders; 1992:1528.
2. Clemente CD (ed): Gray's Anatomy, 30th ed. Philadelphia, Lea & Febiger; 1985:648.
3. Gardin JM, Henry WL, Savage DD, et al. Echocardiographic measurements in normal subjects: Evaluation of an adult population without clinically apparent heart disease. J Clin Ultrasound. 1979;7:439–447.
4. Sahn DJ, Allan H, McDonald G, et al. Real-time cross-sectional echocardiographic diagnosis of coarctation of the aorta: A prospective study of echocardiographic–angiographic correlations. Circulation. 1977;56:762–769.
5. Mintz GS, Kotler MN, Segal BL, et al. Two-dimensional echocardiographic recognition of the descending thoracic aorta. Am J Cardiol. 1979;44:232–238.
6. Peterson TA, Todd B, Edwards JE. Supravalvular aortic stenosis. J Thorac Cardiovasc Surg. 1968;50:734–739.
7. Friedman WF. Aortic stenosis. *In* Adams FH, Emmanouilides GC, Riemenschneider TA (eds): Heart Disease in Infants, Children, and Adolescents, 4th ed. Baltimore, Williams & Wilkins; 1989:224.
8. Williams JCP, Barratt-Boyes BG, Lowe JB. Supravalvular aortic stenosis. Circulation. 1961;24:131–136.
9. Campbell M, Polani PE. Etiology of coarctation of the aorta. Lancet. 1961;1:463–467.
10. Becker AE, Becker MJ, Edwards JE. Anomalies associated with coarctation of the aorta. Circulation. 1970;41:1067–1075.
11. Tawes RL, Berry CL, Aberdeen E. Congenital bicuspid aortic valves associated with coarctation of the aorta in children. Br Heart J. 1969;31:127–132.
12. Perloff J. Coarctation of the aorta. *In* Perloff JK (ed): The Clinical Recognition of Congenital Heart Disease, 3rd ed. Philadelphia, WB Saunders; 1994:125.
13. Titus JL, Kim H-S. Blood vessels and lymphatics. *In* Kissane JM (ed): Anderson's Pathology, 9th ed. St Louis, CV Mosby; 1990:752.
14. Edwards JE, Burchell HB. Specimen exhibiting the essential lesion in aneurysm of the aortic sinus. Proc Staff Meet Mayo Clin. 1956;31:407.
15. Perloff J. Congenital aneurysms of the sinuses of valsalva. *In* Perloff JK (ed): The Clinical Recognition of Congenital Heart Disease, 3rd ed. Philadelphia, WB Saunders; 1994:526.
16. Sakakibara S, Konno S. Congenital aneurysms of the sinus of valsalva. Anatomy and classification. Am Heart J. 1962;63:405–423.
17. van Son JAM, Danielson GK, Schaff HV, et al. Long-term outcome of surgical repair of ruptured sinus of Valsalva aneurysm. Circulation. 1994;90(part 2):II-20–II-29.
18. Desai AG, Sharma S, Kumar A, et al. Echocardiographic diagnosis of unruptured aneurysm of right sinus of Valsalva: An unusual case of right ventricular outflow obstruction. Am Heart J. 1985;109:363–364.
19. Perloff J. Congenital aneurysms of the sinuses of Valsalva. *In* Perloff JK (ed): The Clinical Recognition of Congenital Heart Disease, 3rd ed. Philadelphia, WB Saunders; 1994:526.
20. Peters P, Juziuk E, Gunther S. Doppler color flow mapping detection of ruptured sinus of Valsalva aneurysm. J Am Soc Echocardiogr. 1989;2:195–197.
21. Eliot RS, Wallbrink A, Edwards JE. Congenital aneurysm of the left aortic sinus. A rare lesion and a rare cause of coronary insufficiency. Circulation. 1963;28:951–953.
22. Pyeritz RE, McKusick VA. The Marfan syndrome: Diagnosis and management. N Engl J Med. 1979;300:772–777.
23. Marsalese DL, Moodie DS, Vaconte M, et al. Marfan's syndrome: Natural history and long-term follow-up of cardiovascular involvement. J Am Coll Cardiol. 1989;14:422–428.
24. Murdoch JL, Walker BA, Halpern BL, et al. Life expectancy and causes of death in the Marfan syndrome. N Engl J Med. 1972;286:804–808.

25. Lima SO, Lima JAC, Pyeritz RE, et al. Relation of mitral valve prolapse to ventricular size in Marfan's syndrome. Am J Cardiol. 1985;55:739–743.

26. Child JS, Perloff JK, Kaplan S. The heart of the matter: Cardiovascular involvement in Marfan's syndrome. J Am Coll Cardiol. 1989;14:429–431.

27. Crawford ES, Coselli JS. Marfan's syndrome: Combined composite valve graft replacement of the aortic root and transaortic mitral valve replacement. Ann Thorac Surg. 1988;45:296–302.

28. Gott VL, Pyeritz RE, Magovern GJ, et al. Surgical treatment of aneurysms of the ascending aorta in the Marfan syndrome: Results of composite graft repair in 50 patients. N Engl J Med. 1986;314:1070–1074.

29. Pyeritz RE. Genetics and cardiovascular disease. *In*: Braunwald E (ed): Heart Disease. A Textbook of Cardiovascular Medicine, 4th ed. Philadelphia, WB Saunders; 1992:1622.

30. Jaffe AS, Geltman EM, Rodey GE, et al. Mitral valve prolapse. A consistent manifestation of type IV Ehler's-Danlos syndrome. Circulation. 1981;64:121–125.

31. Pyeritz RE. Maternal and fetal complications of pregnancy in the Marfan syndrome. Am J Med. 1981;71:784–787.

32. Svensson LG, Crawford ES. Aortic dissection and aortic aneurysms surgery: Clinical observations, experimental investigations, and statistical analyses. Part III. Curr Prob Surg. 1993;30:1–172.

33. Eagle KA, De Sanctis RW. Diseases of the aorta. *In* Braunwald E (ed): Heart Disease. A Textbook of Cardiovascular Medicine, 4th ed. Philadelphia, WB Saunders; 1992:1528.

34. Collins JJ, Koster JK, Cohn LH, et al. Common aortic aneurysms: When to intervene. J Cardiovasc Med. 1983;8:245–248.

35. Wheat MW. Pathogenesis of aortic dissection. *In* Doroghazi RM, Slater EE (eds): Aortic Dissection. New York, McGraw-Hill; 1983:55.

36. Roberts WC. Aortic dissection: Anatomy, consequences, and causes. Am Heart J. 1981;101:195–202.

37. Pumphrey CW, Fay T, Weir I. Aortic dissection during pregnancy. Br Heart J. 1986;55:106–109.

38. Nienaber CA, Spielmann RP, von Kodolitsch Y, et al. Diagnosis of thoracic aortic dissection. Magnetic resonance imaging versus transesophageal echocardiography. Circulation. 1992;85:434–447.

39. Cigarroa JE, Isselbacher EM, DeSanctis R, et al. Diagnostic imaging in the evaluation of suspected aortic dissection. Old standards and new directions. N Engl J Med. 1993;328:35–43.

40. Nienaber CA, von Kodolitsch Y, Nicolas V, et al. The diagnosis of thoracic aortic dissection by noninvasive imaging procedures. N Engl J Med. 1993;328:1–9.

41. Khanderia BK. Aortic dissection. The diagnostic dilemma resolved. Chest. 1992;101:303–304.

42. Ballal RS, Nanda NC, Gatewood R, et al. Usefulness of transesophageal echocardiography in assessment of aortic dissection. Circulation. 1991;84:1903–1914.

43. Goldstein SA, Mintz GS, Lindsay J. Aorta: Comprehensive evaluation by echocardiography and transesophageal echocardiography. J Am Soc Echocardiogr. 1993;6:634–659.

44. Erbel R, Daniel W, Visser C, et al. Echocardiography in diagnosis of aortic dissection. Lancet 1989;1:457–461.

45. Williams DM, Joshi A, Dake M, et al. Aortic cobwebs: An anatomic marker identifying the false lumen in aortic dissection. Imaging and pathologic correlations. Radiology. 1994;190:167–174.

46. Khanderia BK, Seward J, Tajik AJ. Transesophageal echocardiography. Mayo Clin Proc. 1994;69:856–863.

47. Silvey SV, Stoughton TL, Pearl W, et al. Rupture of the outer partition of aortic dissection during transesophageal echocardiography. Am J Cardiol. 1991;68:286–287.

48. Tunick PA, Kronzon I. Protruding atherosclerotic plaque in the aortic arch of patients with systemic embolization. A new finding by transesophageal echocardiography. Am Heart J. 1990;120:658–660.

49. Tunick PA, Perez JL, Kronzon I. Protruding atheromas in the thoracic aorta and systemic embolization. Ann Intern Med. 1991;115:423–427.

50. Karalis DG, Chandrasekaran K, Victor MF, et al. Recognition and embolic potential of intraaortic atherosclerotic debris. J Am Coll Cardiol. 1991;17:73–78.

51. Kronzon I, Tunick PA. Transesophageal echocardiography as a tool in the evaluation of patients with embolic disorders. Prog Cardiovasc Dis. 1993;36:39–60.

52. Katz ES, Tunick PA, Rusinek H, et al. Protruding aortic atheromas predict stroke in elderly patients undergoing cardiopulmonary bypass: Experience with intraoperative transesophageal echocardiography. J Am Coll Cardiol. 1992;20:70–77.

53. Wareing TH, Davila-Roman VG, Barzilai B, et al. Management of the severely atherosclerotic ascending aorta during cardiac operations. A strategy for detection and treatment. J Thorac Cardiovasc Surg. 1992;103:453–462.

54. Craig WR, Dressler FA, Vaughn LM, et al. Aortic debris in patients with unexplained systemic embolus: Influence of plaque morphology on efficacy of anticoagulation (abstract). J Am Soc Echocardiogr. 1995;8:368.

55. Glock Y, Massabuau P, Puel P. Cardiac damage in non-penetrating chest injuries. J Cardiovasc Surg. 1989;30:27–30.

56. Parmley LF, Manion WC, Mattingly TW. Non-penetrating traumatic injury of the heart. Circulation. 1958;18:371.

57. Godwin JD, Tolentino CS. Thoracic cardiovascular trauma. J Thorac Imag. 1987;2:32.

58. Cohn PF, Braunwald E. Traumatic heart disease. *In* Braunwald E (ed): Heart Disease. A Textbook of Cardiovascular Medicine, 4th ed. Philadelphia, WB Saunders; 1992:1517.

59. Smith MD, Cassidy JM, Souther S, et al. Transesophageal echocardiography in the diagnosis of traumatic rupture of the aorta. N Engl J Med. 1995;332: 356–362.

60. Seward JB, Khanderia B, Edwards WD. Biplanar transesophageal echocardiography: Anatomic correlations, image orientation, and clinical applications. Mayo Clin Proc. 1990;65:1193–1213.

PART XII

The Profession of Diagnostic Cardiac Sonography

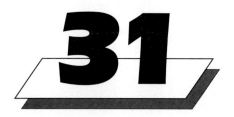

Quality Assurance: Performance Testing and Preventive Maintenance

MARVEEN CRAIG

Introduction

This chapter is being written at a time when medical procedures and the delivery of health care have come under increasing public and private scrutiny regarding their effectiveness, advisability, and costliness. The fundamental questions about when and whether to order echocardiographic studies are increasingly expanding to include concerns about the competence of those performing and interpreting echocardiograms (see Chapter 32) and the reliability of the equipment producing them. Echocardiographers should expect to include designing and executing systematic testing to their current duties to determine whether equipment is working to its maximum efficiency.

The types of tests, testing devices, and measurements useful in evaluating an ultrasound system's function, and what corrective action to take if quality falls below optimum, are described in this chapter.

Definition

The expected end product of any ultrasonic scan is an image with diagnostic potential. Because image quality is greatly dependent on a properly function-

ing diagnostic ultrasound machine, the best method to guarantee consistent optimal image quality is to conduct periodic monitoring of the performance characteristics of the ultrasound system. No ultrasound system is perfect, and even experienced sonographers may not detect day-to-day variations in equipment function. But such variations can affect the performance of ultrasound studies, the critical measurements made, and, ultimately, the diagnostic confidence of the physician interpreting them. Early recognition of such problems, while they are minor, minimizes downtime and reduces the number of times a scan must be repeated. In many of today's echocardiographic laboratories, by the time a problem is detected and a decision made to call in a service representative, valuable time has been wasted trying to make the ultrasound system perform adequately.

The American Institute of Ultrasound in Medicine (AIUM) defines quality assurance (QA) as follows:

- Daily maintenance and optimal operation and care of equipment.
- Periodic testing and assessment of equipment for early detection of image degradation and system performance.

- Documentation of equipment problems and any corrective actions taken.
- Maintenance of accurate records.[1]

In theory, every ultrasound laboratory should develop and carry out QA procedures; unfortunately, in practice, very few do.

Acceptance Testing

Usually, the first test of a new unit is the acceptance test: the initial trial of equipment immediately following installation to determine whether it is operating properly, whether it meets the specifications of the company or purchaser, or both. Such testing establishes an acceptable baseline performance level and ensures a basis for comparison at later dates.[4,5]

Acceptance testing uses the same variety of commercially available test objects and phantoms that should be used daily in echocardiographic laboratories.[4] It is advisable that sonographers and sonologists witness the performance of this postinstallation test before accepting any new ultrasound system.

Most hospitals have a biomedical testing program whose function is to carry out initial and then annual testing of all new electrical equipment to detect any substandard electrical performance. In private office and mobile ultrasound settings this type of safeguard is less likely to exist, particularly if the practice has not purchased a service contract. The importance of routine electrical and safety checks should not be overlooked.

In-House QA Programs

Once a newly installed ultrasound unit has passed a performance evaluation, the burden of maintaining the same level of image quality falls on the user. Initially, the thought of developing a QA program can be daunting, and many sonographers resist the idea. That is why it is important to design a simple testing program that takes no more than 20 min to perform to avoid frustration, boredom, or abandonment. Any individual operating an ultrasound system today should have the necessary background in quality control to be able to troubleshoot problems as they appear. Education, training, and consistent practice play major roles in preparing sonographers and sonologists to establish and maintain suitable QA programs.[6]

Testing Equipment

The passive devices used for measuring modern ultrasound system performance are called *test objects* or *testing phantoms*. Test objects are usually constructed of hydro-gel materials that duplicate or mimic the velocity of ultrasound in tissue (1540 m/sec) or of rubber-based material calibrated for a sound velocity of 1540 m/sec. Some measurements are common to both phantoms and test objects, while others are unique to one or the other.[1,2,4,6,7]

The first test objects were developed in the 1970s and were designed to evaluate A-mode and static B-mode scanners. They were cumbersome and prone to toppling over or leaking. Later models were completely self-contained, fluid-filled, ready to use, and leakproof.

Next to be developed was the *SUAR* (*S*ensitivity, *U*niformity, *A*xial *R*esolution) test object, consisting of a rectangular acrylic block containing a wedge-shaped cavity that could be filled with water. The SUAR object was suitable only for QA testing; it was inappropriate for acceptance testing.[4,6,7]

The introduction of higher-resolution real-time systems in the mid-1970s demanded more advanced testing and led to the development of a *tissue equivalent* phantom containing media that simulated the attenuation, scattering characteristics, and velocity propagation of liver parenchyma. These devices were the forerunners of modern *tissue-mimicking phantoms* that contain embedded "lesions" to simulate clinical scanning situations more closely.[1,4–6]

The most commonly used in-house test device today is the *tissue-mimicking phantom*. These instruments contain water-based gels laced with microscopic graphite particles and are the only type to successfully mimic both the velocity and attenuation characteristics of sound in tissues. In addition to distorting ultrasonic pulses and sound beams in a manner similar to that of tissue, such devices provide an excellent test for transducers of varying frequencies.

Embedded within the device are an assortment of cylinders: low-attenuating cylinders that approximate the echo-free appearance of cysts; high-attenuating cylinders that mimic the appearance of solid lesions; and an additional control cylinder. Additional nylon or wire reflecting targets are distributed in specific clusters or alignments to provide testing of both scanner geometry and spatial resolution (Fig. 31-1A,B).

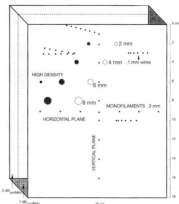

TARGETS:
Material:Nylon
Monofilament Wire Diameter:
0.1mm

VERTICAL PLANE TARGETS
Number of Groups: 1
Number of Targets Per
Group: 10
Depth Range: 18CM
Spacing: 2CM

**HORIZONTAL PLANE
TARGETS**
Number of Groups: 1
Number of Targets: 7
Depth Range: 9CM
Spacing: 2CM

RESOLUTION TARGETS
Number of Arrays: 3
Depths: 3cm and 10cm
Intervals Axial: 0.5, 1 ,
2, 3, 4, and 5mm
Intervals Horizontal:
1, 2, 3, 4, and 5mm

ANECHOIC TARGETS
Number of Targets: 4
Diameter of Targets: 2, 4, 6 and
8mm
Depth of Targets: 2, 4,
6, and 8cm

HIGH CONTRAST TARGETS
Number of Targets: 4
Diameter of Targets:
2, 4, 6 and 8mm
Depth of Targets 2, 4,
6, and 8cm
Contrast of Targets:
11 db over background

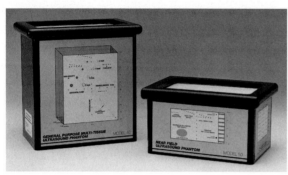

A

B

Figure 31-1. **(A)** Tissue-mimicking phantom. Suspended within a medium that simulates the ultrasound characteristics of human liver tissue are nylon and monofilament wires arranged in vertical and horizontal planes and interval clusters for assessing linearity, resolution, depth calibration, and so on. Additional anechoic and high-contrast targets simulate the ultrasonic characteristics associated with cystic and solid lesions. [General Purpose Multi-Tissue Ultrasound Phantom (Model 40) and Near Field ultrasound phantom (model 50)] **(B)** Schematic of embedded details of a general-purpose multitissue ultrasound phantom. (Courtesy of CIRS, Computerized Imaging Reference Systems, Inc., Norfolk, VA)

Several types of commercially available Doppler phantoms are available to evaluate a Doppler system's ability to detect the location and direction of flow, flow velocity, and sensitivity. Several different models exist; most are constructed of rubber-based tissue-mimicking material.

One popular model, a *cardiac Doppler flow phantom*, contains four flow channels of varying diameter to simulate deep vasculature such as cardiac and abdominal vessels. The device's two fixed-angle scan surfaces maintain a constant angle between the sound beam and the test fluid flowing through the channels (Fig. 31-2). The scanning surfaces of these test objects vary and may range from 5 to 56 degrees, permitting continuous scanning at depths of 3 to 18 cm.[1,4] *Doppler flow directional discrimination* devices are phantoms designed to test color Doppler flow imaging systems. They monitor the ability of the system to discriminate the direction of flow in small vessels at close proximity positioned

at varying depths. One type of tissue-mimicking phantom contains four pairs of 2-mm flow channels (Fig. 31-3). Edge-to-edge spacing between the flow channels within each pair increases progressively

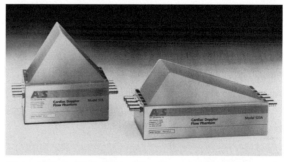

Figure 31-2. Doppler cardiac flow phantoms. These tissue-mimicking phantoms are useful for evaluating flow rate, sensitivity, and depth of penetration of Doppler ultrasound imaging systems. They offer a choice of flow channel diameters. (Courtesy of ATS Laboratories, Inc., Bridgeport, CT)

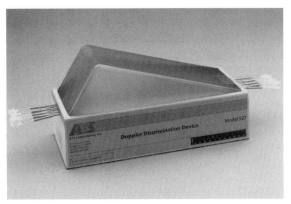

Figure 31-3. Doppler flow directional discrimination phantom. Designed to test color Doppler flow imaging systems, this device monitors the system's ability to discriminate the direction of flow in small vessels at close proximity and at varying depths. (Courtesy of ATS Laboratories, Inc., Bridgeport, CT)

from 1 to 4 mm. If greater distances are desired, a combination of two flow channel pairs can be used. This particular device also requires the use of a Doppler flow controller and a pumping system (Fig. 31-4). The fixed-angle scan surface of the Doppler flow discrimination device also provides a constant angle between the sound beam and the test fluid

flowing through the phantom at 18 to 56 degrees, permitting continuous scanning at depths ranging from 3 to 17 cm. Testing parameters include directional discrimination, flow velocity, sensitivity at varying depths, maximum penetration, and location of flow.[1]

The latest advance in Doppler testing systems offers the advantage of testing both Doppler and B-mode ultrasound systems with a single unit (Fig. 31-5). In addition to containing tissue-mimicking material, the flow phantom offers embedded discrete line reflectors and anechoic cystic targets. Two 5-mm vessel modes can be used to test flow rate accuracy. One vessel runs parallel to the scanning surface at 2 cm to simulate a carotid artery, while the other vessel descends in an angled fashion through the phantom to be used for measuring Doppler sensitivity and developing scanner techniques. A microprocessor-based flow controller produces accurate flow rates, and a total of 10 programmable test options exist for continuous flow and preset pulsatile flow patterns (Fig. 31-6).

Testing Parameters

The key components of an ultrasound system that should be routinely tested are the ultrasound scan-

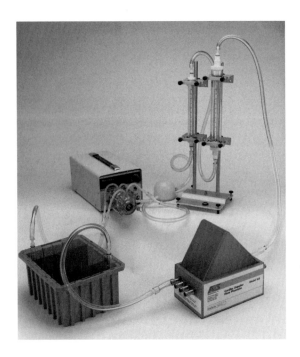

Figure 31-4. Doppler flow controller and pumping system. These instruments are designed to test the ability of Doppler imagers to detect and display sensitivity, maximum penetration, flow velocity, location of flow, and directional discrimination. They permit the continuous monitoring of flow rates and will remain air bubble free over hours of continuous use. (Courtesy of ATS Laboratories, Inc., Bridgeport, CT)

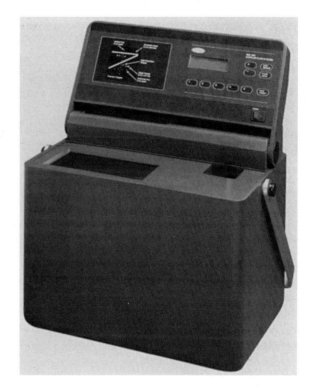

Figure 31-5. Combined Doppler and B-mode testing system. This device contains tissue-mimicking material, simulated cystic and vascular targets, and blood-mimicking fluid. An electronic flow control system allows assessment of maximum signal penetration; channel isolation or directional discrimination; registration accuracy of duplex sample gates and similarities between B-mode and color flow images; and flow rate readout accuracy for various angles, beam directions, and operating modes. (OPTIMIZER Ultrasound Image Analyzer Courtesy of Gammex RMI, Middleton, WI)

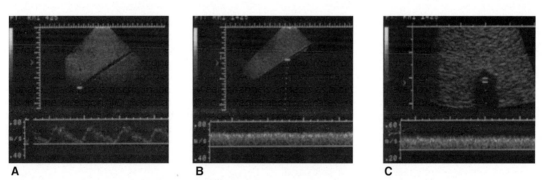

A   B   C

Figure 31-6. (A) Depth of penetration. Displays the weakest echo signal detectable above electronic noise. **(B)** Directional discrimination. Flow away from or toward the transducer is determined by forming Doppler signals into two different electrical channels 90 degrees out of phase. Inadequate discrimination between channels appears as bidirectional even though flow is in one direction. **(C)** Registration of flow. Registration indicates the position accuracy of the sample volume cursor of a Doppler image. The strongest and highest-velocity signal should appear at the center of a vessel. Whenever the sample volume position is inaccurate, the strongest signal will appear off-center. (*A–C* Courtesy of Gammex RMI, Middleton, WI)

TABLE 31-1. IMAGER TESTING PARAMETERS

- Horizontal depth calibration perpendicular to the beam axis
- Vertical depth calibration parallel to the beam axis
- Maximum depth of visualization
- Image uniformity
- Resolution
- Dynamic range (gray-scale level)

ner, the transducers, image displays, and image recording devices (Table 31-1).

ULTRASOUND SCANNING SYSTEMS

Depth Calibration

Vertical and horizontal distance measurement errors on ultrasound images can easily go unnoticed. In the practice of echocardiography, it is critical to ensure that distance indicators are accurate because echocardiographic studies rely heavily on measurements of the heart and all of its internal structures.

Test objects contain rows of reflectors with known spatial distances to test the vertical and horizontal accuracy of the scanner's calipers and 1-cm distance markers. These nylon targets are spaced at 1-cm intervals in columnar form and at 3-cm intervals in a row. During a test scan, electronic calipers are positioned to measure the distance between the reflecting targets. Measurements should be within 1–2% of the actual distance.[1–4,6,7]

Horizontal Distance Measurements

Measurements obtained perpendicular to the beam axis are frequently less accurate because of beam-width artifacts. Horizontal test measurements should be within 3 mm or 3% (whichever is less) of the actual phantom distances.[7]

Sensitivity and Penetration

The ability of an ultrasound system to detect and display echoes from weakly reflecting interfaces and scatterers is called *sensitivity*. This feature is most often affected by electronic noise within the system or by interference from other nearby electrical devices, making it important to keep track of instrument sensitivity and noise levels to see whether they change over time. The point at which usable tissue information disappears indicates the maximum depth of visualization.[1]

Spatial Resolution

The spatial resolution of an ultrasound scanner, which is sometimes called *reflector resolution*, involves lateral and axial resolution as well as slice or scan thickness. These parameters require careful standardization of sensitivity and gain settings to achieve meaningful results. This standarization is often carried out by manufacturers during acceptance testing of scanners and when developing performance specifications for their equipment.[7]

Dynamic Range

It is critical to know how well a system is able to distinctly display two nearly equal degrees of brightness in the same view. The gray scale processing section of an ultrasound system controls the level of contrast by adjusting the amplitude of the echoes received to vary the degree of brightness of the displayed image. The amount of adjustment required to go from a just noticeable (lowest contrast) displayed echo signal to maximum echo brightness is referred to as the *displayed dynamic range*.[7]

Clinically, the ability of a system to distinguish and display structures of similar contrast levels as separate structures is extremely important, since some cystic or solid lesions within an organ like the heart may have very similar levels of brightness and may potentially go undetected.

Contrast resolution test phantoms are also useful in testing functional resolution, definition fill-in, and gray scale. By using the same instrument settings established during the acceptance test, it is possible to determine if any changes in target shape or in the system's ability to distinguish among varying degrees of contrast have occurred. The tissue-mimicking phantom is the most comprehensive testing device and is recommended for contemporary real-time ultrasound system evaluation. It is not uncommon to find either one or a combination of test devices used in QA testing of modern cardiac ultrasound equipment.[4,7]

TRANSDUCERS

Standard Transducers

Every transducer is subjected to sophisticated electronic testing and evaluation before being released to a customer. All of the important information about a transducer can be found in the description of each transducer's imaging characteristics, which is called a *beam profile* and either accompanies each transducer or is available upon request from the manufacturer.

According to Powis and Powis,[6] whenever a new transducer is introduced into an ultrasound lab, its beam profile should be studied to determine the following:

1. The location of its focal point (the narrowest and most intense portion of the sound beam).
2. The rate of focus and defocus (the way amplitudes increase into the focal point and decrease on the way out of the focal point).
3. Any lack of symmetry in the beam geometry (which signifies misalignment of the transducer element).
4. Evaluation of transducer bandwidth (usually expressed as a percentage of the center operating frequency) and its "dot" size or resolution capabilities.

When properly cared for, most transducers offer few, if any, imaging problems and remain remarkably stable over time. But improper handling can result in transducer failure and possible risks to patient safety. Transducer failure can occur because of rough handling of the connectors and cord or long-term use of improper coupling agents. Dropping a transducer may result in a cracked housing or decreased output of some of the individual elements. Following such occurrences, a test object scan should be carried out before returning the transducer to routine scanning.

Because prolonged exposure to organic solvents will damage the transducer, most manufacturers recommend cleansing the transducer face with a clean cloth after the scan of each noninfected patient. Some manufacturers also advocate the use of alcohol as a mild disinfectant, while others warn that alcohol may contribute to delamination of the surface layers of the transducer.[1] When scanning infectious patients, it is important to cleanse and/or disinfect the transducer, the scanner, and the cables according to the manufacturer's recommendations and your institution's infection control policies after each study. A wide array of disinfectants are available, and most manufacturers provide lists of those agents acceptable for use with their products[1] (Table 31-2).

Intracavitary Transducers

Specialized transducers, such as those used for transesophageal or intravascular studies, may require spe-

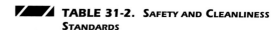

TABLE 31-2. SAFETY AND CLEANLINESS STANDARDS

SAFETY
Cords/cables: loosening or fraying?
Transducers: cracks/delamination of scan surface?
Wheel locks: in working condition?
Mounted accessories: fastened securely to the unit?

CLEANLINESS
Transducers: cleansed after each use?
Image monitors: free of oil, gel, fingerprints, dust?
Air filters: clean?
Gel warmers/dispensers: clean?

cial cleansing or disinfecting. Although intravascular transducers can be effectively sterilized for reuse, most manufacturers do not recommend the practice. Currently, all intravascular transducer combinations are for single use only. Transducers used for endoscopic studies are usually an integral part of an endoscope, and are cleansed and disinfected by using the same procedures applied to other endoscopic instruments: cleansing followed by soaking in an appropriate disinfecting liquid.[1]

IMAGING STORAGE DISPLAYS

In contemporary ultrasound laboratories there are three types of image displays: live video displays (the scanning system's video monitors), hard-copy images (transparency film, Polaroid film, black-and-white or color paper printers), and workstation displays (computer monitors).[1]

Most manufacturers provide an image display monitor, usually a standard television set, for constant viewing during and after the creation of a scan. A second display is available for use in recording images. These displays are usually mounted internally within the scanner system, and either the manufacturer or a maintenance contractor provides installation, connection, and maintenance of the image storage components. After acceptance testing of an ultrasound unit, the brightness, contrast, and horizontal and vertical control settings of the viewing monitor should be noted and a hard-copy image of a clinical scan recorded and saved for future reference.

Problems related to image focus are usually so subtle that the only sign of the problem may be an unacceptably fuzzy echo display. The appearance of "ghosting" at the corners of the image or the presence of double images generally points to an electrical problem in the connector between the scanning system and the hard-copy recording device or within either of the instruments themselves.[1]

Internal image degradation can result from "noise," lack of uniformity, or changes in background density and/or internal image speckling. Noise artifacts are commonly caused by radiofrequency interference nearby or within the scanner itself, and will appear on both the display and the hard-copy image. The echo speckles reflecting from within the focal zone of the transducer should always appear sharp and crisp on the display monitor. If elongated echoes are seen, they are indicative of poor lateral resolution, while widening of the echoes indicates poor axial resolution.[1–4,6,7]

External image degradation can result from inadequate electrical power or nearby radiofrequency interference. Intermittent scanner "lock-ups" during operation of the ultrasound system indicate the need to contact the manufacturer and possibly to monitor the power line to determine if noise exists. Once the source of the noise is isolated, if it cannot be overcome by using special filters or by isolating the ultrasound equipment, a dedicated power line may be needed.[1]

Qualitative evaluations should be made daily to detect any signs of image degradation (Table 31-3). If any problems are noted, a quantitative evaluation, using a test phantom, should be carried out to compare the current images with the initial reference image. Comparison testing not only identifies the problem but can also be used to document the result of any corrective action.[1]

HARD-COPY IMAGING DEVICES

Current image recording devices fall into two categories: (1) hard-copy devices, consisting of a visible image on material such as paper or transparent plastic, and (2) soft-copy devices that store information in computer memory for retrieval and translation into an image displayed on a TV monitor or similar device.

Polaroid Cameras

Some ultrasound systems, particularly color-flow units, are equipped with Polaroid cameras that allow direct photography of one of the system's monitors. Polaroid images can be made in either black and white or color; they provide good-resolution reproductions and require little equipment. The primary disadvantages of Polaroid imaging are the limited gray scale of Polaroid film and the relatively high cost.[1,5]

Multiformat Film Cameras

More commonly used in radiology-based ultrasound settings, multiformat film cameras are small enough to be incorporated into or onto the ultrasound imager. As many as six images can be recorded on an 8×10-in. transparency film sheet. The advantages of this type of film are its ability to display a wider range of gray scale and the lower cost per image.[1]

Laser Cameras

The transparency film used in laser cameras is similar to that mentioned above. However, it is exposed by scanning it with a laser beam modulated according to a digital image stored in the laser camera's memory. The advantage of using laser cameras is that they generally use larger (14×17-in.) transparency film capable of recording up to 18 images per film sheet in a format that improves the gray-scale sensitivity of the eye and provides a higher degree of resolution. The most significant disadvantage of laser cameras is that they are not portable because they must be coupled directly to a film processor.[1]

Regardless of what type of camera and film are used to acquire images, the following features and potential flaws should be evaluated:

1. A black background is favored for ultrasonic imaging. It should be dark enough to prevent the loss of any echoes within the gray-scale range and should be uniform. Nonuniformity of the background may indicate the presence of dirty optical components or problems with a laser

TABLE 31-3. KEY SIGNS OF IMAGE DEGRADATION

Image noise or artifacts
Image uniformity
Image background density
Image dot size and resolution
Image focus
Electronic marker distortion/inaccuracy

camera's imaging system or a multiformat camera's monitor.[1]

2. Resolution and distortion are serious and common potential imaging problems. The simplest way to routinely assess photography settings involves observing the gray bar pattern that appears at the edge of most image displays and checking to see that the brightness displayed on the viewing monitor matches that of the hard-copy image.

3. Artifacts appearing only on the photographic film's hard copy can be caused by static electric discharges, hair, and dust adhering to the film emulsion.

4. The presence of foreign objects is usually the cause of any obstruction of the light path within the camera.

Thermal Paper Gray-Scale Recorders

These recording devices provide instant display of images on thermally sensitive paper without the need of a film processor. Better known as *strip-chart recorders*, these systems produce a continuous recording of cardiac events over long periods of time utilizing a long roll of paper. They are excellent for M-mode recordings and can reproduce very high resolution images even at very expanded recording scales. The disadvantages of paper systems are their limited gray-scale reproducibility, the high cost of the paper and its storage (due to bulk), and the fact that the images will fade over time unless they are well protected from heat/light. Because it is necessary to freeze the image before recording, the product has lower image resolution than an unprocessed continuous strip-chart recording.[1,5]

Color Thermal Printers

High-resolution color images can be printed on paper using a thermal dye transfer process. Although both the cost of the printer and the per print cost are relatively high, the image quality is excellent. The costs can be reduced by including up to four images per sheet, but only by sacrificing some degree of resolution. Pressure or heat marks on heat-sensitive paper can produce artifacts.[1]

Video Page Printers

These systems accept a video format image that has already been processed through the system scan converter and print out high-resolution copies for a few pennies per page. Printer costs vary, depending on size, print quality, and whether the unit produces black-and-white or color prints. Because they have their own memory, some printers permit recording without freezing the image, which helps lessen the examination time.

All hard-copy images represent the interaction of sound with tissue that appears on the display screen. Regardless of what medium is used to capture hard-copy images, they should always be compared to the displayed images. Any drift in the ultrasound imager, hard-copy cameras, printing devices, or in film processing can reduce image quality to such an extent that significant subtle variations in echo signal amplitude can be lost. As we enter the era of networking image displays from various workstations, the importance of monitoring the quality of the images emanating from these workstations can only increase.

SOFT-COPY IMAGING DEVICES

There are basically two categories of soft-copy devices: video tape or digital tape and magnetic or optical disks.

Videotape

The most universally used imaging device in the echocardiography setting is the videotape recorder based on the VHS system of recording. Super VHS (SVHS) and high-definition television (HDTV) produce the highest-quality videotape recordings. Industrial-quality recorders are preferred for their tolerance of a great deal of stop, play, and rewind activity, as well as long periods in the PAUSE mode between recordings. Many systems offer a SEARCH feature that allows searching for a particular location on the videotape and stopping automatically. In the long run, they are very cost effective from the standpoint of time saving and cost per image. Audio outlets are provided for Doppler units and are sometimes recorded in stereo.[5]

If the VCR output is fed to a video hard-copy or storage device, the stationary images produced with the system in the PAUSE mode cannot be captured by the hard-copy storage device. Scanners that provide digital freeze frame options can circumvent this problem.[1]

For those using videotape archiving, it is essential that the tape deck heads be routinely cleansed

Quality Assurance Worksheet

Fiber/Cylinder Type Phantom

Test Date _____

Machine Description:
Make & Model _____
Serial No. _____
Room No. _____

Phantom Description:
Make & Model _____

Transducer Description:
Name _____ Serial No. _____
Type: Mechanical ☐ Single Element
☐ Annular Array
Electronic ☐ Linear Array
☐ Curvilinear Array
☐ Phased Array
Elevational Focusing Yes ☐ No ☐

Transducer Inspection:	Yes	No	Corrective Action
Cords, Frayed or Cracked	☐	☐	_____
Housing, Cracked or Damaged	☐	☐	_____
Face, Cracked or Delaminated	☐	☐	_____
Missing Lines of Sight	☐	☐	_____

For Mechanical Transducers:

Air bubbles present	none	< 5 mm	≥ 5 mm	_____
Vibration or noise	none	mild	severe	_____
Image flicker	none	mild	severe	

General Cleanliness:	Yes	No	Mechanical:		Yes	No
Monitor Screen	☐	☐	Wheels: Fastened Securely		☐	☐
Keyboard and Knobs	☐	☐	Rotate Easily		☐	☐
Transducer Holders	☐	☐	Locks Working		☐	☐
and Connectors:			Accessories Fastened Securely			
Machine Housing	☐	☐	(camera, VCR, printers, etc.)		☐	☐
Air Filters	☐		Power Cord			
Transducers (cleaned		☐	Plugged Securely into Wall Outlet	☐		☐
normally after each use)	☐	☐	Attached Securely to Machine	☐		☐
			Accessory Cords			
			Attached Securely to Machine		☐	☐

Hard Copy Imaging:
Gray Scale (Either A or B)
A. Continuous Gray Scale Bar
   Length of Black-to-White Transition on Monitor _____
   Length of White-to-Black Transition on Hard Copy _____
B. Discrete Gray Scale Bars
   Number of Gray Scale Bar Steps on Monitor _____
   Number of Gray Scale Bar Steps on Hard Copy _____

	Yes	No	Corrective Action
Discrepancy (Hard Copy Versus Monitor)	☐	☐	_____

Alphanumeric Characters and Centimeter Markers:	Yes	No	Corrective Action
Sharp	☐	☐	_____
Ghost Free	☐	☐	_____
Uniform Brightness Throughout Image	☐	☐	_____
Low-Level Echoes on Monitor Recorded on Hard Copy	☐	☐	_____

Machine Settings:

Depth of Field: _____ cm   Gain: _____   Power: _____
Focal Zone(s): _____ cm _____ cm _____ cm _____ cm _____ cm
Dynamic Range: _____ Preprocessing: _____ Postprocessing: _____
Other (e.g., TGC settings): _____

Tissue-Mimicking Phantom Measurement:

Maximum Depth of Visualization:
   Low-Level Echos _____ cm
   Baseline Value From Acceptance Tests (see page 39) _____ cm
   Discrepancy (Absolute value should be less than 1 cm.) _____ cm

Image Uniformity:	Yes	No
Is brightness near the edge same as in the middle?	☐	☐
Is there shadowing possibly from element dropout (array scanners)?	☐	☐
If multiple focus, are there brightness transitions between focal zones?	☐	☐

Vertical (Axial) Distance Measurement Accuracy:
   Caliper distance between 2 reflectors lying on a vertical line _____ cm
   Actual distance between reflectors _____ cm
   Discrepancy _____ cm
   Discrepancy/(distance between reflectors) × 100 = _____ % (Should be less than 2%)

Horizontal (Lateral) Distance Measurement Accuracy:
   Caliper distance between 2 reflectors lying on a horizontal line _____ cm
   Actual distance between reflectors _____ cm
   Discrepancy _____ cm
   Discrepancy/(distance between reflectors) × 100 = _____ % (Should be less than 3%)

Axial Resolution (Do A or B):
A. Number of targets separated far enough axially to be resolved _____
   Baseline number from acceptance tests (see page 39) _____
   Discrepancy (should be 0) _____
   Target depth _____ cm

B. Target size in the axial direction _____ mm
   Baseline target size from acceptance tests (see page 39) _____ mm
   Discrepancy _____ mm
   Target depth _____ cm

Lateral Resolution:
   Target depth _____ cm
   Target size in lateral direction _____ mm
   Baseline target size from acceptance tests (see page 39) _____ mm
   Discrepancy (should be 0) _____ mm

Action Taken to Correct Problems   Date Completed

_____ _____

_____

_____

_____

_____

_____

_____

_____

_____

_____

Attach All Hard Copies.

Figure 31-7. Example of a QA worksheet. (Reprinted with the permission of the American Institute of Ultrasound in Medicine from AIUM Quality Assurance Manual for Gray-Scale Ultrasound Scanners, available from The American Institute of Ultrasound in Medicine, 14750 Sweitzer Lane, Suite 100, Laurel, MD 20707-5906; phone: 301/498-4100; 800/638-5352; fax 301/498-4450)

with a swab dipped in alcohol to remove the buildup of tape residue that naturally occurs with constant stop–start–rewind activities.

Digital Tape

Less commonly used than analog VHS videotape recording, digital tape systems produce digital images in which pixel gray levels are recorded numerically. This allows measurements of Doppler velocities, distance, and so on to be made from the image. A disadvantage of this imaging format is that it is currently impossible to interchange the units of one manufacturer with those of another manufacturer.[1]

Magnetic Disks

Magnetic hard disks can store digital images and are often used for temporary storage prior to transfer to optical storage devices (optical disks). Their greatest drawback is that the typical ultrasound image requires approximately 200 KB of disk space per image, making storage of large numbers of clinically generated images impractical.[1]

Optical Disks

The increased storage capacity of optical disks (128 MB to 2 GB per disk) makes this technology a very cost-effective way to store large numbers of images in permanent form. Despite their current cost ($600 to $3000), optical disk drives are growing in favor because they can be equipped with units that allow for the transfer of images to separate workstations. Picture archiving systems, which are typically found in large imaging departments, are capable of accessing 10 or more optical disks to carry out both recording and retrieval functions. However, the quid pro quo of optical disks drives is that they have a much slower data access time than magnetic disks.[1]

Recordkeeping

In any QA program, it is important to maintain detailed records to detect changes in equipment performance. A log book should be kept to record the result of each test performed, along with the date and transducer identification (Fig. 31-7). Such recordkeeping makes it very easy to look back and compare any transducer's past performance with its present condition or to identify any negative trends that may be occurring. Both written and photographic documentation of perceived problems, service calls, repairs, and regularly scheduled preventive maintenance should also be included in the log.

Conclusion

The obvious fact that image quality is largely dependent on proper equipment function, coupled with the strong moves being made in the direction of laboratory accreditation, make the QA issue more timely than ever. Monitoring the performance characteristics of an ultrasound system with routine QA programs makes it possible not only to verify that an ultrasound system is functioning satisfactorily, but also to document the performance of a specific unit over time. That is the primary reason for structuring a simple, quick QA program that can be consistently maintained rather than establishing an overambitious schedule of testing that is soon abandoned.

Sonographers and sonologists interested in obtaining comprehensive information and step-by-step protocols for QA testing and recordkeeping are strongly advised to obtain a copy of the *AIUM Quality Assurance Manual for Gray-Scale Ultrasound Scanners,* which is available from the American Institute of Ultrasound in Medicine (AIUM).[1]

REFERENCES

1. AIUM Technical Standards Committee. AIUM Quality Assurance Manual for Gray-Scale Ultrasound Scanners. (Stage 2). Laurel, MD, American Institute of Ultrasound in Medicine; 1995.
2. Banjavic RA. Design and maintenance of a quality assurance program for diagnostic ultrasound equipment. Semin Ultrasound. 1983;4(1):10–25.
3. Hussey M. Basic Physics and Technology of Medical Diagnostic Ultrasound. New York, Elsevier; 1985.
4. Hykes DL, Hedrick WR, Starchman DE. Ultrasound Physics and Instrumentation. New York, Churchill Livingstone; 1985.
5. Lichtenberg GS. Echocardiography instruments and principles. *In* Craig M (ed): Diagnostic Medical Sonography. A Guide to Clinical Practice, Vol 2. Philadelphia, JB Lippincott; 1991.
6. Powis RL, Powis WJ. A Thinker's Guide to Ultrasonic Imaging. Baltimore, Urban & Schwarzenberg; 1984.
7. Zagzebski JA. Physics and instrumentation. *In* Sabbagha RE (ed): Diagnostic Ultrasound Applied to Obstetrics and Gynecology, 3rd ed. Philadelphia, JB Lippincott; 1994.

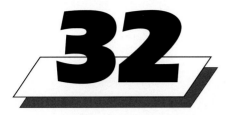

Echocardiography: Education and Training

MARVEEN CRAIG

Introduction

The recognition of echocardiography as a valuable clinical tool is neither automatic nor guaranteed. It is earned by maintaining quality control with positive results in clinical diagnosis, a goal that is obtainable only when high educational standards are met in the production of cardiac sonographers and sonologists.[1]*

    The primary purpose of this chapter is to define the role of cardiac sonographers and their level of professional practice. An integral part of that task must involve the current recommendations of the American Society of Echocardiography (ASE) and other collaborating organizations concerning the art and technique of cardiac sonography, as well as a discussion of the education- and training-related issues affecting cardiac sonographers today.

Education Versus Training

There is a significant difference between education and training. Education involves the process of developing knowledge as well as skills through formal schooling. Training involves subjecting a candidate to certain exercises and instructions in order to de-

velop proficiency at a specific task. The serious nature of cardiac sonography requires individuals who wish to become cardiac sonographers to be exposed to both disciplines if they are to assume the responsibilities required of them in a quality cardiac ultrasound setting. Nevertheless, sonography educational programs and training courses exist as entirely separate entities, each convinced that their methods are more valuable and desirable than those of the other. While there are some exceptions, the chief complaint about hiring graduates of an echocardiography education program is that while they have an admirable grasp of theoretical knowledge, their scanning skills and their ability to integrate into a busy clinical setting are often lacking. According to Anne Dempsey, supervisor of Boston University Medical Center's echocardiography lab, it takes *at least* 6 to 9 months to bring their skills up to the standards required in her institution.[2] These numbers may represent the minimum time required, as other institutions' estimates range from 12 to 18 months.

    The reverse complaint is lodged when comparing the performance of recent graduates of short-term training programs. They may have the manual dexterity and eye–hand coordination to step up to the act of scanning, but many lack the clinical knowledge necessary to make independent judgments about the need to extend or expand an ultrasound study based on the patient's clinical complaints and their ultrasound results.

---

* *Sonologist*: This term refers to the physician who interprets the results of and/or personally performs echocardiographic studies.

Sonographers employed in laboratories offering specialized echocardiographic procedures are often examining patients who have been administered powerful medications and who must be monitored for intolerance to stress echocardiographic sessions or transesophageal examinations. Few training programs prepare students to function under the pressures of this type of duty. Blending the best of both teaching methods would achieve the best results for the student, the institution, and the patient.

The Cardiac Sonographer

In the United States, most echocardiograms are performed by cardiac sonographers, requiring an exceptional level of skill, knowledge, and experience unique among diagnostic procedures performed by nonphysicians. Unquestionably, the results of such studies are sonographer dependent.[7]

Because the cardiac sonographer is the initial examiner, an interpretive interchange between the sonographer and the interpreting physician is vital. Such a collegial relationship helps foster learning, reinforces the understanding of cardiac principles, and can only benefit all involved (particularly the patient). It (1) allows critical assessment of the techniques of each study, (2) helps to achieve and maintain even higher standards, and (3) requires physicians who interpret echocardiograms to also be skilled in examination techniques to ensure that the technical quality of studies is optimal.[6,7]

Cardiac sonographers must possess a keen understanding of ultrasound physics and instrumentation, plus the manual dexterity to manipulate a transducer. To produce diagnostically adequate documentation of all the anatomic malformations that can accompany heart disease requires familiarity with cardiac anatomy, physiology, and blood flow hemodynamics, as well as the clinical aspects of cardiology.[7] But cardiac sonographers must also be analytical and possess independent judgment and critical thinking skills if they expect to solve the problems that arise in daily operations.

Education and Training Recommendations for Sonographers

The ASE has consistently played a major role in ensuring quality patient care, fostering a professional level of echocardiographic practice through comprehensive specialized education, and leading to the credentialing of cardiac sonographers. It has developed well-respected guidelines for cardiac sonographer education.

ROLE AND LEVEL OF PRACTICE

The primary role of the cardiac sonographer is to obtain diagnostic recordings of cardiac ultrasound images and Doppler hemodynamic data. Because the technique is so operator dependent, optimal performance requires:

- Ability to continuously integrate known clinical information, ultrasound image content, and related physiologic data.
- Continuous application of principles of ultrasound physics and instrumentation during the examination.
- Independent judgment, knowledge of clinical cardiology, and problem-solving skills.
- Thorough understanding of cardiac and thoracic anatomy, physiology, hemodynamics, embryology, and sectional anatomy and pathophysiology.
- Ability to recognize abnormalities, extend the scope of the exam, and correlate the information obtained from the echocardiographic exam with other data.
- Capable of applying the techniques of cardiopulmonary resuscitation if necessary.
- Ability to obtain pertinent clinical information from patients, referring physicians, and patient's records.
- Skill in interacting with patients: able to explain procedures to patients but to refrain from discussing clinical findings of the examination.
- Complete understanding of the physical principles of ultrasound, the operation of diagnostic instruments, and the bioeffects of ultrasound.
- Cognizance of patient exposure to ultrasonic energy and its effects on human tissue systems to ensure patient safety without sacrificing exam quality.
- Capable of performing routine quality assurance (QA) and safety checks on the ultrasound equipment.
- Understanding of echocardiographic data and quantitation of derived parameters.

Cardiac sonographers should always work under the supervision of a *qualified* physician and should participate with the supervising physician in the interpretive review of the examination to provide input in the evaluation of data and to contribute relevant technical information.[3,10]

RECOMMENDED CURRICULUM

Recognizing that quality education and credentialing of cardiac sonographers is important to the future of the field, the ASE recommends that educational institutions provide a standardized curriculum to promote uniform quality for the education of the cardiac sonographer. Such a curriculum should include both comprehensive and rigorous didactic instruction and a supervised clinical internship. Prospective sonography students should have completed the following college-level prerequisite courses:

- Anatomy and physiology
- Pathophysiology
- Algebra and trigonometry
- Basic sciences (e.g., biology, chemistry, and physics to provide the foundation necessary to understand more advanced concepts)

Student cardiac sonographers should complete a Committee on Allied Health Education and Accreditation (CAHEA)-accredited program consisting of a *minimum* of 6 months (960 hours) of didactic instruction and a *minimum* of 6 months of clinical instructions. The total didactic and clinical experience should amount to at least 12 months of full-time echocardiography education (1920 hours). An additional 6 months of clinical instruction in a primary pediatric setting is recommended for more comprehensive training in pediatric echocardiography.[3,10]

ASE-RECOMMENDED EDUCATIONAL CURRICULUM FOR CARDIAC SONOGRAPHERS

To provide quality education requires commitment on the part of educators as well as students and challenges them to provide the degree of difficulty and types of educational experiences necessary to ensure competence and a professional level of practice. The ASE recommendations are *guidelines* and, as such, cannot be all-encompassing. Curriculum guidelines are primarily of interest to educators wishing to design or update a course, but students can also derive benefits by comparing the curriculum of their selected institution with the well-written and very complete ASE guidelines[10] (Table 32-1).

Credentialing

The recognition of cardiac sonography as a special diagnostic field has been a milestone for the profession. Unlike other allied health professionals, sonographers are not required to be certified or licensed; credentialing is voluntary.[1,4] Credentials enhance professional status, ultimately improving the quality of patient care. Credentials not only constitute visible proof of a cardiac sonographer's abilities but may also increase remuneration and career benefits.[1]

Cardiac sonographers are fortunate to have the special resources offered by membership in professional organizations devoted to establishing and maintaining high standards, bridging gaps between physicians and sonographers, alerting sonographers to proposed legislation, and lobbying on their behalf.

Continuing Education

Formal, continuing education at local, regional, and national levels is required to maintain the competence of both the physician and the sonographer in today's rapidly changing environment of echocardiography. Currently, registered diagnostic cardiac sonographers must accrue 30 hr of continuing education over a 3-year period. It is recommended that sonologists accrue 50 hr of echocardiography credits over a 3-year period.

It is also vital that practicing echocardiographic professionals sustain a case volume sufficient to maintain their skills and competence (a case volume of 100 cases per year is recommended). Periodic reviews of both study performance and interpretation should be carried out at regular intervals[8-10] (Tables 32-2 and 32-3).

Professional Status

Sonography requires direct participation in the diagnostic decision-making process. Consequently, cardiac sonographers, like their counterparts in the other specialty areas, must have a relatively high degree of knowledge about numerous cardiac diseases

(Text continues on p. 634)

▰▰ **TABLE 32-1. ASE EDUCATIONAL CURRICULUM RECOMMENDATIONS FOR CARDIAC SONOGRAPHERS**

I. Didactic curriculum
  A. Physical principles of ultrasound
    1. Basic ultrasound physics
    2. Doppler ultrasound physics
    3. Principles of ultrasound instrumentation
      a. Transducers
      b. Acoustics
      c. Instrument design and function
      d. Bioeffects and concepts of minimum acoustic exposure
      e. Quality assurance (diagnostic equipment)
  B. Cardiac anatomy and physiology (assumes college-level anatomy and physiology)
    1. Gross cardiac anatomy
    2. Cross-sectional anatomy (echocardiographic planes)
    3. Electrophysiology
      a. Anatomy and physiology of the conduction system
      b. Basic ECG interpretation
    4. Normal cardiac hemodynamics
    5. Basic cardiac pharmacology
    6. Embryology
  C. Cardiac pathology and pathophysiology (assumes college-level pathophysiology)
    1. Congenital heart disease
      a. Neonate/infant
      b. Adult
    2. Acquired heart disease
      a. Ischemic heart disease
      b. Valvular heart disease
      c. Myocardial disease
      d. Pericardial disease
      e. Diseases of the aortic root
      f. Cardiac masses, tumors
      g. Descriptors of altered cardiac performance
  D. Basic history-taking and cardiac physical examination
    1. Cardiac history review
    2. Auscultatory examination
      a. Normal and abnormal heart sounds
      b. Blood pressure measurement
      c. Differential diagnosis
  E. Special procedures
    1. Cardiopulmonary resuscitation techniques
    2. Isolation techniques
    3. HIV/AIDS/hepatitis B and other communicable disease precautions
    4. Sterile technique (surgical suite environment)
  F. Echocardiography: techniques and applications
    1. Two-dimensional and M-mode echocardiography
    2. Doppler echocardiography
    3. Echocardiographic evaluation using provocative maneuvers
    4. Stress echocardiography
    5. Contrast echocardiography
    6. Echocardiography-assisted pericardiocentesis
    7. Transesophageal echocardiography
    8. Intraoperative echocardiography
    9. Intraluminal echocardiography
    10. Myocardial perfusion
    11. Three-dimensional echocardiography
    12. Intracardiac imaging
    13. Intravascular imaging
    14. Non-Doppler flow imaging

(continued)

▰▰▰ TABLE 32-1. *(Continued)*

  G. Echocardiographic quantitative methods
    1. Chamber dimensions: measurement and calculation
    2. Two-dimensional echocardiographic quantitation
    3. Doppler echocardiographic calculation and quantitation
  H. Basic interpretation and understanding of other cardiac diagnostic methods
    1. Invasive techniques
      a. Cardiac catheterization (including coronary arteriography and ventriculography)
      b. Electrophysiology testing
      c. Digital radiographic techniques
    2. Noninvasive techniques
      a. Electrocardiography, Holter monitoring
      b. Phonocardiography, pulse recording
      c. Exercise treadmill testing (with or without thallium imaging)
    3. Other cardiac assessment procedures
      a. Chest x-ray
      b. Chest computed tomographic (CT) scanning
      c. Magnetic resonance imaging (MRI)
      d. Radionuclide imaging
  I. Understanding of cardiovascular therapeutic technique and intervention; echocardiographic evaluation
    1. Valve replacement and surgical repair
    2. Balloon valvuloplasty
    3. Coronary artery bypass grafting (CABG), percutaneous transluminal coronary angioplasty (PTCA)
    4. Cardiac surgical repair and reconstruction
    5. Congenital surgical repair and reconstruction
  J. Determinants of echocardiographic image quality
    1. Evaluation of dynamic images
    2. Ultrasonic imaging artifacts
    3. Doppler ultrasound artifacts
    4. Recording techniques
  K. Research techniques and statistical analysis
    1. In vitro studies
    2. Animal research
    3. Human research
    4. Epidemiological studies
    5. Research statistics and design
    6. Developing diagnostic protocols
  L. Medical ethics and legal issues
  M. Professionalism, health care delivery
    1. Professional interaction, communications skills
    2. Health care administration
    3. Sterile technique
    4. Quality assurance (diagnostic procedure, examination results)
  N. Continuing professional development
    1. Professional organizations and societies
    2. Current literature and review
II. Clinical internship

    The clinical internship portion of the curriculum should be a minimum of 6 months (960 hours) of full-time supervised instruction. During this clinical training portion, the cardiac sonographer student should perform complete echocardiography examinations (i.e., "hands-on" scanning incorporating two-dimensional and M-mode imaging as well as cardiac Doppler velocity recordings) including measurement and preliminary impressions on a minimum of 40 patients per month (two per day), with an additional 240 echocardiograms (two per day) observed and reviewed. The optimal clinical internship should extend for 12 months and include a minimum of 480 patients examined (two per day, "hands-on" scanning), with an additional 480 echocardiograms (two per day) observed and reviewed with the supervising physicians.[3,10]

Source: Guidelines for cardiac sonographer education. J Am Soc Echocardiogr. 1992;5:635–639. Reprinted with permission.

◤◢◤◢ **TABLE 32-2. LEVELS OF TRAINING IN ECHOCARDIOGRAPHY**

	Objectives	Duration	No. of Cases
PHYSICIANS IN CARDIOLOGY TRAINING PROGRAMS			
Level 1	Introductory experience	3 months	150 2-D/M-mode examinations 75 Doppler examinations
Level 2	Sufficient experience to take independent responsibility for echocardiographic studies	3 additional months (beyond level 1)	150 2-D/M-mode examinations 150 Doppler examinations
Level 3	Sufficient expertise to direct an echocardiography laboratory	6 additional months (beyond level 2)	450 examinations (using both imaging and Doppler)
PHYSICIANS' POST-CARDIOLOGY TRAINING			
	Responsibility for performance and interpretation of echocardiograms	variable; level of achievement equivalent to level 2 above	250–300 patients (2-D/M-mode and Doppler examinations)
	Direct echo laboratory in hospital or large group practice	variable; level of expertise equivalent to level 3 above	450 patients (2-D/M-mode and Doppler examinations)
2-D = 2-dimensional			

Source: Pearlman AS, Gardino JM, Martin RP, et al. Guidelines for optimal physician training in echocardiography: Recommendations of the American Society of Echocardiography Committee for Physician Training in Echocardiography. Am J Cardiol. 1987;60:158–163. Copyright by Excerpta Medica, Inc.

and their physiologic manifestations. They must demonstrate independent judgment case by case and tailor each examination to answer the clinical questions. They must simultaneously consider other diagnostic possibilities and be prepared to pursue them for the maximum benefit of the patient. In some clinical settings, sonographers are asked to report diagnostic impressions and are required to train physicians in sonographic techniques and interpretation.[5] The totality of these virtually unparalleled roles makes sonography unique, differentiating it from other allied health occupations. Yet, this alone has not been sufficient to qualify sonography as a profession.

The road to professional recognition is both tedious and laborious. It begins with the development of educational and training standards, a process usually addressed by individual sonographers and their professional societies. The next step is to develop a certification process and a method of demonstrating

◤◢◤◢ **TABLE 32-3. RECOMMENDED MINIMUM CASELOADS OF COMPREHENSIVE STUDIES PER MONTH TO BE CONSIDERED A LEVEL III ECHOCARDIOGRAPHIC SERVICE**

Type of Study*	Physicians**		Sonographers**
	Perform	Interpret	Perform***
Chest wall	4~	50	50
Nonoperative TEE	4	4	NA
Intraoperative TEE/epicardial	4	4	NA
Stress	4	4	8

TEE, Transesophageal echocardiography.
* If services are available. It is recognized that not all echocardiographic laboratories provide all of the above services.
** Physicians and sonographers dealing with both adult and pediatric patients should achieve minimum levels in both adult and pediatric patients. Physicians and sonographers not specifically trained or experienced in treating heart disease in the young should not perform and interpret such studies. Modifications may be made for those involved in teaching and supervision.
*** This assumes that sonographers are employed and meet the minimum requirement of 50 studies per month. These numbers also assume that individuals performing TEE or epicardial or stress studies also are qualified from the chest wall.
Source: Recommendations for continuous quality improvement in echocardiography. J Am Soc Echocardiogr 1995;8 (Part 2, suppl): 1–28. Used with permission.

continual maintenance of proficiency through mandatory continuing education programs. Next, physician and institutional employers must recognize, respect, and require these professional and occupational accomplishments, providing in return opportunities for advancement, as well as educational and monetary incentives. The final, and as yet untaken, step to achieving professional status and recognition lead to the development of a baccalaureate degree entry-level standard. Such a maneuver to elevate the profession will likely be a hotly debated topic on the cardiac sonography agenda well into the next century. Unfortunately, because of the lack of *mandatory* standards, not all practicing echocardiographers have completed each of these steps. Until cardiac sonographers universally achieve similar status via appropriate training, certification, and competency maintenance, they will remain simply a collection of individuals who perform echocardiographic examinations.[4,5]

Physician Training

Echocardiography has flourished because of the valuable contributions it makes to cardiac diagnosis and treatment and also because it is inexpensive, portable, safe, and operates without any regulatory interference. Leaders within the echocardiography community have expressed concern that as a result of its easy accessibility, cardiac ultrasound may attract individuals without sufficient education or training. According to Kisslo, the practice of echocardiography and Doppler has become so complex that it is difficult for physicians without prior formal training in these techniques to simply enter the field and provide high-quality services with ease. He believes that it takes years to achieve an adequate level of practice.[4,5]

Both the ASE and the American College of Cardiology (ACC) have published standards for physician training. The ASE recommends three levels of training in echocardiography for cardiology fellows: introductory, intermediate, and advanced. A minimum of 3 months of formal training solely in ultrasound techniques has been recommended for fellowship programs to serve as a simple baseline. Physicians who ultimately wish to interpret echocardiograms at the conclusion of their training are advised to log an additional 6 months of formal training. For physicians who wish to establish independent practices, including their own echocar-

diographic laboratory, a minimum of 1 year is required[3,4,8–10] (Table 32-2).

Practicing physicians often find it very difficult to take time away from their clinical practices for advanced education and training. It is recommended that physicians in practice optimally perform and interpret echocardiographic studies in at least 250 to 300 patients before considering themselves proficient to make independent diagnostic judgments. Some of that training may take place in their own institutions, but it would be desirable if most of their patient studies were performed and interpreted under the supervision of an experienced physician-echocardiographer (sonologist)[3,8–10] (Table 32-3).

Just like sonographer training standards, physician training standards have become more stringent with the passage of time. The formation of a separate, cross-specialty certification board for sonologists was suggested at least a decade ago. It was hoped that such a body would help make substandard exams less likely by having users demonstrate a minimum level of skill before being certified. Hopefully, the existence of such a certifying agency would encourage the development of more training and fellowship programs and would encourage a second level of reimbursement for ultrasound exams done by users who are specifically trained. Given the current health reform climate and the tying of reimbursement to certification or accreditation in other ultrasound specialties, it seems only a matter of time before the same practices will prevail in echocardiography.

Conclusion

It has taken more than four decades for echocardiography to develop into a highly respected and valuable method of evaluating cardiac disease. A large part of its success is due to the collaborative action of cardiac sonographers and sonologists. But while it is satisfying to look back on the progress that has been made, it is vitally important to keep pace with the constant technical innovations in cardiac ultrasound and the changes in health care delivery that can affect it. Exciting new advanced teaching tools such as ultrasound training simulators hold the promise of revolutionizing preclinical education, advanced specialized training, and continuing medical education. Such units are already available for abdominal and obstetric/gynecologic applications.

Both cardiac and peripheral vascular modules should be available soon. As users of one of medicine's most accessible imaging instruments, the cardiac community must constantly focus on training for both sonographers and physicians, and must discourage the involvement of individuals who lack sufficient knowledge and experience to perform or interpret echocardiographic studies.

Establishing training guidelines for physicians and sonographers, and working to help cardiac sonographers achieve professional status and recognition, strengthens the field and satisfies the dual responsibilities of protecting and advancing it. We are indeed fortunate to have professional specialty organizations acting as both information resources and guardians willing to take primary responsibility for developing the skills of their members.

This chapter has focused on the tangible elements of echocardiographic education and training, but there is much more to the creation of a good sonographer. Patience, tenacity, intellectual curiosity, enthusiasm, and warmth are only a few of the intangible qualities that cannot be taught. These traits are the mark of a true professional.

Acknowledgment

It is only through the generous cooperation of the following organizations that we have been able to present the information contained in this chapter. These organizations should be looked on as valuable resources, not only for medical writers but for potential and practicing cardiac sonographers.

American Cardiology Technologists Association (ACTA)
American College of Cardiology (ACC)
American College of Chest Physicians (ACCP)
American College of Radiology (ACR)
American Institute of Ultrasound in Medicine (AIUM)
American Medical Association (AMA)
American Registry of Diagnostic Medical Sonographers (ARDMS)
American Society of Echocardiography (ASE)
American Society of Radiologic Technologists (ASRT)
Canadian Society of Diagnostic Medical Sonographers (CSDMS)
Cardiovascular Credentialing International (CCI)

Joint Review Committee on Education in Cardiovascular Technology (JRC CVT)
Joint Review Committee on Education in Diagnostic Medical Sonography (JRC DMS)
National Alliance of Cardiovascular Technologists (NACT)
National Society of Cardiovascular Technologists (NSCT)
Society of Diagnostic Medical Sonographers (SDMS)
Society of Non-Invasive Vascular Technology (SNIVT)
Society for Vascular Surgery/International Society for Cardiovascular Surgery (SVS/ISCS)

REFERENCES

1. Adams D, Kisslo KB, Kisslo J. Credentialing of the cardiac sonographer: The need for unification. J Am Soc Echocardiogr. 1988;1:100–102.
2. Personal communication: Anne Dempsey, MEd, RDCS, RDMS.
3. Guidelines for cardiac sonographer education: Report of the American Society of Echocardiography Sonographer Education and Training Committee. J Am Soc Echocardiogr. 1992;6:635–639.
4. Kisslo J. Crises in echocardiography. J Am Soc Echocardiogr. 1988;3:235–239.
5. Kisslo J. The Illusion of professional status (guest editorial). J Diagn Med Sonogr. 1983;2:9–10.
6. Kisslo J, Millman DS, Adams DB, et al. Interpretation of echocardiographic data: Are physicians and sonographers violating the law? J Am Soc Echocardiogr. 1988;1:95–99.
7. Mazer MS. What constitutes a good cardiac echo lab: The "team" approach (guest editorial). J Diagn Med Sonogr. 1985;2:47.
8. Pearlman AS, Gardin JM, Martin RP, et al. Guidelines for optimal physician training in echocardiography: Recommendations of the American Society of Echocardiography Committee for Physician Training in Echocardiography. Am J Cardiol. 1987;60:158–163.
9. Pearlman AS, Gardin JM, Martin RP, et al. Guidelines for physician training in transesophageal echocardiography: Recommendations of the American Society of Echocardiography Committee for Physician Training in Echocardiography. J Am Soc Echocardiogr. 1992;5:187–194.
10. Recommendations for continuous quality improvement in echocardiography. J Am Soc Echocardiogr. 1995;8 (Part 2, suppl):1–28.

Index

Numbers followed by an "f" indicate a figure; "t" following a page number indicates tables or displays.